Thieme

Cosmetic Breast Surgery

Sameer A. Patel, MD, FACS
Interim Chief and Program Director
Plastic and Reconstructive Surgery
Temple University
Interim Chief
Division of Plastic and Reconstructive Surgery
Fox Chase Cancer Center
Philadelphia, Pennsylvania, USA

C. Bob Basu, MD, MBA, MPH, FACS
Founder and Managing Director
Basu Aesthetics + Plastic Surgery
Houston, Cypress, The Woodlands, Texas, USA

277 illustrations

Thieme
New York • Stuttgart • Delhi • Rio de Janeiro

Library of Congress Cataloging-in-Publication Data

Names: Patel, Sameer A., editor. | Basu, C. Bob, editor.
Title: Cosmetic breast surgery / [edited by] Sameer A. Patel, C. Bob Basu.
Description: New York : Thieme, [2020] | Includes bibliographical references and index.
Identifiers: LCCN 2020000703 (print) | LCCN 2020000704 (ebook) | ISBN 9781626235281 (hardback) | ISBN 9781626235298 (ebook)
Subjects: MESH: Breast–surgery | Reconstructive Surgical Procedures–methods | Breast Diseases–surgery
Classification: LCC RD539.8 (print) | LCC RD539.8 (ebook) | NLM WP 910 | DDC 618.1/9059–dc23
LC record available at https://lccn.loc.gov/2020000703
LC ebook record available at https://lccn.loc.gov/2020000704

Important note: Medicine is an ever-changing science undergoing continual development. Research and clinical experience are continually expanding our knowledge, in particular our knowledge of proper treatment and drug therapy. Insofar as this book mentions any dosage or application, readers may rest assured that the authors, editors, and publishers have made every effort to ensure that such references are in accordance with **the state of knowledge at the time of production of the book.**

Nevertheless, this does not involve, imply, or express any guarantee or responsibility on the part of the publishers in respect to any dosage instructions and forms of applications stated in the book. **Every user is requested to examine carefully** the manufacturers' leaflets accompanying each drug and to check, if necessary in consultation with a physician or specialist, whether the dosage schedules mentioned therein or the contraindications stated by the manufacturers differ from the statements made in the present book. Such examination is particularly important with drugs that are either rarely used or have been newly released on the market. Every dosage schedule or every form of application used is entirely at the user's own risk and responsibility. The authors and publishers request every user to report to the publishers any discrepancies or inaccuracies noticed. If errors in this work are found after publication, errata will be posted at www.thieme.com on the product description page.

Some of the product names, patents, and registered designs referred to in this book are in fact registered trademarks or proprietary names even though specific reference to this fact is not always made in the text. Therefore, the appearance of a name without designation as proprietary is not to be construed as a representation by the publisher that it is in the public domain.

Thieme Publishers New York
333 Seventh Avenue, New York, NY 10001 USA
+1 800 782 3488, customerservice@thieme.com

Thieme Publishers Stuttgart
Rüdigerstrasse 14, 70469 Stuttgart, Germany
+49 [0]711 8931 421, customerservice@thieme.de

Thieme Publishers Delhi
A-12, Second Floor, Sector-2, Noida-201301
Uttar Pradesh, India
+91 120 45 566 00, customerservice@thieme.in

Thieme Revinter Publicações Ltda.
Rua do Matoso, 170 – Tijuca
Rio de Janeiro RJ 20270-135 - Brasil
+55 21 2563-9702
www.thiemerevinter.com.br

Cover design: Thieme Publishing Group
Typesetting by Thomson Digital, India

Printed in the United States of America
by King Printing Co., Inc.

5 4 3 2 1

ISBN 978-1-62623-528-1

Also available as an e-book:
eISBN 978-1-62623-529-8

Dedicated to my mentors, past and present, and to the numerous residents and fellows I have had the privilege of mentoring; to Chrissy and Vivian, whose sacrifices have allowed me to grow personally and professionally; to my father Anil for his support through years of school and training; and to my mother Nikunj, whose absence from this earth continues to be felt every day.

—Sameer A. Patel

I would like to dedicate this textbook to my parents, Tapan K. Basu and Manju Basu, to my beloved wife Dr. Sugene Kim, and to my boys Devan and Dylan. My work is possible because of your unconditional love and support. And to my mentors who have cultivated my continued professional growth.

—C. Bob Basu

Contents

Preface

We are excited to present this comprehensive textbook on aesthetic breast surgery. We have assembled plastic surgeons who not only have extensive clinical experience but who are internationally recognized for their clinical work and research in various aspects of aesthetic breast surgery. This textbook has been written for the plastic surgeon who remains the constant student—the resident, junior attending, mid-career, or seasoned senior surgeon. The topics were selected both to provide a contemporary update on long-standing topics associated with breast augmentation, lift, reduction, and revisional surgery as well as to present chapters on relatively new topics. Recognizing that the human body changes over time and the potential for unpredictability in any elective surgery, we have dedicated several chapters on revisional surgery focusing on the management and correction of the undesirable result. This includes a novel chapter utilizing an internal bra technique in the context of weak breast tissue or poor soft tissue support. And we provide a contemporary update on capsular contracture and biofilms with evidence-based insights on prevention and treatment. In addition, our expert faculty provide a timely update on breast implant associated anaplastic large cell lymphoma. Equally important is the chapter on managing and mitigating risk in aesthetic breast surgery. With the increasing demand for aesthetic procedures from men, we have included expert perspectives on male chest aesthetics and relevant aesthetic procedures. We are also proud to include a valuable chapter on transgender breast surgery. Last but not least, we provide valuable insights on how to market a cosmetic breast surgery practice in the evolving digital ecosystem including social media. We hope that this textbook provides an expansive collection of diverse and recently emerging topics that will leave you with extra pearls and seasoned wisdom from our esteemed faculty and that will help you enhance your skillset to achieve the best results and outcomes for your patients.

Sameer A. Patel, MD, FACS
C. Bob Basu, MD, MBA, MPH, FACS

Contributors

C. Bob Basu, MD, MBA, MPH, FACS
Founder and Managing Director
Basu Aesthetics + Plastic Surgery
Houston, Cypress, The Woodlands, Texas

Ethan Baughman, MD, PhD
Resident Surgeon
Division of Plastic & Reconstructive Surgery
Washington University School of Medicine
St. Louis, Missouri

Bradley P. Bengtson, MD, FACS
Founder and CEO
Bengtson Center for Aesthetics and Plastic Surgery
Assoicate Professor
Department of Surgery
Michigan State University
Grand Rapids, Michigan

Donald W. Buck II, MD, FACS
Assistant Professor of Plastic Surgery
Division of Plastic & Reconstructive Surgery
Washington University School of Medicine
St. Louis, Missouri

Alexandra Bucknor, MD
Plastic Surgeon
Queen Victoria Hospital
East Grinstead, United Kingdom

Katherine H. Carruthers, MD, MS
Resident
West Virginia University
Department of Surgery
Division of Plastic Surgery
Morgantown, West Virginia

Akash Chandawarkar, MD
Resident Physician
Department of Plastic and Reconstructive Surgery
John Hopkins University
Baltimore, Maryland

R. Brannon Claytor, MD, FACS
Chief of Plastic Surgery
Main Line Health
Claytor/Noone Plastic Surgery
Bryn Mawr, Pennsylvania

Mark W. Clemens, MD, FACS
Associate Professor of Plastic Surgery
MD Anderson Cancer Center
University of Texas
Houston, Texas

Sharona Czerniak, MD
Plastic and Reconstructive Surgeon
Head and Body Contouring Service
Assuta Ashdod Academic Medical Center
Ashdod, Israel

Anand K. Deva, BSc(Med), MBBS(Hons), MS, FRACS
Head, Cosmetic Plastic and Reconstructive Surgery
Macquarie Plastic & Reconstructive Surgery
Surgical Infection Research Group
Faculty of Medicine and Health Sciences
Macquarie University
Australia

Berry Fairchild, MD
Resident
General Surgery
University of Texas Health Science Center at Houston
Houston, Texas

Megan Fracol, MD
Plastic Surgery Resident
Northwestern Memorial Hospital
Chicago, Illinois

Heather J. Furnas, MD, FACS
Adjunct Assistant Professor
Stanford University School of Medicine
Private Practice
Santa Rosa, California

Renee Gasgarth, MD
Private Practice
West Palm Beach, Florida

James C. Grotting, MD, FACS
Clinical Professor
Division of Plastic Surgery
University of Alabama
Birmingham, Alabama

Jeffrey A. Gusenoff, MD
Associate Professor
Plastic Surgery
University of Pittsburgh
Pittsburgh, Pennsylvania

Elizabeth J. Hall-Findlay, MD, FRCSC
Plastic Surgeon
Private Practice
Banff, Alberta
Canada

Ziyad S. Hammoudeh, MD
Private Practice
Marina Plastic Surgery
Marina del Rey, California

Kent K. "Kye" Higdon, MD, FACS
Associate Professor
Program Director
Department of Plastic Surgery
Vanderbilt University Medical Center
Medical Center North
Nashville, Tennessee

Matthew P. Jenkins, MD
Clinical Assistant Professor
Reconstructive Plastic Surgery
Jefferson University Hospital
Philadelphia, Pennsylvania

Christodoulos Kaoutzanis, MD
Assistant Professor
Plastic and Reconstructive Surgery
Division of Plastic & Reconstructive Surgery
UCHealth University of Colorado Hospital
Aurora, Colorado

Jordan Kaplan, MD
Resident
Division of Plastic Surgery
Baylor College of Medicine
Houston, Texas

Ergun Kocak, MD
Private Practice
Midwest Breast and Aesthetic Surgery
Gahanna, Ohio

Bernard T. Lee, MD, MPH, MBA, FACS
Professor of Surgery
Harvard Medical School
Chief
Plastic and Reconstructive Surgery
Beth Israel Deaconness Medical Center
Boston, Massachusetts

Samuel J. Lin, MD, MBA
Associate Professor of Surgery
Harvard Medical School
Program Director
Beth Israel Deaconess Medical Center
Harvard Medical School Plastic Surgery Residency
Boston, Massachusetts

Michele Ann Manahan, MD, MBA, FACS
Associate Professor of Plastic and Reconstructive Surgery
Department of Plastic and Reconstructive Surgery
Johns Hopkins Hospital
Baltimore, Maryland

Munique Maia, MD
Private Practice
Mclean, Virginia

Alan Matarasso, MD, FACS
Immediate Past President
American Society of Plastic Surgeons (ASPS)
Clinical Professor of Surgery
Hofstra University/Northwell School of Medicine
Hempstead, New York

Raja Mohan, MD
Chief Resident
Plastic and Reconstructive Surgery
Johns Hopkins
Department of Plastic and Reconstructive Surgery
Dallas, Texas

Maurice Y. Nahabedian, MD, FACS
Professor of Plastic Surgery
VCU-College of Medicine: Inova Branch
National Center for Plastic Surgery
McLean, Virginia

Marilyn Ng, MD, MSc
Assistant Professor
Northwell Health-Staten Island University Hospital
Department of Surgery
Division of Plastic Reconstructive and Hand Surgery
Staten Island, New York

Ash Patel, MD, MBChB, FACS
The Chao Family Distinguished Professor of Plastic Surgery
Chief
Division of Plastic Surgery
Residency Program Director
Albany Medical Center
Albany, New York

Nirav Bipin Patel, MD, MS, JD
Plastic and Cosmetic Surgeon
Marietta Plastic Surgery
Marietta, Georgia

Sameer A. Patel, MD, FACS
Interim Chief and Program Director
Plastic and Reconstructive Surgery
Temple University
Interim Chief
Division of Plastic and Reconstructive Surgery
Fox Chase Cancer Center
Philadelphia, Pennsylvania

Pratik Rastogi, MBBS (Hons 1), GDAAD, MS
Plastic Surgery Resident
Macquarie University Hospital
Sydney, New South Wales, Australia

Neal R. Reisman, MD
Private Practice
Houston, Texas

Kristen Rezak, MD, FACS
Assistant Professor of Surgery
Division of Plastic, Maxillofacial, and Oral Surgery
Duke University Medical Center
Durham, North Carolina

Rod J. Rohrich, MD
Plastic Surgeon
Dallas Plastic Surgery Institute
Dallas, Texas

J. Peter Rubin, MD
Professor
University of Pittsburgh
Department of Plastic Surgery
Pittsburgh, Pennsylvania

Justin Sacks, MD, MBA
Assistant Professor
Plastic & Reconstructive Surgery
Director Oncological Reconstruction
Johns Hopkins Department of Plastic and Reconstructive Surgery
Baltimore, Maryland

Loren S. Schechter, MD, FACS
Clinical Professor of Surgery
The University of Illinois at Chicago
Attending Surgeon
Rush University Medical Center
Director
The Center for Gender Confirmation Surgery
Weiss Memorial Hospital
Chicago, Illinois

Clark Schierle, MD, PhD, FACS
Plastic Surgeon
Northwestern Specialists in Plastic Surgery
Chicago, Illinois

Alan Serure, MD
Private Practice
Miami, Florida

M. Shuja Shafqat, MD
Assistant Clinical Professor
Division of Plastic & Reconstructive Surgery
Department of Surgical Oncology
Fox Chase Cancer Center
Philadelphia, Pennsylvania

Sumner A. Slavin, MD
Private Practice
Chestnut Hill, Massachusetts

Joseph R. Spaniol, MD
Resident
Plastic and Reconstructive Surgery
Temple University Hospital
Philadelphia, Pennsylvania

Douglas S. Steinbrech, MD, FACS
Private Practice
New York, New York

W. Grant Stevens, MD, FACS
Clinical Professor of Surgery
USC - Keck School of Medicine
Division of Plastic Surgery
Director
USC Aesthetic Surgery Fellowship American Society of Aesthetic Plastic Surgery
Past President Orange Twist, Co-Founder and CMO
Los Angeles, California

John T. Stranix, MD
Assistant Professor
Plastic and Maxillofacial Surgery
University of Virginia School of Medicine
Charlottesville, Virginia

Pankaj Tiwari, MD
Private Practice
Midwest Breast and Aesthetic Surgery
Gahanna, Ohio

Emily Van Kouwenberg, MD
Assistant Professor of Surgery
Division of Plastic and Reconstructive Surgery
Rutgers Robert Wood Johnson Medical School
New Brunswick, New Jersey

Eric Weiss, MD
PGY5 General Surgery Resident
Einstein Healthcare Network
Philadelphia, Pennsylvania

Paul R. Weiss, MD
Clinical Professor of Surgery
Division of Plastic Surgery
Albert Einstein College of Medicine
New York, New York

Julian Winocour, MD
Assistant Professor
Department of Plastic Surgery
Vanderbilt University Medical Center
Medical Center North
Nashville, Tennessee

Steven G. Woodward, MD
General Surgery Resident
Thomas Jefferson University Hospital
Department of Surgery
Philadelphia, Pennsylvania

Part I

Anatomy of the Breast

I

1 Anatomy of the Breast

Ethan Baughman and Donald W. Buck II

Summary

Surgery of the breast requires a detailed understanding of the anatomy and embryology of the breast. A knowledge of the anatomy and development of the breast is important in understanding many of the conditions that plastic and reconstructive surgeons treat. This chapter will focus on the anatomy of the breast and conditions that may arise with aberrant development of the breast.

Keywords: breast anatomy, breast development, breast embryology

1.1 Introduction

The appearance and function of the breast are important to both men and women. Female breasts appear in adolescence, are typically larger than male ones, and serve an important role in child-rearing (lactation), distinguishing feminine body image, clothing wear, and courting a mate. Male breasts, on the other hand, lack glandular tissue, are smaller, and help to maintain a masculine body image.

In addition, breast appearance and shape are of chief importance to plastic and reconstructive surgeons, as they are routinely asked to restore or augment the normal shape and function of breasts. In fact, it is no surprise that the breast is one of the most common areas operated on by plastic surgeons. In this chapter, we will review normal breast development and anatomy and highlight the contrast with abnormal breast conditions that surgeons commonly encounter.

1.2 Embryology

The first sign of breast development in mammals occurs with the appearance of the milk lines (mammary ridges, mammary crests), which are a pair of ventral ectodermal ridges that initially extend from the axilla to the inguinal region at 4 to 6 weeks gestation.[1] The ectoderm gives rise to the ventral breast skin and the lactiferous ducts, while the mesenchyme gives rise to the fascia, or connective tissue stroma, and vascularity. By the fifth or sixth week, the ectodermal skin layer penetrates into the mesodermal layer to form the ducts. At 10 weeks the milk line normally atrophies proximally and distally to the pectoral region, leaving a pair of mammary glands. The areola is often visible by 5 months gestation.

Mammary gland formation and hypertrophy are driven by maternal hormones, specifically prolactin. The nipple is typically everted at birth due to local relative abundance of mesenchymal tissue.[2] Neonatal breast buds at birth may secrete small amounts of cloudy fluid similar to milk due to maternal hormonal exposure in utero, which normally wanes in the first weeks after birth. Any deviation in or persistence of early embryologic stages of development will result in congenital breast malformations and abnormalities, which will be described later in further detail. It is important to note that male and female breast development in utero and up to the point of puberty are essentially identical.

1.3 Development

With the onset of puberty, sex hormones drive secondary development of distinguishing breast characteristics. In males, testosterone and relative lack of estrogen increases androgen-responsive traits, including increased muscle mass and hair growth with decreases in body fat, including, but not limited to the breast. Male breast ductal tissue remains hypoplastic and incapable of lactation under these hormonal conditions. In females, estrogen and relative lack of testosterone drive lobular hypertrophy as well as ductal extension into the submammary fat pad. Specifically, this lobular hypertrophy results in lactiferous ducts increasing their branching and acini at the proximal duct. The final result of this hypertrophy is the development of 16–24 terminal duct lobular units, which are arranged radially from the nipple areolar complex (NAC; ▶ Fig. 1.1[3]). Each lobular unit is organized along a main lactiferous duct, which is fed by hundreds of acini and terminates in the nipple. The developing female nipple and areolar skin are secondarily enlarged by parenchymal hypertrophy.

In puberty, mammary gland, nipple, and areola development follows stages first described by British pediatrician James Tanner. Tanner staging describes genital, breast, and pubic hair changes in both male and female adolescents. Except for female breast development, most of the Tanner staging is beyond the scope of the plastic surgeon.

Up to typically 10 years of age, girls are at Tanner stage I, with no mammary glandular development and the areola slightly elevated. The presence of a breast bud with areolar widening heralds Tanner stage II, which typically occurs by age 11 years. Tanner stage III, characterized by the breast bud widening beyond the borders of the areola, usually occurs by age 13. By age 15 years, most girls enter Tanner stage IV, marked by a secondary mound of the NAC projecting from the breast mound. Breast development continues until adult size is attained, with elimination of this secondary NAC projection (Tanner stage V).

Multiple factors can impact the timing of each Tanner stage, including end-organ responsiveness to sex hormones, familial early onset of puberty, ethnicity, and body fat percentage, all of which can globally impact estrogen production in the peripheral tissues. Dysregulation of adolescent breast development requires a multidisciplinary team approach and will be discussed further in more detail. Breast aging and senescence will also be described later.

1.4 Pregnancy and Lactation

During pregnancy, breast parenchyma growth occurs under the influence of progesterone, estrogen, prolactin, placental lactogen, and chorionic gonadotropin. During the postpartum period, elevated prolactin promotes milk secretion, while oxytocin promotes milk letdown and ejection. These hormones are

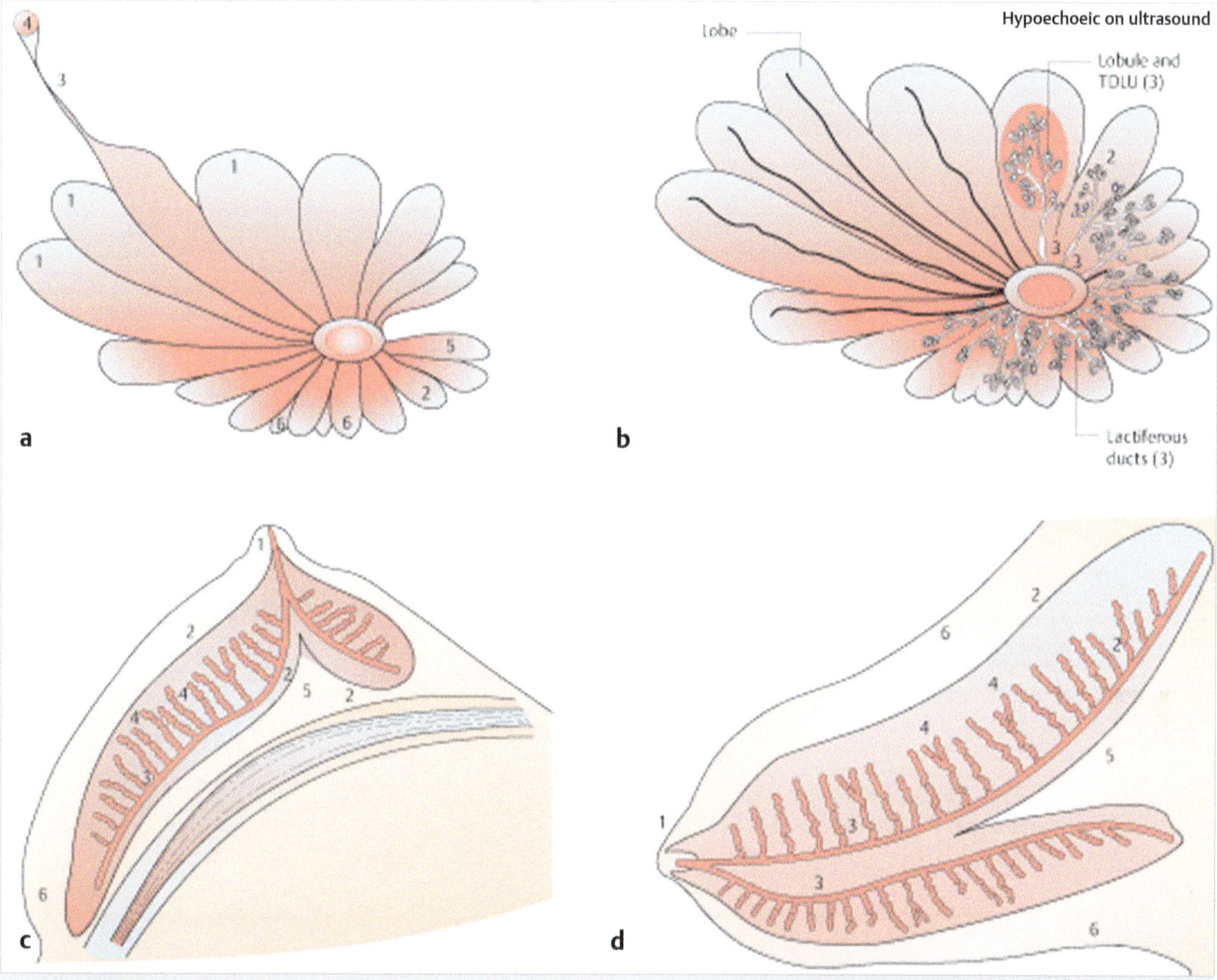

Fig. 1.1 (a,b) The breast parenchyma contains 16 to 24 terminal duct lobular units, which are arranged radially from the nipple areolar complex (NAC). **(c,d)** Tuberous breasts have narrow base width, high inframammary fold, and herniation of parenchyma into the NAC. (Reproduced from Barth V. Diagnosis of Breast Diseases: Integrating the Findings of Clinical Presentation, Mammography, and Ultrasound. Stuttgart, Germany: Thieme Medical Publishers; 2011.)

often persistently elevated through breastfeeding. Once the stimulation for prolactin and oxytocin is eliminated, the levels fall, milk production ceases, and the gland atrophies.

1.5 Landmarks

There are numerous anatomic landmarks of the breast that are critical to the plastic surgeon for preoperative evaluation and operative planning (▶ Fig. 1.2).[3] The midline is often marked from the sternal notch to the umbilicus. With the patient standing, the nipple-to-midline and nipple-to-nipple distances are often measured. The breast meridian, a line from the midclavicle through the NAC, is also marked bilaterally. The sternal notch–to-nipple distance is measured bilaterally, and differences are noted. The inframammary fold (IMF) is marked bilaterally, and the distance from the nipple to the IMF is measured and recorded. The upper breast border is often marked at the edge of the breast parenchyma superiorly (▶ Fig. 1.3a), along with the anterior axillary fold and lateral breast border. Each breast base width is measured from medial to lateral parenchyma and recorded.

1.6 Basic Breast Anatomy

Surgical techniques around the breast are grounded in a foundation of basic breast anatomy and physiology. The majority of the mammary gland lies directly superficial to the pectoralis major muscle (▶ Fig. 1.3b).[4] Breast parenchyma, which is predominantly made up of glandular tissue and fat, may extend to the sternum medially, the clavicle superiorly, the IMF inferiorly, and the lateral border of the pectoralis major laterally. The parenchyma is suspended by Cooper's ligaments (pectineal ligaments), connective tissue in the breast that maintains structural integrity and extends from the clavicle and deep fascia of the upper chest to the dermis. Perforating branches of the internal mammary arteries and vein are the major blood supply medially (▶ Fig. 1.4). Additionally, a rich collateral vascular supply is available from the intercostal, lateral thoracic, and

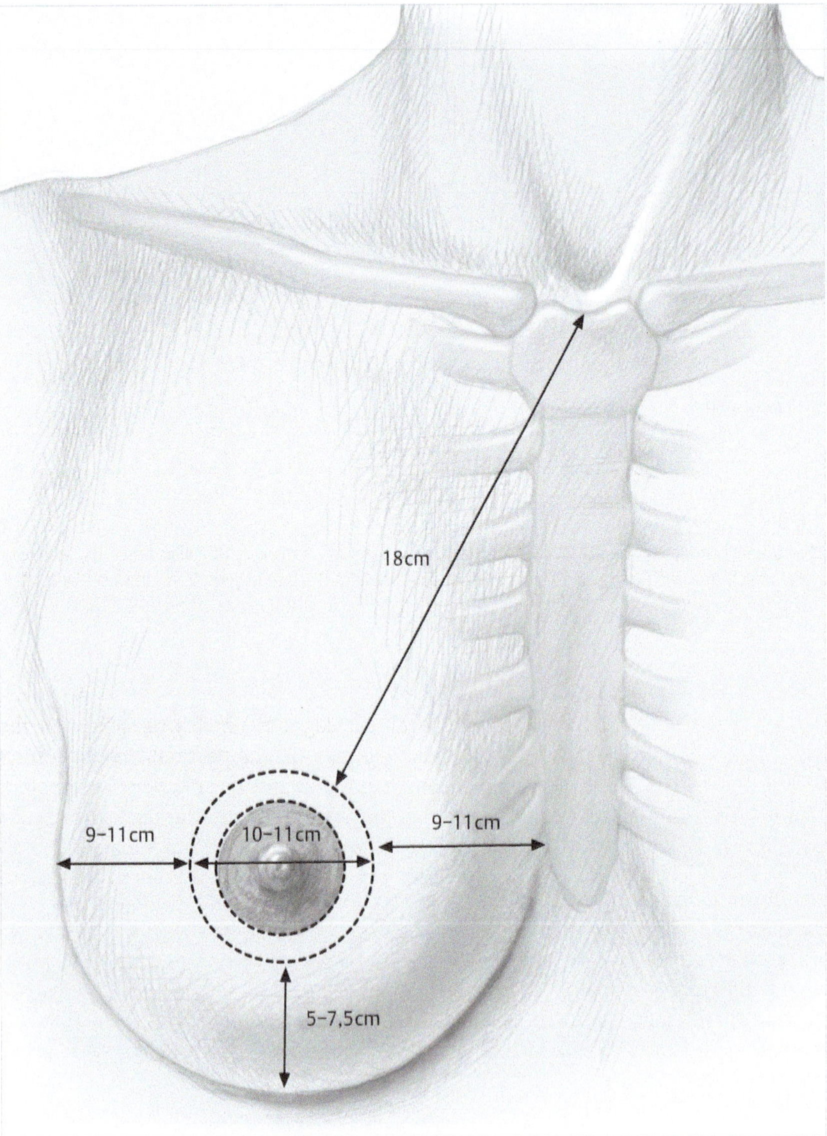

Fig. 1.2 Ideal measurements are on average sternal notch-to-nipple distance of 18 cm, midline-to-nipple distance of 9–11 cm, lateral border of breast gland-to-nipple distance of 9–11 cm, and nipple-to-inframammary fold distance of 5–7.5 cm. (Reproduced from Wallwiener D, Becker S, Veronesi U. Atlas of Breast Surgery. Stuttgart, Germany: Thieme Medical Publishers; 2015.)

thoracoacromial perforators. Most lymphatic drainage is via level 1 axillary lymph nodes. Most of the breast sensory fibers are derived from medial and lateral intercostals. Greater breast anatomic detail will be described in the following paragraphs.

1.6.1 Aesthetic Subunits of the Female Breast

The aesthetic breast maintains natural size and shape with ideal NAC position (▶ Fig. 1.2). The ideal NAC is positioned naturally on the most projecting aspect of the breast mound, centered over the parenchyma halfway between the sternum and anterior axillary line and above the IMF.[5] The ideal breast parenchyma has less upper pole fullness, an upper pole-to-lower pole ratio of approximately 45 to 55%, a full lower pole, with upward nipple angulation of approximately 20° (▶ Fig. 1.3b). Approximate ideal dimensions are sternal notch-to-nipple distance of 18–21 cm, internipple distance of 18–21 cm, and nipple-to-IMF distance of 5–8 cm (▶ Fig. 1.2). Breast symmetry is ideal but uncommon in the general population. The aging process and its effect on breast shape will be described in greater detail in a subsequent section of this chapter.

1.6.2 Vascular Supply

The plastic surgeon can take advantage of the rich vascular network of the breast when choosing a pedicle for parenchymal reduction and/or rearrangement. Medially, the blood supply to the breast is derived from the internal mammary artery and vein. Superiorly, branches of the thoracoacromial trunk perfuse the breast. Intercostal vessels perforate the pectoralis fascia laterally but medially as well. The superficial dermal plexus provides important venous drainage of the breast (▶ Fig. 1.5). As evident by its rich vascular supply, redundant collateral circulation of the breast allows inferiorly, medially, superiorly, and superomedially based pedicle design.

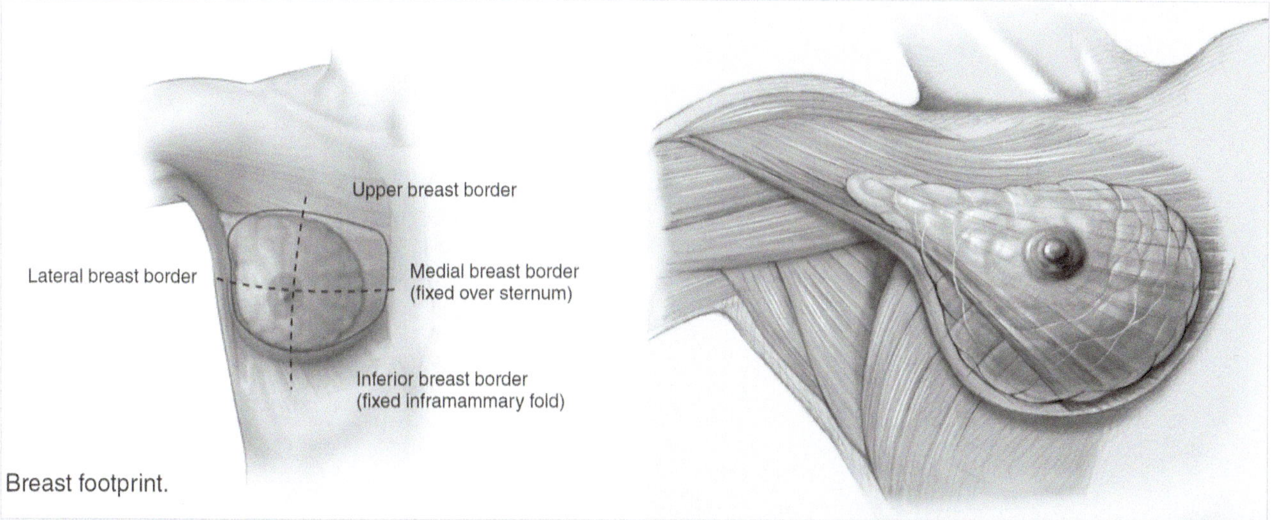

Fig. 1.3 **(a)** The breast footprint is marked by the upper breast border, inframammary fold, sternocostal junction, and anterior axillary fold. **(b)** Most of the glandular tissue of the breast overlies the pectoralis major muscle. (Reproduced from Janis JE. Essentials of Plastic Surgery. 2nd ed. New York, NY: Thieme Medical Publishers; 2014.)

1.6.3 Sensory Innervation

Breast paresthesias are often the result of incision design. The majority of the breast receives cutaneous nerves from lateral and medial branches of the intercostal nerves (▶ Fig. 1.6). A few cutaneous nerves reach the breast superiorly from the supraclavicular nerves. The NAC receives terminal fibers from the third and fourth thoracic intercostal nerves. Surgical damage to the T3–4 cutaneous nerves can result in temporary or permanent nipple paresthesias. The intercostobrachial nerve is commonly injured during axillary surgery and can result in medial upper arm numbness and/or discomfort. Axonal regeneration in cutaneous nerves is not time limited and can occur approximately 1 mm/day from the site of injury under ideal conditions.

1.6.4 Lymphatic Drainage

Advanced breast cancer spreads via the lymphatic system. Thus, an understanding of breast lymphatic drainage is critical to the staging and treatment of breast cancer. The lymphatic drainage of the breast occurs predominantly into the level 1 axillary lymph nodes, which are located below the lower edge of the pectoralis minor muscle (▶ Fig. 1.7). Level II axillary lymph nodes lie underneath the pectoralis minor, while the level III nodes are located above this muscle. The superior aspect of the breast also drains into the supraclavicular node basin, and medial portions of the breast can drain into retrosternal lymph nodes as well.

1.6.5 Musculature

Several key muscles are located near the breast and are important for the plastic surgeon. The most common muscle coverage for implant placement is the pectoralis major. The pectoralis major muscle originates superiorly on the sternal aspect of the clavicle, medially on the anterior aspect of the sternum, and inferiorly on the costal cartilages of ribs 2 through 6 and the anterior rectus abdominis sheath. The pectoralis major inserts on the greater tubercle of the humerus for shoulder adduction and chest press. The vascular supply to the pectoralis major muscle is via the thoracoacromial artery and vein, which run along the deep surface of the muscle at the medial border of the pectoralis minor.

The pectoralis minor originates from the costochondral junctions of ribs 2 through 6, inserts on the coracoid process of the scapula, and functions to depress the shoulder. Pectoralis major and minor innervation are via the medial and lateral pectoral nerves, originating from the medial and lateral cords of the brachial plexus, respectively.

The serratus anterior muscle lies along the lateral chest and is sometimes utilized in submuscular coverage of tissue expanders during breast reconstruction procedures. It originates from the surface of the first through the eighth ribs and inserts along the medial border of the scapula. It functions to support the scapula and pull it forward around the thorax during arm motion. The muscle is innervated by the long thoracic nerve, which can be injured during axillary surgery. Damage to the long thoracic nerve can result in a winged scapula.

1.7 Breast Aging and Breast Ptosis

Breast aging is caused by changes in the skin, the gland, and Cooper's ligaments. The Cooper's ligaments and breast skin elasticity attenuate with increasing breast size, age, lactation, and parity. As the ligaments attenuate, they stretch and no longer maintain the breast parenchyma in its anatomic position on the chest wall, resulting in drooping, or breast ptosis. It is important to note that augmentation of breast volume with implants may exacerbate breast ptosis because of the additional weight of the implants on the skin envelope.

Breast ptosis is graded with the Regnault classification, based on the position of the NAC relative to the IMF (Table 1.1).

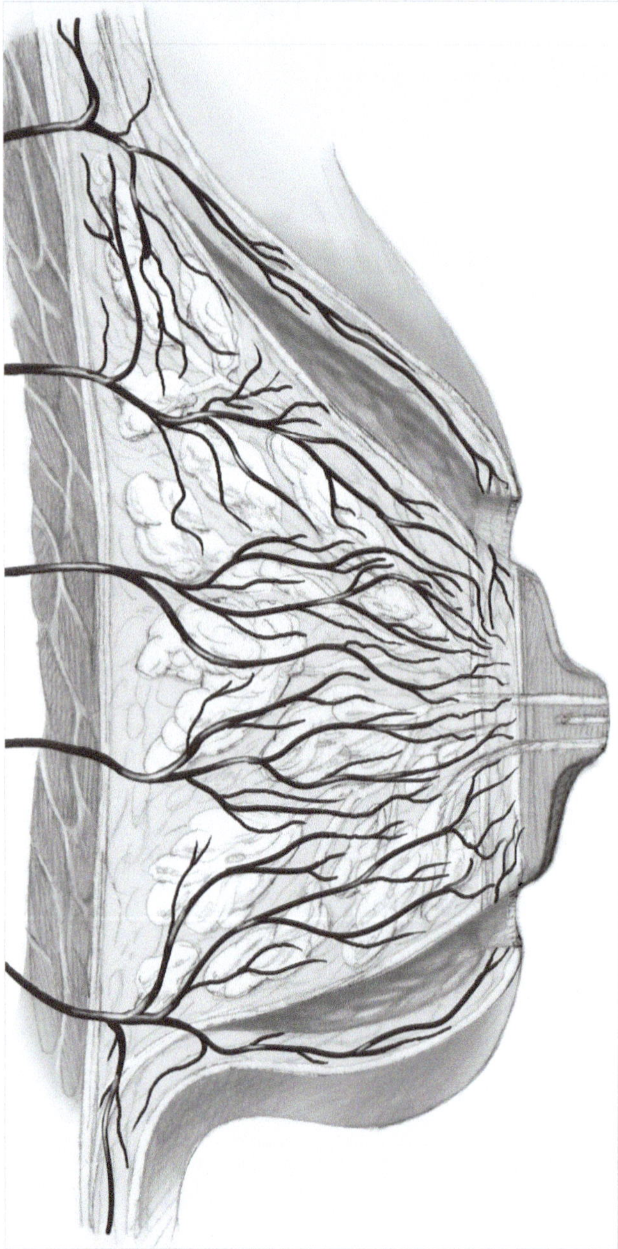

Fig. 1.4 Parasagittal section of breast blood supply shows perforating branches of the internal mammary artery projecting anteriorly through the pectoralis major muscle and through the breast gland parenchyma toward the nipple areolar complex. (Reproduced from Wallwiener D, Becker S, Veronesi U. Atlas of Breast Surgery. Stuttgart, Germany: Thieme Medical Publishers; 2015.)

Pseudoptosis consists of inferior pole glandular ptosis below the IMF with the NAC above the IMF. In first-degree, or mild, breast ptosis the NAC is at or less than 1 cm below the IMF. Second-degree breast ptosis is moderate, with the NAC 1 to 3 cm below the IMF but above the lower border of the breast (▶ Fig. 1.8, ▶ Fig. 1.9). Third-degree breast ptosis is severe, with the NAC at the lowest point of the breast.

The technique employed to correct breast ptosis largely depends upon the degree of ptosis. For example, first-degree breast ptosis can be corrected with crescent mastopexy, which allows up to 1 cm nipple areolar complex elevation, or augmentation. First degree and mild second-degree breast ptosis can be treated with periareolar (▶ Fig. 1.9) or circumvertical (▶ Fig. 1.10) mastopexy, which allows 1–2 cm nipple areolar complex elevation, or occasionally augmentation. Moderate second- and third-degree breast ptoses are often treated with an inverted-**T** skin incision, where the horizontal incision reduces vertical inferior pole skin excess and NAC-to-IMF distance, while the vertical incision reduces breast base diameter (▶ Fig. 1.11).

1.8 Anatomic Concepts in Cosmetic Breast Surgery

The anatomy and landmarks of the breast described so far are critically important for evaluation and operative planning in cosmetic breast surgery. While these topics will be covered in more detail in their respective chapters, we will highlight a few examples here to demonstrate the importance of breast anatomy to cosmetic breast surgery and surgical outcome. For example, to achieve a more natural augmentation, the existing breast base width should not be exceeded by implant width. Likewise, significant laxity of the skin envelope, or ptosis, and a correspondingly long nipple-to-IMF distance often requires a combined or staged augmentation–mastopexy procedure to restore aesthetic form.

The upper breast pole parenchyma thickness, as determined by the "pinch test," often determines the plane in which an implant is placed.[6] Inadequate pinch thickness, often characterized by a thickness of < 2 cm, often results in a subpectoral or dual-plane (part submuscular, part subglandular) implant placement. Total submuscular implant placement with pectoralis and serratus muscles places the implant higher and increases upper breast pole fullness, with increased risk of high implant malposition and animation deformity. Dual-plane implant placement with pectoralis inferior border release reduces pressure on lower implant pole, reducing risk of high or lateral malposition. Adequate pinch thickness (2 cm or greater) will allow subglandular implant placement. A potential advantage of subglandular implant placement includes minimal implant animation deformity.

1.9 Abnormal Breast Anatomy

There are many causes of abnormal breast anatomy, and the complete list is too numerous to mention within the confines of this text. However, a few situations are frequently encountered by the cosmetic breast surgeon and are thus mentioned for completeness. Specific technical details for these conditions will be highlighted in respective chapters; thus, the conditions are mentioned here only as a precursor to more detailed information found later in this text.

As previously mentioned, asymmetry in breast volume, position, and shape is relatively normal in the general population. These often subtle differences must be identified and incorporated into operative plans to achieve optimal operative results and ultimately greater patient satisfaction. By

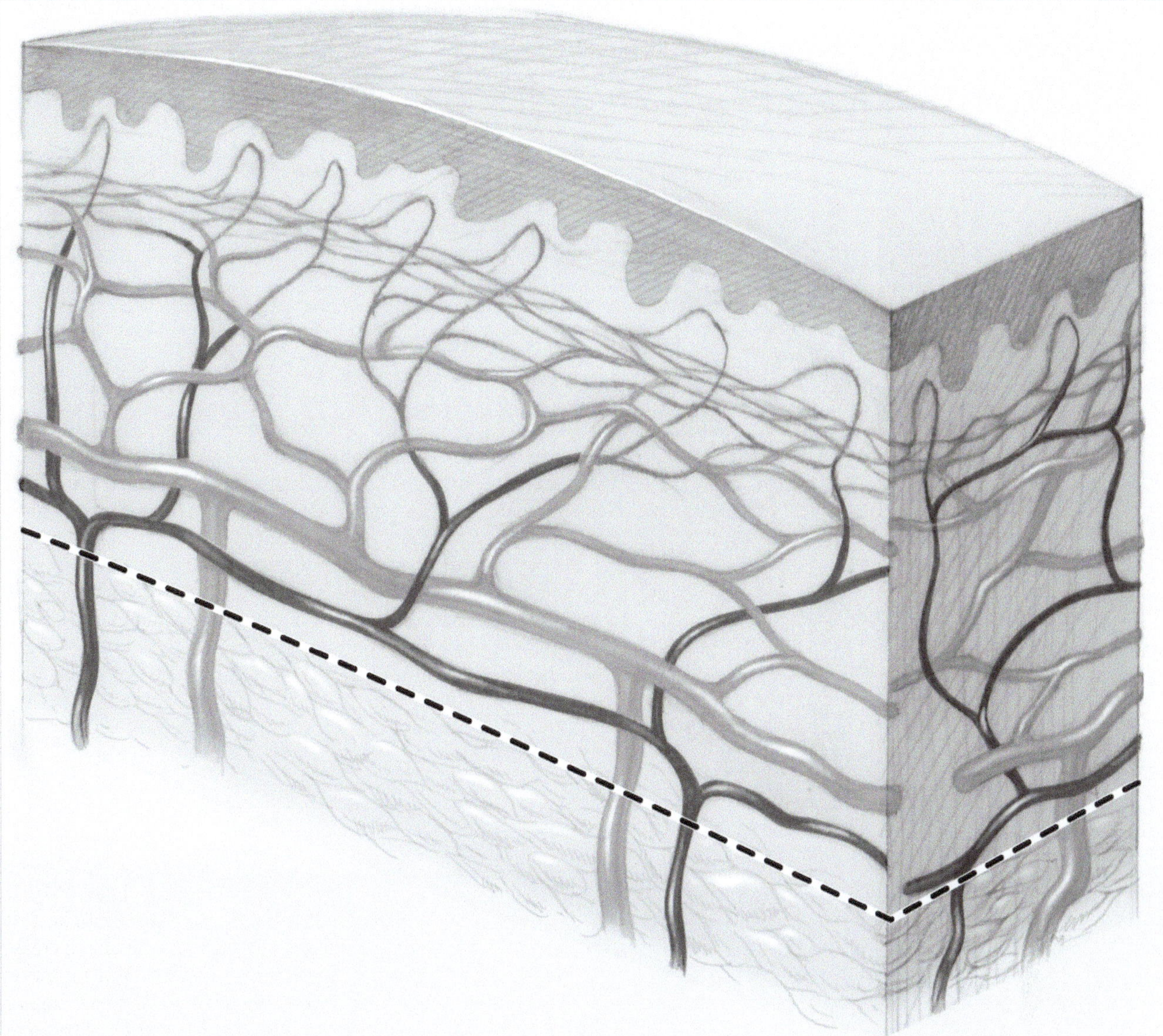

Fig. 1.5 The subcutaneous and dermal plexus is the primary blood supply to the remaining skin and nipple areolar complex after mastectomy. (Reproduced from Wallwiener D, Becker S, Veronesi U. Atlas of Breast Surgery. Stuttgart, Germany: Thieme Medical Publishers; 2015.)

systematically evaluating the anatomic landmarks previously described, as well as the aesthetic norm of the breast, the surgeon should be able to identify and account for these differences quite easily.

Common abnormal breast conditions include hypomastia, macromastia, and gynecomastia. Hypomastia is simply postpubertal underdevelopment of female breast tissue. Women with hypomastia frequently seek consultation for augmentation mammoplasty procedures. Macromastia is defined as postpubertal overdevelopment and hypertrophy of female breast tissue. Macromastia is often characterized by significant breast volume, associated with long sternal notch–to nipple distances, long NAC-to-IMF distances, shoulder strap grooves, IMF intertrigo, and back/neck pain. Women with macromastia are often seen in consultation for reduction mammoplasty procedures. Gynecomastia is a characterized by postpubertal overdevelopment of male breast tissue. This overdevelopment can be mild, moderate, or severe and include parenchymal hypertrophy alone or in combination with breast ptosis. Treatment of gynecomastia is discussed in detail in Chapter 18.

Although congenital breast abnormalities are not as prevalent, plastic surgeons are often consulted for assistance with them, including tuberous breasts and Poland syndrome. Breasts with constricted lower poles, or tuberous breasts, which are characterized by narrow base width, high IMF, and herniation of parenchyma into the NAC, offer a unique set of challenges for the cosmetic breast surgeon (▶ Fig. 1.1d). Radial release of internal "constriction" bands and/or concentric scoring of parenchyma is often required to widen the base width and redistribute parenchyma via a periareolar incision. With optimal parenchyma redistribution, placement of an implant can improve breast size and shape.

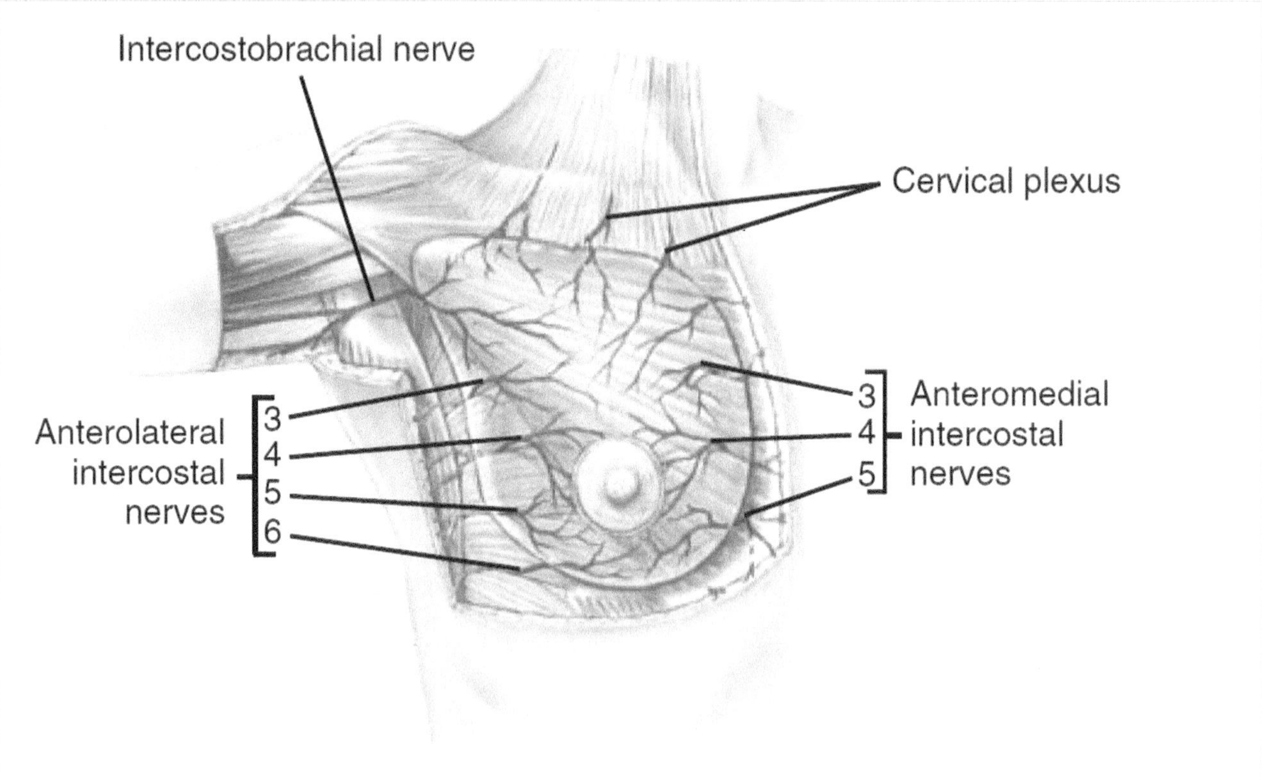

Fig. 1.6 Nipple areolar complex sensation is derived from the fourth intercostal nerve. (Reproduced from Janis JE. Essentials of Plastic Surgery, 2nd edition. New York, NY: Thieme Medical Publishers; 2014.)

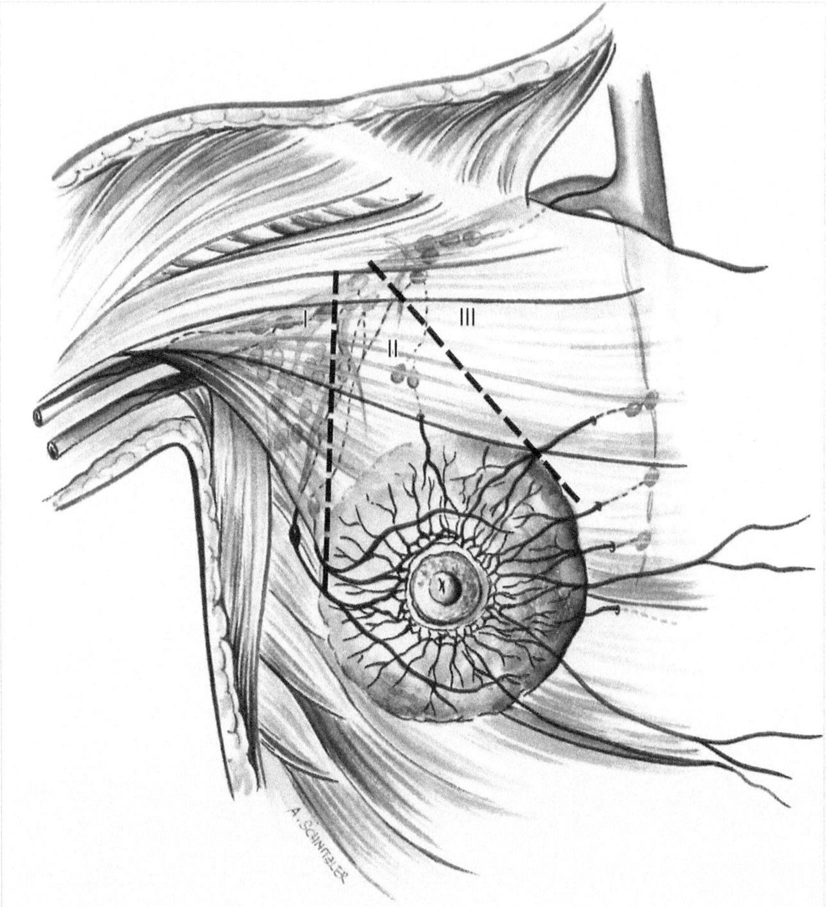

Fig. 1.7 The lymphatic drainage of the breast includes level 1, 2, and 3 lymph nodes. Level 1 lymph nodes are lateral and inferior to the pectoralis minor muscle. Level 2 nodes are directly posterior to the pectoralis minor. Level 3 nodes are medial to the pectoralis minor. (Reproduced from Wallwiener D, Becker S, Veronesi U. Atlas of Breast Surgery. Stuttgart, Germany: Thieme Medical Publishers; 2015.)

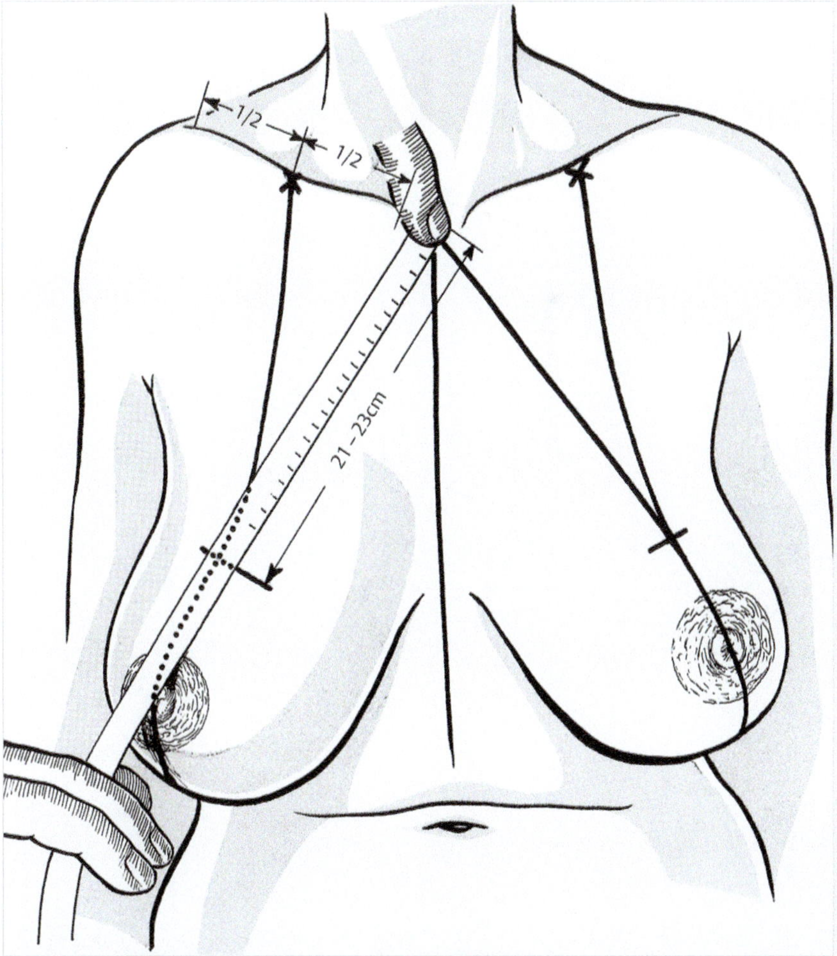

Fig. 1.8 In planning mastopexy, new position of the nipple should be on the most anteriorly projected portion of the breast parenchyma and above the inframammary fold. The patient depicted shows second-degree breast ptosis. (Reproduced from Wallwiener D, Becker S, Veronesi U. Atlas of Breast Surgery. Stuttgart, Germany: Thieme Medical Publishers; 2015.)

Table 1.1 Degrees of breast ptosis

Ptosis severity	Definition
Pseudoptosis	NAC above IMF
Mild (first-degree)	NAC at or < 1 cm below IMF
Moderate (second-degree)	NAC 1–3 cm below IMF
Severe (third-degree)	NAC at inferior position of breast

Poland syndrome is characterized by congenital underdevelopment or absence of the pectoralis muscle with associated breast and NAC abnormalities. This defect can also be associated with chest wall abnormalities, rib defects, and occasionally shortened (brachydactyly) or webbed (syndactyly) fingers. It is often unilateral in presentation. Treatment of Poland syndrome is challenging and often requires staged reconstructive procedures.

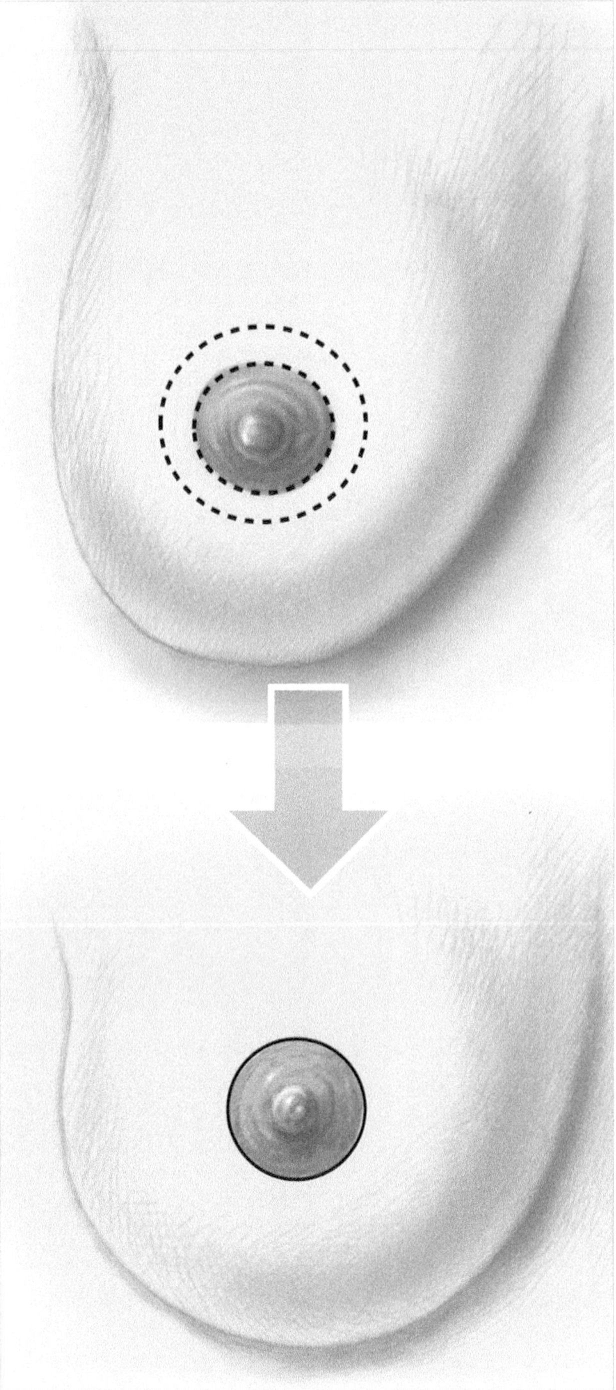

Fig. 1.9 Periareolar incision allows elevation of nipple up to 1 cm. (Reproduced from Wallwiener D, Becker S, Veronesi U. Atlas of Breast Surgery. Stuttgart, Germany: Thieme Medical Publishers; 2015.)

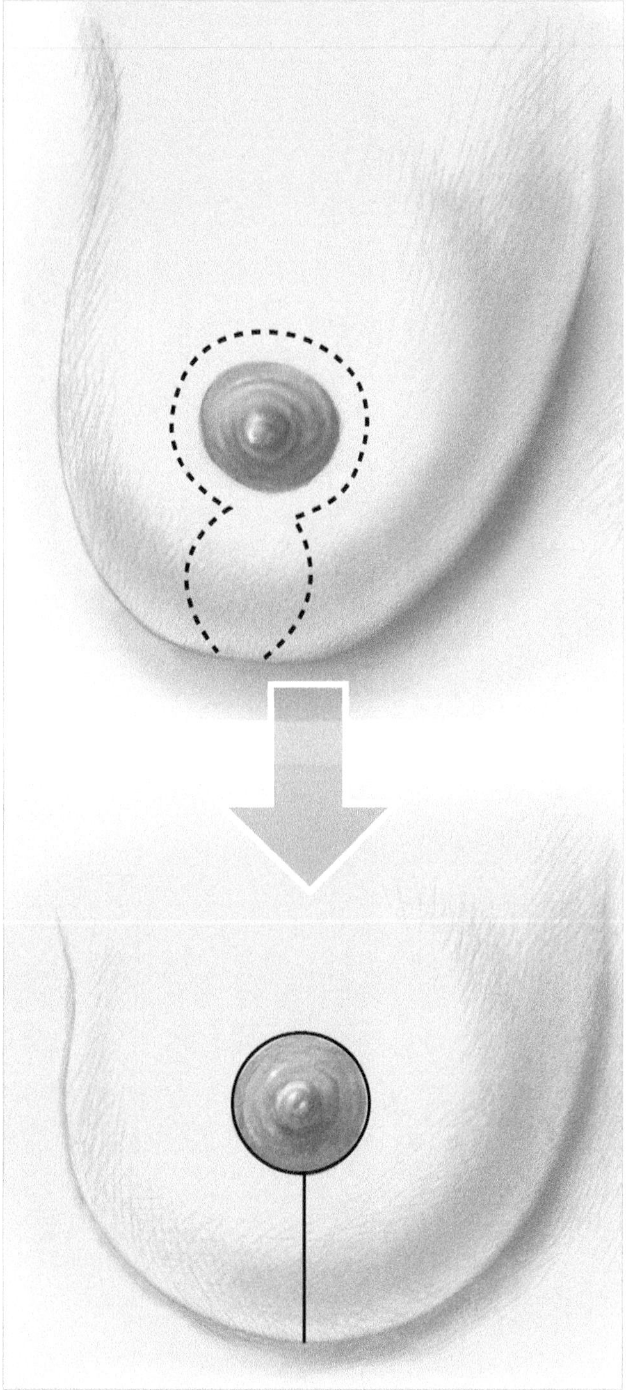

Fig. 1.10 Circumvertical incision allows elevation of the nipple greater than 1 cm while narrowing the breast inferior pole width. (Reproduced from Wallwiener D, Becker S, Veronesi U. Atlas of Breast Surgery. Stuttgart, Germany: Thieme Medical Publishers; 2015.)

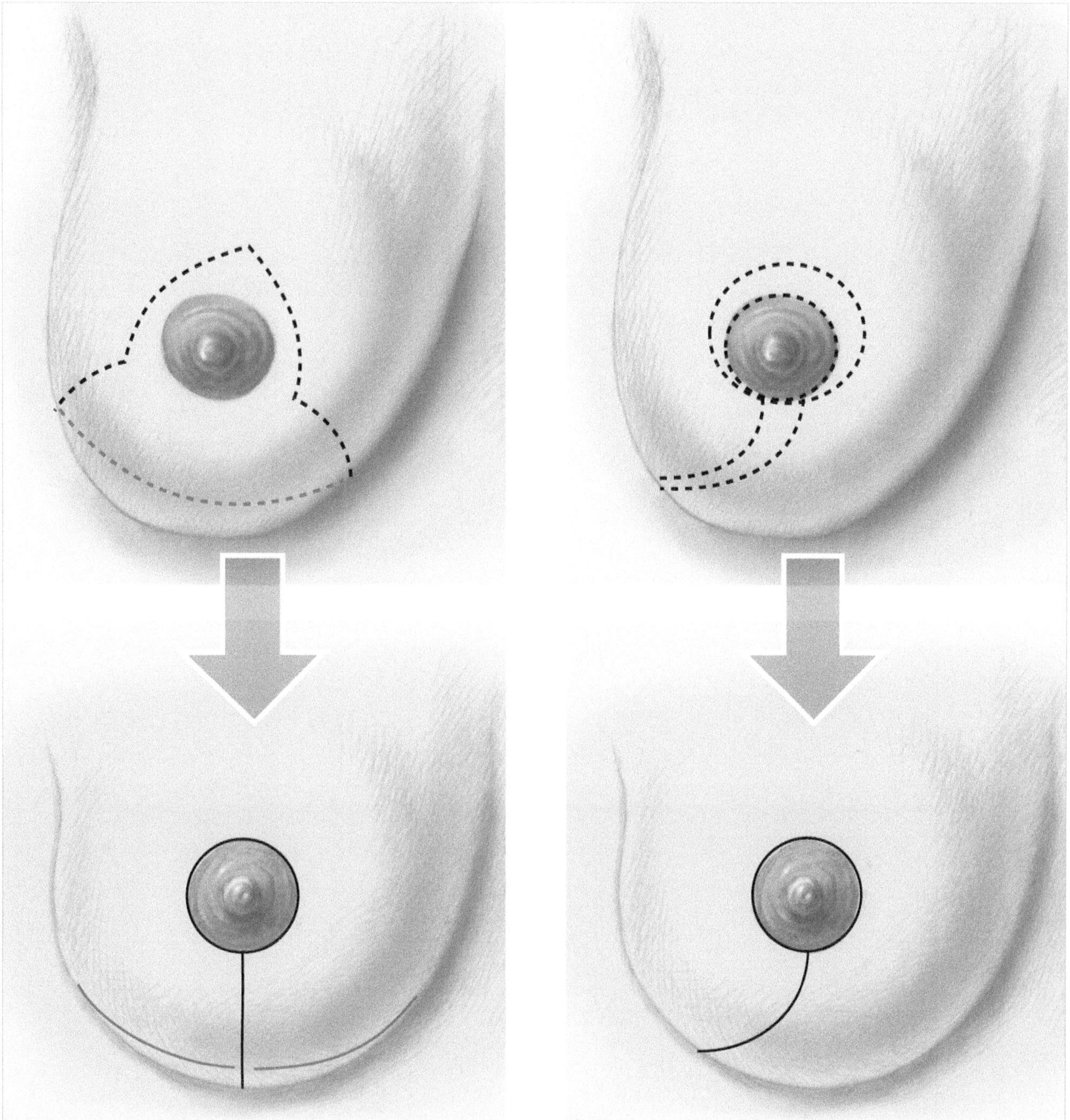

Fig. 1.11 Inverted T (Wise)-pattern incision allows elevation of the nipple, reduction of nipple-to-inframammary fold vertical skin excess, and narrowing of breast base width. (Reproduced from Wallwiener D, Becker S, Veronesi U. Atlas of Breast Surgery. Stuttgart, Germany: Thieme Medical Publishers; 2015.)

1.10 Conclusion

The plastic surgeon's grasp of breast anatomy and aesthetic subunits provides the foundation of understanding surgical techniques. Breast appearance is of great concern to both men and women as well as to the plastic and reconstructive surgeon who deals in matters of restoring and augmenting normal shape and function of the breast. By understanding breast development, basic anatomy, and critical landmarks, the plastic surgeon can identify specific abnormalities and/or deficiencies, thereby optimizing operative planning and ultimately surgical outcome.

Key Points

- Assessment of commonly accepted anatomical landmarks is important for any surgical procedure on the female or male breast.
- The rich vascular supply and redundant collateral circulation of the breast allows for inferiorly, medially, superiorly, and superomedially based pedicle design.

References

[1] Buck DW. Breast anatomy, embryology, and congenital defects. In: Buck DW, ed. Review of Plastic Surgery. New York, NY: Elsevier; 2016:75–82

[2] Crosby MA, Mahabir RC. Breast anatomy and embryology. In: Janis JE, ed. Essentials of Plastic Surgery. 2nd ed. New York, NY: Thieme; 2014:509–517

[3] Wallwiener D, Becker S, Veronesi U, eds. Preliminary remarks about the region. In: Wallwiener D, Becker S, Veronesi U, eds. Atlas of Breast Surgery. Stuttgart, Germany: Thieme; 2015:1–18

[4] Buck DW. Noncancer breast surgery. In: Buck DW, ed. Review of Plastic Surgery. New York, NY: Elsevier; 2016: 91–95

[5] De la Torre JE, Davis MR. Anatomy for plastic surgery of the breast. In: Neligan PC, Grotting JC, eds. Plastic Surgery, Vol 5: Breast. 3rd ed. New York, NY: Elsevier; 2012:1–12

[6] Hammond DC. Applied anatomy. In: Hammond DC, ed. Atlas of Aesthetic Breast Surgery. St Louis, MO: Saunders; 2009:1–10

Part II

Primary Breast Augmentation

II

2 Made to Match: The Essence of Breast Implant Selection

Bradley P. Bengtson

Summary
State-of-the-art breast implant–related surgery in primary augmentation, revision, or reconstruction requires the patient and plastic surgeon to navigate a number of critical decisions involving multiple factors. Implant selection and the patient education process this entails is the most critical and most challenging part of the surgical process. It involves evaluating patient expectations including reported bra cup size; optimally, three-dimensional imaging and simulation; and tissue-based planning, leading up to a sequence and algorithm assessing the specific indication for the procedure, the shape of the device, soft tissue assessment, implant softness and cohesivity, and, finally, implant style and size. This sequential, straightforward implant selection process is the essence of breast implant surgery and should assist the surgeon and patient who are navigating the important process of accurate patient assessment and implant selection so that they are truly Made to Match.

Keywords: breast augmentation, silicone breast implants, tissue-based planning, biodimensional planning, implant selection, patient selection, breast implant cohesivity, three-dimensional imaging and simulation, bra cup sizing

2.1 Introduction

Breast augmentation is a process, not simply a procedure. The key components as outlined by Adams[1] are comprehensive patient education and informed consent; tissue-based operative planning; refined surgical technique with rapid recovery; and detailed postoperative education. By far the most important of these processes are the first two: patient education and operative planning. In fact, if these first two critical steps are neglected, the surgeon may have performed a technically successful procedure, but the result may be deemed a failure by the patient.

With the advance of social media, the Internet, TV shows, and marketing as well as our profession itself, it is becoming increasingly difficult to meet a patient's expectations, and it all begins with patient education. Surgeons have to make some very fundamental decisions when it comes to breast surgery and plastic surgery in general. Among the first is, "Am I looking to perform an augmentation to restore volume and shape and create a natural, proportional outcome based on the patient's tissues, or not?" As we must decide whether we are going to place fat in the breast anywhere except the subcutaneous fatty plane, surgeons need to decide on how they will approach breast augmentation patients and whether they will use tissue-based planning techniques to determine implant selection, or not. This chapter will make several assumptions. The first is that the plastic surgeon interested in this chapter and approach uses current, tissue-based planning principles in selecting breast implants and educates patients to what this approach delivers. In general, it is advisable not to augment less than or greater than 1 cm of the patient's breast base width. This principle creates a range of about 150–250 cc based on the implant's projection. There is not one implant size or style that will work for any given patient. In fact, there are probably 10 to 15 implants that may work. The goal is to achieve a size that is best for the patient's body to obtain a great outcome, but not so large or so small that it creates a complication, malposition, asymmetry, or suboptimal aesthetic result. Next, the patient's cup size is standardized, and the patient is then shown three-dimensional (3D) imaging and simulation of the expected outcome.[2] If the surgeon's recommendations and the patient's desires do not align, the surgeon should try to educate the patient further or should consider avoiding operating on the patient.

Next, the surgeon should match the implant style and specific gel characteristics to each patient. There are hundreds of different styles of available implants on the market today. The benefit of having so many different implant styles, projections, shells, and gel cohesivities is that the surgeon can match the patient's desires very well and even correct minor asymmetries. The challenge of having all of these possibilities is deciding which implant to use. One current implant manufacturer has over 900 implant options, and the product line continues to grow.[3] It is no wonder that what patients desire and demand as an acceptable outcome is becoming an increasingly difficult target to hit. The intent of this chapter is to arm the reader with the tools, techniques, and approaches to help simplify and navigate these core critical decisions that need to be made with the patient to achieve a successful outcome.

2.2 Bra Cup Sizing

A great deal has been written on patient education and informed consent, and one cannot overemphasize its critical importance in the entire education process. Trying to determine what a patient is looking to achieve and then educating that patient on what is or is not possible, cutting through all of the misinformation and myth, is a challenging task. Informed consent is not just a document. It is a process that walks the patient through the procedure in detail, including details of the procedure, options and alternatives to achieve the desired goal, the anticipated course and potential outcomes, and all potential complications in detail. One of the most difficult aspects of adequate breast augmentation informed consent is that there is no standard.

One of the challenges of standardizing outcomes is that bra sizing is variable and often times not reproducible. The author has developed a method to standardize breast cup size, and although still imperfect, it adds an incredible educational benefit for the patient–surgeon relationship and helps to create a standard starting point and endpoint with one simple measurement.[2] Most importantly, it enables the surgeon and the patient to begin the discussion on size. This, along with patient imaging, will enable the surgeon to come to an agreement on the range of outcomes for the patient. The bra cup can be standardized with one hemi-circumference measurement over the maximum apex of the breast, supporting the breast if it is ptotic. These measurements were determined from evaluation

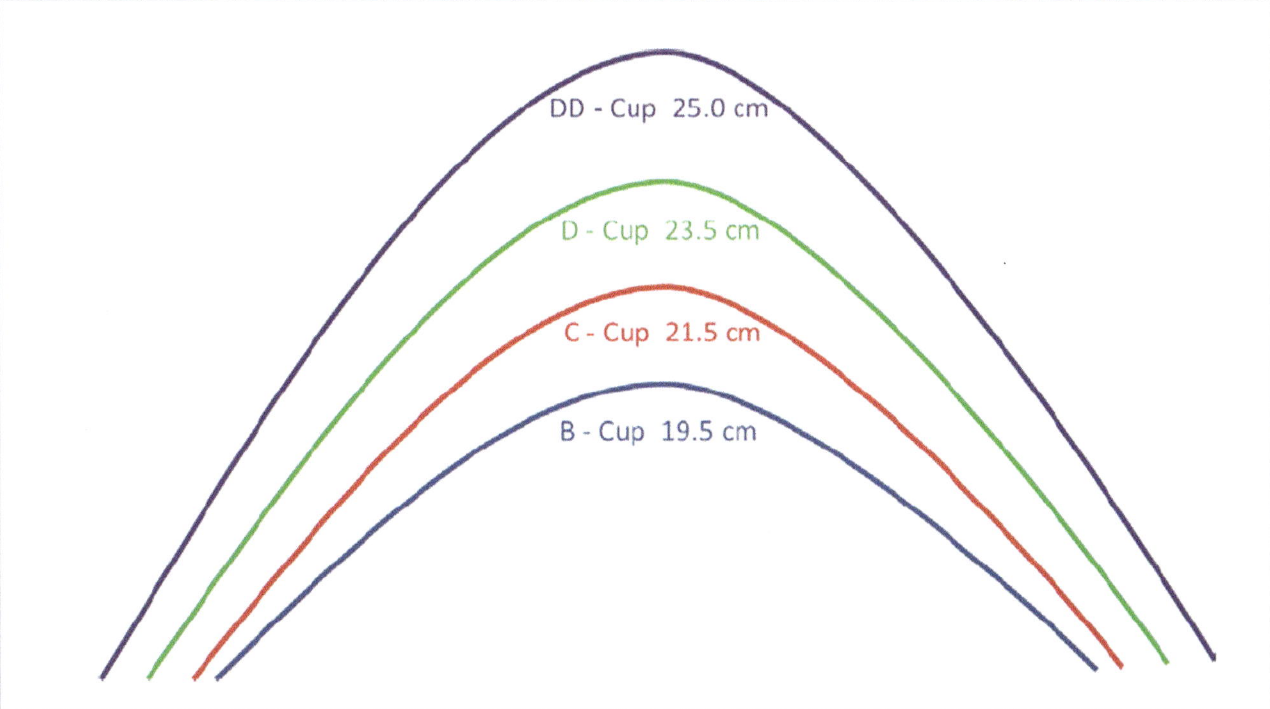

Fig. 2.1 Standardization of the bra cup can be based on one measurement: the breast hemicircumference. It is based on measuring the medial-to-lateral breast inflection points, which represent the take-off points where the breast attaches to the cheast wall. The average bra cup size measurement between the largest single-surgeon cohort and total group cohort is shown here.

of over 6,000 patients and have been confirmed in over 3,000 more. Assessing and setting the bra cup measurement as a standard at the consult is an excellent educational tool that puts the surgeon and patient on the same starting page concerning size and allows for standardization for the outcome both as an objective measurement and visually when 3-D imaging and simulation are added. Once the bra cup size is established, adding approximately 200 cc raises the bra cup incrementally by one size. Bra cup sizing, along with the 3D imaging and simulation discussed in the following section, enable patients to visualize and experience their outcome before surgery. In the author's experience, use of 3D imaging and simulation allows for the best visual for setting expectations and limiting the need for revisional surgery (▶ Fig. 2.1, ▶ Fig. 2.2).

2.3 Three-Dimensional Imaging and Simulation

Along with the new cohesive implant options, imaging and simulation has been one of the most significant technical enhancements in the author's practice in the past 10 years. It is not just a great marketing tool (although it certainly is that). It enables the patient to visualize the outcome. In addition, it is an incredible educational and planning tool, enabling the surgeon to determine volume and projection differences specifically from side to side. In striving for as much symmetry as possible, over 60% of the author's patients receive implants that are asymmetric in volume or profile to achieve the best symmetry possible, because native breasts are often asymmetric to some degree. This technology is quite reliable; outcomes average less than 2% different from the simulation at 1 year (Fig. 2.3).[4,5] Mastopexy and augmentation–mastopexy procedures can also be simulated and used to walk patients visually through these procedures. The author is currently working on reduction and revision modules to simulate the removal of specific volumes or known implant volumes and subsequently adding volume back in or lifting the breast.[6]

2.4 Implant Characteristics and Implant Selection

Implant selection using tissue-based planning principles has been very well documented, and the author currently uses a modification of the "High-Five" principles as outlined by Tebbetts and Adams.[7,8] The importance of using exam and measurements in selecting the implant range for each patient cannot be overemphasized. Each surgeon will need to decide how to help patients select a range of implants that match their breast and body. Key critical factors and assessments for general selection include the following:

1. Determine the patient's breast base width (BBW). BBW is the actual breast width minus the soft tissue thickness (on average 1.5 cm). The actual breast width is measured as the transverse width from the medial to lateral inflection points of the breast, which represent the breast borders (▶ Fig. 2.4a). This BBW is critical and determines the overall range of implants. The author chooses implants with a diameter or width within 1 cm of the BBW.

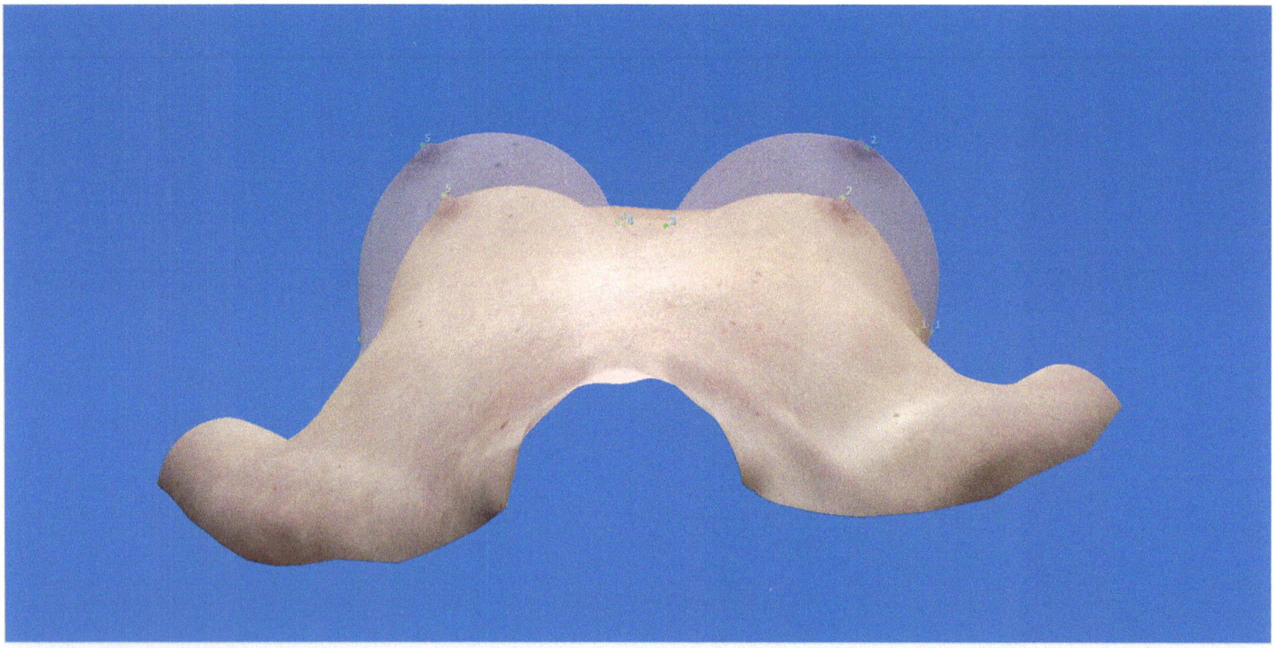

Fig. 2.2 Vectra imaging shows the medial and lateral inflection points where the skin meets the chest wall. The hemicircumference is then measured over the apex of the breast maximum arc. This single measurement then correlates to the bra cup size, with a 21.5-cm hemicircumference measuring out to a middle or C- cup.

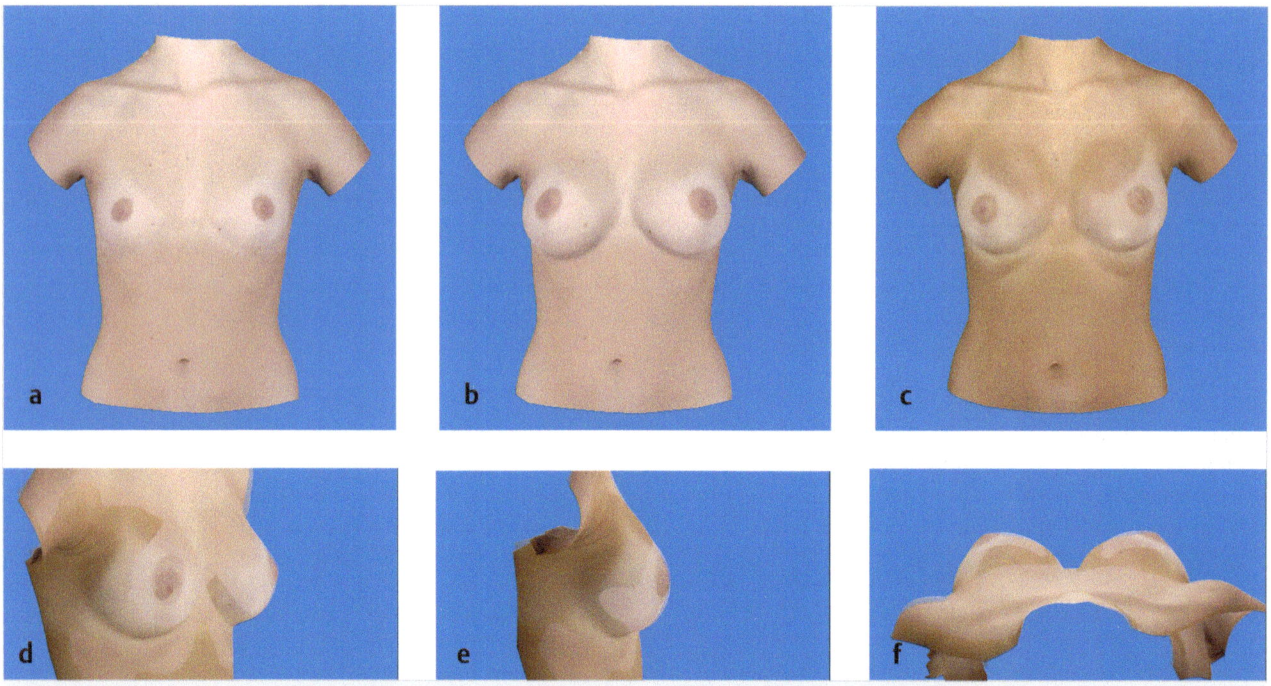

Fig. 2.3 Simulation sequence of a primary augmentation patient who selected Style 410, 335-cc MF implants, showing **(a)** her preoperatively, along with **(b)** her 3D simulation with Canfield Vectra system with Style 410 MF, followed by **(c–f)** her actual 1-year postoperative outcome with this same device style and size. These images show that there is minimal variation between the simulated view and the actual 1-year outcome. Even though we inform patients that there are no guarantees and that their outcome will differ from the simulation, in reality, barring any rare capsular contracture or complications, it is extremely accurate.

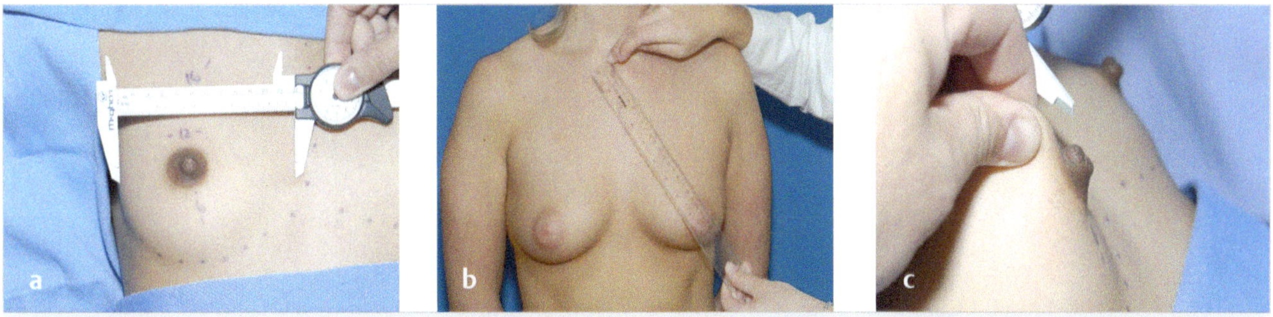

Fig. 2.4 **(a)** Breast base width (BBW), **(b)** SN-to-N distance, and **(c)** elasticity are the three critical assessments that need to be measured and help determine the implant range, height/diameter, and implant projection.

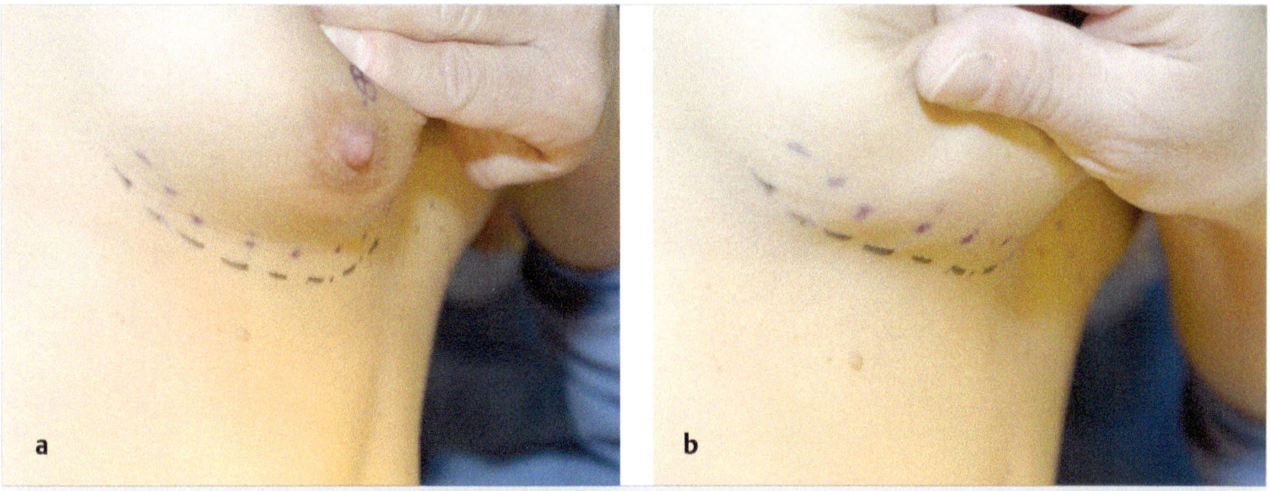

Fig. 2.5 **(a)** Resting versus **(b)** actual or true inframammary fold. The resting fold shows what the lower breast inflection point is at rest versus the actual or true fold, where the base of the implant will eventually set. This is why in a full mastopexy or breast reduction the patient will have her lower breast incision ride up on the lower pole of the breast if the incision is made in the resting fold following a tight closure.

2. Determine the sternal notch (SN)-to-nipple (N) (▶ Fig. 2.4b) and nipple-to-inframammary fold (IMF) distances. If the patient has a short SN-to-N distance, shorter-height and smaller-diameter implants are chosen, or alternatively, the IMF needs to be adjusted. N-to-IMF distance also affects implant diameter and height selection.
3. Determine breast type and compliance or elasticity. This helps to determine implant projection. This can be determined objectively or subjectively and, in general, can be classified as tight, average, or loose. The looser the skin envelope, the more projecting the implant needs to be, or, alternatively, mastopexy and skin reduction will be required to match the breast and implant volume (Box 2.1 and ▶ Fig. 2.4c).

Box 2.1 Basic Principles of Implant Selection

- Breast base width (BBW) helps determine implant range
- Sternal notch–to-nipple (SN-to-N) distance and nipple-to-IMF determine implant height
- Breast type and compliance-elasticity
  - Tight 0–2 cm, average 2–3 cm, loose 3–4 cm
  - Help determine implant projection
- Select implant and set IMF

A note on the IMF is important. The IMF is the key foundation of the breast. The author has written and presented a great deal on the IMF and would refer the reader to these papers.[9,10] It is vital to understand one key concept of the IMF: the resting versus the actual fold. Surgeons tend to mark patients in the standing or sitting position, and if the inferior inflection point is ascertained by simply pushing the breast down and marked, the resting fold is demarcated (▶ Fig. 2.5a). However, this is not the true IMF. If the breast is slightly lifted off the chest and forced down with pressure, the true IMF is elucidated (▶ Fig. 2.5b). This actual or true fold may be 1.5 to 2 cm lower than the resting fold and needs to be considered. This is where the new IMF will be and where the incision should be placed when the IMF incisional approach is utilized.

The reason for this fold variation has been studied extensively by Acland and colleagues and is ascribed to the fascial fibers extending down at an oblique angle, allowing for the inferior descent of the device to the lower true fold.[11]

2.5 Made to Match

After the patient has been assessed and implant dimensions selected, the final and increasingly critical piece is selecting the implant cohesivity and fill characteristics that are best for the patient and surgical application. First, the surgical application should be considered: augmentation, revision, or reconstruction. This is extremely difficult to address and discuss in any semblance of order, unless the selection is broken down into an easy-to-understand format. The author uses an approach for selecting the actual implant characteristics that are best suited for each patient, embodied in an algorithm titled *Made to Match*. It does make several assumptions, one being that wrinkling and rippling along with accompanying increased palpability is the most common complication observed in implant surgery and the most difficult to fix. As such, the author prioritizes implants with the greatest fill and cohesivity in the following patients: reconstruction patients, many revision patients, and even a subset of primary augmentation patients who are extremely thin. This may not be how some surgeons look at or assess patients, but the author encourages the reader to use some of these principles to help navigate this critical implant selection process.

Implant cohesivity is playing an increasingly important role in implant selection. It also increases the complexity of implant selection, with over 900 implant style and shape options for each patient. Every patient presents with specific characteristics of coverage, elasticity, ptosis, or soft tissue constriction that need to be the driving force and priority in the implant selection process (▶ Fig. 2.6).[12]

So, with so many options, how can one simplify this selection process? The *Made to Match* algorithm summarizes the essence of breast implant surgery with the following six factors: surgical application, shape, soft tissue quality, softness, style, and size (▶ Fig. 2.7).

The initial decision is to determine what type of procedure the patient is actually having. Is the patient having a primary augmentation, breast revision, or breast reconstruction (▶ Fig. 2.8)? There are certain assumptions that this introduces, but generally, breast reconstruction patients have poor to extremely poor soft tissue coverage. Because soft tissue coverage trumps all other factors, the author prioritizes using the implant with the greatest fill and cohesivity in patients with minimal soft tissue coverage. New highly cohesive round or shaped implant options with increased form stability are chosen in thin patients to minimize wrinkling, rippling, and palpability issues. This removes 80% of the other less cohesive, lower-fill devices and simplifies implant selection. The focus can then shift to the next level of selection.

The second step is to choose the implant shape. Patients who desire more of a rounded upper pole are better suited for a round, more highly cohesive device. Sufficient soft tissue support, however, is required to hold the device in position, and the cohesivity of the device needs to be great enough to hold the implant volume up versus collapsing into the lower pole of the device. The amount of soft tissue coverage and elasticity of the soft tissue are also critical. Older implant styles with low cohesivity will fall into more of a shaped look, depending on the soft tissue support, the amount of coverage, and, most importantly, the soft tissue laxity. The negative aspect is a much greater degree of shell wrinkling and rippling. However, the new highly cohesive devices are form-stable enough to maintain the overall implant shape: either a shaped or a round implant with minimal shell collapse and irregularity (▶ Fig. 2.9).

Step three is a very critical evaluation and involves the determination of the patient's soft tissues (▶ Fig. 2.10). This is a critical step, as wrinkling and rippling are the most common adverse events in implant-based surgery and the most difficult to correct. The degree of visible implant wrinkling and rippling is dependent upon the patient, the implant, and the surgeon. The patient's soft tissue thickness and elasticity, making up the breast type, is a primary critical factor. Thin tissue coverage and greater elasticity lead to greater implant visibility. The greater the potential there is for visibility, the more cohesive the device should be. The surgeon factors are the plane chosen, with the submuscular pocket having the greatest coverage, and whether secondary procedures such as fat grafting or additional lower pole scaffold support is utilized. In breast revision patients with wrinkling and rippling, the best current options include using the implant with the greatest cohesivity, placing the device in the submuscular plane, and consideration for fat grafting and scaffold support in severe cases.

We have initiated a study to evaluate the current implant styles in vitro and in position postoperatively in the sitting and standing position with high-resolution ultrasound (HRUS). Our early findings confirm that the higher the degree of cohesivity, the less the wrinkling and rippling secondary to shell collapse. Again, the pocket is important in that, if it is significantly tight, the pressure can smooth out the surface. In the clear majority of patients, however, the pocket is elastic enough to allow the implant characteristics to be visible. This is the same process with significant capsular contracture. The implant wrinkling may be completely blocked by a stiff capsule and patients may even complain of wrinkling of the implant after successful treatment of a capsular contracture patient when a less cohesive device is used. ▶ Fig. 2.11, ▶ Fig. 2.12, and ▶ Fig. 2.13, respectively, show patients requiring devices of progressively increasing cohesivity, along with their upright images on ultrasound. As anticipated, the greater the degree of cohesivity, the less visible the implant wrinkling and rippling, both clinically and on ultrasound in the upright position.

The fourth factor in the algorithm deals with the implant softness compared to the patient's breast parenchyma. This aspect in the *Made to Match* decision tree is for the patient and the surgeon to make together. In patients with adequate soft tissue coverage and relatively normal laxity, the surgeon and patient can choose to match the patient's breast parenchyma characteristics to the implant characteristics. For patients with soft, fatty breasts, a less cohesive device may be chosen. For patients with extremely firm, dense breasts or with tight skin envelopes or for patients with true breast constriction, highly cohesive round or shaped devices may be used (▶ Fig. 2.14).

The fifth decision is implant style or projection. This aspect was discussed in Section 2.1 and is based upon the soft tissue laxity. Tight skin envelopes can accommodate less projecting devices, whereas loose skin envelopes require more projecting implants to fill the volume. This measurement may be subjective or objective (▶ Fig. 2.15, ▶ Fig. 2.16).

The final implant size range, as discussed in Section 2.1, is then selected based on the patient's breast base width. The breast base width, again, is the overall breast width minus the soft tissue thickness. Ultimately, the breast base width should closely match the implant width. This is the essence of tissue-based planning (▶ Fig. 2.17, ▶ Fig. 2.18).

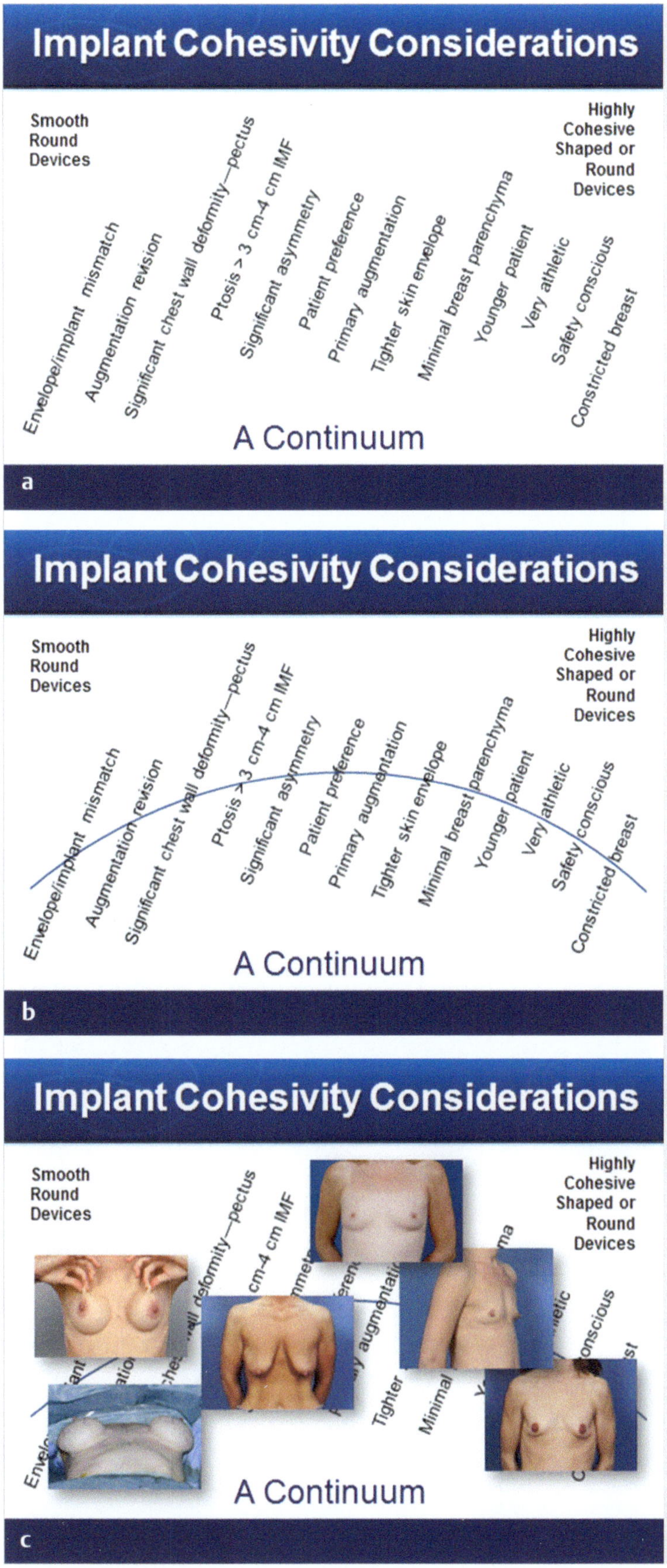

Fig. 2.6 (a–c) Implant cohesivity is playing an increasingly important role in implant selection. It also increases the complexity of implant selection now with over 900 implant style and shape options for each and every patient. Each patient presents with specific characteristics of coverage, elasticity, ptosis, or soft tissue constriction that needs to be the driving force and priority in the implant selection process.

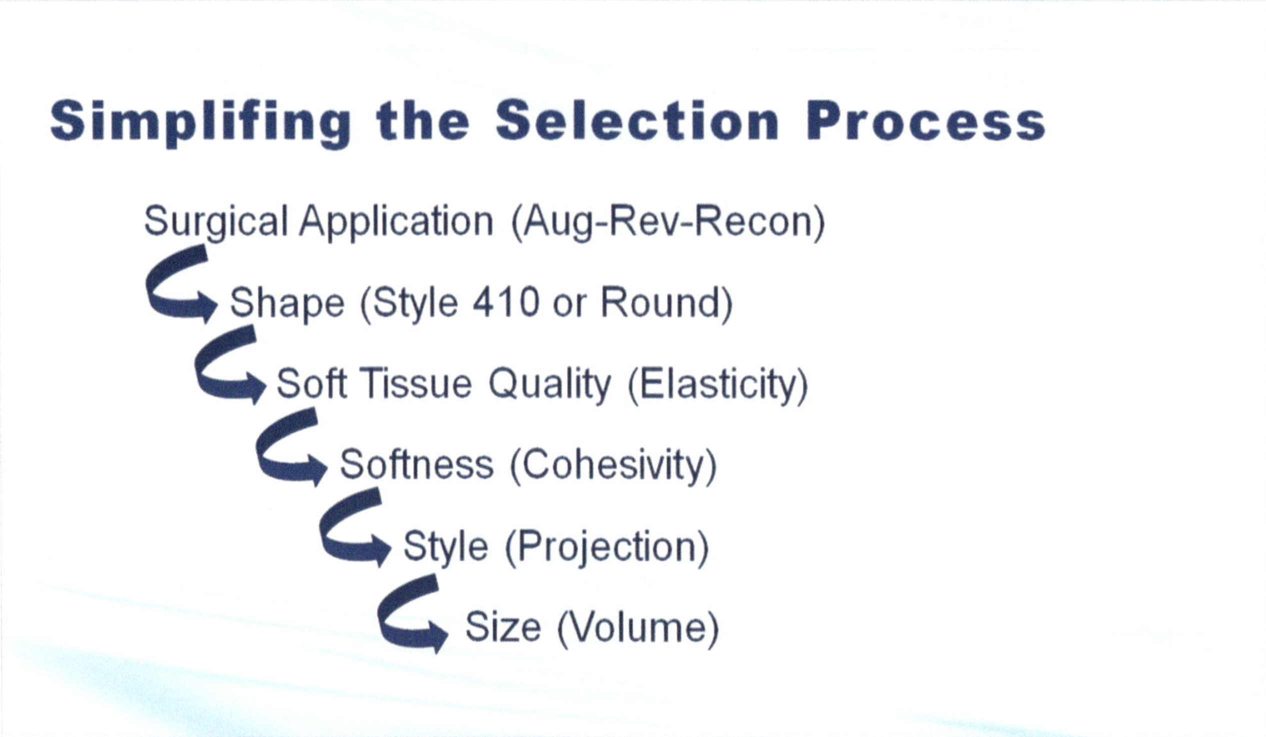

Fig. 2.7 The author's current algorithm to simplify the implant selection conundrum.

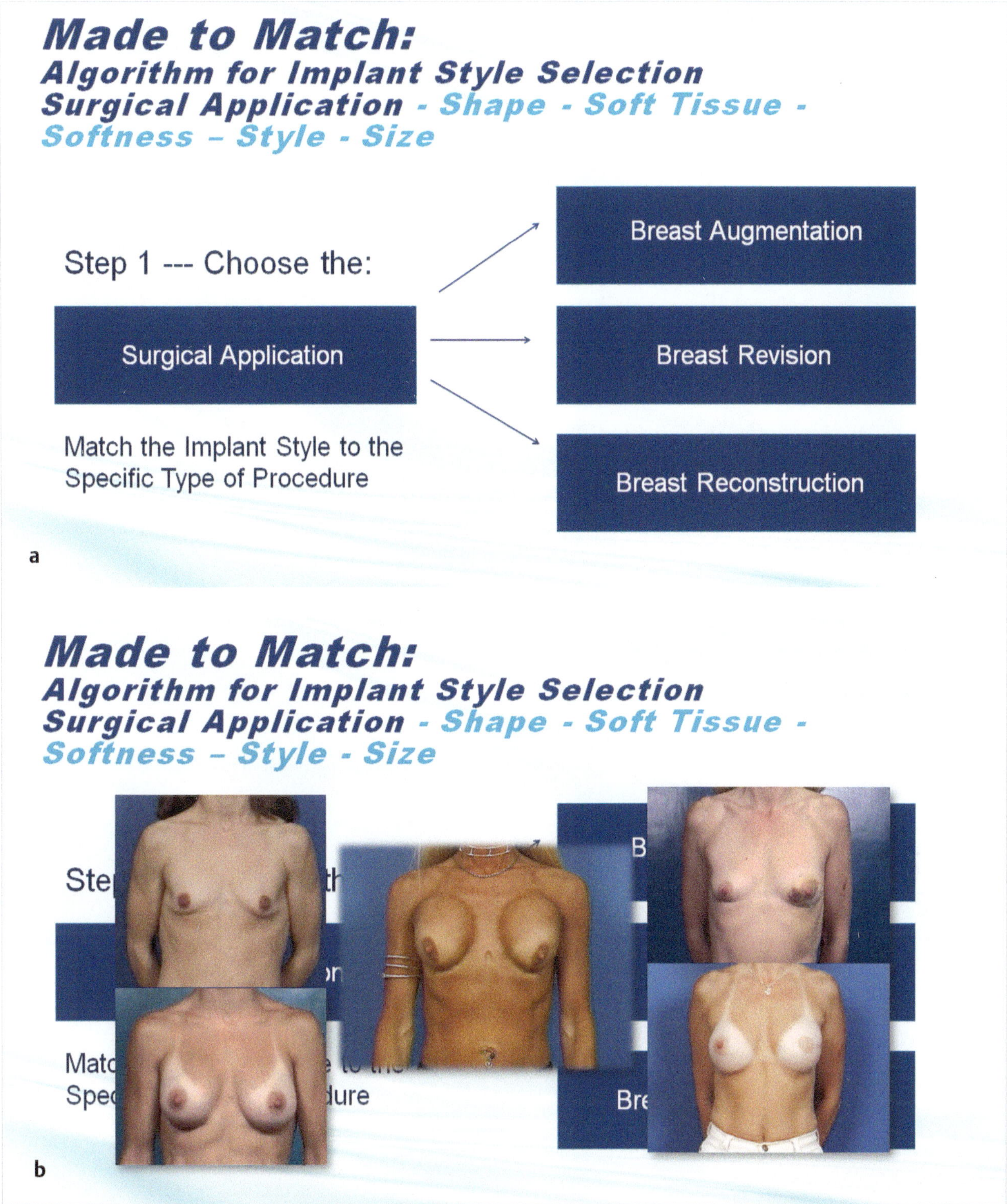

Fig. 2.8 **(a)** The first step in the *Made to Match* algorithm is to choose the specific surgical application that will be performed. **(b)** Is the patient having a primary augmentation (left), breast revision (center), or breast reconstruction (right)?

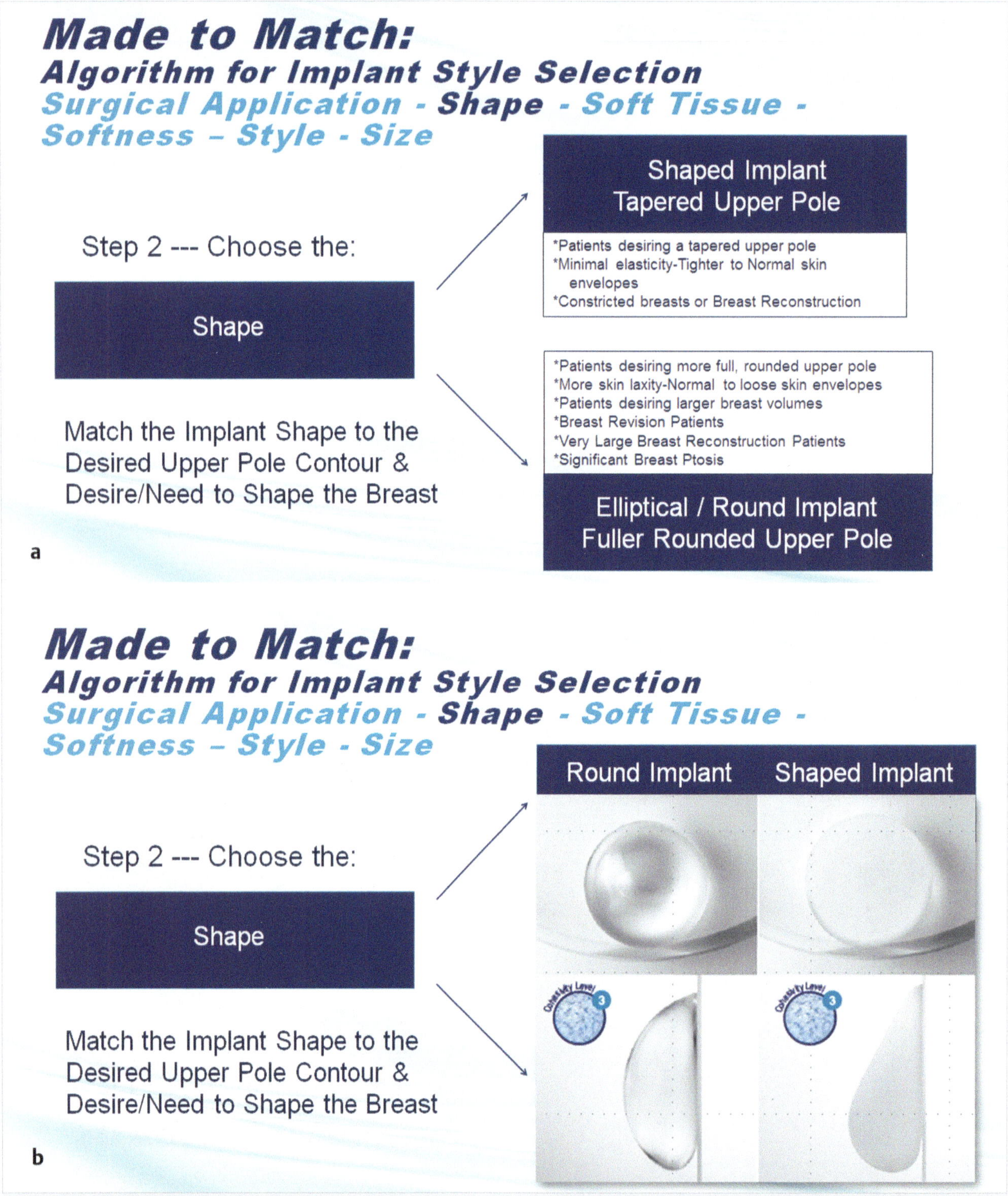

Fig. 2.9 (a,b) The second step in the *Made to Match* algorithm is to choose the implant shape. Shape retention is dependent on the breast type: how elastic the skin is and the amount of soft tissue coverage as well as the cohesivity of the gel filler. The more cohesive the gel, the less the gel collapses into the lower pole of the device when the patient is upright, and the better shape retention.

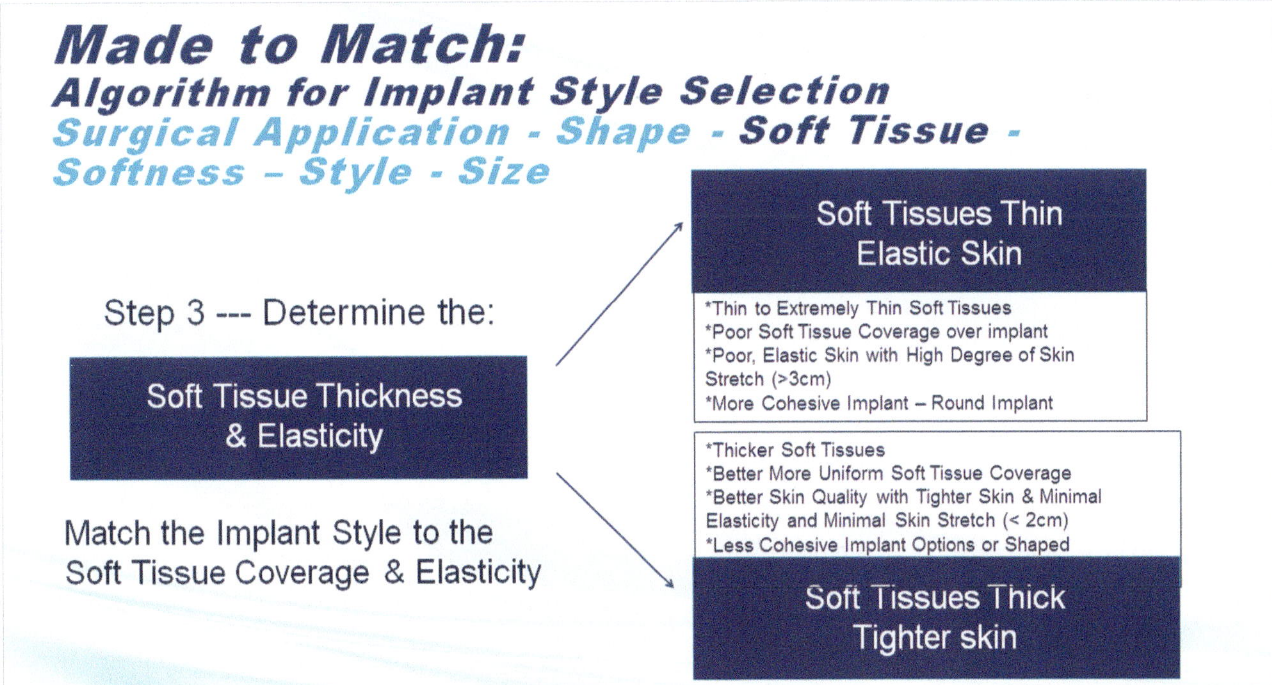

a

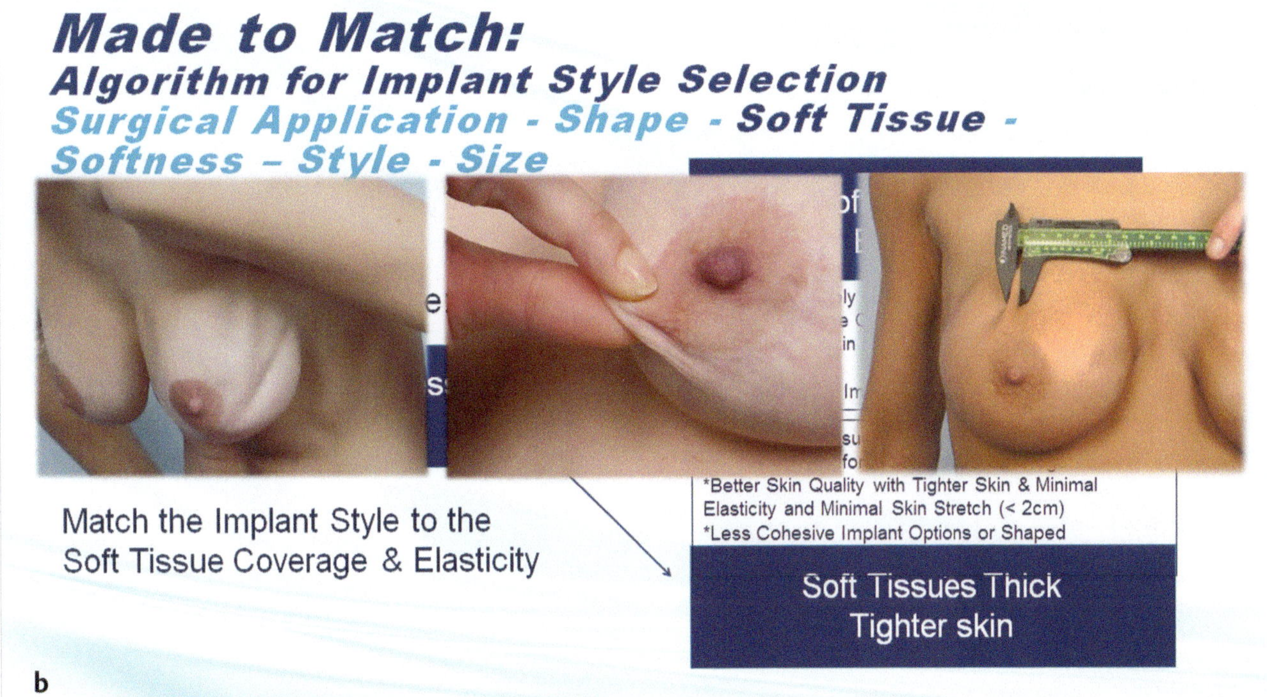

b

Fig. 2.10 (a,b) Step three in the *Made to Match* algorithm is a very critical evaluation and involves the determination of the patient's soft tissues.

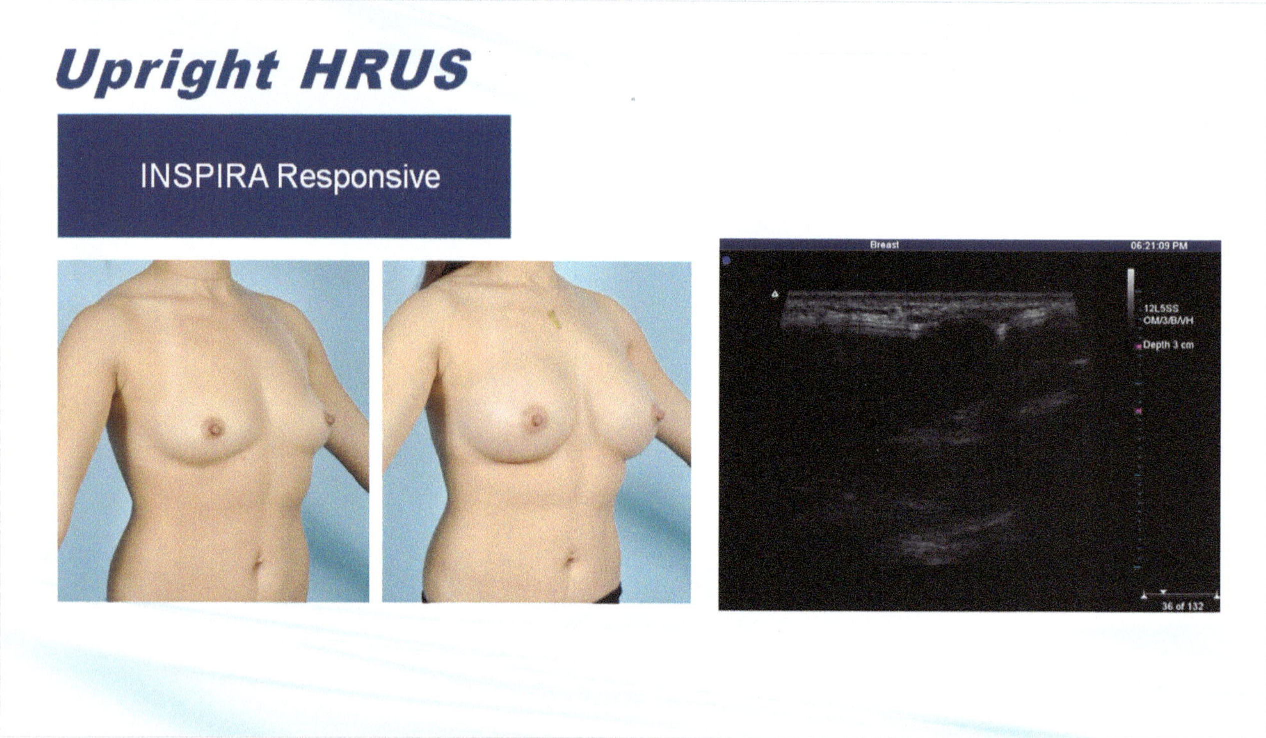

Fig. 2.11 Patient with a 397-cc, Style 15, responsive gel, noncohesive device clinically (pre- and postoperative) and on ultrasound. In the submuscular position and with 3 cm of pinch thickness, the patient has no clinical wrinkling or rippling, but it is visible on ultrasound in the upper pole.

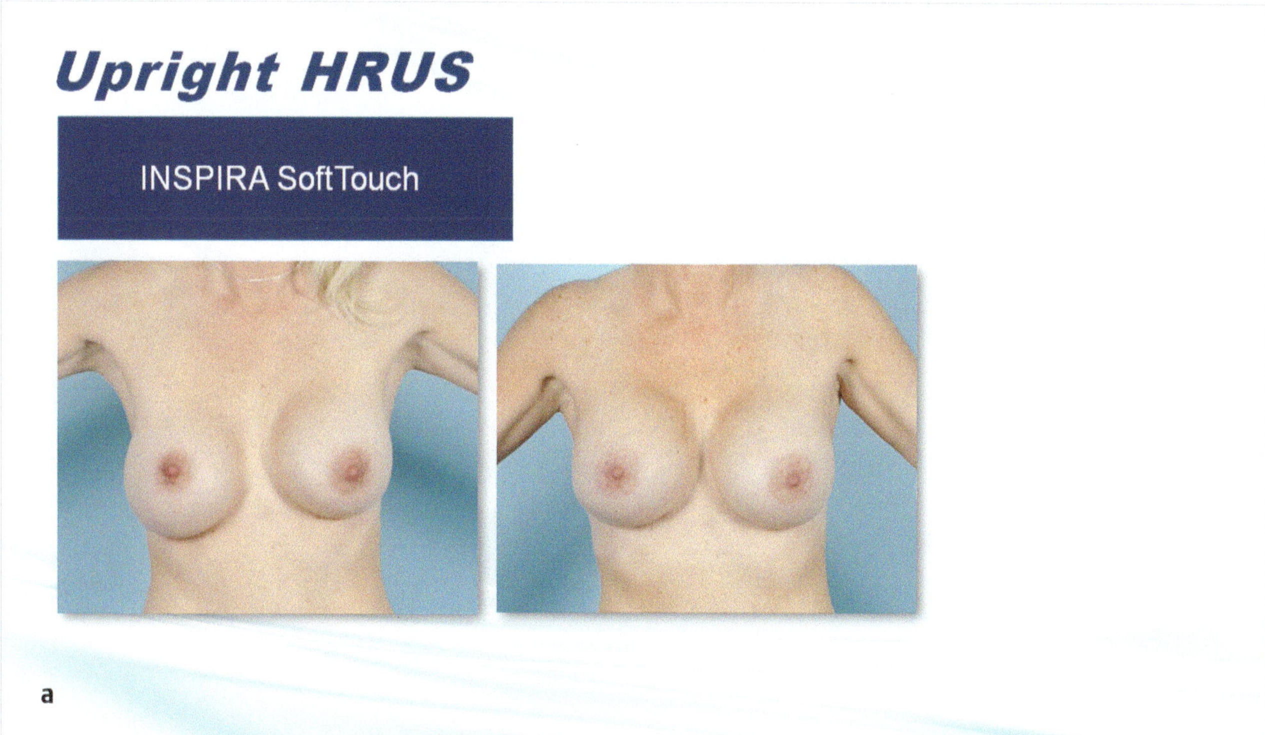

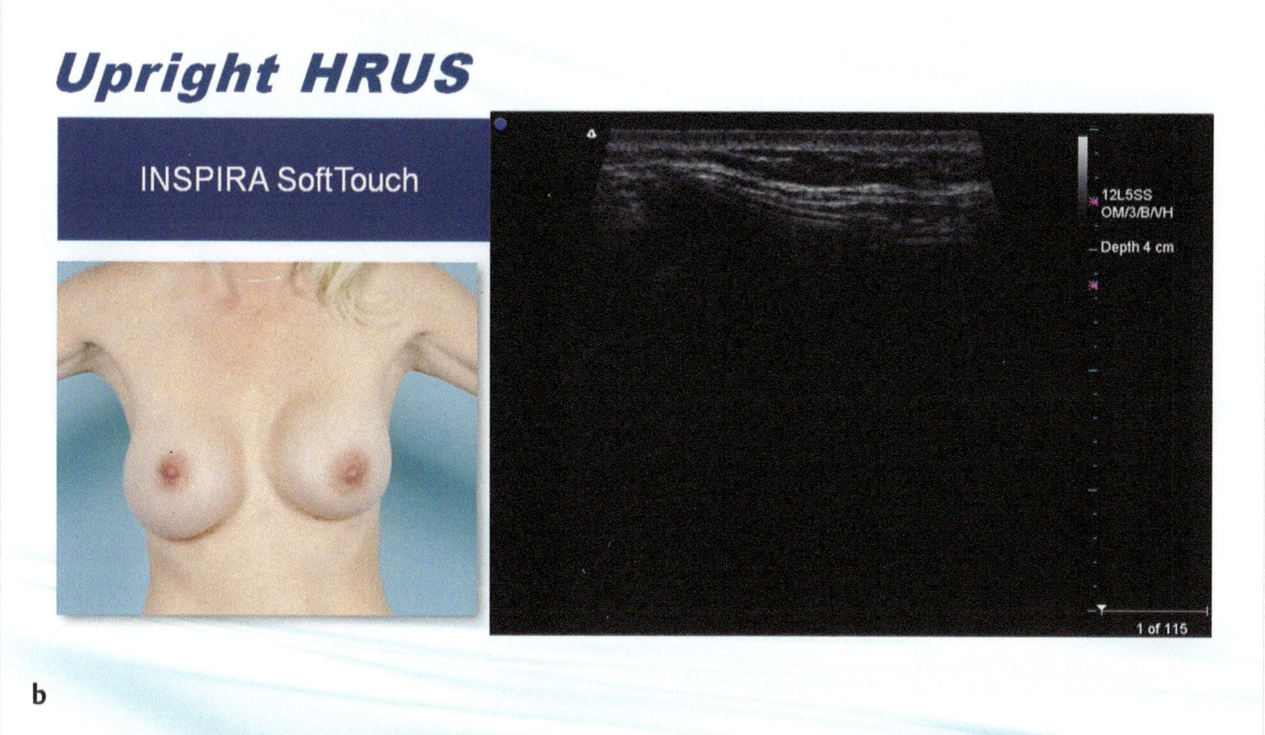

Fig. 2.12 **(a)** Revision patient exchanging saline implants with asymmetry and fold malposition for Allergan Inspira Soft Touch cohesive implants, with **(b)** only gentle waviness on ultrasound of the upper pole.

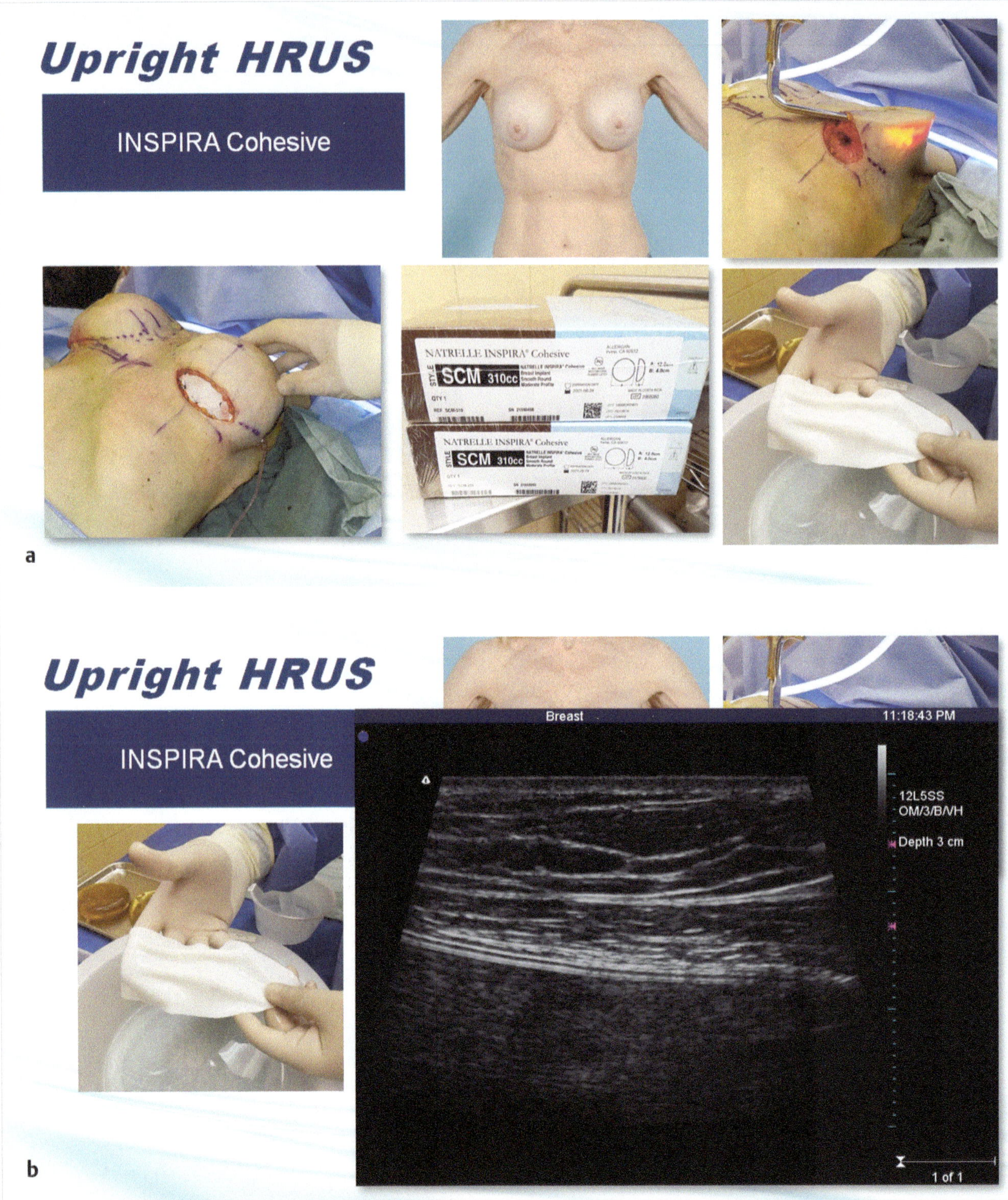

Fig. 2.13 Severe bilateral capsular contracture (a) preoperatively and revised with highly cohesive devices and an acellular dermal matrix bilaterally, along with (b) the patient's postoperative ultrasound showing a completely smooth upper pole contour postoperatively.

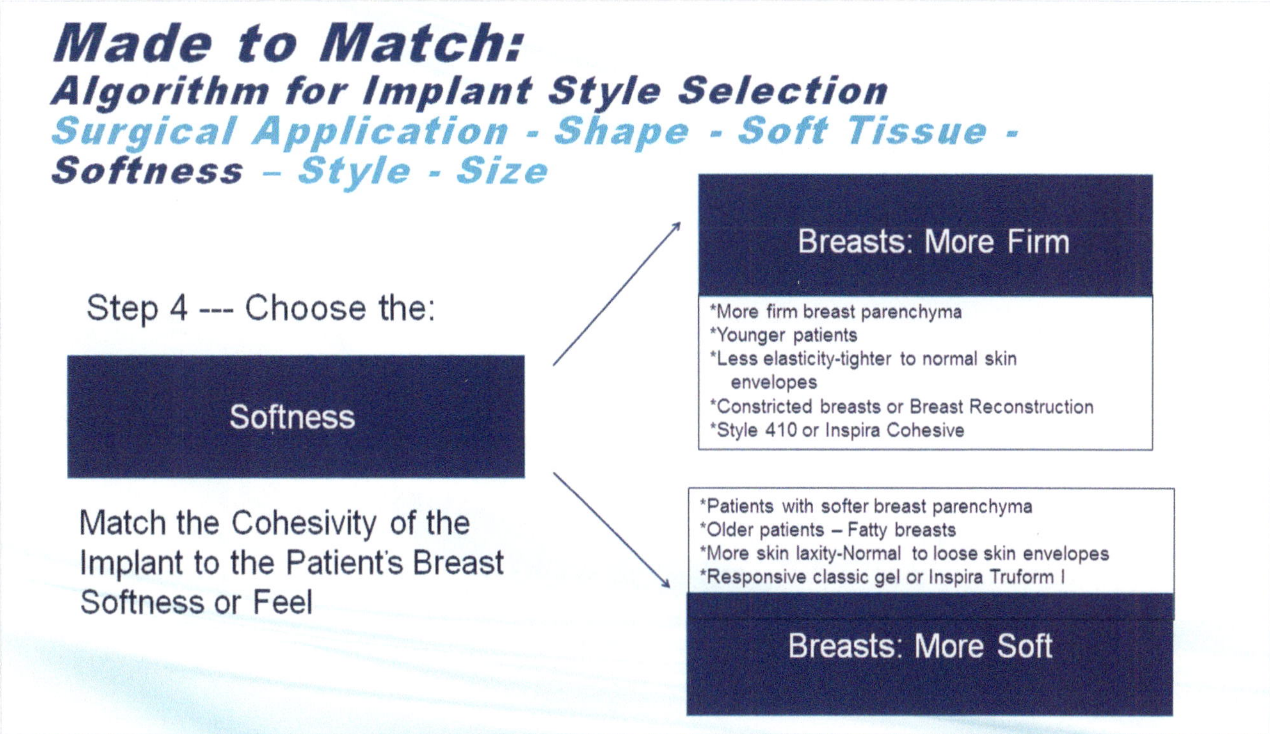

Fig. 2.14 The fourth factor in the *Made to Match* algorithm deals with the implant softness compared to the patient's breast parenchyma.

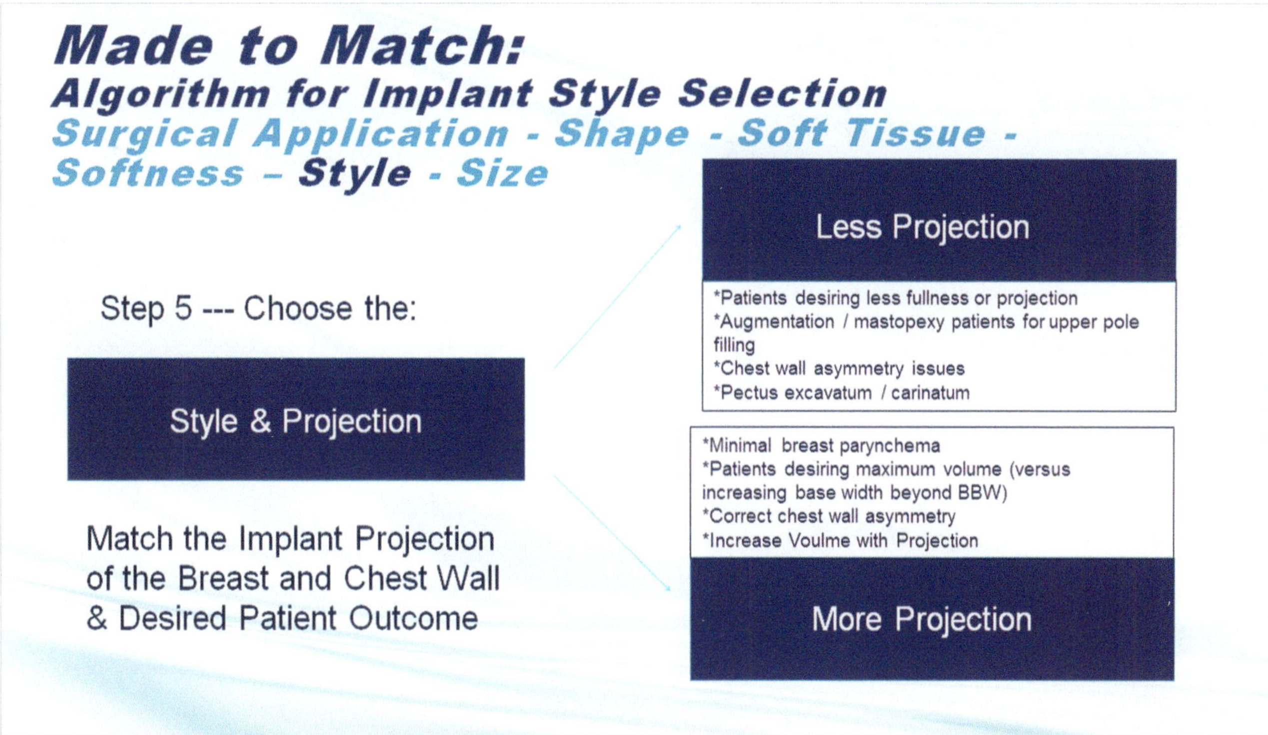

Fig. 2.15 The fifth decision in the *Made to Match* algorithm is implant style or projection.

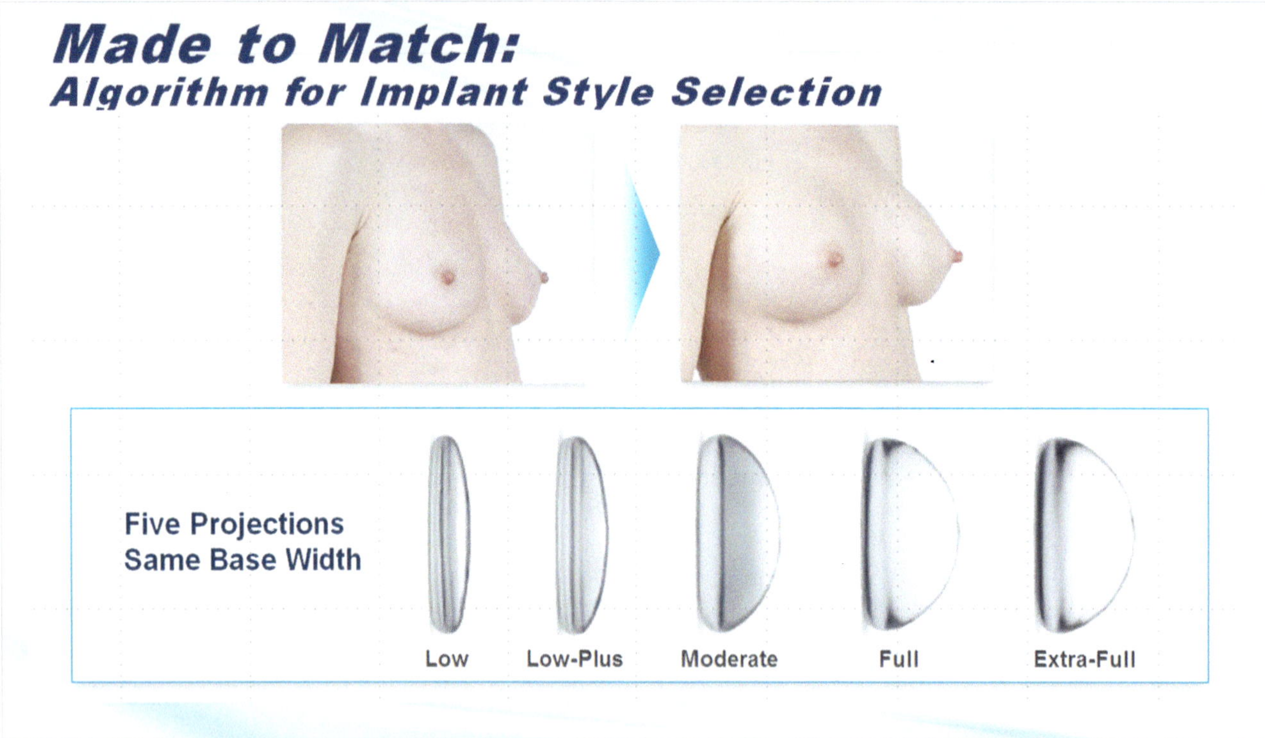

Fig. 2.16 Greater laxity in the skin envelope requires a more projecting implant to fill the implant pocket.

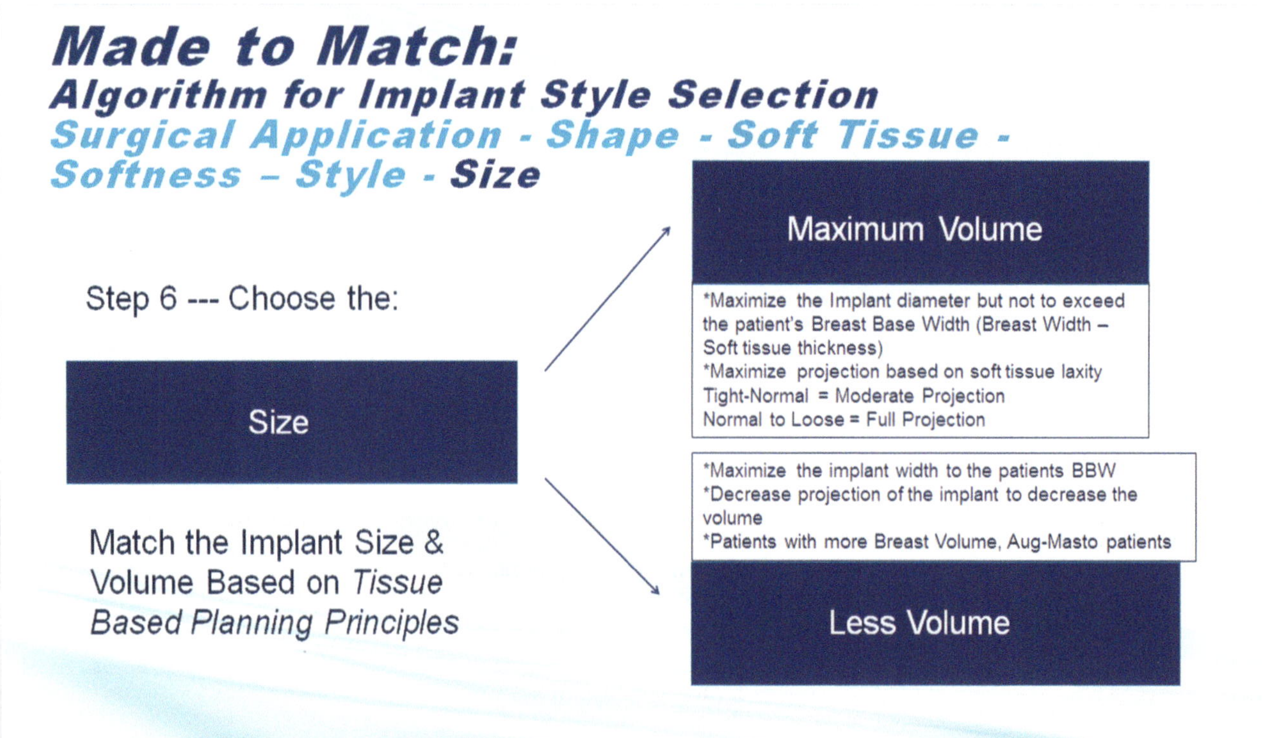

Fig. 2.17 The final implant size range is then selected based on the patient's breast base width.

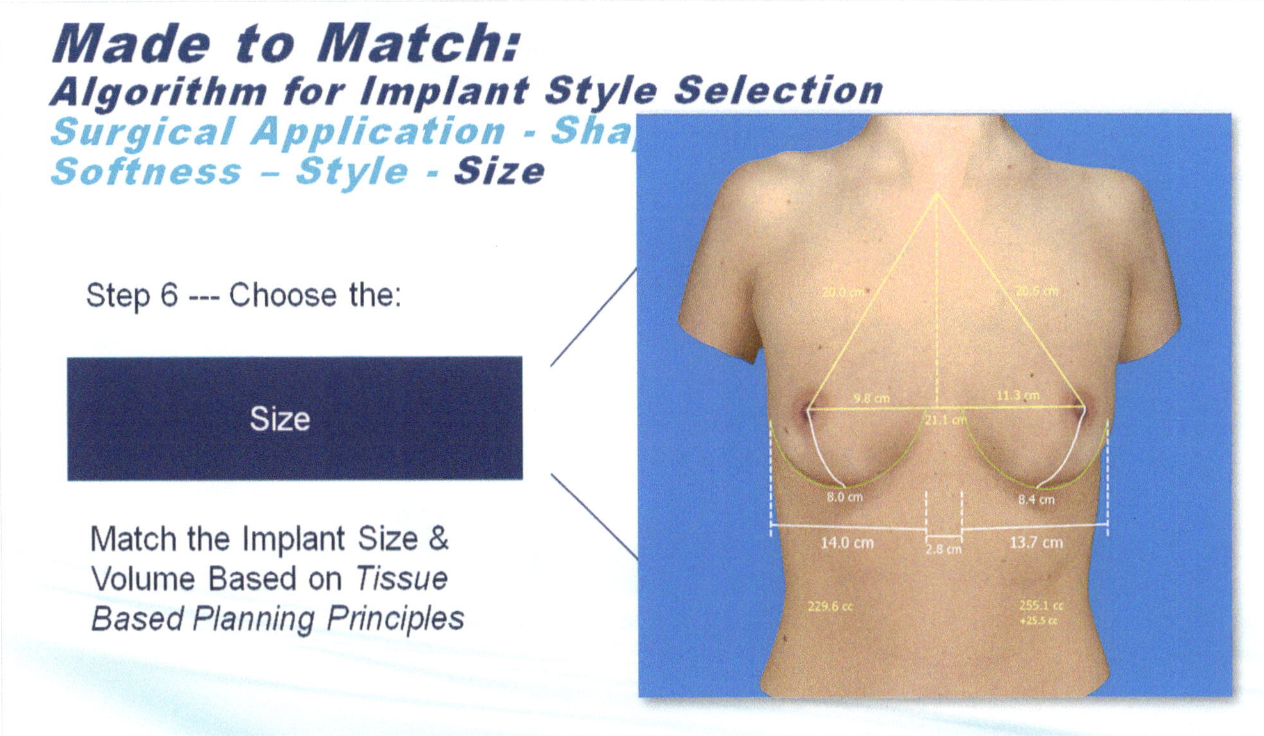

Fig. 2.18 Selection of the implant size is the sixth and final step in the *Made to Match* implant selection algorithm.

2.6 Conclusion

Optimizing aesthetics in implant-related breast surgery requires a careful analysis of patient-related factors, patient expectations and desires, implant-related variables, and the surgeon's approach and experience. Use of 3D imaging and simulation can provide patients and surgeons with a valuable tool for achieving ideal outcomes and minimizing elective revisions for size change. Only through careful preoperative planning, understanding patients' expectations, intraoperative considerations, and careful selection of the most appropriate implant for each patient can these outcomes be consistently achieved.

Key Points

- Breast augmentation is a process, not a procedure. The key components are comprehensive patient education and informed consent, tissue-based operative planning, refined surgical technique with rapid recovery, and detailed postoperative education.
- The author's approach is to determine the patient's breast base width (BBW), which is the actual breast width minus the soft tissue thickness (on average 1.5 cm). The actual breast width is measured as the transverse width from the medial to lateral inflection points of the breast, which represent the breast borders. This BBW is critical and determines the overall range of implants. The author recommends choosing implants with a diameter or width within 1 cm of the BBW.
- It is vital to understand one key concept of the inframammary fold (IMF): the resting versus the actual fold. The actual or true fold is where the implant will settle and rest. It is 1.5 to 2 cm lower than the resting fold and needs to be taken into account. This is where the new IMF will be and where the incision should be placed when the IMF incisional approach is utilized.
- After the patient has been assessed and implant dimensions selected, the final and increasingly critical piece is selecting the implant cohesivity and fill characteristics that are best for each patient and surgical application: augmentation, revision, or reconstruction.

References

[1] Adams WP, Jr. The process of breast augmentation: four sequential steps for optimizing outcomes for patients. Plast Reconstr Surg. 2008; 122(6):1892–1900

[2] Bengtson BP, Glicksman CA. The standardization of bra cup measurements: redefining bra sizing language. Clin Plast Surg. 2015; 42(4):405–411

[3] Allergan. Natrelle® Silicone-Filled Breast Implants: Physician Labeling: Directions for Use (DFU). Markham, Ontario: Allergan; 2011. URL: https://www.allergan.com/miscellaneous-pages/allergan-pdf-files/ca_natrelle_silicone_dfu_en. Accessed July 7, 2019

[4] Roostaeian J, Adams WP, Jr. Three-dimensional imaging for breast augmentation: is this technology providing accurate simulations? Aesthet Surg J. 2014; 34(6):857–875

[5] Weissler JM, Stern CS, Schreiber JE, Amirlak B, Tepper OM. The evolution of photography and three-dimensional imaging in plastic surgery. Plast Reconstr Surg. 2017; 139(3):761–769

[6] Epstein MD, Scheflan M. Three-dimensional imaging and simulation in breast augmentation: what is the current state of the art? Clin Plast Surg. 2015; 42(4):437–450

[7] Tebbetts JB, Adams WP. Five critical decisions in breast augmentation using five measurements in 5 minutes: the High Five decision support process. Plast Reconstr Surg. 2005; 116(7):2005–2016

[8] Tebbetts JB. A system for breast implant selection based on patient tissue characteristics and implant-soft tissue dynamics. Plast Reconstr Surg. 2002; 109(4):1396–1409, discussion 1410–1415

[9] Maclin MM , II, Deigni OA, Bengtson BP. The laminated nature of the pectoralis major muscle and the redefinition of the inframammary fold: clinical implications in aesthetic and reconstructive breast surgery. Clin Plast Surg. 2015; 42(4):465–479

[10] Bengtson BP. The inframammary fold: histologic and anatomic description, classification and definitions, and options for repair and reinforcement. In Spear SL, ed. Surgery of the Breast: Principles and Art. 2nd ed. Philadelphia, PA: Lippincott Williams & Wilkins; 2011:1510–1515

[11] Muntan CD, Sundine MJ, Rink RD, Acland RD. Inframammary fold: a histologic reappraisal. Plast Reconstr Surg. 2000; 105(2):549–556, discussion 557

[12] Bengtson BP. The highly cohesive, Style 410 form-stable gel implant for primary breast augmentation. In: Spear SL, ed Surgery of the Breast: Principles and Art. 2nd ed. Philadelphia, PA: Lippincott Williams and Wilkins; 2011:1346–1365

3 Implant Options

Marilyn Ng, M. Shuja Shafqat, and Sameer A. Patel

Summary
Implant options for breast augmentation have evolved and improved significantly over the last several decades. Plastic surgeons have many different implants from which to choose based on volume, surface type, and shape.

Keywords: breast implant, breast augmentation, implant selection, saline implant, silicone implant

3.1 Implant Background

Breast augmentation is the most common cosmetic surgical procedure performed in the United States, with over 300,000 procedures performed in 2018.[1] Plastic surgeons presently have a large assortment of breast implants to achieve desired aesthetic goals and improve quality of life. We will briefly review the evolution of breast implants and the different implant characteristics available when choosing an implant.

3.2 Implant Evolution

Vincenz Czerny performed the first breast augmentation in 1895, transferring a lipoma to replace a resection defect.[2] Subsequently, surgeons experimented with various solid alloplastic implant materials, such as polyurethane, polytetrafluoroethylene (PTFE), and spongelike material, but patients experienced suboptimal results.[3,4] The use of silicone in breast augmentation began disastrously with free silicone injection for breast soft tissue augmentation and resulted in disfiguring long-term effects.[5] In response to complications from free silicone injection, Thomas Cronin and Frank Gerow developed the first silicone implant in 1962 using a thin, smooth silicone elastomer shell surrounding the silicone gel filling materal.[6,7] Saline implants were created in 1965 as an alternative to solid silicone implants. Since then, silicone gel–filled implants have undergone several technical and physical modifications. All generations of silicone implants are composed of polydimethylsiloxanes (PDMS), a group of polymers that determines gel cohesiveness with varying degrees of cross-linking.

3.3 Silicone Implants

See ▶ Table 3.1 for an overview of five generations of silicone breast implants.

3.3.1 Generations of Silicone Implant

First Generation (1960s)

The first silicone implant was an anatomically shaped (teardrop) implant with several Dacron fixation patches on the posterior aspect to maintain implant position in situ. The shell was a thick, smooth two-piece silicone elastomer envelope with a peripheral seam enclosing a moderately viscous shell. This implant generation was associated with a relatively high contracture rate secondary to the shell properties and the lack of gel cohesivity (▶ Fig. 3.1).

Second Generation (1970s)

A round implant with a thinner, seamless elastomer shell without Dacron fixation patches was developed to reduce the rate of capsular contracture.[8] A less viscous silicone gel filling of this implant generation provided a "natural feel." Unfortunately, these implants were associated with "gel-bleed" as the low viscosity of the gel permitted diffusion of microscopic silicone molecules through the thin, permeable shell.[9] An oily, sticky residue surrounding the implant within the periprosthetic capsule is characteristic during explantation of second-generation implants. Device shell failure was also higher in this implant generation.[10,13]

Third Generation (1980s)

Gel bleed and device shell failure were reduced in third-generation implants, when a more viscous gel and a thicker, multilayer silicone elastomer shell with barrier layer were introduced. For the first time, textured surfacing was added to implants as an attempt to decrease the capsular contracture rate. From 1992 to 2006, the FDA placed a moratorium on third-generation implants due to an unfounded claim that silicone caused

Table 3.1 Five generations of silicone breast implants

Generation	Period	Shell	Silicone fill	Texturing	Shape	Implant concerns
First	1960s	Thick	Viscous	No	Anatomic	Posterior Dacron patch
Second	1970s	Thin	Less viscous	No	Round	Gel bleed
Third	1980s	Thick	Viscous	Yes	Round	FDA safety recall
Fourth	1990s–present	Thick	Viscous	Yes	Anatomic	Stricter manufacturing standards
Fifth	1990s–present	Thick	Cohesive	Yes	Anatomic	–

Adapted from Henderson PW, Nash D, Laskowski M, Grant R. Objective comparison of commercially available breast implant devices. Aesth Plast Surg. 2015;39:724–732.
Additional data from Maxwell GP, Gabriel A. The evolution of breast implants. Plast Reconstr Surg 2014;134(1 Suppl):12S–17S; Maxwell GP, Gabriel A. The evolution of breast implants. Clin Plast Surg 2009;36(1):1–13; O'Brien J. History of breast prostheses. Plast Surg Nurs 1999;19(2):59–61, 107.

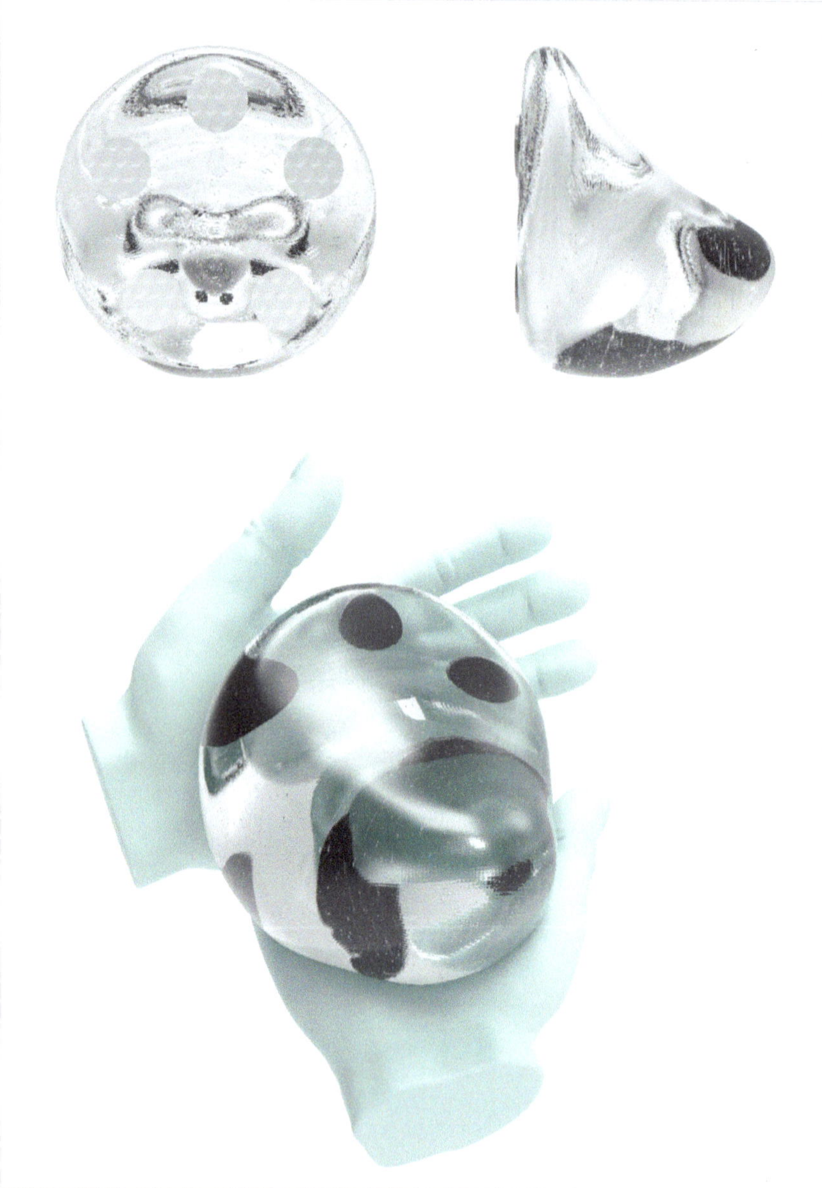

Fig. 3.1 First-generation permanent silicone implant developed by Cronin and Gerow and manufactured by Dow Corning in 1963. The tear-shaped device featured posterior Dacron patches to affix it in the implant pocket.

cancer.[11,12] They were also still subject to rupture and contracture (▶ Fig. 3.2).

Fourth Generation (1990s to Present)

These implants improved on the previous generation by being manufactured under stringent FDA quality control and criteria for device shell thickness and greater gel viscosity.[13] Implants were also made available in a greater variety of textures and shapes.

Fifth Generation (1990s to Present)

These "form-stable" implants were produced to provide a natural contour, unlike the fullness created with round implants.[14,15,16] Fifth-generation implants are also defined by greater gel cohesion and textured surface (▶ Fig. 3.3).[17]

3.3.2 Indications

Breast augmentation with permanent silicone implants is indicated in women at least 22 years old who acknowledge the FDA-required recommendation of magnetic resonance imaging (MRI) surveillance 3 years postimplantation and then every 2 years thereafter.

3.3.3 Shape and Projection

The goal of breast augmentation is to achieve aesthetically pleasing proportion, shape, and volume. To that end, implant selection is just one of a number of decisions, which include preoperative evaluation (Chapter 17), selection of surgical approach (Chapter 4), and implant placement (Chapter 5). The

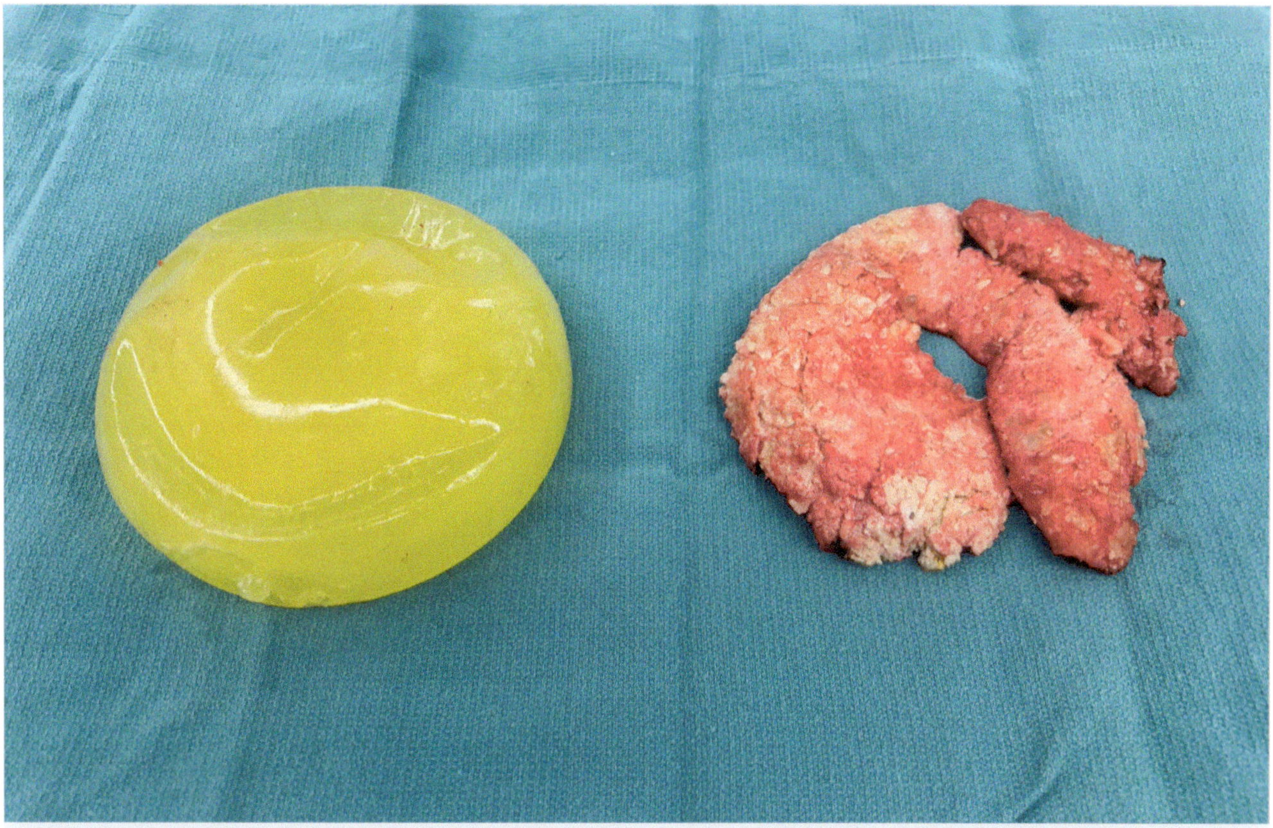

Fig. 3.2 Third-generation permanent silicone implant that was removed secondary to rupture and severe capsular contracture. Note the oily residue covering the implant surface and the yellow discolored silicone "bleeding" through the device shell. To the right, the periprosthetic capsule is thick and calcified.

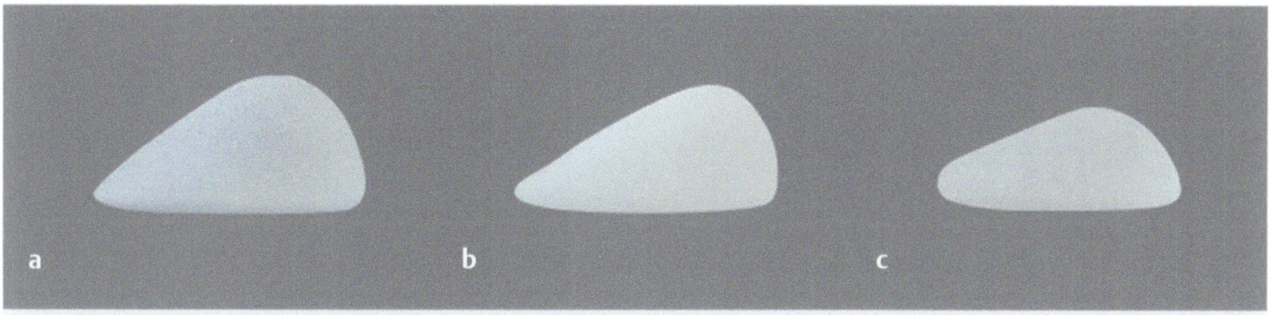

Fig. 3.3 Fifth-generation permanent silicone implants. Profiles of **(a)** Sientra High-Strength Cohesive+, **(b)** Allergan 410, and **(c)** Mentor Contour Profile Gel "form-stable" cohesive gel implants.

decision regarding implant shape selection is influenced by factors that include implant cohesivity, degree of implant overfilling, projection, breast analysis including upper and lower pole breast parenchyma coverage of the implant, and proposed vertical placement of the implant.[18,19]

Another component of implant shape selection is determined by three additional components: patient's desires, anatomy, and surgical history. The importance of understanding the subjective appearance the patient desires cannot be underestimated. It may be prudent to show photographs of results of other patients or use three-dimensional imaging tools to align expectations of the patient and the surgeon. A patient who desires a natural appearance, one that has a linear or slightly concave upper pole, may prefer an anatomic-shaped implant to mimic the normal breast. The anatomic-shaped implants provide the desired contour owing to their "form stable" silicone formulations. Generally, the implant is tapered at the top, and there is more projection at the bottom. For patients who request an "augmented" appearance, round implants will provide greater volume for a given base width and tend to provide upper pole fullness. In both cases, the patient's anatomy must be considered during implant selection.

Anatomic factors that influence implant shape selection are breast shape and soft tissue coverage, lower pole constriction, breast asymmetries, chest wall deformities, and ptosis. Broadly speaking, round implants are indicated when a patient has a good baseline breast shape and adequate soft-tissue coverage (> 2 cm) to camouflage the implant edge. Aesthetic outcomes may not vary greatly according to implant shape, particularly when low- or moderate-profile implants are placed. In comparison, anatomic-shaped implants are indicated when one or more of the following conditions is present:[20]

1. Lack of breast shape or thin soft tissue coverage (< 2 cm).
2. Lower pole constriction or tuberous breast, to expand the lower pole and minimize double-bubble deformity.
3. Breast and chest wall asymmetries in which differential customization can correct shape and volume.
4. Ptosis that can be corrected with an anatomical implant to elevate the nipple areolar complex (NAC) and augment the lower pole, given the array of implants with different height and projection combinations.

The last consideration is the patient's surgical history. Round implants should be used in cases of recurrent implant rotation, situations where precise implant pocket control cannot be obtained, and instances that require low-cohesive implants to mold into the implant pocket after capsular contracture correction.

Altogether, implant shape selection is dependent on several factors that rely on preoperative assessment and combined patient- and surgeon-directed goals. In the United States, surgeons may chose round and anatomic-shaped implants made by Allergan, Mentor, and Sientra. Each company offers implants in a range of different base width diameters that permit custom sizing (▶ Fig. 3.4). As a response to early round implants, higher-profile options were created to achieve greater projection (▶ Fig. 3.5). Thus, for a given base width diameter, the greater projection profiles allowed fill volume to increase with each implant device. All three companies offer anatomic-shaped implants with different projection profiles (▶ Fig. 3.6). Similarly, these companies produce implants with taller and lower heights relative to the base width. However, Sientra is the only company that offers a round-based anatomic implant.

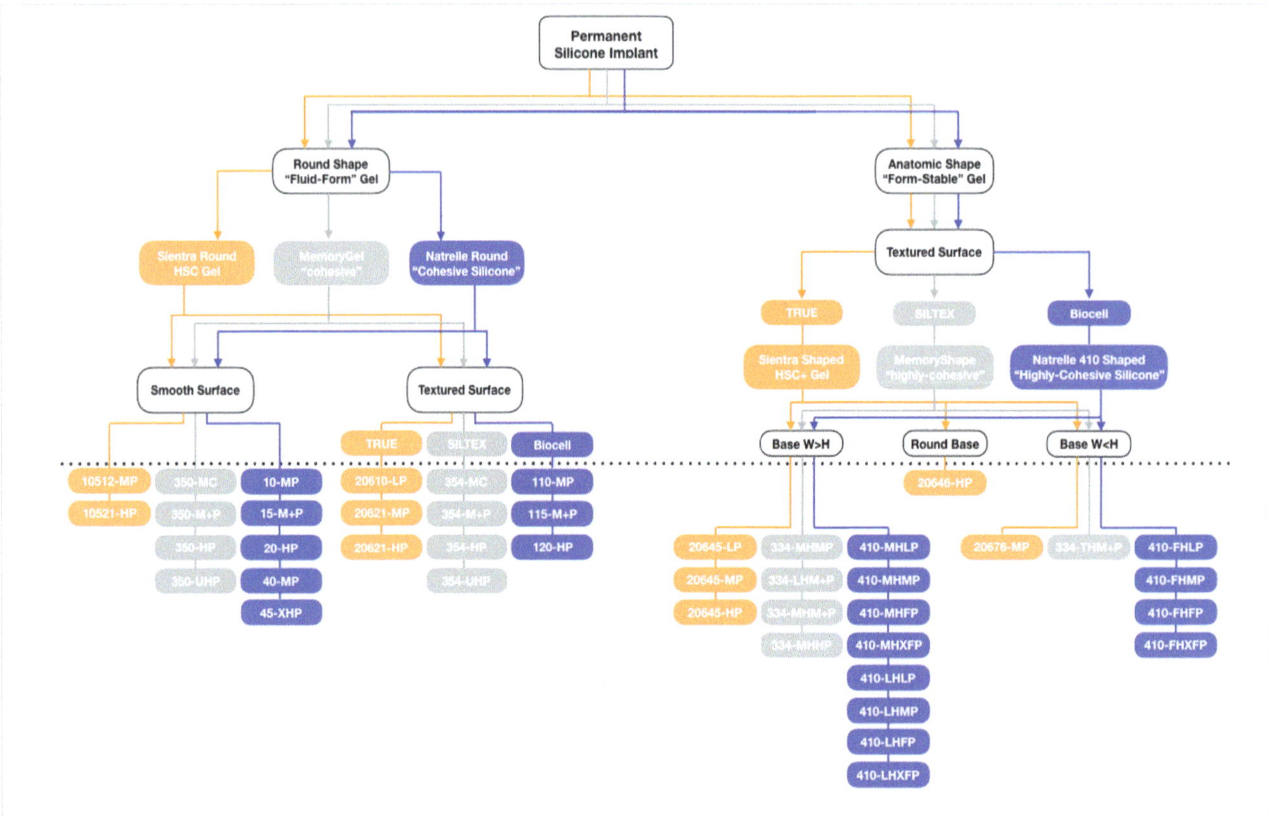

Fig. 3.4 Currently available FDA-approved silicone permanent breast implants. (Adapted from Henderson P, Nash D, Laskowski M, Grant RT. Objective comparison of commercially available breast implant devices. Aesth Plast Surg 2015; 39(5):724–732.)

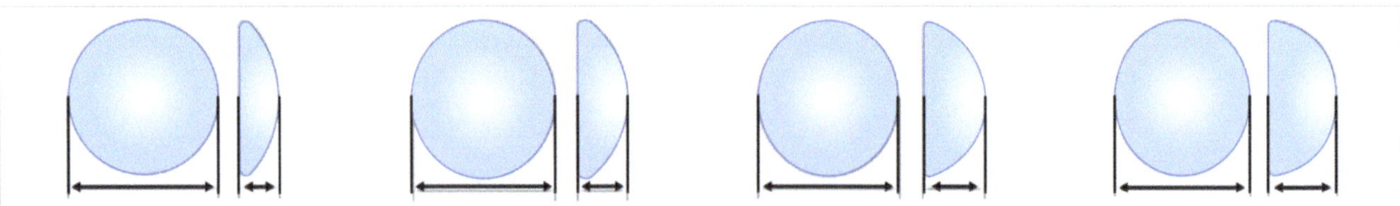

Fig. 3.5 Round silicone implant devices with different projection options. Each U.S.-based company offers a selected number of profile projections and varying implant base width diameters.

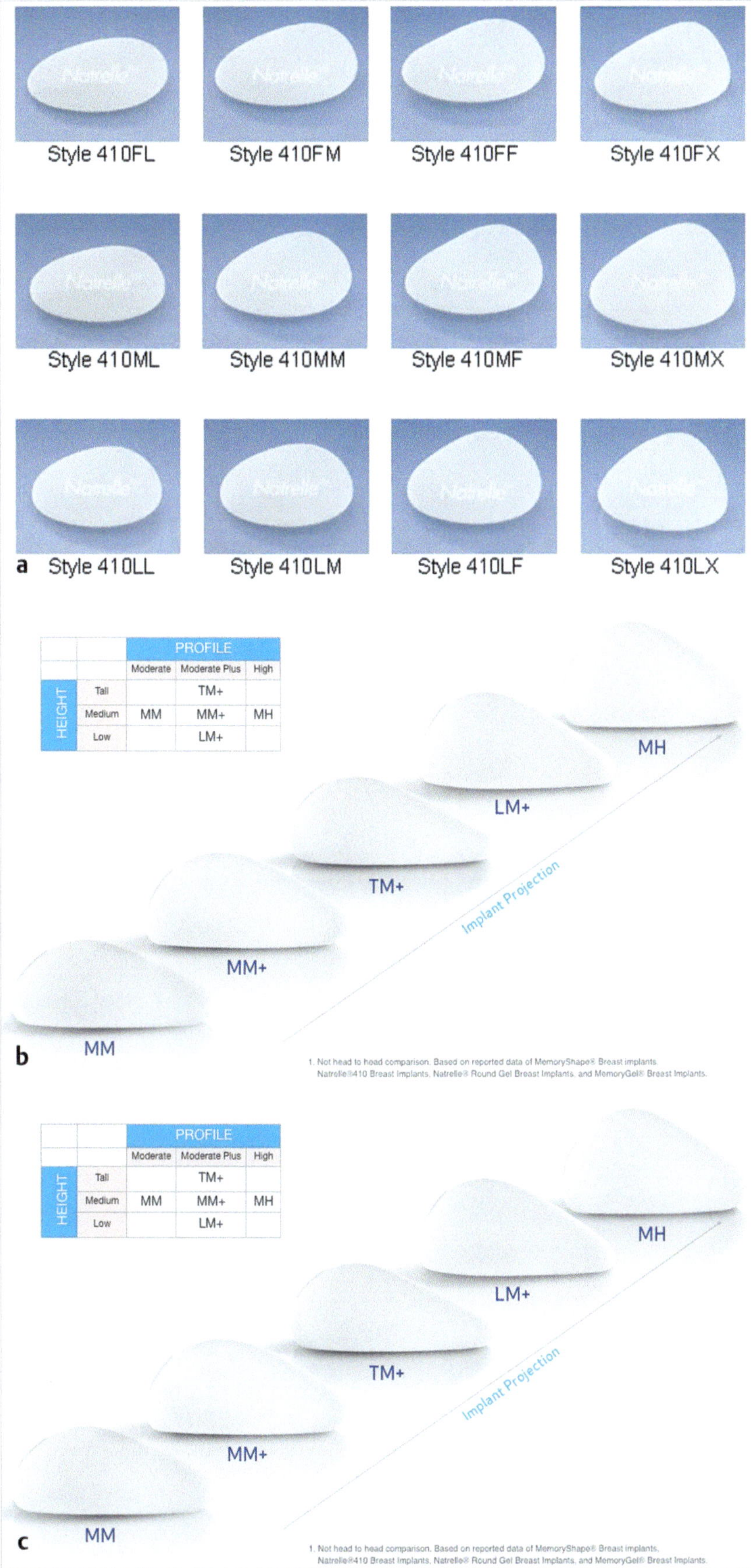

Fig. 3.6 Anatomic-shaped implant devices that are FDA-approved in the United States. **(a)** Allergan *Natrelle* 410. **(b)** Mentor MemoryShape. **(c)** Sientra High-Strength Cohesive + .

3.3.4 Texturing

The decision to choose a textured implant is primarily based on minimizing capsular contracture when placed in a subglandular plane.[21,22] Round implants are available as smooth-surfaced and textured implants. Anatomic implants are all textured to minimize malrotation within the breast pocket. Compared to textured implants, smooth implants are less firm and form a thinner periprosthetic capsule.

Different manufacturing processes create textured implants (▶ Fig. 3.7).[2,6,23] The Biocell (Allergan, Irvine, CA) texture is created using a "loss-salt" technique in which a salt crystal layer is covered by a thin coat of silicone and cured in a laminar flow oven.[23] The Siltex (Mentor, Santa Barbara, CA) texture is created using an "imprint stamping," where the uncured silicone surface is pushed into polyurethane foam and the imprint is finalized with pressure.[23] TRUE Texture (Sientra, Santa Barbara, CA) is created with small, hollow pores with minimal thin cell webbing and does not employ sodium chloride or pressure stamping in the manufacturing process.[23]

3.4 Saline Permanent Implants

3.4.1 Indication

Breast augmentation with saline-filled implants is indicated in women who are at least 18 years old. Patients may request saline-filled implants, as they remain the gold standard of safety, eliminating the worry of silicone implant rupture or gel exposure. Saline implant deflation (rupture) is visible and is innocuous, as the soft tissue absorbs the saline solution. Other indications include patients who desire smaller incisions through which the noninflated implant is delivered.[24]

Of particular importance is to discuss the potential negative outcomes associated with saline implants, such as "scalloping" along the prosthetic edge, unnatural firmness, and the risk of deflation. Also inherent with the low viscosity of saline is the difficulty to control implant fill distribution to shape the adjacent breast tissue. Thus, a saline implant may be better suited in patients with good breast shape and adequate soft tissue coverage.

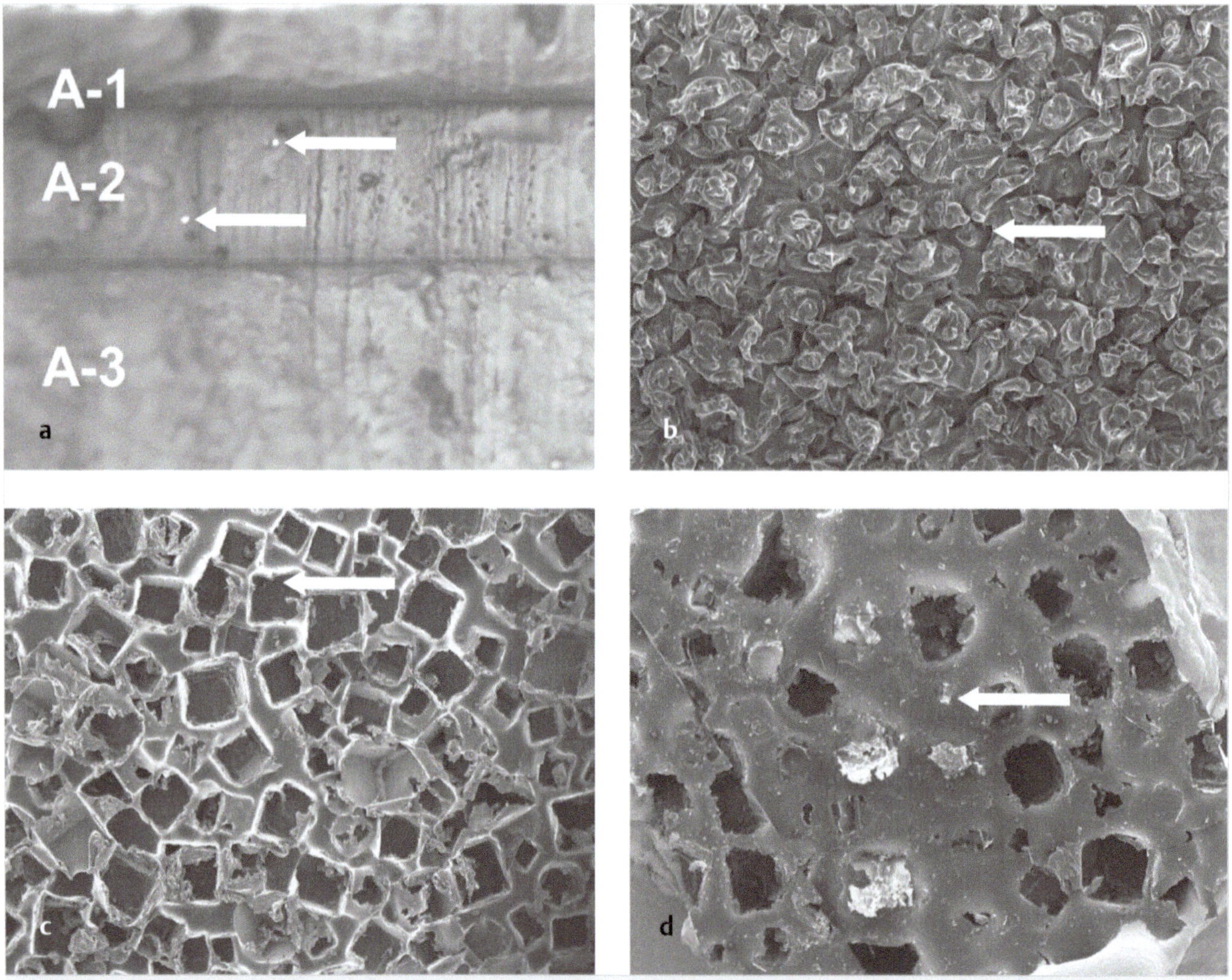

Fig. 3.7 Scanning electron microscopic images of silicone implant devices. **(a)** Cross-section of smooth-surface silicone implant (original magnification, x 25); **(b)** Mentor Siltex textured shell surface (original magnification, x25); and **(c,d)** Silimed TRUE Texture, Allergan Biocell shell surface (original magnification, x 25) of unused device and device explantation. (Reproduced from Cohen M, Thaller S. The Unfavorable Result in Plastic Surgery: Avoidance and Treatment. 4th ed. New York, NY: Thieme Medical Publishers; 2018.)

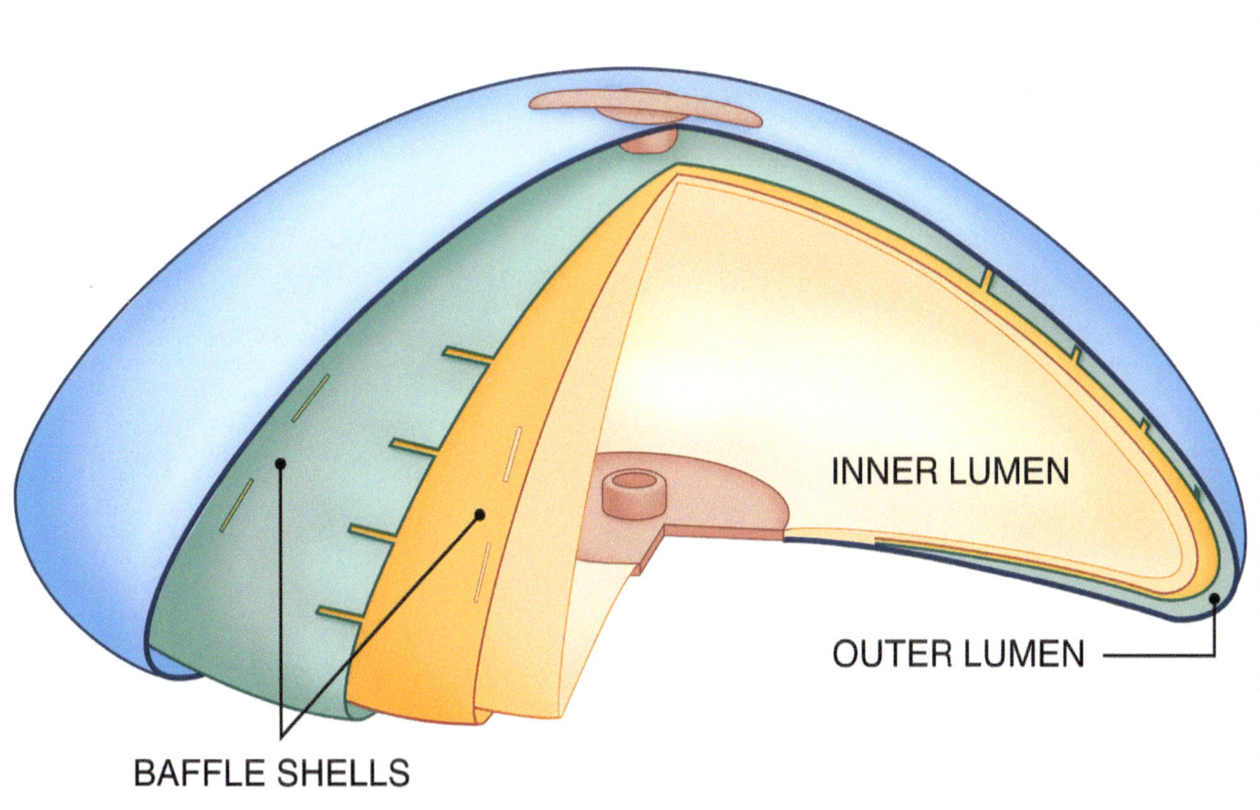

Fig. 3.8 Construct schematic view of the Ideal Implant saline-filled breast implant (Ideal Implant Incorporated, Irving, TX). Smaller sizes have one baffle shell, medium sizes have two baffle shells, and larger sizes have three baffle shells.

3.4.2 Saline Implant Options

Only two companies, Allergan and Mentor, market permanent saline implants. The assortment of shape in saline implants is limited compared to the selection of permanent silicone implants. Most saline implants are filled to their final volume in the operating room.

However, Mentor has created postoperatively adjustable round saline implants and anatomic-shaped saline implants, referred to as the Spectrum and Contour Profile Spectrum lines, respectively.

Nonadjustable, round saline implants are available in smooth and textured surfaces from both Allergan and Mentor. Anatomic-shaped saline implants are available only in a textured surface.

While the majority of saline implants placed in patients are single-lumen implants, in 2015 the FDA approved a double-lumen saline implant marketed as Ideal Implant (Ideal Implant Incorporated, Irving, TX) for use in the United States and Canada. The Ideal Implant contains a baffle structure that provides internal support to the implant edge and controls saline movement (▶ Fig. 3.8, ▶ Fig. 3.9). In an outcome study, the Ideal Implant demonstrated less wrinkling and capsular contracture compared to reported data on single-lumen saline implants and also had high patient-reported and surgeon-reported satisfaction.[25]

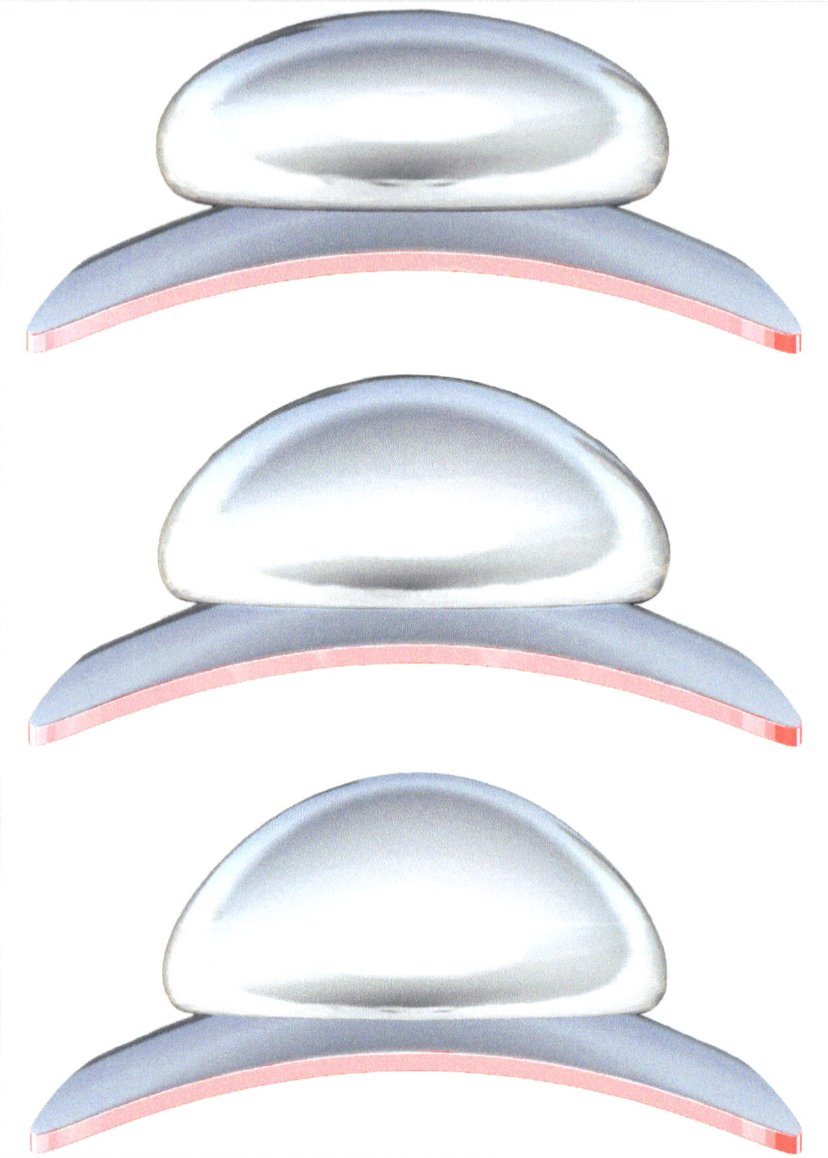

Fig. 3.9 Implants on a convex surface simulating the chest wall. **(a)** Mentor MemoryGel implant, moderate plus profile (Mentor Worldwide LLC, Santa Barbara, CA), 350 cc. **(b)** Allergan Natrelle implant, Style 15, moderate profile (Allergan, Inc., Irvine, CA), 371 cc. **(c)** Ideal Implant (Ideal Implant Incorporated, Irving, TX) at minimum fill volume, 405 cc. The edges of the Natrelle implant and Ideal Implant are lower relative to the convex surface, so they contour better to the simulated chest wall and have a more natural, tapered shape than the Mentor implant, which has a more globular shape.

3.5 Conclusion

The silicone and saline implant devices discussed are currently FDA-approved and serve as the basis of safe and ethical options. With both technical and aesthetic implant advancements, plastic surgeons now have a substantial variety of options to offer a carefully selected implant device that fits the needs and desires of a cosmetic breast augmentation patient.

Key Points

- Breast implant augmentation is a common aesthetic procedure.
- Saline implant devices are indicated in women who are at least 18 years old.
- Silicone implant devices have evolved over the past six decades and include expanded options for cohesivity, volume, shape, and texture.

References

[1] American Society of Plastic Surgeons. New plastic surgery statistics reveal trends toward body enhancement. Arlington Heights, IL: American Society of Plastic Surgeons; 2019. URL: https://www.plasticsurgery.org/news/press-releases/new-plastic-surgery-statistics-reveal-trends-toward-body-enhancement. Accessed July 8, 2019

[2] Czerny V. Plastic replacement of the breast with a lipoma [in German]. Chir Kong Verhandl. 1895; 24:216–217

[3] Glatt BS, Afifi G, Noone RB. Long-term follow-up of a sponge breast implant and review of the literature. Ann Plast Surg. 1999; 42(2):196–201

[4] Maxwell GP, Gabriel A. The evolution of breast implants. Plast Reconstr Surg. 2014; 134(1) Suppl:12S–17S

[5] Chasan PE. The history of injectable silicone fluids for soft-tissue augmentation. Plast Reconstr Surg. 2007; 120(7):2034–2040, discussion 2041––2043

[6] Cronin TD, Gerow FJ. Augmentation mammaplasty: a new "natural feel" prosthesis. Paper presented at: Transactions of the Third International Congress of Plastic Surgery; 1964; Amsterdam

[7] Cronin TD, Brauer RO. Augmentation mammaplasty. Surg Clin North Am. 1971; 51(2):441–452

[8] Young VL, Watson ME. Breast implant research: where we have been, where we are, where we need to go. Clin Plast Surg. 2001; 28(3):451–483, vi

[9] Barker DE, Retsky MI, Schultz S. "Bleeding" of silicone from bag-gel breast implants, and its clinical relation to fibrous capsule reaction. Plast Reconstr Surg. 1978; 61(6):836–841
[10] Marotta JS, Goldberg EP, Habal MB, et al. Silicone gel breast implant failure: evaluation of properties of shells and gels for explanted prostheses and meta-analysis of literature rupture data. Ann Plast Surg. 2002; 49(3):227–242, discussion 242--247
[11] Cohen IK. Impact of the FDA ban on silicone breast implants. J Surg Oncol. 1994; 56(1):1
[12] Bondurant S, Ernster V, Herdman R, eds. Safety of Silicone Breast Implants. Washington, DC: Institute of Medicine;1999
[13] Guidoin R, Rolland C, Fleury D, et al. Physical characterization of unimplanted gel filled breast implants. Should old standards be revisited? ASAIO J. 1994; 40(4):943–958
[14] Hammond DC, Migliori MM, Caplin DA, Garcia ME, Phillips CA. Mentor Contour Profile Gel implants: clinical outcomes at 6 years. Plast Reconstr Surg. 2012; 129(6):1381–1391
[15] Unger JG, Carreras JM, Nagarkar P, Jeong HS, Carpenter W. Allergan Style 410 implants for breast reconstruction: a prospective study in efficacy, safety, and symmetry. Plast Reconstr Surg. 2016; 138(3):548–555
[16] Stevens WG, Calobrace MB, Harrington J, Alizadeh K, Zeidler KR, d'Incelli RC. Nine-year core study data for Sientra's FDA-approved round and shaped implants with high-strength cohesive silicone gel. Aesthet Surg J. 2016; 36(4): 404–416
[17] Calobrace MB, Capizzi PJ. The biology and evolution of cohesive gel and shaped implants. Plast Reconstr Surg. 2014; 134(1) Suppl:6S–11S
[18] Tebbetts JB, Adams WP. Five critical decisions in breast augmentation using five measurements in 5 minutes: the High Five decision support process. Plast Reconstr Surg. 2005; 116(7):2005–2016
[19] Hedén P, Montemurro P, Adams WP, Jr, Germann G, Scheflan M, Maxwell GP. Anatomical and round breast implants: how to select and indications for use. Plast Reconstr Surg. 2015; 136(2):263–272
[20] Hidalgo DA, Weinstein AL. Intraoperative comparison of anatomical versus round implants in breast augmentation: a randomized controlled trial. Plast Reconstr Surg. 2017; 139(3):587–596
[21] Headon H, Kasem A, Mokbel K. Capsular contracture after breast augmentation: an update for clinical practice. Arch Plast Surg. 2015; 42(5):532–543
[22] Barnsley GP, Sigurdson LJ, Barnsley SE. Textured surface breast implants in the prevention of capsular contracture among breast augmentation patients: a meta-analysis of randomized controlled trials. Plast Reconstr Surg. 2006; 117(7):2182–2190
[23] Barr S, Hill E, Bayat A. Current implant surface technology: an examination of their nanostructure and their influence on fibroblast alignment and biocompatibility. Eplasty. 2009; 9:e22
[24] Regnault P, Baker TJ, Gleason MC, et al. Clinical trial and evaluation of a proposed new inflatable mammary prosthesis. Plast Reconstr Surg. 1972; 50(3):220–226
[25] Nichter LS, Hamas RS. Two-year outcomes with a novel, double-lumen, saline-filled breast implant. Aesthet Surg J. 2012; 32(7):861–867

4 Selection of the Surgical Approach

Ziyad S. Hammoudeh and W. Grant Stevens

Summary

Breast augmentation with implants may be accomplished through various surgical incisions. These include the inframammary, periareolar, transaxillary, and transumbilical approaches. This chapter will discuss these various options and discuss technical considerations as well as advantages and disadvantages of the different techniques.

Keywords: breast augmentation, augmentation, implant, approach, incision

4.1 Introduction

Selection of incision location is an important component of the breast augmentation consultation that must be discussed between the patient and the plastic surgeon. Available options include inframammary, periareolar, transaxillary, and transumbilical approaches. Each technique has its own advantages and disadvantages. The plastic surgeon should be well informed about each to select the approach that is best suited for each individual patient (▶ Fig. 4.1). For all incision types, the surgeon must balance the desire for an inconspicuous scar with the need for adequate exposure for dissection that will accommodate the implant and minimize the chance of complications. This chapter will focus on the technical aspects of each technique, favorable/unfavorable patient anatomy for each approach, effect on nipple sensation and breastfeeding, and rate of capsular contracture associated with each approach.

4.2 Approaches

4.2.1 Inframammary Fold Breast Augmentation

Most published literature regarding breast augmentation involves the use of the inframammary incision. Therefore, it is certainly the best-studied approach and is the incision of choice for most plastic surgeons.[1] A 4- to 5-cm transverse incision is made in the skin parallel to the inframammary fold (IMF) with

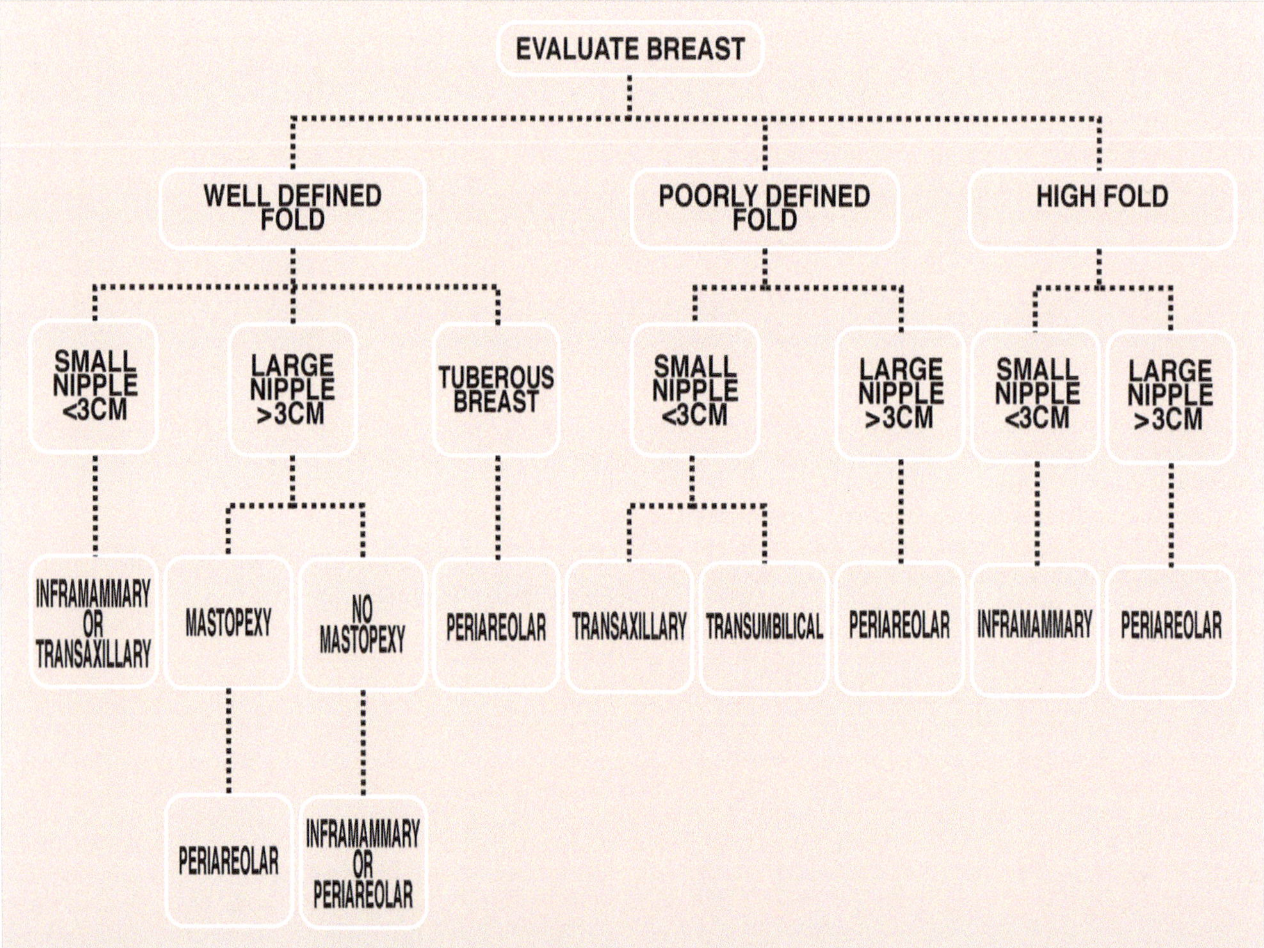

Fig. 4.1 Algorithm for selection of approach for breast augmentation.

a scalpel. For ideal aesthetics, the inframammary incision should be centered over a vertical line marking the meridian of the breast or shifted slightly laterally. A medially shifted incision tends to be more visible and thus less desirable. Electrocautery is used to dissect through the superficial fascia of the breast at a 45° angle until the pectoralis major muscle fascia is reached. The surgeon can then elect to develop either a subpectoral, a subglandular, or a subfascial pocket for implant insertion.

Special attention must be given to asymmetry of the native IMFs when planning the inframammary incision. In the majority of patients, the left IMF is located slightly more superiorly.[2] The difference in IMF position can be more easily visualized by drawing a horizontal tangent line from each IMF to the midline. Differences in IMF position can be managed by lowering the more superiorly positioned IMF to a more inferior level by placing the skin incision at the more inferior horizontal tangent level bilaterally. However, this will not correct asymmetry in craniocaudal position of the nipple areola complex (NAC). For instance, if both the IMF and NAC are positioned more superiorly in the left breast, lowering the left IMF to the same level as the right IMF will not change the more superior position of the left NAC compared to the right NAC. Therefore, the nipple-to-incision distance will not be the same bilaterally even though the new IMF and breast mound positions will appear more symmetric.

Compared with the other approaches, careful planning of the exact location for the inframammary incision is critical so that it lies precisely in the IMF at the end of the operation (▶ Fig. 4.2). Insertion of an implant stretches the breast skin to accommodate the increased volume, often recruiting abdominal skin onto the breast mound and thus lowering the IMF to a more inferior position. Therefore, in patients with relatively short nipple-to-IMF distances undergoing augmentation using an implant with a wide base width, the incision should be made inferior to the native IMF on the abdominal wall such that the incision will ultimately lie in the IMF after the implant is inserted and the IMF is lowered by the implant. Effective lowering of the IMF by an implant is a product of tissue shifting such that structural integrity of the lower border of the breast is maintained and should not be confused with iatrogenic violation of the IMF, as the latter can lead to a double-bubble deformity and inferior malposition of the implant.

Various calculations have been proposed for selecting the precise location of the inframammary incision based on implant dimensions and nipple-to-IMF distance. The Randquist formula is a simple approach that has been effective in the authors' practice (▶ Table 4.1).[3] The Randquist[3] and High Five[4] systems are commonly used formulas but have been criticized as basing their calculations on inconsistent measurements such as skin stretch.[5] Recently, the ICE principle was introduced, which relates the implant dimensions (*I*), the capacity of the breast (*C*), and the excess tissue needed to accommodate the implant (*E*), equal to the difference between *I* and *C*.[6] The authors showed greater than 99% accuracy of scar placement in the IMF through calculations based on implant dimensions and nipple-to-IMF distance.[6]

After placement of the implants, the inframammary incisions should be closed in three layers (superficial fascia, deep dermal, and subcuticular). Some authors have advocated the placement of three-point sutures between the superficial fascia of the breast, superficial fascia of the IMF, and deep fascia of the IMF in select patients to prevent inferior malposition over time.[7] When implants are placed in a subpectoral pocket, the IMF is subjected to repeated downward force by the implant from contraction of the overlying pectoralis major, with progressive instability of the IMF.

Table 4.1 Randquist formula for inframammary incision placement based on implant base width

Implant width (cm)	New nipple-to-IMF distance (cm)*
11.0	7.5
11.5	8.0
12.0	8.5
12.5	9.0
13.0	9.5

*If the patient has a tight or firm envelope that does not stretch, 0.5 cm should be added. If the patient has loose or overstretched skin, 0.5 cm should be subtracted.
Abbreviation: IMF, inframammary fold.

Advantages and Disadvantages

Advantages of the inframammary approach include an easier learning curve with direct visualization of the breast for precise pocket dissection and potentially less risk of contamination. In a thorough analysis of the literature, Namnoum et al found a lower relative risk of capsular contracture, moderate to severe malposition, and secondary procedures with the inframammary approach compared to the periareolar and transaxillary approaches.[8]

The primary disadvantage of the inframammary approach is a more visually noticeable scar from a basilar view of the breasts and in patients with a poorly defined IMF. A well-placed scar in the IMF should not be visible in an upright position. In patients who preoperatively have adequately sized breasts and a prominent IMF crease, the inframammary scar is well hidden as gravity allows the inferior pole of the augmented breast to descend over the fold. Pre- and postoperative photos of two patients who underwent breast augmentation via the IMF are shown in ▶ Fig. 4.3 (anatomic implant) and ▶ Fig. 4.4 (round implant).

4.2.2 Periareolar and Transareolar Breast Augmentation

Periareolar (PAr) Approach

Jones and Tauras first described the periareolar (PAr) approach to breast augmentation in 1973.[9] An advantage of the PAr approach is that it offers direct visualization of the IMF from a cephalad direction within the pocket. As opposed to the inframammary approach, the PAr approach allows for a more controlled manipulation of the IMF when desired; it also affords maintenance of the IMF via avoidance of dissection of the fold (when desired), which could lead to instability of the fold. It is considered by some to be the most versatile approach because it allows central access to the breast with the greatest ability to lower the IMF.[10,11] Easy access to all four quadrants of the breast

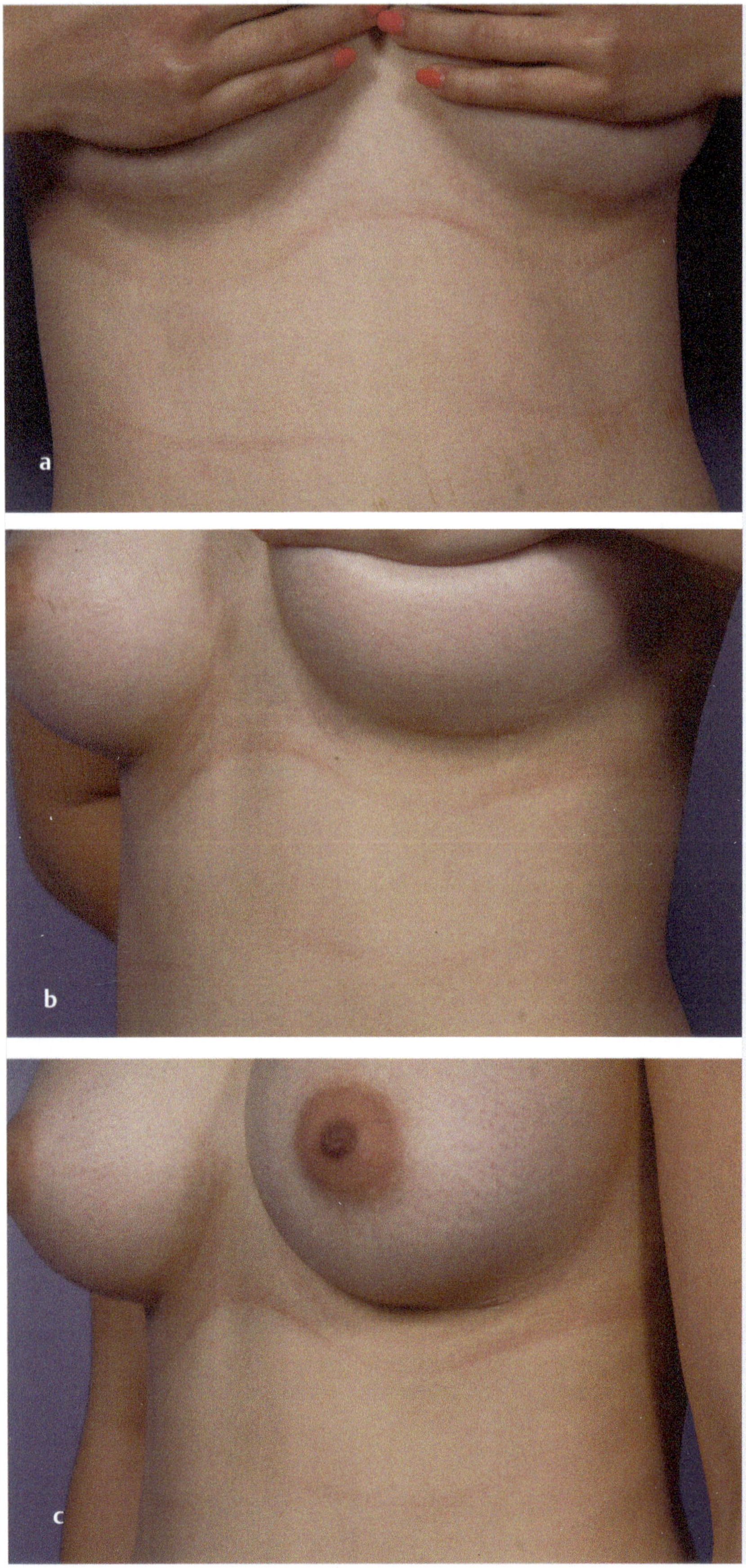

Fig. 4.2 **(a–c)** Inframammary incision well healed at 4 years postoperatively.

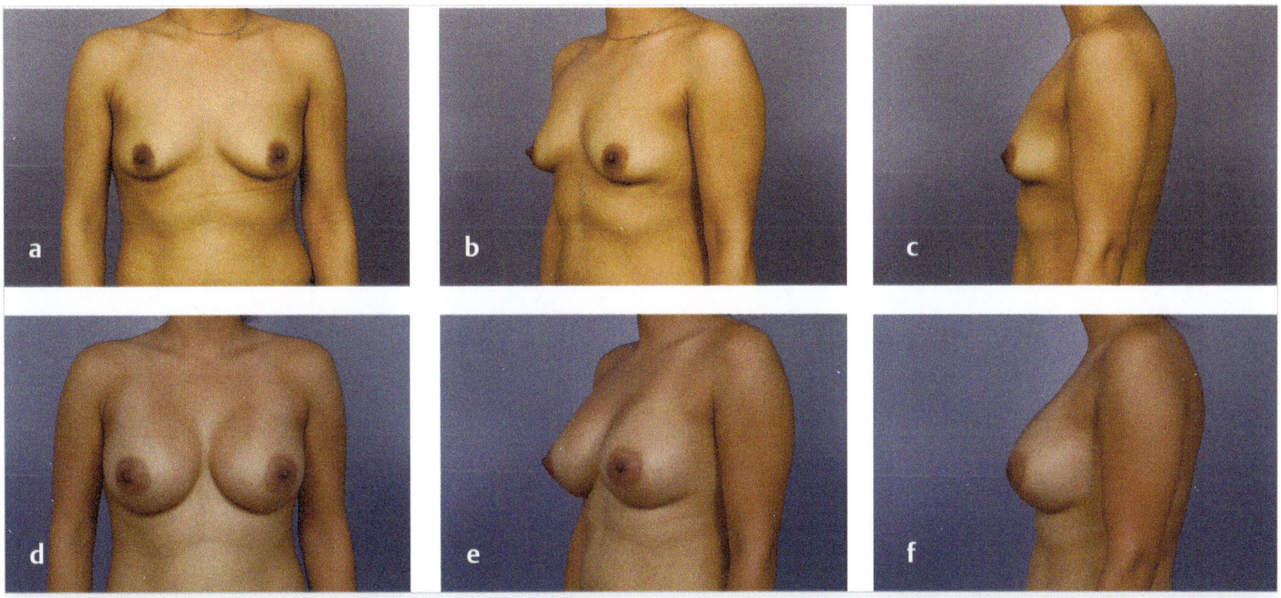

Fig. 4.3 Breast augmentation via inframammary fold incision with anatomic implants in a subfascial plane (375 cc bilateral). **(a–c)** Preoperative. **(d–f)** Postoperative.

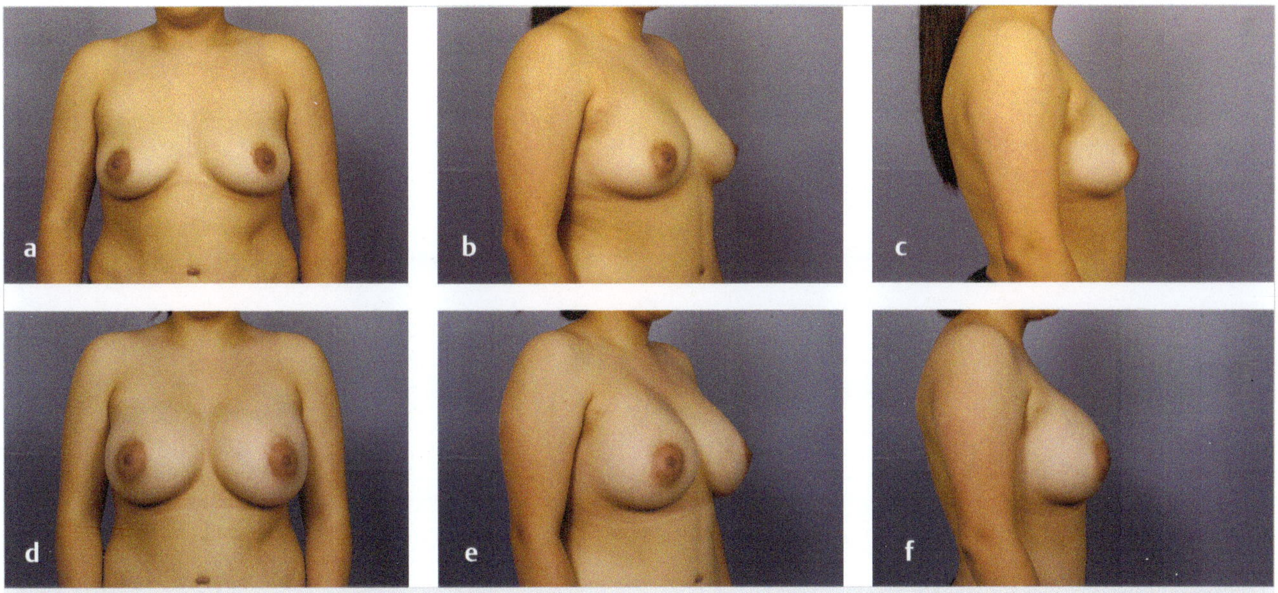

Fig. 4.4 Breast augmentation via inframammary fold incision with round implants in a subfascial plane (485 cc bilateral). **(a–c)** Preoperative. **(d–f)** Postoperative.

offers the greatest ease in performing secondary procedures such as capsulectomy.

After the PAr skin is incised, there are two possible paths of dissection that can be used to reach the pectoralis major muscle (▶ Fig. 4.5). The first option is a transparenchymal dissection in which electrocautery is used to go directly straight down posteriorly through the breast parenchyma (transparenchymal approach). The second option is to leave the breast parenchyma undisturbed by first dissecting caudad toward the IMF, raising a flap of inferior pole skin at the level of the superficial fascia, and then dissecting cephalad along the chest wall toward the pectoralis major muscle (periparenchymal approach).[12] The advantage of raising a flap of inferior pole skin is that it allows for more effective release of superficial bands in the case of a constricted breast, but the disadvantage is thinness of the tissue, which can lead to a flattened lower pole contour in some patients after healing. The advantage of the transparenchymal route is an easier, more direct dissection with less chance of devascularizing the lower pole skin, but the disadvantage is a theoretically greater risk of bacterial release from division of breast ducts.[12]

The size of the PAr incision is determined mainly by the size of the areola. The surgeon has little ability to increase incision

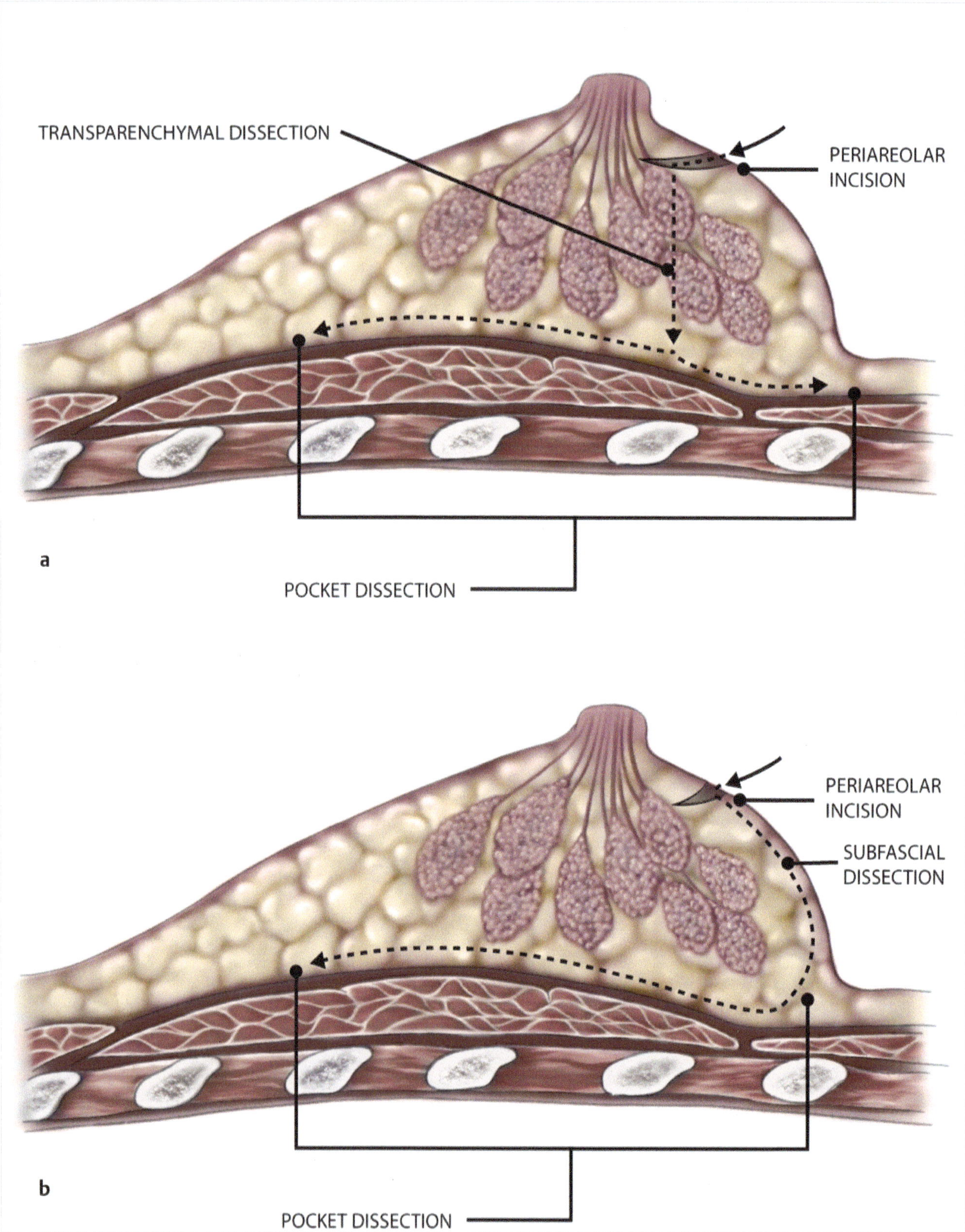

Fig. 4.5 **(a)** Transparenchymal and **(b)** periparenchymal approaches via a periareolar incision. (Adapted from Hammond DC. The periareolar approach to breast augmentation. Clin Plast Surg 2009;36:45–48.)

length intraoperatively if exposure is inadequate and still stay within the confines of the areola. In patients with large areolas, the PAr technique can be advantageous. A large areola allows the surgeon to create a longer incision in the shape of a semicircle for better exposure during dissection while still maintaining a well-hidden scar at the inferior areolar border (▸ Fig. 4.6a). If areola reduction or circumareolar mastopexy is to be performed concomitantly, the PAr approach may be preferable to avoid an additional scar. As such, this approach is especially useful in patients with tuberous breasts who have large, herniating areolas and high (superiorly positioned) IMFs with short nipple-to-IMF distances. In patients with small areolas, use of the PAr approach limits exposure and thus makes dissection more difficult. The PAr approach can still be used in patients with small areolas with the addition of omega extensions beyond the pigmented border of the areola, but this produces a more visible scar. The PAr approach has been shown to have good outcomes in Asian women.[13] Asian patients often have small areolas, and thus the use of a zigzag incision that straddles the areolar border has been described.[14] The proposed advantages of the PAr zigzag include extension of the effective incision length and a multidirectional incision for less scar contracture (▸ Fig. 4.6b).

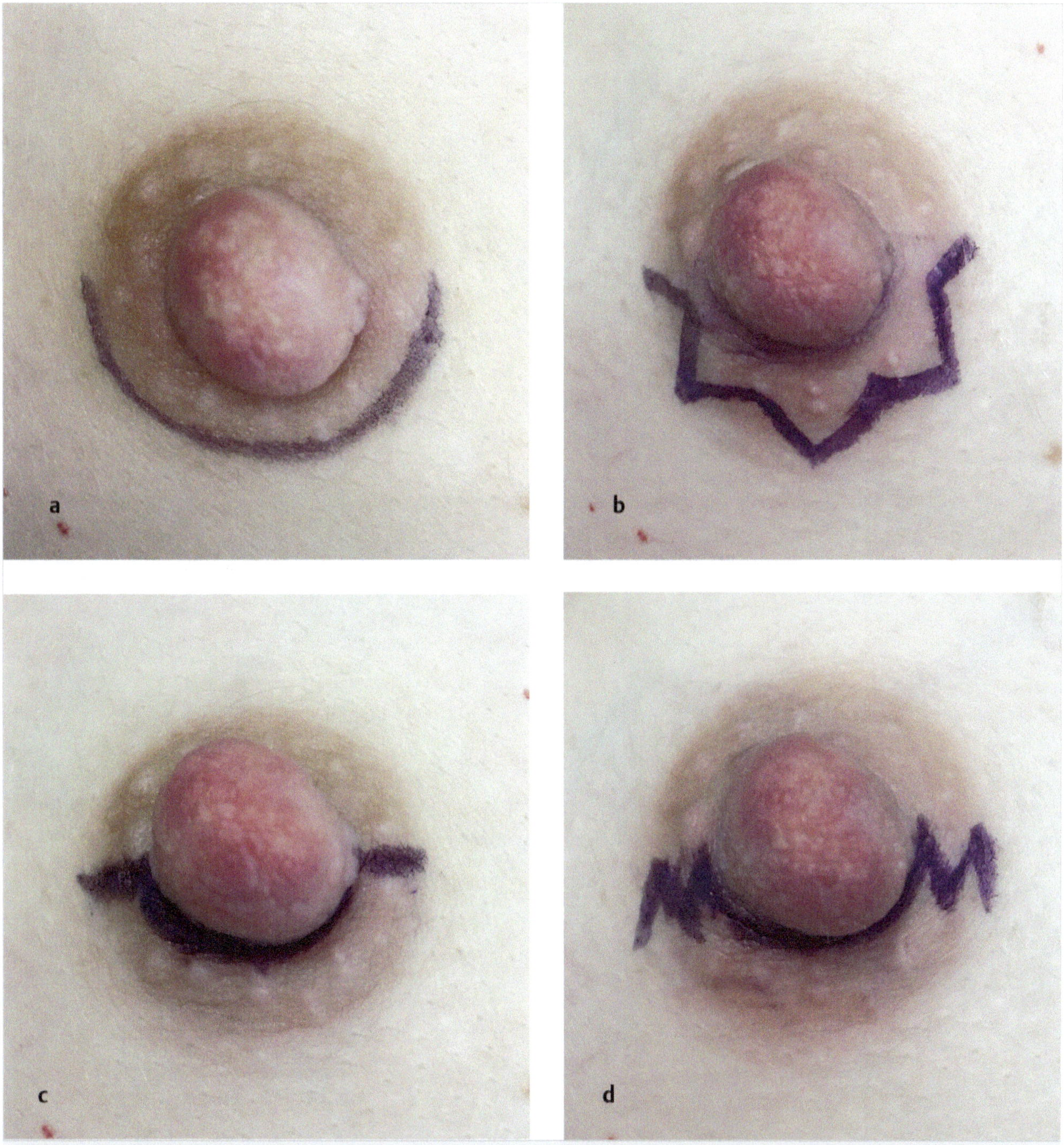

Fig. 4.6 **(a)** Periareolar traditional incision. **(b)** Periareolar zigzag incision. **(c)** Transareolar traditional incision. **(d)** Transareolar zigzag incision.

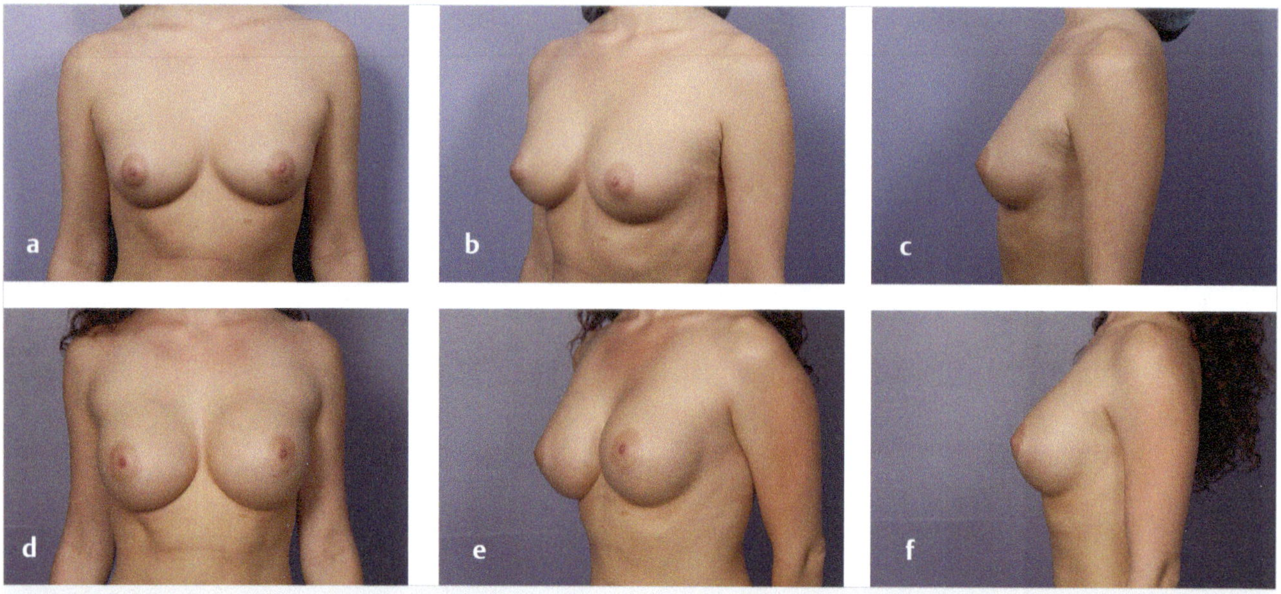

Fig. 4.7 Breast augmentation via periareolar incision with round implants in a subpectoral plane (375 cc bilateral). **(a–c)** Preoperative. **(d–f)** Postoperative.

Transareolar (TAr) Approach

The transareolar (TAr) approach, also known as the perinipple approach, is a similar alternative to the PAr approach with a few small differences that make it better suited for certain patients who desire augmentation via the NAC.[15,16,17] TAr incisions are maintained within the body of the areola but can be less camouflaged because they are not at the natural breast skin–areola junction. The TAr incision is marked in a transverse direction from the 3 o'clock to 9 o'clock positions of the areola or angled slightly obliquely; the incision is continued along the inferior edge of the nipple in the central areola (▶ Fig. 4.6c). The medial and lateral extensions within the areola on each side of the nipple can also be performed in a zigzag pattern (▶ Fig. 4.6d); this zigzag pattern can be used to extend the length of the incision for greater access for dissection in the case of a small areola.[17] In patients with darkly pigmented areolas with distinct margins, a PAr scar may be preferable to a TAr scar because of the potential for hypopigmentation when the TAr scar matures within the dark skin of the areola. Conversely, in patients with lightly colored areolas with indistinct margins, a PAr scar may be more noticeable; therefore, a TAr approach may be preferable in patients with these physical characteristics.[10,11]

Advantages and Disadvantages

Disadvantages of the PAr and TAr approaches include a scar that is visible at the central focal point of the breast (the NAC) with violation of the lactiferous ducts and breast parenchyma during dissection. The PAr/TAr scar is best concealed in scant clothing or swimwear compared to the other approaches, but the scar is the most noticeable in the upright position in the absence of clothing. This can be an important consideration for models and actresses whose occupation requires nudity or in the setting of intimate relationships. The PAr scar is preferable to the TAr scar if a mastopexy is later performed for ptosis as the patient ages because the mastopexy incisions can be placed through the previous PAr scar. Microscopic analysis of samples obtained during TAr breast augmentations have shown the presence of skin flora.[18] This presence of bacteria in the region of the areola has been hypothesized to influence development of capsular contracture. However, Stoff-Khalili et al found that the rate of complications such as capsular contracture with the subglandular approach through a PAr incision are reduced by the subfascial approach to a rate similar to the subpectoral approach without the postoperative discomfort and muscle animation.[19] ▶ Fig. 4.7 and ▶ Fig. 4.8 demonstrate pre- and postoperative photos of two patients who underwent breast augmentation via the PAr approach.

4.2.3 Transaxillary (TAx) Breast Augmentation

Transaxillary (TAx) breast augmentation was first introduced in the early 1970s[20,21,22,23] and was advanced by the introduction of the endoscope in the early 1990s.[24,25] With both the endoscopic and nonendoscopic (blind) techniques, a 4- to 5-cm horizontal incision is made just lateral to the lateral border of the pectoralis major muscle through a crease as cephalad as possible in the axilla to allow it to be better concealed with the shoulder abducted to 90 degrees. Dissection is performed in a subcutaneous plane to avoid axillary lymphatics and intercostobrachial nerves until the pectoralis major fascia is reached.[26,27,28] Intercostobrachial nerve injury has been reported to be a common complication if dissection is performed deeper than in a subcutaneous plane prior to reaching the pectoralis major muscle.[29] The subglandular, subpectoral, or subfascial plane of dissection is then selected. The pectoralis major fascia is thicker on the cephalad portions of the muscle compared to at the IMF, making the subfascial plane of dissection a little easier to get started through this approach compared to the inframammary

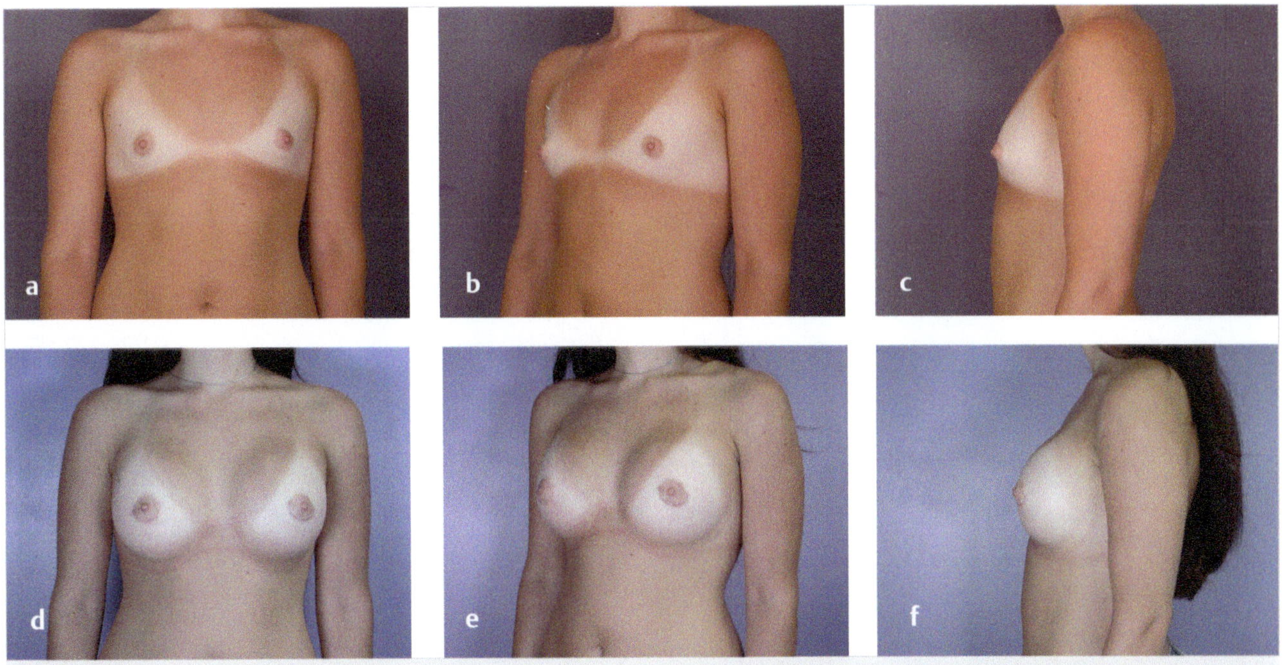

Fig. 4.8 Breast augmentation via periareolar incision with round implants in a subpectoral plane (385 cc bilateral). **(a–c)** Preoperative. **(d–f)** Postoperative.

approach. Pereira reported similar satisfaction rates in a comparison of various planes of dissection with the transaxillary approach.[30] The transaxillary approach is a little more challenging in patients with a long torso and a low breast footprint, and thus patients with a short torso and high breast footprint are considered more favorable candidates.[10]

With the *blind* technique, an Agris-Dingman dissector[31] is passed bluntly in the selected plane to create the pocket. Blunt dissection via this technique works well in the subpectoral plane, with avulsion of the inferomedial attachments of the pectoralis major muscle to the chest wall (▶ Fig. 4.9a). A long, straight retractor and long electrocautery tip with sharp dissection are more effective than the Agris-Dingman dissector for the subfascial approach because the pectoralis major muscle fascia does not separate bluntly from the muscle very well. With the *endoscopic* technique, a 10-mm, 30° endoscope is inserted (▶ Fig. 4.9b).[32,33] In theory, use of an endoscope allows precise pocket dissection, especially at the IMF, and meticulous hemostasis compared to the blind approach.[34] However, debate exists about whether these assumptions are adequately supported by data or more theoretical in nature. Roxo et al have reported significantly longer operative times without improved safety or better outcomes with the endoscopic approach.[35] In a 20-year experience of 1,682 patients utilizing the blind approach, Huang et al reported the need for secondary procedures in 13% of patients with low rates of malposition (3.0%), hematoma (0.1%), and capsular contracture (1.9%).[36]

Advantages and Disadvantages

Advantages of transaxillary breast augmentation include no visible scars on the breast and excellent concealment of the scar in one of the natural creases of the axilla (▶ Fig. 4.10). Therefore, this technique is ideal in patients desiring silicone augmentation who scar poorly or are averse to scars. It is also a good option in patients with small breasts that do not descend over the IMF or have poorly defined IMFs that would make an inframammary scar more pronounced. For these reasons, it is often the preferred technique in patients of Asian descent.[37] Despite this preference in Asian patients, scar assessment of the transaxillary approach compared to the inframammary approach showed comparable cosmetic results.[38] Because of the difficulty of pocket dissection relative to the inframammary and periareolar approaches, the transaxillary approach is also a good option in patients who already have sizable breasts and want only a small augmentation.[10] Disadvantages of the transaxillary approach include a difficult learning curve, less precise pocket dissection that can lead to asymmetry, potential for superior or inferior implant malposition, and inability to perform all reoperations through the same axillary incision. Operatively raising the IMF, advanced capsular contractures, plane change, ptosis, and complicated pocket revision are difficult or impossible to correct through the same axillary incision.[36]

Inferior implant malposition or "bottoming-out" of the implant due to excessive release of the IMF is a major concern with the transaxillary approach. Conversely, superior implant malposition is also a common occurrence resulting from inadequate release of the prepectoral fascia. Improvements in the blind technique to prevent malposition have been described, including disruption of the extended pectoral fascia.[39] To combat a bottomed-out implant, postoperative techniques have also been developed.[40,41,42] Mills et al developed the shoelace breast cast to reinforce the IMF until sealing of the pocket occurs and the capsule matures with the implants in the appropriate position.[42] With concerns about technical control, many surgeons prefer to use round implants with the transaxillary approach.[34]

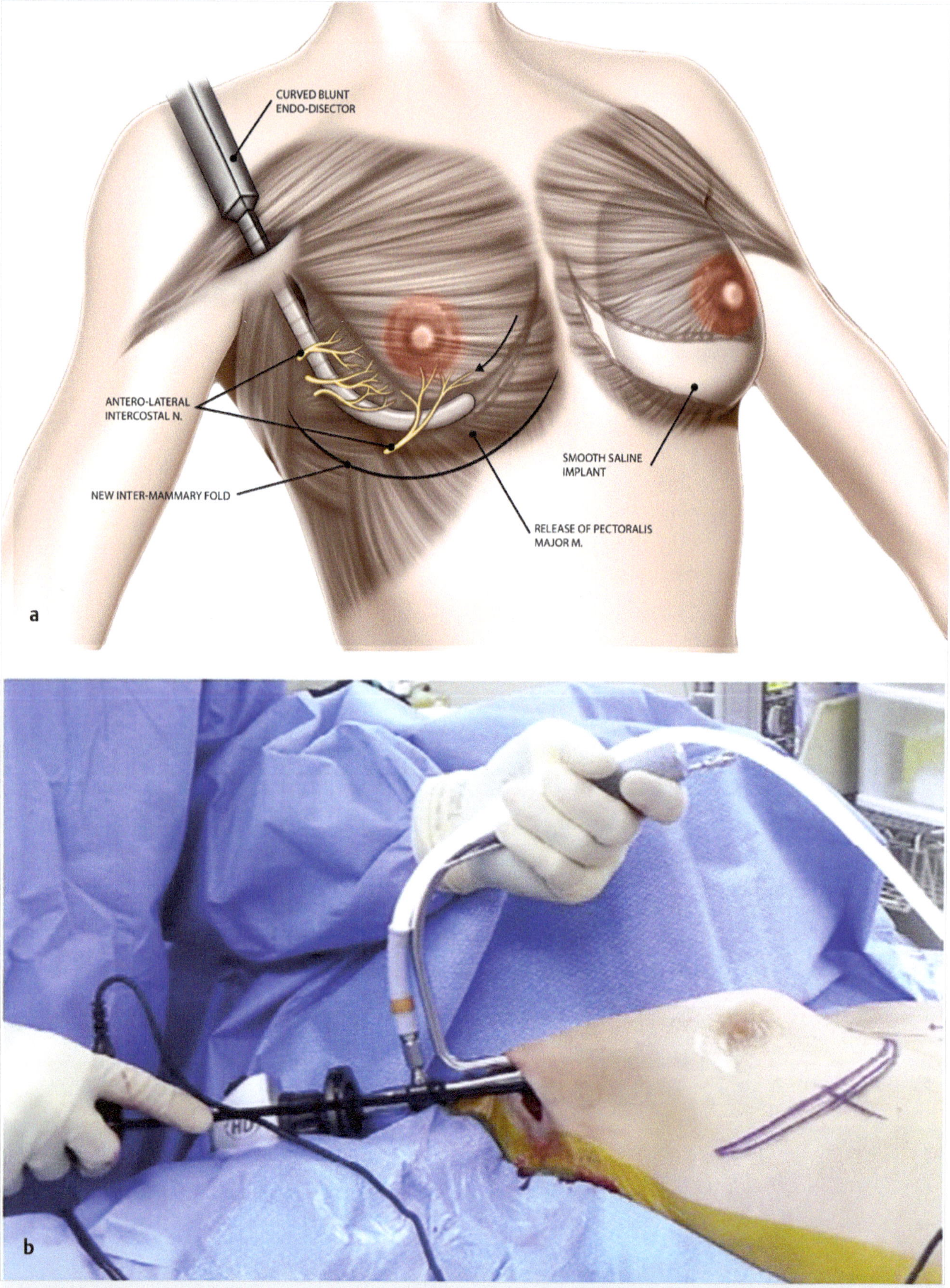

Fig. 4.9 (a,b) Transaxillary blind approach via Agris-Dingman blunt dissection of a subpectoral pocket. (Adapted from Day CR, Nahai F. Transaxillary endoscopically assisted subpectoral augmentation mammoplasty. Oper Tech Plast Reconstr Surg 2000;7:107–115.)

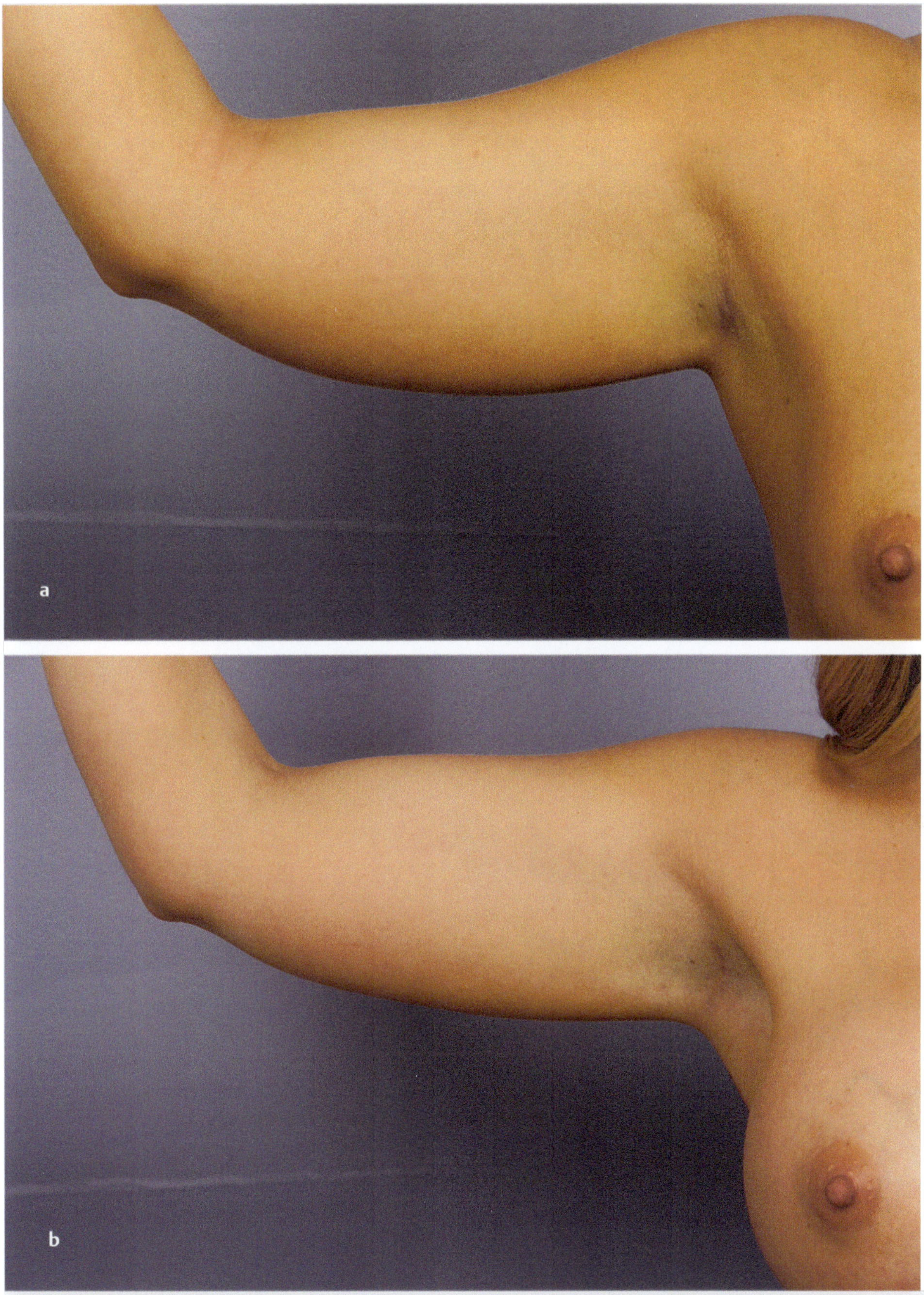

Fig. 4.10 Axilla of a patient who underwent transaxillary breast augmentation **(a)** preoperatively and **(b)** at 3 months postoperatively with incision positioned as cephalad as possible in the axilla.

However, other authors have reported success with the use of anatomic implants.[43,44]

The transaxillary approach has also met criticism regarding potential interference with sentinel lymph node biopsy (SLNB) later in life due to disruption of axillary lymphatics.[45,46] This is a legitimate concern, considering that augmentations are mainly performed in young women and breast cancer develops in 1 out of 8 women over their lifetime. Studies by Sado et al and Weck Roxo et al in which lymphoscintigraphy was performed preoperatively, within 1 month postoperatively, and 6 months postoperatively following transaxillary augmentation found that some patients may experience a transient reduction in lymphatic flow that later returns to normal. They suggested that there might be pressure on the lymphatics from edema or the implant in the early postoperative period, with normalization or adaptive/regenerative capacity of lymphatic pathways in the late postoperative period rather than permanent obstruction by cicatricial fibrosis of lymphatic vessels.[47,48]

High satisfaction has been reported with the transaxillary approach.[49,50] Momeni et al reported higher satisfaction with the transaxillary approach compared to the inframammary approach.[49] Many of the available studies reporting complications are from authors who infrequently perform the transaxillary approach. Authors with greater experience report lower rates of complications. In over 2,500 transaxillary augmentations, Gelfant recalled only seven hematomas and one infection requiring explantation with a capsular contracture rate around 1%.[51] ▸ Fig. 4.11 and ▸ Fig. 4.12 demonstrate pre- and

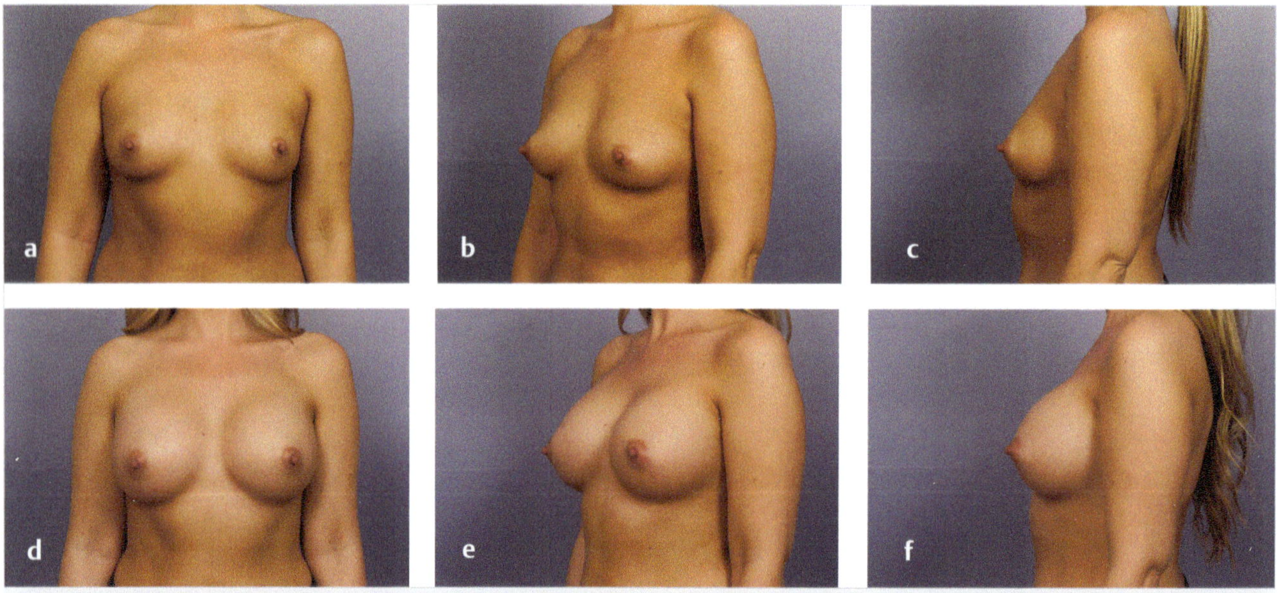

Fig. 4.11 Breast augmentation via transaxillary incision with round implants in a subpectoral plane (355 cc bilateral). **(a–c)** Preoperative. **(d–f)** Postoperative.

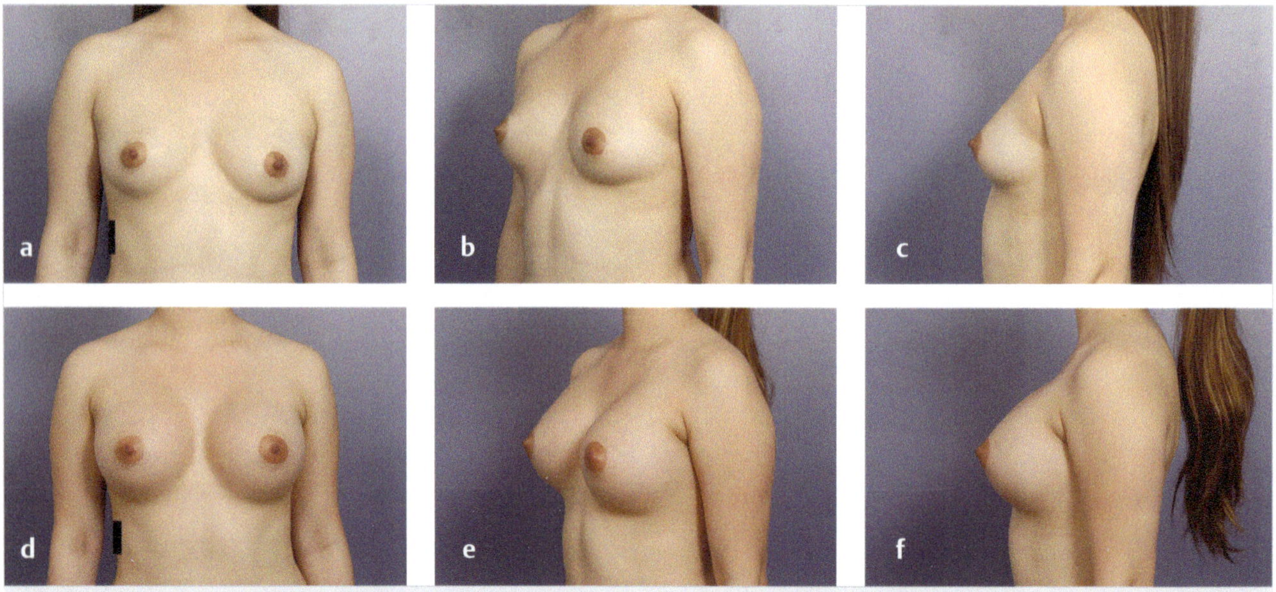

Fig. 4.12 Breast augmentation via transaxillary incision with round implants in a subpectoral plane (385 cc on the right, 355 cc on the left). **(a–c)** Preoperative. **(d–f)** Postoperative.

postoperative photos of two patients who underwent breast augmentation via the transaxillary approach.

4.2.4 Transumbilical Breast Augmentation (TUBA)

The TUBA technique was first introduced in 1993 by Johnson and Christ.[52] It takes advantage of the fact that inflatable saline implants can be inserted through small, remote incisions, which is not normally possible with prefilled silicone implants. The implants can be placed in either the subglandular or subpectoral planes.[53,54,55,56,57]

The procedure is performed using an instrument called a mammascope or endotube. The mammascope has the basic configuration of a sigmoidoscope (10 mm, 0° endoscope) but is longer (30 cm) and has an enlarged handle on the obturator for better control during passage through the tissue and ability to span the longer distance to the breast. The path of dissection is marked by drawing a line starting from the umbilicus that passes tangentially along the medial edge of the areola bilaterally (▶ Fig. 4.13). The lateral edge of the pectoralis major is lateral to this line. An incision is made around the rim of the umbilicus, and the mammascope with internal obturator is inserted through this incision. The mammascope with obturator is tunneled through the deep layer of the subcutaneous tissue just superficial to the abdominal wall fascia (in a manner analogous to a liposuction cannula) to just above the NAC (▶ Fig. 4.14a). The nondominant hand is used to lift the subcutaneous tissue and breast away from the abdominal wall and chest wall musculature, respectively, while passing the cannula. The obturator is then removed and the mammascope is used to inspect the plane of dissection to confirm a bloodless field (▶ Fig. 4.14b), followed by removal of the mammascope for implant loading. A subglandular plane is illustrated, as the technique was originally described.

The saline implant is cigar-rolled around its fill tube, the fill tube is attached to an extension tube through the mammascope, and the implant is loaded into the mammascope (▶ Fig. 4.15). The implant-loaded mammascope is then pushed through the previously created tunnel into the breast, with the fill tube facing the underlying fascia. The deflated implant is then deployed by gently rocking the mammascope free and withdrawing the mammascope from the body, making sure not to dislodge the fill tube prematurely (▶ Fig. 4.16a). If the fill tube dislodges prematurely, the surgeon can milk the implant

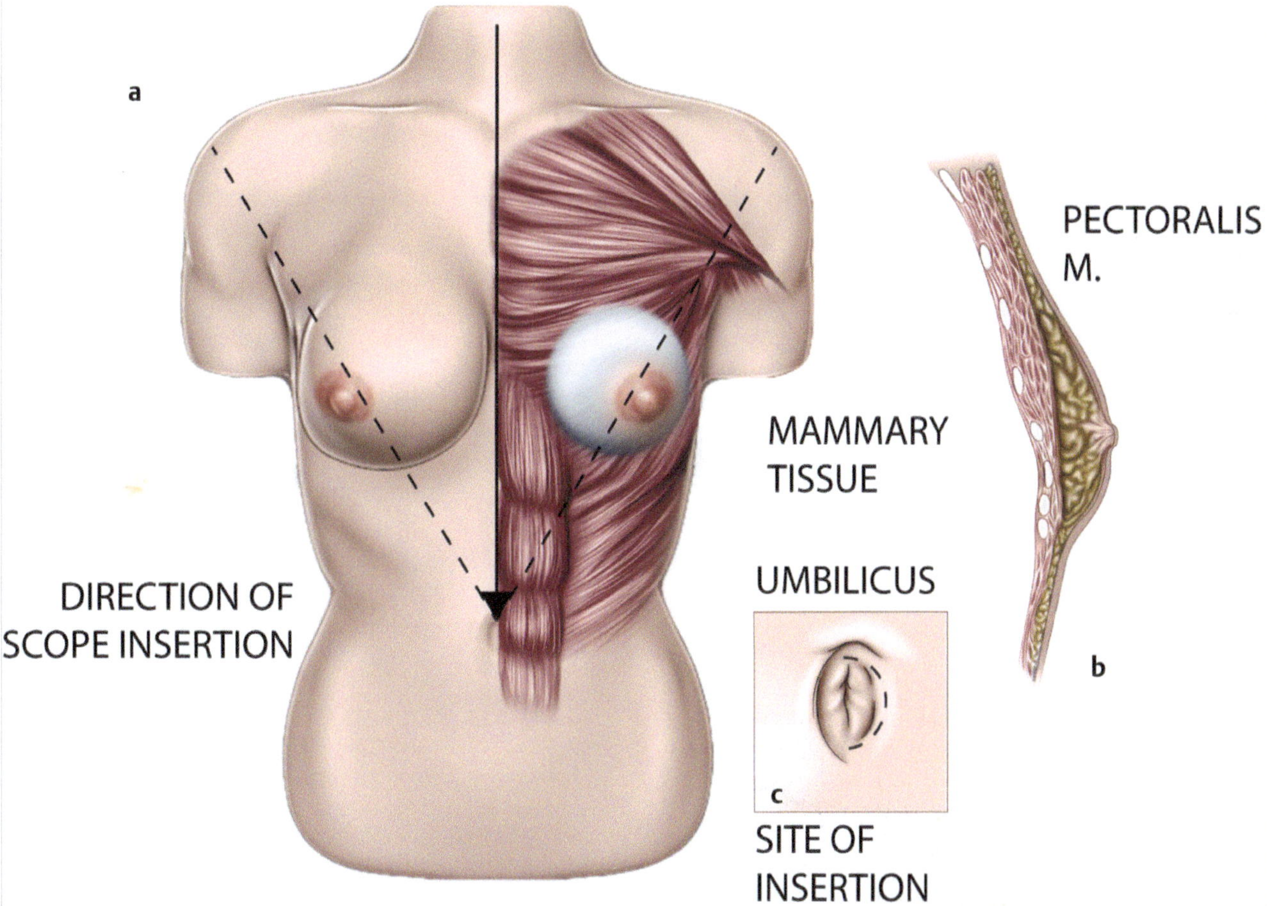

Fig. 4.13 **(a)** Path of the dissection from the superior edge of the umbilicus to the medial border of the nipple-areola complex. **(b)** Cross section of the breast when viewed laterally. **(c)** Incision at the umbilicus. (Adapted from Johnson GW, Christ JE. The endoscopic breast augmentation: the transumbilical insertion of saline-filled breast implants. Plast Reconstr Surg 1993;92:801–808.)

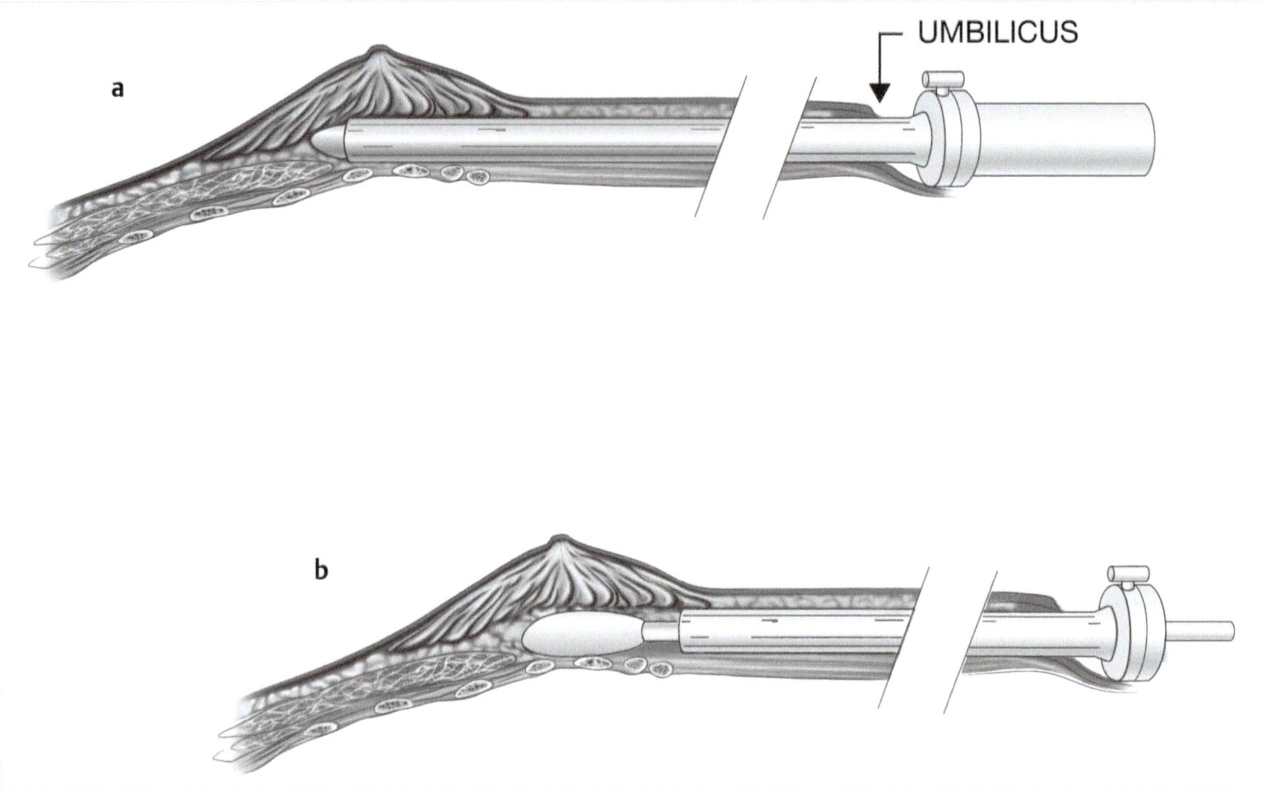

Fig. 4.14 **(a)** Tunneling of the mammascope subcutaneously and suprafascially from the umbilical insertion site to the subglandular plane. **(b)** Removal of the obturator; endoscopic view of the field should confirm that it is dry. (Adapted from Johnson GW, Christ JE. The endoscopic breast augmentation: the transumbilical insertion of saline-filled breast implants. Plast Reconstr Surg 1993;92:801–808.)

retrograde out the umbilical opening, reattach the implant to the fill tube, and reinsert it with the mammascope. The implant is overfilled with saline inside the pocket (▶ Fig. 4.16b), and the pocket dissection is adjusted by manually manipulating the implant extracorporally. The same procedure is repeated for the contralateral breast, and the fill tubes are removed by manual traction once the breast volumes are deemed symmetric (▶ Fig. 4.16c). If the fill tube is dislodged while the implant is only partially filled, the implant must be sacrificed by intentional deflation so that it can be removed and a new implant used.

Advantages and Disadvantages

TUBA does offer the least conspicuous scar that is farthest from the breast. However, the transumbilical approach has the distinct disadvantage of traditionally requiring saline implants. Like axillary augmentation, TUBA has the disadvantage of imprecise pocket creation due to the remote access to the breast and near impossibility of revision for complications through the umbilicus. A unique disadvantage of TUBA is development of contour deformities in the form of track marks; however, this is minimized in experienced hands.[58,59] The presence of an epigastric hernia is a relative contraindication due to the potential for bowel injury. Scars from previous surgery in the epigastric region also potentially make the dissection more difficult when performed through the umbilicus. Alternatively, these scars can be used for insertion.

TUBA was once a popular approach when saline implants were the predominant implant material used for primary augmentations. Following removal of the moratorium on silicone breast implants that lasted from 1992 to 2006, this technique has fallen out of favor by many surgeons. Therefore, TUBA is mainly considered to be of historical importance at this point because of the renewed popularity of silicone implants. However, a group in South Korea has recently described the placement of round silicone implants via the transumbilical approach.[60]

4.3 Capsular Contracture

Capsular contracture is the most common complication following breast augmentation. The incidence has been reported to be around 4% to 5% during the first 2 years postoperatively,[61,62] and it increases to 11% to 18% at 9 years postoperatively.[63] Some studies have shown higher rates of capsular contracture as the time from augmentation increases,[62,63,64] but others have shown that greater than 90% of contractures occur within the first year.[61] The exact etiology is not completely understood, but the infection theory is currently the leading hypothesis.[65] Exposure to bacteria through incisions at different anatomic locations could lead to the development of biofilms on implants and contribute to the development of capsular contracture. Some authors have hypothesized that bacteria in the ducts around the nipple could be associated with higher rates of

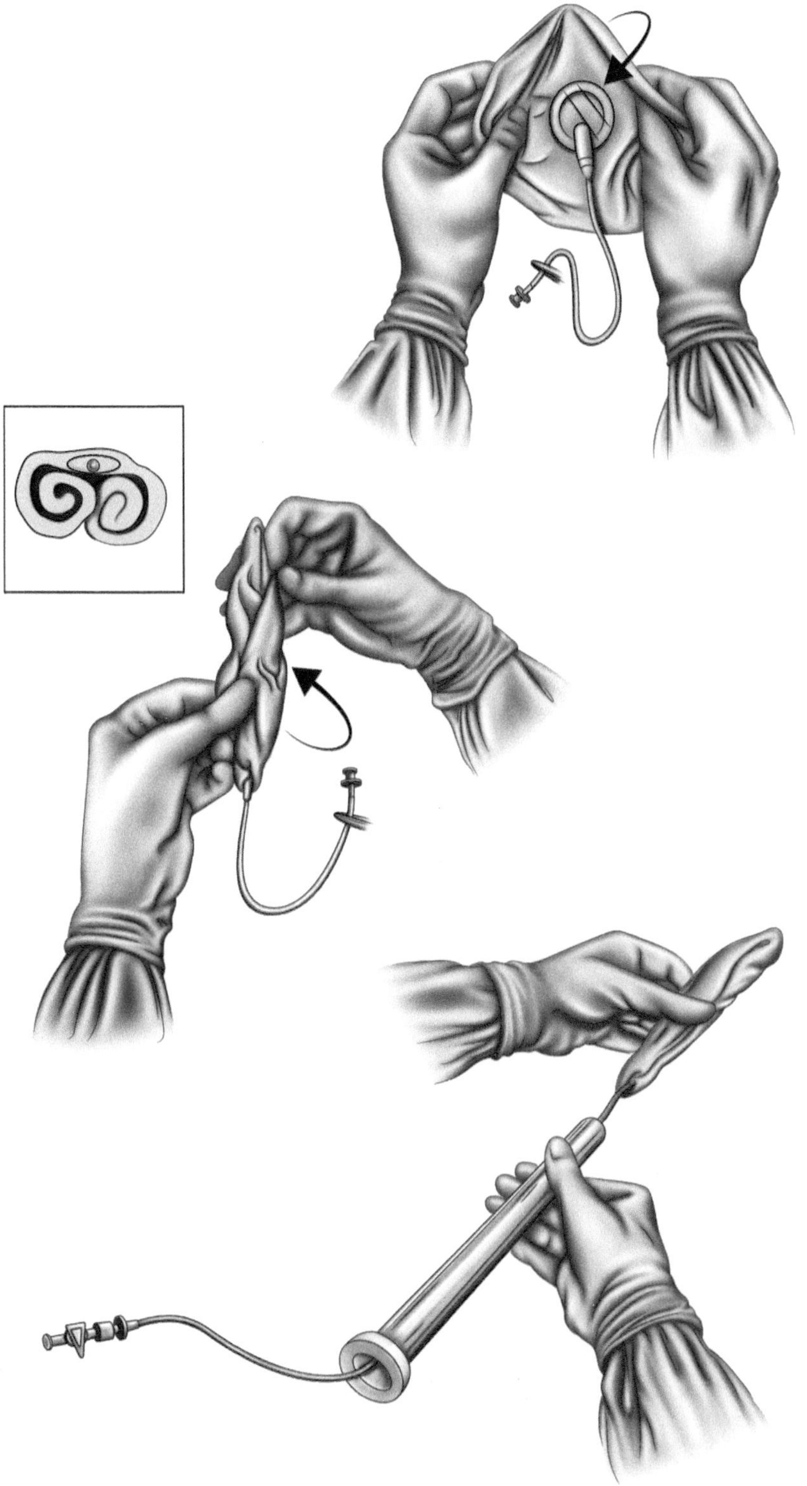

Fig. 4.15 The medial and lateral edges of the deflated saline implant are rolled posteriorly with the fill-tube positioned posteriorly. The deflated implant is then loaded into the mammascope for insertion. (Adapted from Johnson GW, Christ JE. The endoscopic breast augmentation: the transumbilical insertion of saline-filled breast implants. Plast Reconstr Surg 1993;92:801–808.)

contracture when implants are placed through a periareolar incision.[12]

As previously discussed, Namnoum et al found a lower relative risk of capsular contracture with the inframammary approach than with the periareolar and transaxillary approaches.[8] Jacobson et al reported an overall rate of capsular contracture of 1.8% in 336 augmented breasts with a mean follow-up of over 1 year. They found a statistically significant higher rate of capsular contracture with transaxillary incisions than with periareolar or inframammary incisions.[66] They suggested a possible increased rate of capsular contracture with the periareolar approach compared to the inframammary approach that did not reach statistical significance. In most studies comparing rates of capsular contractures through different incision types, the transaxillary approach is the least frequently used, with added operative time and difficulties during

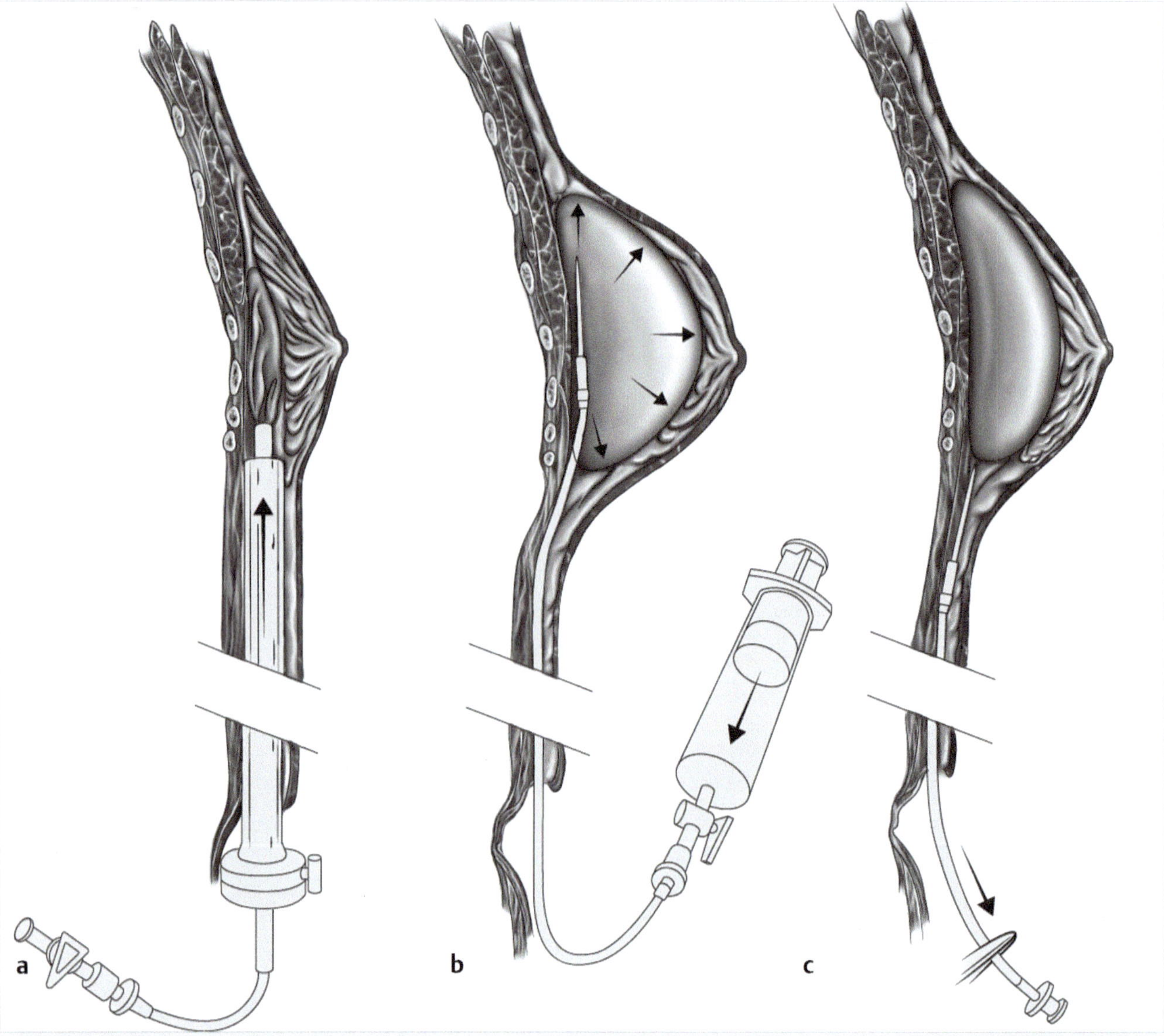

Fig. 4.16 **(a)** Once the implant-loaded mammascope is appropriately positioned in the breast, the deflated implant is deployed by gently rocking the mammascope free and withdrawing it. **(b)** Saline is injected into the implant with a 60-mL syringe to the desired volume. **(c)** The fill tube is removed by manual traction. (Adapted from Johnson GW, Christ JE. The endoscopic breast augmentation: the transumbilical insertion of saline-filled breast implants. Plast Reconstr Surg 1993;92:801–808.)

the operation leading to increased exposure of bacteria into the pocket and subsequent capsular contractures.

In a comparison of inframammary and periareolar augmentations, Wiener reported a statistically significant higher rate of capsular contracture with the periareolar approach.[67] Stutman et al found no statistically significant difference in complications such as capsular contracture, rippling, implant rupture, hematoma, or infection based on incision location in 1,238 augmented breasts.[68] Consequently, the literature has mixed evidence regarding the differences in capsular contracture with the various approaches.

4.4 Nipple Sensation and Breastfeeding

In 1976, Courtiss and Goldwyn reported decreased sensation following various plastic surgery procedures of the breast, including breast augmentation.[69] There is a theoretical concern that due to the proximity of the incision to the NAC, patients are at increased risk of impaired NAC sensation with the periareolar approach compared to other approaches for breast augmentation. Only three studies have made a direct comparison between inframammary and periareolar approaches, so each is discussed here in detail. Mofid et al quantitatively measured cutaneous pressure thresholds for the NAC in 20 women who had undergone augmentation and 9 women who had not, finding that there was a statistically significant negative effect on sensory outcomes in the augmentation patients, but there was no difference in sensory outcomes between inframammary and periareolar approaches.[70] In a prospective study, Okwueze et al found no significant difference in quantitive measures of sensation of the NAC between the inframammary and periareolar approaches at 6 months postoperatively; however, they did find decreased sensation in the lower pole with the inframammary approach compared to the periareolar approach.[71] Araco et al retrospectively studied the subjective assessment of 1,222 augmentation patients (15.5% periareolar) and found no sensory alteration in 95% of patients; however, contrary to the previous studies, the rate of impaired NAC sensation and pain was significantly higher by threefold in the periareolar than in the inframammary group.[72]

Studies in the obstetrics literature from the 1990s associated periareolar incisions with impaired lactation,[73,74] but due to small sample sizes and study designs, the conclusions were not considered definitive.[11] In 2010, Cruz and Korchin found that the success rate of breastfeeding significantly decreased by 25% and the need to supplement breastfeeding increased by 19% after augmentation, but there was no significant difference between periareolar and inframammary incisions. They also reported loss of nipple sensation in 2% of patients, with no significant difference between the periareolar and inframammary approaches.[75]

Therefore, there is no strong evidence to suggest that the periareolar incision negatively impacts breastfeeding compared to the other approaches and limited, mixed evidence to suggest that the periareolar approach impairs nipple sensation compared to the other approaches.

4.5 Conclusion

Breast augmentation can be performed through various approaches including the inframammary, periareolar, transareolar, transumbilical, and transaxillary approaches. Consideration of patient desires as well as the advantages and disadvantages of these various approaches should be considered when discussing breast augmentation with patients.

Key Points

- Available options include inframammary, periareolar, transaxillary, and transumbilical approaches. Each technique has its own advantages and disadvantages.
- For all incision types, the surgeon must balance the desire for an inconspicuous scar with the need for adequate exposure for dissection that will accommodate the implant and minimize the chance of complications.
- The exact etiology of capsular contracture is not completely understood, but the infectious theory is currently the leading hypothesis. Exposure to bacteria through incisions at different anatomic locations could potentially lead to the development of biofilm on implants and contribute to the development of capsular contracture. Some authors have hypothesized that bacteria in the ducts around the nipple could be associated with higher rates of contracture when implants are placed through a periareolar incision.
- The literature has mixed evidence regarding the differences in capsular contracture with the various approaches.
- Inframammary breast augmentation is the most popular approach with an easy learning curve and direct visualization of the pocket, but it may produce a more noticeable scar. Careful preoperative planning must be done to ensure the incision will lie in the IMF after the augmentation has been performed.
- Periareolar or transareolar approaches have a scar on the focal point of the breast and may limit visualization through a smaller incision, but there are multiple ways to conceal the scar and extend the access. It may be the preferable incision in constricted breasts, as it allows direct visualization of the IMF, or in patients who may also require a mastopexy.
- Transaxillary augmentation can be done blindly or with an endoscope. There are no visible scars on the breast, and this approach may be used in patients with a history of poor scarring, those who want to avoid any scars on the breast, and Asian patients. The learning curve is more difficult, there may be a higher risk of implant malposition, and it may be more difficult to perform secondary revisions.
- The transumbilical approach offers the least noticeable scar, but it can be done only with saline implants, and it suffers from difficulty with control of the pocket and inability to perform secondary revisions through the same approach.
- Capsular contracture can be reduced through a number of methods, but the literature is not conclusive on which approach is best.
- Additionally, there is no conclusive evidence on periareolar approaches affecting sensation or breastfeeding in the future.

References

[1] Teitelbaum S. The inframammary approach to breast augmentation. Clin Plast Surg. 2009; 36(1):33–43, v--vi

[2] Yeslev M, Braun SA, Maxwell GP. Asymmetry of inframammary folds in patients undergoing augmentation mammoplasty. Aesthet Surg J. 2016; 36(2): 156–166

[3] Randquist C, Gribbe O. Highly cohesive textured form stable gel implants: principles and technique. In: Hall-Findlay EJ, Evans GRD, eds. Aesthetic and reconstructive surgery of the breast. Edinburgh, UK: Elsevier Ltd; 2010:339–355

[4] Tebbetts JB, Adams WP. Five critical decisions in breast augmentation using five measurements in 5 minutes: the High Five decision support process. Plast Reconstr Surg. 2005; 116(7):2005–2016

[5] Atiyeh BS, Dibo SA, Nader M, Papazian NJ. Preoperative assessment tool for the planning of inframammary incision and implant profile in breast augmentation. Aesthetic Plast Surg. 2014; 38(5):878–886

[6] Mallucci P, Branford OA. Design for natural breast augmentation: the ICE principle. Plast Reconstr Surg. 2016; 137(6):1728–1737

[7] Campbell CF, Small KH, Adams WP, Jr. The inframammary fold (IMF) fixation suture: proactive control of the IMF in primary breast augmentation. Aesthet Surg J. 2016; 36(5):619–623

[8] Namnoum JD, Largent J, Kaplan HM, Oefelein MG, Brown MH. Primary breast augmentation clinical trial outcomes stratified by surgical incision, anatomical placement and implant device type. J Plast Reconstr Aesthet Surg. 2013; 66(9):1165–1172

[9] Jones FR, Tauras AP. A periareolar incision for augmentation mammaplasty. Plast Reconstr Surg. 1973; 51(6):641–644

[10] Hidalgo DA. Breast augmentation: choosing the optimal incision, implant, and pocket plane. Plast Reconstr Surg. 2000; 105(6):2202–2216, discussion 2217–2218
[11] Spear SL, Bulan EJ, Venturi ML. Breast augmentation. Plast Reconstr Surg. 2004; 114(5):73E–81E
[12] Hammond DC. The periareolar approach to breast augmentation. Clin Plast Surg. 2009; 36(1):45–48, vi
[13] Sohn BK, Chung YJ, Kim G, Yoon WJ. Submuscular periareolar approach to augmentation mammoplasty in Korean women. Aesthetic Plast Surg. 2000; 24(6):455–460
[14] Zelken J, Huang JJ, Wu CW, Lin YL, Cheng MH. The transareolar-periareolar approach. Plast Reconstr Surg Glob Open. 2016; 4(9):e1020
[15] Atiyeh BS, Al-Amm CA, El-Musa KA. The transverse intra-areolar infra-nipple incision for augmentation mammaplasty. Aesthetic Plast Surg. 2002; 26(2): 151–155
[16] Kompatscher P, Schuler C, Beer GM. The transareolar incision for breast augmentation revisited. Aesthetic Plast Surg. 2004; 28(2):70–74
[17] Han HH, Kim KK, Lee KH, et al. Transareolar-perinipple (areolar omega) zigzag incision for augmentation mammaplasty. Plast Reconstr Surg. 2015; 135 (3):517e–525e
[18] Jianu DM, Săndulescu O, Streinu-Cercel A, et al. Microbiologic safety of the transareolar approach in breast augmentation. Aesthet Surg J. 2016; 36(1): 51–57
[19] Stoff-Khalili MA, Scholze R, Morgan WR, Metcalf JD. Subfascial periareolar augmentation mammaplasty. Plast Reconstr Surg. 2004; 114(5):1280–1288, discussion 1289–1291
[20] Troques R. Implantation of mammary prosthesis by axillary incision [in French]. Nouv Presse Med. 1972; 1(36):2409–2410
[21] Hoehler H. Breast augmentation: the axillary approach. Br J Plast Surg. 1973; 26(4):373–376
[22] Eiseman G. Augmentation mammaplasty by the trans-axillary approach. Plast Reconstr Surg. 1974; 54(2):229–232
[23] Wright JH, Bevin AG. Augmentation mammaplasty by the transaxillary approach. Plast Reconstr Surg. 1976; 58(4):429–433
[24] Ho LC. Endoscopic assisted transaxillary augmentation mammaplasty. Br J Plast Surg. 1993; 46(4):332–336
[25] Price CI, Eaves FF, III, Nahai F, Jones G, Bostwick J, III. Endoscopic transaxillary subpectoral breast augmentation. Plast Reconstr Surg. 1994; 94 (5):612–619
[26] Tebbetts JB. Transaxillary subpectoral augmentation mammaplasty: long-term follow-up and refinements. Plast Reconstr Surg. 1984; 74(5):636–649
[27] Tebbetts JB. Transaxillary subpectoral augmentation mammaplasty: a 9-year experience. Clin Plast Surg. 1988; 15(4):557–568
[28] Tebbetts JB. Axillary endoscopic breast augmentation: processes derived from a 28-year experience to optimize outcomes. Plast Reconstr Surg. 2006; 118 (7) Suppl:53S–80S
[29] Ghaderi B, Hoenig JM, Dado D, Angelats J, Vandevender D. Incidence of intercostobrachial nerve injury after transaxillary breast augmentation. Aesthet Surg J. 2002; 22(1):26–32
[30] Pereira LH, Sterodimas A. Transaxillary breast augmentation: a prospective comparison of subglandular, subfascial, and submuscular implant insertion. Aesthetic Plast Surg. 2009; 33(5):752–759
[31] Agris J, Dingman RO, Wilensky RJ. A dissector for the transaxillary approach in augmentation mammaplasty. Plast Reconstr Surg. 1976; 57(1):10–13
[32] Day CR, Nahai F. Transaxillary endoscopically assisted subpectoral augmentation mammoplasty. Oper Tech Plast Reconstr Surg. 2000; 7:107–115
[33] Strock LL. Transaxillary endoscopic silicone gel breast augmentation. Aesthet Surg J. 2010; 30(5):745–755
[34] Pacella SJ, Codner MA. The transaxillary approach to breast augmentation. Clin Plast Surg. 2009; 36(1):49–61, vi
[35] Roxo AC, Marques RG, De Castro CC, Aboudib JH. Utility of video-assisted endoscopy in transaxillary breast augmentation. Aesthet Surg J. 2015; 35(3): 265–272
[36] Huang GJ, Wichmann JL, Mills DC. Transaxillary subpectoral augmentation mammaplasty: a single surgeon's 20-year experience. Aesthet Surg J. 2011; 31(7):781–801
[37] Sun J, Liu C, Mu D, et al. Chinese women's preferences and concerns regarding incision location for breast augmentation surgery: a survey of 216 patients. Aesthetic Plast Surg. 2015; 39(2):214–226
[38] Sun J, Mu D, Liu C, et al. Scar assessment after breast augmentation surgery with axillary incision versus inframammary fold incision: long-term follow-up in Chinese patients. Aesthetic Plast Surg. 2016; 40(5):699–706
[39] Barnett A. Transaxillary subpectoral augmentation in the ptotic breast: augmentation by disruption of the extended pectoral fascia and parenchymal sweep. Plast Reconstr Surg. 1990; 86(1):76–83
[40] Troilius C. Correction of implant ptosis after a transaxillary subpectoral breast augmentation. Plast Reconstr Surg. 1996; 98(5):889–895
[41] Troilius C. A ten-year evaluation following corrections of implant ptosis subsequent to transaxillary subpectoral breast augmentation. Plast Reconstr Surg. 2004; 114(6):1638–1641, discussion 1642–1643
[42] Mills DC, II, Ereso AQ, Engle C, Cessna LE. Shoelace breast cast. Aesthet Surg J. 2014; 34(5):776–781
[43] Aygit AC, Basaran K, Mercan ES. Transaxillary totally subfascial breast augmentation with anatomical breast implants: review of 27 cases. Plast Reconstr Surg. 2013; 131(5):1149–1156
[44] Sim HB, Sun SH. Transaxillary endoscopic breast augmentation with shaped gel implants. Aesthet Surg J. 2015; 35(8):952–961
[45] Munhoz AM, Aldrighi C, Ono C, et al. The influence of subfascial transaxillary breast augmentation in axillary lymphatic drainage patterns and sentinel lymph node detection. Ann Plast Surg. 2007; 58(2):141–149
[46] Prado A, Andrades P, Leniz P. Implications of transaxillary breast augmentations: lifetime probability for the development of breast cancer and sentinel node mapping interference. Aesthetic Plast Surg. 2007; 31:317–319
[47] Sado HN, Graf RM, Canan LW, et al. Sentinel lymph node detection and evidence of axillary lymphatic integrity after transaxillary breast augmentation: a prospective study using lymphoscintography. Aesthetic Plast Surg. 2008; 32 (6):879–888
[48] Weck Roxo AC, Aboudib JH, De Castro CC, De Abreu ML, Camões Orlando MM. Evaluation of the effects of transaxillary breast augmentation on sentinel lymph node integrity. Aesthet Surg J. 2011; 31(4):392–400
[49] Momeni A, Padron NT, Föhn M, et al. Safety, complications, and satisfaction of patients undergoing submuscular breast augmentation via the inframammary and endoscopic transaxillary approach. Aesthetic Plast Surg. 2005; 29 (6):558–564
[50] Gryskiewicz J, LeDuc R. Transaxillary nondendoscopic subpectoral augmentation mammoplasty: a 10-year experience with gel vs saline in 2000 patients —with long term-patient satisfaction measured by the BREAST-Q. Aesthet Surg J. 2014; 34(5):696–713
[51] Gelfant BM. Misconceptions of capsular contracture, operative times, and complications in the transaxillary breast augmentation literature. Aesthet Surg J. 2016; 36(5):NP190
[52] Johnson GW, Christ JE. The endoscopic breast augmentation: the transumbilical insertion of saline-filled breast implants. Plast Reconstr Surg. 1993; 92 (5):801–808
[53] Pound EC, Pound EC. Trans-umbilical breast augmentation (TUBA): Technique for pre-pectoral and post-pectoral placement of implants. Oper Tech Plast Reconstr Surg. 2000; 7:116–124
[54] Pound EC, III, Pound EC, Jr. Transumbilical breast augmentation (TUBA): patient selection, technique, and clinical experience. Clin Plast Surg. 2001; 28 (3):597–605
[55] Sudarsky L. Experience with transumbilical breast augmentation. Ann Plast Surg. 2001; 46(5):467–473
[56] Songcharoen S. Endoscopic transumbilical subglandular augmentation mammaplasty. Clin Plast Surg. 2002; 29(1):1–13
[57] Brennan WA, Haiavy J. Transumbilical breast augmentation: a practical review of a growing technique. Ann Plast Surg. 2007; 59(3):243–249
[58] Dowden RV. Dispelling the myths and misconceptions about transumbilical breast augmentation. Plast Reconstr Surg. 2000; 106(1):190–194, discussion 195--196
[59] Dowden RV. Transumbilical breast augmentation is safe and effective. Semin Plast Surg. 2008; 22(1):51–59
[60] Lee W, Choi BK, Bang SI, Yang EJ. Augmentation mammoplasty with silicone implant using transumbilical approach at a subpectoral level. Ann Plast Surg. 2014; 73(3):268–274
[61] Henriksen TF, Hölmich LR, Fryzek JP, et al. Incidence and severity of short-term complications after breast augmentation: results from a nationwide breast implant registry. Ann Plast Surg. 2003; 51(6):531–539
[62] Handel N, Cordray T, Gutierrez J, Jensen JA. A long-term study of outcomes, complications, and patient satisfaction with breast implants. Plast Reconstr Surg. 2006; 117(3):757–767, discussion 768--772
[63] Stevens WG, Calobrace MB, Harrington J, Alizadeh K, Zeidler KR, d'Incelli RC. Nine-year core study data for Sientra's FDA-approved round and shaped implants with high-strength cohesive silicone gel. Aesthet Surg J. 2016; 36(4): 404–416

[64] Araco A, Gravante G, Araco F, Delogu D, Cervelli V, Walgenbach K. A retrospective analysis of 3,000 primary aesthetic breast augmentations: postoperative complications and associated factors. Aesthetic Plast Surg. 2007; 31(5):532–539
[65] Adams WP, Jr. Capsular contracture: what is it? What causes it? How can it be prevented and managed? Clin Plast Surg. 2009; 36(1):119–126, vii
[66] Jacobson JM, Gatti ME, Schaffner AD, Hill LM, Spear SL. Effect of incision choice on outcomes in primary breast augmentation. Aesthet Surg J. 2012; 32 (4):456–462
[67] Wiener TC. Relationship of incision choice to capsular contracture. Aesthetic Plast Surg. 2008; 32(2):303–306
[68] Stutman RL, Codner M, Mahoney A, Amei A. Comparison of breast augmentation incisions and common complications. Aesthetic Plast Surg. 2012; 36(5): 1096–1104
[69] Courtiss EH, Goldwyn RM. Breast sensation before and after plastic surgery. Plast Reconstr Surg. 1976; 58(1):1–13
[70] Mofid MM, Klatsky SA, Singh NK, Nahabedian MY. Nipple-areola complex sensitivity after primary breast augmentation: a comparison of periareolar and inframammary incision approaches. Plast Reconstr Surg. 2006; 117(6): 1694–1698
[71] Okwueze MI, Spear ME, Zwyghuizen AM, et al. Effect of augmentation mammaplasty on breast sensation. Plast Reconstr Surg. 2006; 117(1):73–83, discussion 84--85
[72] Araco A, Araco F, Sorge R, Gravante G. Sensitivity of the nipple-areola complex and areolar pain following aesthetic breast augmentation in a retrospective series of 1200 patients: periareolar versus submammary incision. Plast Reconstr Surg. 2011; 128(4):984–989
[73] Neifert M, DeMarzo S, Seacat J, Young D, Leff M, Orleans M. The influence of breast surgery, breast appearance, and pregnancy-induced breast changes on lactation sufficiency as measured by infant weight gain. Birth. 1990; 17(1): 31–38
[74] Hurst NM. Lactation after augmentation mammoplasty. Obstet Gynecol. 1996; 87(1):30–34
[75] Cruz NI, Korchin L. Breastfeeding after augmentation mammaplasty with saline implants. Ann Plast Surg. 2010; 64(5):530–533

5 Implant Placement Options

Maurice Y. Nahabedian

Summary

Current approaches to breast augmentation are diverse and controversial. A long-standing topic of discussion is whether to place a breast implant in the subglandular, subfascial, or subpectoral position. Selection of the ideal location is often based on patient and breast characteristics but, interestingly, has geographic variability from a global perspective. Decision making often depends on the size of the natural breast, the patient's degree of physical activity, and an appreciation of patient expectations. With all options, breast enhancement is readily achieved, adverse events are infrequent, and patient satisfaction is high. This chapter will review many of the salient aspects of subglandular, subfascial, and subpectoral breast augmentation with an emphasis on technique and outcomes.

Keywords: breast augmentation, subglandular, subfascial, subpectoral, breast implants, pectoralis major, pectoralis fascia

5.1 Introduction

Deciding upon the ideal plane for breast augmentation has been a long-standing topic of debate and controversy. Options for implant placement include the subglandular, subpectoral, and subfascial locations. Each of these planes has advantages and disadvantages. Clearly, enhancement of volume and contour are achieved with all; however, the plane of implant placement can affect other outcomes such as capsular contracture, animation deformity, rippling, and wrinkling, as well as malposition. The intent of this chapter is to review the options for implant position in cosmetic breast augmentation.

5.2 Anatomy

The relevant anatomy of the breast as it relates to breast augmentation will be reviewed. The natural borders of the breast include the inframammary fold (IMF), anterior axillary line, medial sternal border, and the clavicle. The breast is composed of parenchyma, which includes the lobules and ducts, as well as the subcutaneous layer, which ranges from 1 mm to 3 cm in thickness with a median thickness of 1 cm.[1] The subcutaneous layer gradually and naturally becomes thinner as it approaches the nipple areolar complex (NAC). Other components of the breast include the ligaments of Cooper (pectineal ligaments), the deep and superficial layers of the superficial fascia, as well as the pectoralis major fascia. The diameter of the areola is highly variable and can range from 3 to 8 cm.

The vascularity of the breast is another important concern in considering the planes of dissection. The primary blood supply to the breast is derived from the perforating branches of the internal mammary artery (IMA). Van Deventer has demonstrated that of the six perforators emanating from the medial costal interspaces and arising from the IMA, the third perforator was most commonly seen, followed by the second, the first, and the fourth.[2] Many of these perforators form an anastomotic cluster around the periareolar region and enhance the vascularity to the NAC. These anastomoses are primarily formed from the lateral thoracic and internal mammary perforators. Le Roux demonstrated that the IMA perforators traverse superficially 1 cm under the skin surface.[3] A dominant vessel originates from either the third or the fourth intercostal space with a depth of 10.3 mm at the NAC boundary and 14.2 mm at 3 cm medially. Würinger demonstrated that the second, third, and fourth perforating branches of the IMA coursed within the medial vertical ligament of the breast toward the nipple.[4] The remainder of the vascular supply to the breast is derived from the lateral thoracic, anterior intercostal, thoracoacromial, posterior intercostal, and superficial thoracic arteries. It should be noted that although the vascularity of the breast is generally predictable, embryologic variation could result in vascular unpredictability of the NAC.

Anatomic studies have demonstrated that the innervation to the breast is derived from the first through seventh intercostal nerves and that the innervation to the NAC is derived primarily from the fourth intercostal nerve.[5,6] The dominant innervation of the NAC is derived from the lateral and anterior cutaneous branches of the third, fourth, and fifth intercostal nerves (▶ Fig. 5.1). Schlenz has demonstrated that the most constant innervation patterns were from the fourth lateral (79%) and the third and fourth anterior cutaneous branches (57%).[5] The specific pathways within the breast for these sensory nerves were relatively constant. The anterior cutaneous nerve branch coursed superficially within the subcutaneous tissue and terminated at the medial border of the NAC, whereas the lateral cutaneous branches coursed deep within the pectoral fascia and approached the NAC from its posterior surface.

Beneath the breast parenchyma are the pectoralis fascia and the pectoralis major muscle (▶ Fig. 5.2). The origin of the pectoralis major muscle is from the sternal segment of the clavicle, the anterior surface of the sternum extending to the sixth and seventh ribs, and the aponeurosis of the external oblique muscle. The insertion is to the bicipital groove of the humerus. The medial and lateral pectoral nerves innervate the pectoralis major muscle. Understanding of this innervation is especially important when breast implant–associated animation deformity becomes problematic. The medial and lateral pectoral nerves enter the pectoral space from lateral to medial. The medial pectoral nerve pierces the pectoralis minor muscle before innervating the pectoralis major muscle. The lateral pectoral nerve pierces the pectoralis major muscle directly. Additional anatomic studies have demonstrated that the branches of the lateral and medial pectoral nerves penetrate the pectoralis major several centimeters from the lateral edge of the sternum, thus minimizing the risk of injury to the medial pectoral nerve during breast augmentation.[7]

Anatomic studies depicting the relationship between the pectoralis major and the external oblique muscles have demonstrated that the costal portion of the pectoralis major originates from the fifth (25%), sixth (70%), or seventh rib (5%).[8] The distances from the midclavicular line to the lateral border of the

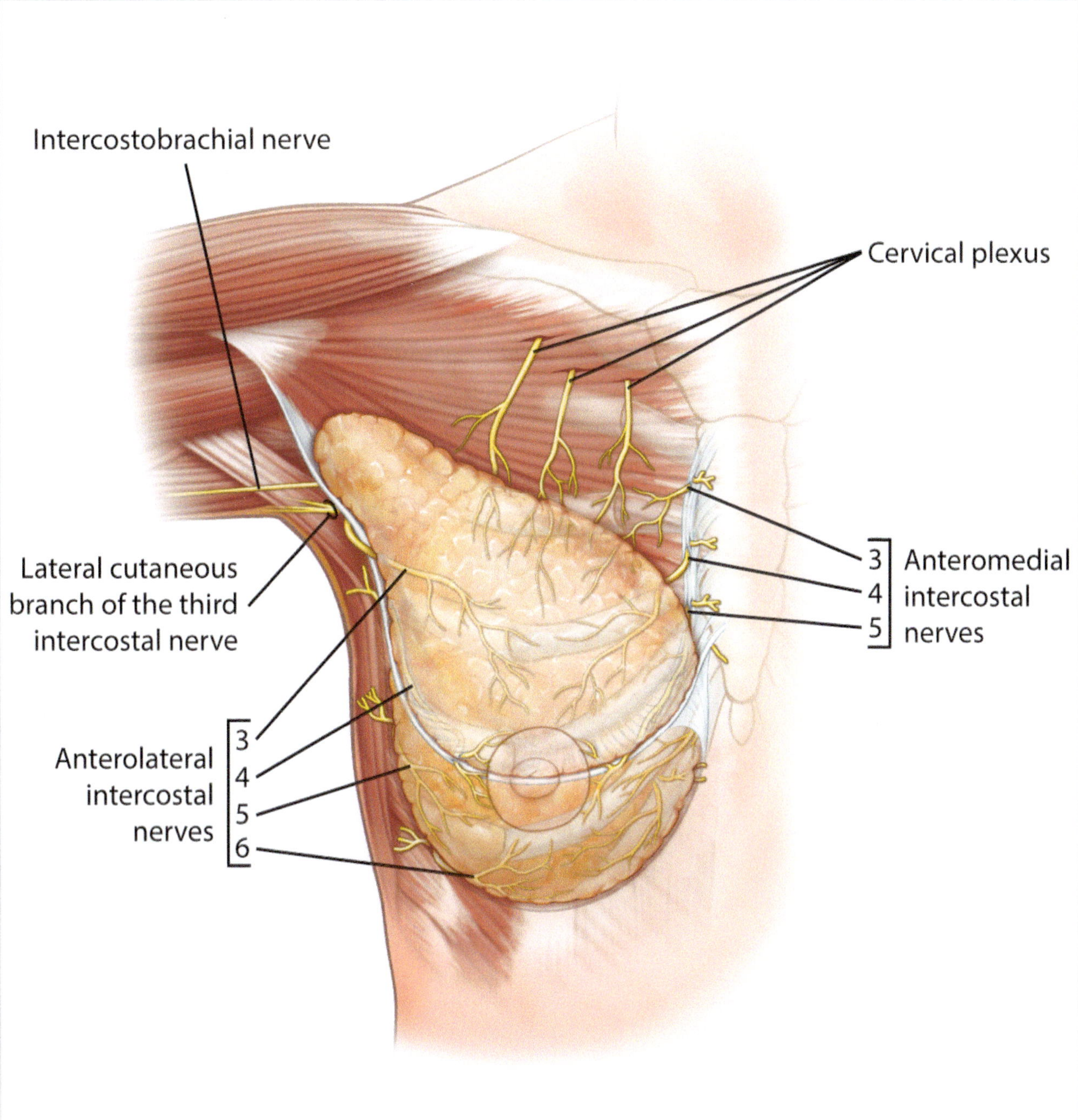

Fig. 5.1 The sensory innervation to the breast and nipple areolar complex is principally derived from the medial and lateral divisions of the second through sixth intercostal nerves. (Reproduced from Nahai F. The Art of Aesthetic Surgery: Principles & Techniques. 2nd ed. New York, NY: Thieme Medical Publishers; 2011.)

pectoralis major muscle at the fourth, fifth, and sixth ribs were 49.8 mm, 30.5 mm, and 6.3 mm, respectively. The pectoralis major and the external oblique muscles overlapped near the midclavicular line in 90% of patients, and the width of the overlap was about 25 mm.

With the advent of subfascial breast augmentation, the anatomy of the pectoral fascia has become important. The benefits of preserving the pectoral fascia–parenchyma interface are several but include retention of the Cooper's ligament attachments as well as the horizontal septum of Würinger. Anatomic studies have demonstrated that the pectoral fascia originates superiorly and medially from the clavicle and sternum and extends over the surface of the muscle.[9] Lin and others have demonstrated that the thickness of the pectoral fascia ranges from 0.2 to 1.1 mm.[9] Tebbetts demonstrated that the thickness ranged from 0.1 to 0.5 mm,[10] whereas Graf found that the thickness of the pectoral fascia was approximately 0.2 mm centrally and 1.0 mm laterally and medially.[11]

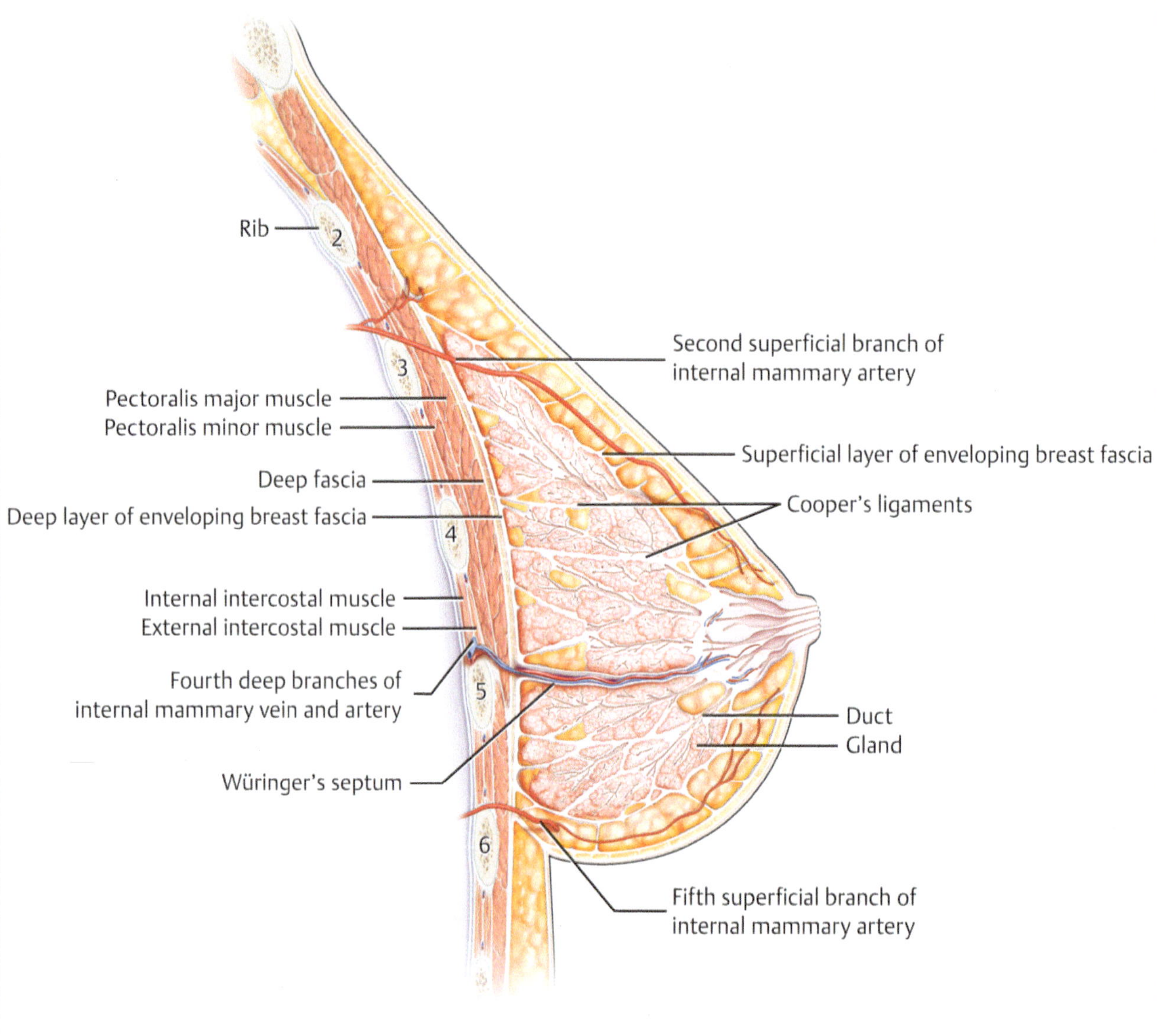

Fig. 5.2 The breast parenchyma as well as the superficial and deep layers of the superficial fascia is depicted. (Reproduced from Hall-Findlay EJ. Aesthetic Breast Surgery: Concepts & Techniques. New York: Thieme Medical Publishers; 2011.)

5.3 Patient Selection

Patient selection for breast augmentation begins with a complete history and physical examination. Included in this are a thorough assessment of patient expectations and an understanding of the risks and benefits. These issues were explained in detail in prior chapters. The discussion relating to the ideal plane of dissection will depend in part on physical examination and surgeon preference. Patient selection for glandular and subfascial device placement are essentially the same because the device is superficial to the pectoralis major muscle for both planes. However, selection criteria for subpectoral placement may differ in some cases. In general, the subpectoral position is typically recommended in patients with a thin body habitus and an upper pole pinch test < 2 cm, whereas the subglandular or subfascial plane can be considered in patients with an upper pole pinch thickness > 2 cm.

5.4 Advantages and Disadvantages

The subglandular position of a breast implant results in ideal projection; however, in thin patients, implant visibility in the form of rippling and wrinkling as well as edge visibility may be problematic.[12,13] When the thickness of the upper pole of the natural breast is > 2 cm, the likelihood of implant visibility and rippling is minimized. The subglandular approach is sometimes recommended in women with larger breasts or in women who are more athletic to minimize distortion and compression associated with pectoralis contraction. With a subglandular dissection plane Cooper's ligaments are divided, and the likelihood of glandular ptosis over time may be increased.

With the advent of the newest generation of silicone gel implants, including the optimally filled and highly cohesive implants, visibility in thin patients can be minimized. There are a variety of anatomic implants that can minimize upper pole visibility and reduce the incidence of rippling and wrinkling, even when in the subglandular position. Because these devices have different handling characteristics than the traditional less cohesive silicone gel implants, their use in the subglandular position may be considered in thinner patients.

The subpectoral position of a breast implant will generally improve the contour of the upper pole of the breast, especially in patients with a pinch test < 2 cm, because the upper pole of the device is naturally compressed by the muscle and less visible. In addition, studies have demonstrated that the incidence of capsular contracture is least when implants are placed in the subpectoral plane; however, the use of a textured-surface device placed in the subglandular position will mimic that of subpectoral position.[14] Studies have also demonstrated that breast imaging, namely mammography, is facilitated when implants are in the subpectoral position because the parenchyma–pectoral muscle interface is more clearly visualized.[15] A limitation of subpectoral implant placement is the development of animation deformity associated with voluntary contraction of the pectoralis major muscle.[16] Other disadvantages associated with subpectoral placement of implants include malposition, distortion, asymmetry, and distortion.[13] Banbury evaluated the function of the pectoralis major muscle in 47 patients following subpectoral augmentation and did not detect any change in muscle flexion, extension, or adduction from preoperative to 3 and 6 months postoperative.[17]

The subfascial position has the advantage of providing improved projection, similar to the subglandular but without the edge visibility, because the upper pole of the implant is under the pectoral fascia. This plane has the additional benefit in that it separates the implant from the breast parenchyma and is associated with a reduced incidence of capsular contracture than in subglandular positioning, with an incidence similar to subpectoral placement.[18] In addition, it has been theorized that since Cooper's ligaments are retained, glandular ptosis over time may be minimized; however, there have been no studies to corroborate this.

5.5 Technique

With all three planes, the markings and the incision locations can be the same. Typical markings include delineation of the sternal midline and the peripheral outline of the breast footprint. The level of the IMF is delineated and extended to the midline to ensure equal position. The distance from the NAC to IMF on and off stretch, as well as the sternal notch-to-NAC distance, are measured. The upper pole pinch test is performed to assess the thickness of the soft tissues and facilitate the decision between subglandular/subfascial and subpectoral placement. In a recent review of 1,067 plastic surgeons in the United States, Hidalgo has demonstrated that the most common pocket locations are the partial submuscular or dual plane (79.5%), complete submuscular (12.7%), subglandular (5.4%), and subfascial (2.4%).[19] These percentages vary globally, as subfascial placement is more common in Europe and South America. The incision choices for subpectoral, subglandular, and subfascial include the inframammary, periareolar, and transaxillary locations. In the Hidalgo review, the most common incision choice in the United States was the inframammary (83.9%), followed by the periareolar (12.6%), transaxillary (3.3%), and periumbilical (0.2%).[19]

5.5.1 Subglandular Augmentation

Cronin and Gerow performed the first breast augmentation procedure with silicone gel implants in 1962 and them in the subglandular position.[20] Although the subglandular placement of implants often results in excellent volume and contour with an easier recovery, disadvantages include implant visibility, especially in patients with thin tissues, and an increased incidence of capsular contracture.[21] Some surgeons have questioned the longevity of the breast shape with implants in the subglandular space, because implant ptosis is a potential problem, as the majority of the connective fibers between the breast parenchyma and the pectoralis fascia are disrupted with the subglandular dissection (Hunstad).[7]

The salient details of the subglandular augmentation technique will be described. With the patient standing, the relevant breast landmarks are delineated and include the breast footprint and the proposed incisions. The incisional approach can be through the periareolar, inframammary, or transaxillary regions. The incision length varies from 3 to 5 cm, depending upon the size of the implant. The inframammary approach is the most common and will be profiled. A scalpel is used to create the incision through the dermis to the subcutaneous fat. Double-pronged skin hooks are used to separate the dermal edges, and electrocautery is used to dissect to the level of the fascia. At the level of the fold, the fascia may be that of the rectus abdominis or the pectoralis major. A narrow 90° retractor is used to elevate the upper soft tissue, and the dissection is continued in a cephalad direction. The inferior edge of the pectoralis major is identified. The dissection continues medially, superiorly, and laterally above the pectoralis major muscle and the pectoralis fascia. The borders of the dissection plane include the medial border of the pectoralis, the upper footprint of the breast parenchyma, and the lateral border of the pectoralis major. All perforating branches within the plane of dissection are identified and cauterized before bleeding occurs. It is important not to expand the pocket excessively but rather to create a space that will result in a hand-in-glove fit with the implant itself. Hemostasis is achieved, and the subglandular space is irrigated with an appropriate solution. ▶ Fig. 5.3 illustrates a patient before and after subglandular augmentation.

5.5.2 Subfascial Augmentation

Graf et al initially described the subfascial technique in 2002.[11] It is important to recognize that the benefit of subfascial placement is not to provide additional thickness between the skin and the implant; its real benefit is twofold, as it provides a barrier function between the breast parenchyma and the implant in addition to providing additional support to the implant by preserving Cooper's ligaments, which attach breast parenchyma to the chest wall. The pectoral fascia essentially functions as an internal bra to support the implant and minimize its inferior migration, which is typically associated with subglandular placement. Advocates claim to achieve an enhanced

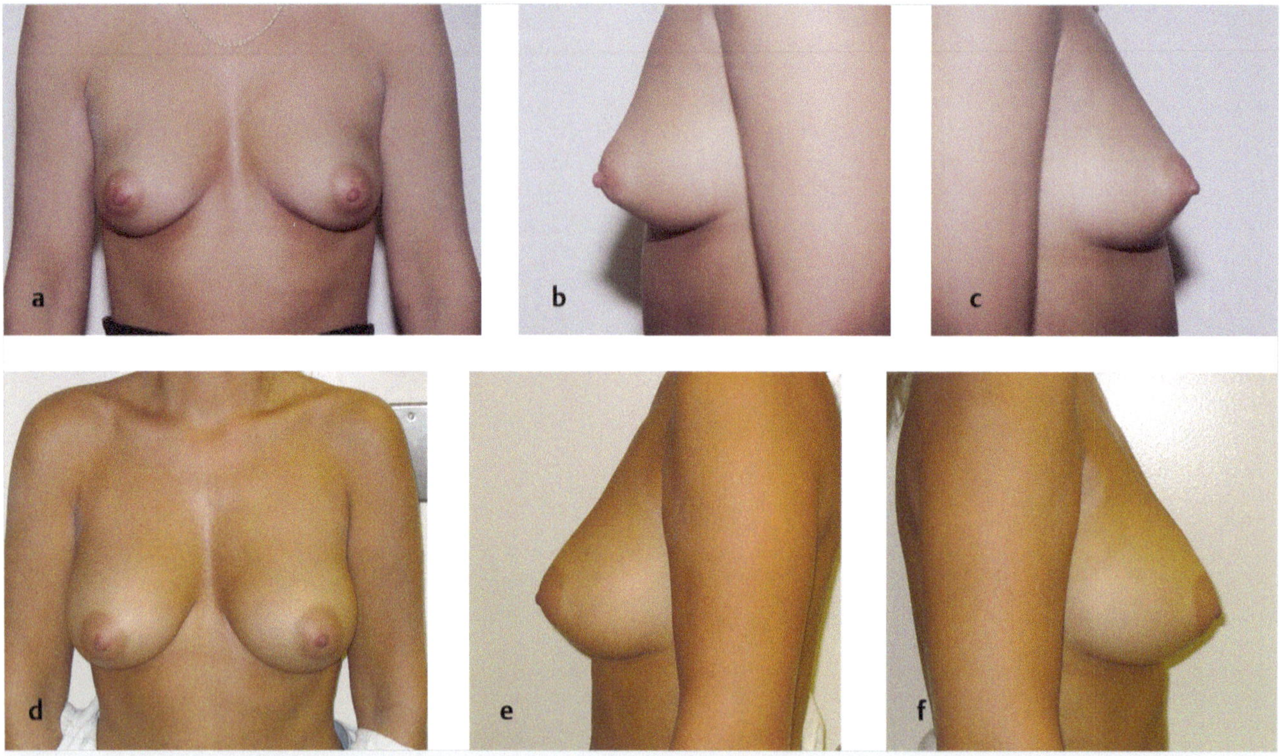

Fig. 5.3 Subglandular breast augmentation using a 300-cc smooth round silicone gel implant, preoperative and 6-year postoperative views. **(a)** Preoperative anterior view. **(b)** Preoperative left lateral view. **(c)** Preoperative right lateral view. **(d)** Postoperative anterior view. **(e)** Postoperative left lateral view. **(f)** Postoperative right lateral view.

aesthetic outcome with less upper pole visibility of the implant, a reduced incidence of capsular contraction, and less animation of the implant.[11,21,22] As previously mentioned, the pectoralis fascia is thin and varies in thickness based on the specific segment. Thickness measurements are 0.49 mm superiorly, 0.68 mm laterally at the margin of the muscle and axillary fascia, and 0.52 mm at its attachments to the sternal margin over the second to fourth ribs. Inferiorly, it condenses into the fascia overlying the latissimus dorsi muscle. Despite the thin nature of the pectoral fascia, it can be dissected as a firm and distinct layer with structural integrity. The dense attachment of the pectoral fascia at the upper aspect of the dissection can prevent upward displacement of the implant, provide compression of the upper pole of the breast, and reduce superior implant visibility.[23]

Graf has described the technical aspects of subfascial breast augmentation based on the location of the incision, which includes the transaxillary, periareolar, and inframammary.[24]

With axillary access, a 4-cm, **S**-shaped incision is created along the axillary fold approximately 1 cm behind the lateral border of the pectoralis major. Care must be exercised to avoid damage to the lymphatics in the region by directing the dissection upward toward the superolateral edge of the pectoralis major. The pectoralis fascia is incised, and the subfascial pocket is dissected using electrocautery. The fascial incision should be created perpendicular to the direction of the pectoral muscle fibers.[21]

When the periareolar incision is selected, it is important to mark the exact location of the proposed incision along the inferior areolar edge with the patient standing.[21,24] Once the patient is supine and prepped and infiltrated with local anesthetic, the areolar edge may be less distinct. The fascial incision is created at the vertical level of the midclavicle a few centimeters away from the NAC to minimize the risk of injury to the sensory nerves.[21] The dissection toward the IMF is directed along the parenchyma–subcutaneous fat plane. The transglandular approach is avoided to minimize injury to the ductal elements of the breast, which often harbor bacteria. The dissection extends to the chest wall and then extends cephalad toward the pectoralis major muscle. The pectoralis fascia is incised at the level of the NAC.

When the inframammary approach is selected, a 3- to 5-cm incision is created along the crease.[24] In cases where the level of the IMF needs adjustment, the location of the incision is modified accordingly such that the final incision lies within the crease. The dissection progresses toward the inferior edge of the pectoralis major muscle. Once the pectoralis fascia is identified, it is incised and the subfascial plane is dissected.

The actual creation of the subfascial pocket requires attention to several salient points.[24] During the undermining process, care should be exercised to avoid fascial injury such as thermal injury and perforation. In cases where it is very thin, inclusion of thin slips of pectoral muscle fibers may be elevated with the fascia. The dissection is performed using a low-set electrocautery device in coagulation mode to minimize any potential bleeding. Finger dissection can also be used to develop the subfascial plane and eventually to allow the insertion of an endoscope to facilitate the dissection.[21] Stoff-Khalili advocates for the dissection of breast tissue to begin at the lateral border of the pectoralis muscle and continue to the level of the pectoral fascia.[18] Once the fascia is identified, it is separated from the muscle using cauterizing scissors. It was noted that the thickness of the fascia increased from approximately 0.1 mm inferiorly to approximately 0.5 mm in the upper third of the pectoralis major muscle. According to Stoff-Khalili, this increase in thickness is sufficient to minimize implant rippling. Other maneuvers to facilitate the dissection include upward traction of the breast. The typical boundaries for the dissection include the second intercostal space superiorly, 1–2 cm from the midsternum medially, 5–8 cm below the NAC, and the anterior axillary line laterally. It is important to avoid dissection beyond the lateral border of the pectoralis major muscle to prevent lateral displacement of the implant.[21] It is also important to ensure hemostasis and to irrigate the pocket prior to implant insertion. ▶ Fig. 5.4 illustrates a patient before and after subfascial augmentation.

5.5.3 Subpectoral Augmentation

Dempsey and Latham were the first to consider the subpectoral position and performed the first subpectoral breast augmentation in 1968.[23] The advantages included less visibility, decreased ptosis, reduced capsular contracture, and increased longevity compared to subglandular placement. Like the subglandular and subfascial techniques, the technique of subpectoral augmentation can also be performed through a variety of access incisions that include the periareolar, transaxillary, and inframammary. Subpectoral augmentation can be performed using a total muscle coverage approach as well as partial muscle coverage. The total submuscular plane has been performed less frequently, primarily because the natural contour of the breast may be compromised and because it sometimes involves elevation of the serratus anterior muscle as well for lateral coverage. Indications for total muscle coverage are few. Partial subpectoral coverage has become far more common. The release of the inferior origin of the pectoralis major muscle allows improved lower pole projection and contour. Another benefit of the subpectoral positioning is that capsular contracture rates are generally lower compared to subglandular placement; however, this will also be dependent upon the surface texturing of the implant.[14]

The evolution of partial subpectoral coverage has been refined and more accurately defined by Tebbetts and is now commonly referred to as dual-plane breast augmentation.[28] Dual-plane augmentation involves the release of the inferior origin of the pectoralis major muscle without release of the muscle along the sternal border, as well as varying degrees of subglandular dissection. The defining characteristics of dual-plane augmentation, according to Tebbetts[26]:

- The breast implant is partially behind the pectoralis major muscle and partially behind the breast parenchyma.
- A specific portion of the origin of the pectoralis major muscle is divided to alter the position of the pectoral muscle relative to the implant, with the ultimate goal of altering the relationship between the implant and breast parenchyma.

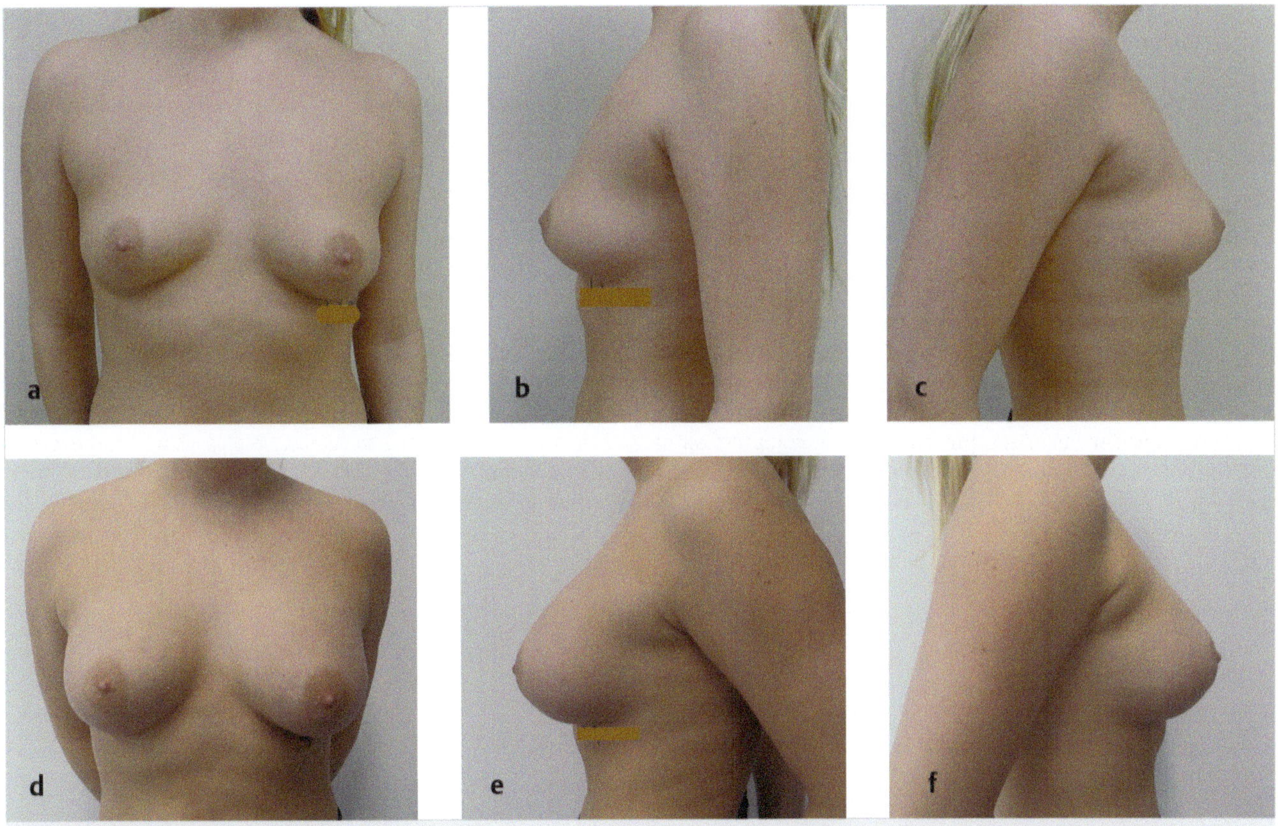

Fig. 5.4 Subfascial breast augmentation using a 350-cc smooth round silicone gel implant, preoperative and 1-year postoperative views. **(a)** Preoperative anterior view. **(b)** Preoperative left lateral view. **(c)** Preoperative right lateral view. **(d)** Postoperative anterior view. **(e)** Postoperative left lateral view. **(f)** Postoperative right lateral view.

- The parenchyma–pectoralis major interface is sufficiently altered to change the dynamic nature of the parenchyma–implant relationship.

Three types of dual-plane breast augmentation have been described.[26] Dual-plane 1 is defined as the release of the inferior pectoral origin of the pectoralis major muscle only and is indicated for patients without glandular ptosis, tight attachments of the parenchyma–muscle interface, and a minimally stretched lower pole (▶ Fig. 5.5). Dual-plane 2 is defined as a release of the inferior origin of the pectoralis major and a subglandular dissection to the level of the inferior border of the areola and is indicated for patients with minimal glandular ptosis, looser attachments of the parenchyma–muscle interface, and a lower pole that has more stretch (▶ Fig. 5.6). Dual-plane 3 is defined as a release of the inferior origin of the pectoralis major and a subglandular dissection to the level of the superior border of the areola and is indicated for patients with glandular ptosis in which more than one-third of the parenchyma is below the desired IMF, loose attachments of the parenchyma–muscle interface, a markedly stretched lower pole, as well as a constricted lower pole (▶ Fig. 5.7). Extensive medial and superior release of the pectoralis major muscle can result in upward retraction of the muscle, known as window-shading, and may lead to animation deformity.[27] Overdissection along the medial origin of the pectoralis major may also result in symmastia as the soft-tissue attachments over the sternum gradually weaken, eventually resulting in implant–implant contact.[27]

The salient aspects of the subpectoral technique are as follows. Preoperative markings are made with the patient standing. As with other implant planes, the incisional approach can be periareolar, transaxillary, or inframammary. When the inframammary approach is selected, the skin and subcutaneous fat are incised and dissected to the level of the deep fascia. Often this is the fascia of the rectus abdominis muscle. The suprafascial dissection is advanced to the inferior edge of the pectoralis major muscle, which is then incised extending from the inferomedial origin to the midclavicular line. ▶ Fig. 5.8 illustrates a patient preceding and following subpectoral augmentation. At this point the three variations of the dual plane dissections are considered.

Dual-Plane 1

The subpectoral plane is entered, leaving a 1-cm cuff of the inferior pectoralis major on the chest wall. The pectoral incision extends from the inferior sternal border of the pectoralis major to the lateral inferior border. The pectoralis major–parenchymal interface is not separated. It is best to enter the subpectoral space along the medial aspect of the areola. The subpectoral dissection is performed with electrocautery. Care must be exercised to identify and cauterize the perforating branches of the

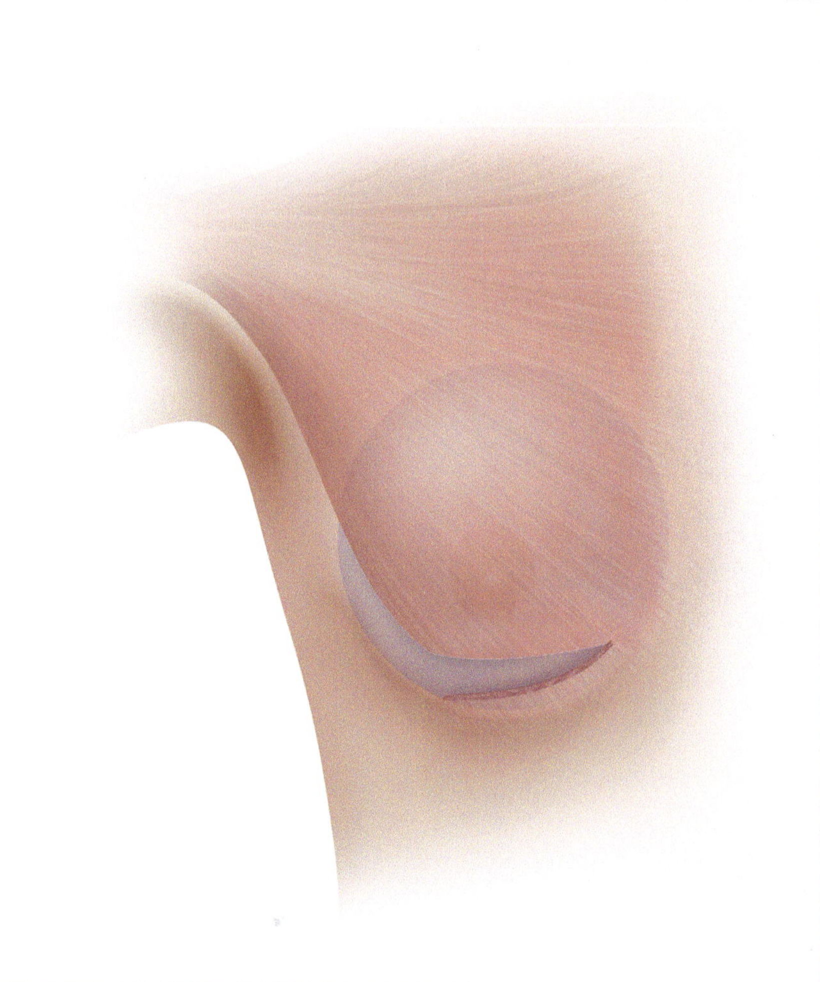

Fig. 5.5 Schematic illustration of a dual-plane 1 subpectoral implant. (Reproduced from Adams WP Jr. Breast Augmentation Video Atlas. 2nd ed. New York, NY: Thieme Medical Publishers; 2019.)

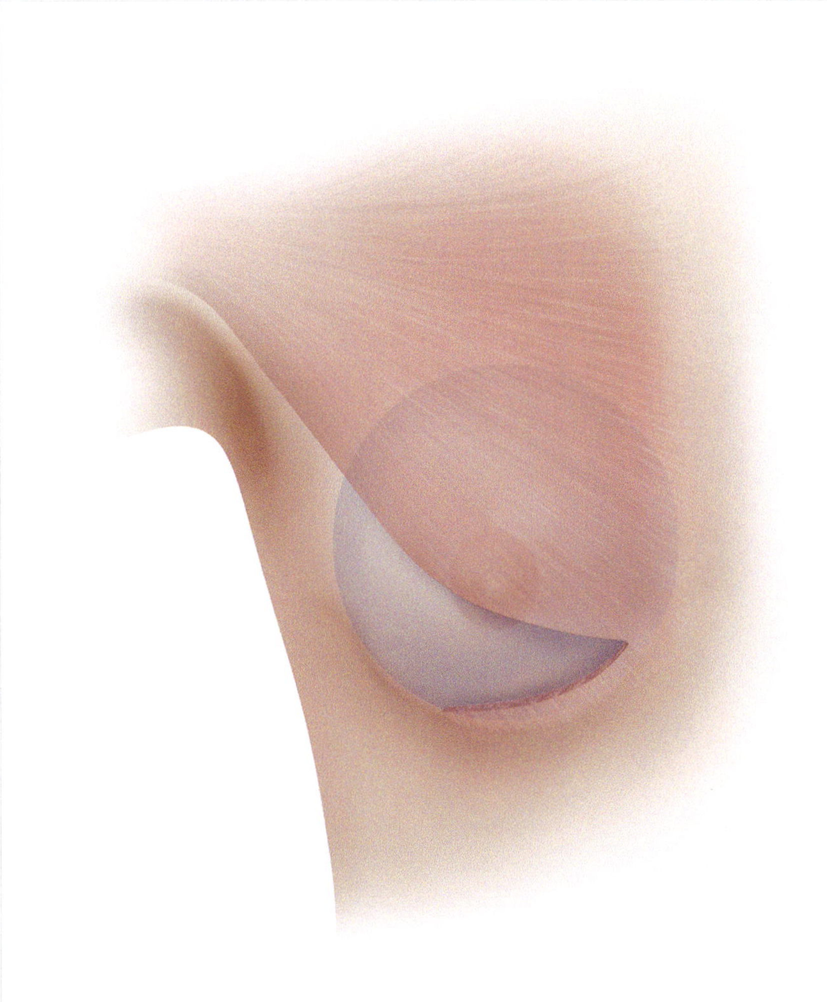

Fig. 5.6 Schematic illustration of a dual-plane 2 subpectoral implant. (Reproduced from Adams WP Jr. Breast Augmentation Video Atlas. 2nd ed. New York, NY: Thieme Medical Publishers; 2019.)

internal mammary artery and vein as they pierce the pectoral fascia and the costal interspaces. The pectoralis major is separated from the pectoralis minor and the serratus anterior muscle using blunt dissection technique. The dimensions or footprint of the created subpectoral pocket should approximate the dimensions of the desired implant. The original description of the dual-plane technique recommended that the superior extent of the dissection proceed to the level of the thoracoacromial vascular pedicle; however, this degree of dissection is no longer recommended. The lateral dissection should not extend beyond the lateral edge of the pectoralis major. The medial dissection should extend to the medial origins of the pectoralis major without complete division to avoid future symmastia.

Dual-Plane 2 and 3

The technique for the dual-plane 1 and 2 procedures begins exactly as it does for dual-plane 1. Once the subpectoral pocket is created, upward traction on the parenchyma is applied and the pectoral–parenchymal interface is identified. An electrocautery device is then used to separate the interface extending from medial to lateral. The lateral limit is the lateral edge of the pectoralis major muscle. With the type 2 dual-plane, the dissection extends approximately to the inferior border of the areola, whereas for the type 3 dual-plane the dissection extends approximately to the superior border of the areola. The muscle–parenchymal interface should be released until no muscle banding is appreciated internally that could potentially restrict implant projection.

5.6 Complications

Adverse outcomes associated with breast augmentation, based on the plane of implant placement, are varied and include capsular contracture, animation deformity, implant malposition, compromised sensation, and soft tissue alterations. The incidence of these adverse outcomes can be influenced by the plane of insertion and must be appreciated. This ensuing section will review these adverse events and how devices placed in the subpectoral, subfascial, and subglandular positions can influence the incidence of these adverse events.

5.6.1 Capsular Contracture

When comparing the subglandular and subpectoral position of breast implants, one of the proposed advantages of subpectoral placement is a reduction in the incidence of capsular

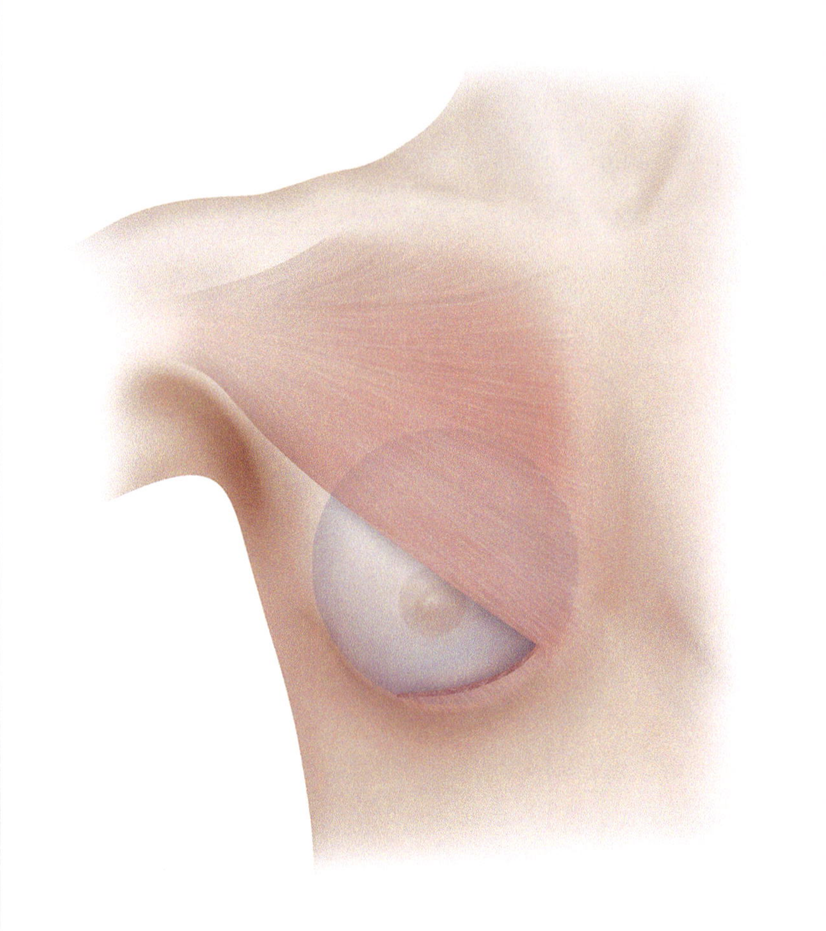

Fig. 5.7 Schematic illustration of a dual-plane 3 subpectoral implant. (Reproduced from Adams WP Jr. Breast Augmentation Video Atlas. 2nd ed. New York, NY: Thieme Medical Publishers; 2019.)

contracture. Although implant location is considered by many to be the most important predictor of this event, the surface characteristics of the implant are also important. In a review of 5,109 breast implants placed in the setting of breast augmentation, the incidence of capsular contracture varied based on plane of insertion and surface texture of the implant.[16] When textured devices were placed, the incidence of capsular contracture was 4.9% for subglandular and 2.1% for subpectoral. When smooth-surfaced implants were used, the incidence of capsular contracture was 21% when subglandular and 5.1% when subpectoral. Numerous studies have demonstrated that subpectoral placement of implants is associated with a reduced incidence of capsular contracture.[9,21,28,29] Although this relation is generally accepted, Codner et al were unable to demonstrate any difference in capsular contracture rates between subglandular and subpectoral placement.[30]

Complications related to subglandular and subpectoral placement of implants have been studied. In a review of 328 patients following breast augmentation, Stoff-Khalili demonstrated that postoperative complications occurred in 49% of patients with subglandular augmentation and in 16% of patients following subpectoral augmentation ($p < 0.001$). On the other hand, from the subpectoral cohort to the subfascial cohort the incidence of complications decreased from 16% to 6.7% ($p < 0.031$). The incidence of Baker grade 3 capsular contracture was 14.35% with textured subglandular implants, 4.5% with textured subpectoral implants, 1.9% with smooth subpectoral implants, and 1.5% with smooth subfascial implants. In the subglandular cohort, revisions were performed in 37% of patients. Eight patients with either a Baker 3 or 4 capsular contracture had explantation, capsulotomy, and no reaugmentation. Also within this subglandular cohort, fourteen patients with Baker grade 3 capsular contracture (13.3%) had explantation, capsulectomy, and a new smooth implant placed in the subpectoral position. In the subpectoral cohort, the rate of secondary revisions was 9.1% compared with 37% for the subglandular cohort ($p < 0.05$).[18] A criticism of this study was that for any comparative study such as this to have scientific validity, patient cohort samples must be similar preoperatively.[31]

The correction of capsular contracture following breast augmentation in the subglandular position has been described. In a review of 85 patients with capsular contracture (54 subpectoral, 31 subglandular) by Spear et al, correction was achieved using a dual-plane strategy.[16] The subglandular contracture patients were managed by pocket conversion to a partial subpectoral space, with the inferior edge of the pectoralis major muscle being stabilized to the overlying skin with marionette sutures. The subpectoral contracture patients were managed by releasing the inferior origin of the pectoralis major muscle and creating a partial subglandular plane that extended to the inferior border of the areola. Three of the 85 patients (3.5%) required reoperation for complications due to implant

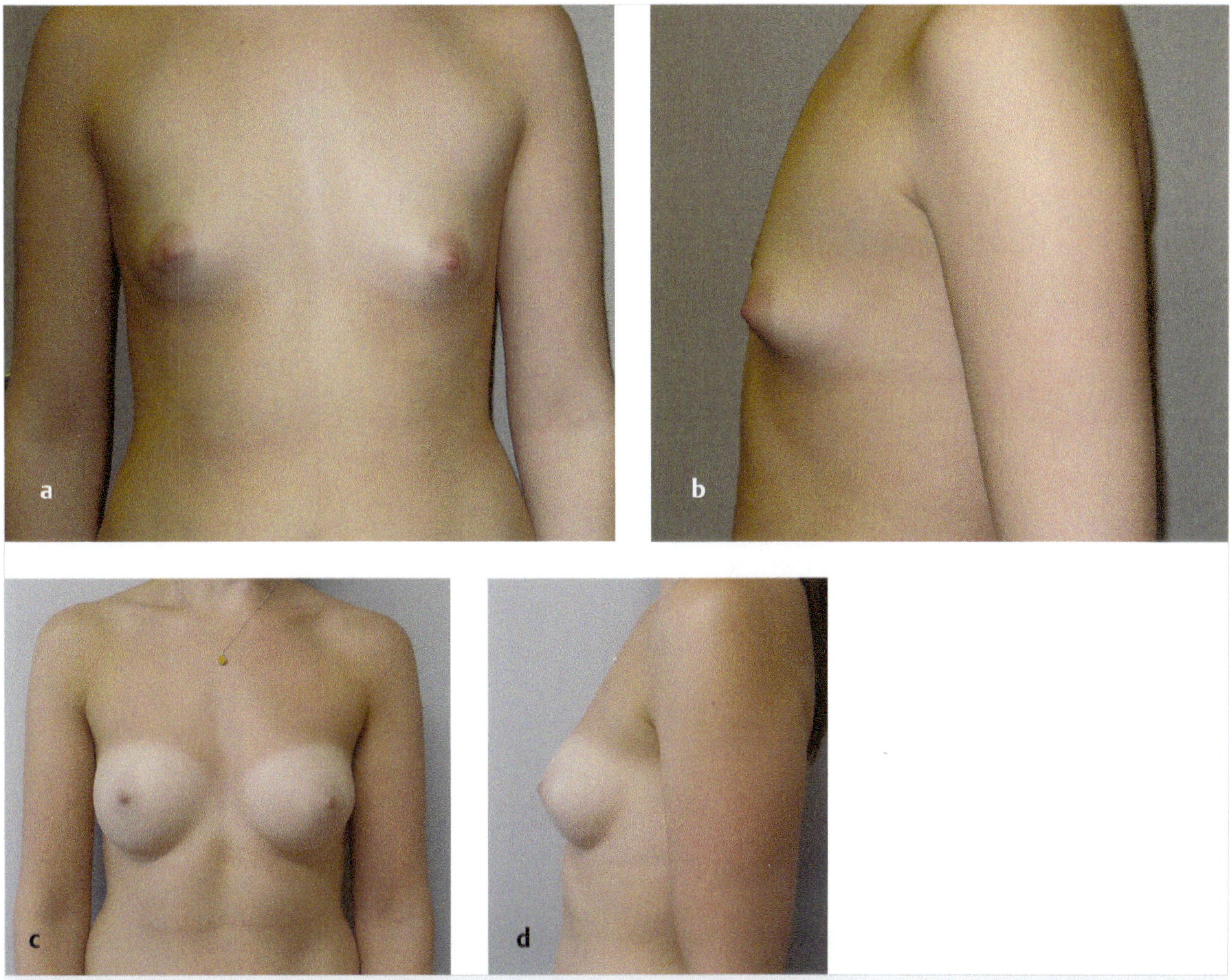

Fig. 5.8 Subpectoral breast augmentation using a 225 cc smooth round silicone gel implant, preoperative and 10-year postoperative views. (a) Preoperative anterior view. (b) Preoperative left lateral view. (c) Postoperative anterior view. (d) Postoperative left lateral view.

malposition. There were no Baker grade 3 or 4 capsular contractures noted in patients who were converted to the dual plane position; however, 2% were graded as Baker grade 2.

Mofid et al described a technique whereby the subglandular implant is removed and a capsulectomy is performed.[32] A dual-plane or subpectoral pocket is created by incising the inferior origin of the pectoralis major muscle, dissecting the subpectoral plane, using an acellular dermal matrix (ADM) to stabilize the position of the pectoral muscle, and placing a new implant. They compared outcomes with this technique to the traditional pocket conversion without ADM described by Spear and demonstrated that adverse events using ADM were significantly fewer based on implant displacement, pain, and need for revision.

5.6.2 Animation Deformity

Animation deformity with pectoral muscle contraction is becoming increasingly appreciated as problematic in patients with subpectoral breast implants. Spear et al, in a review of 40 patients following subpectoral breast augmentation, demonstrated based on photographic analysis that 9 (22.5%) had no distortion, 25 (62.5%) had minimal distortion, 4 (10%) had moderate distortion, and 2 (5%) had severe distortion.[33] In a subsequent questionnaire, 56 patients (82%) described mild to no distortion, 7 patients (10%) described moderate distortion, and 5 patients (7%) described severe distortion. The most common activities exacerbating animation included lifting weights and exercising (24% and 19%, respectively). The authors concluded that in patients who are very active and exercise regularly, subglandular placement should be considered. Adams has stated that animation is reduced with the dual-plane 2 and 3 techniques based on the separation of the pectoralis major muscle and parenchyma.[28] Brown, Graf, and Hunstad have stated that implants placed in the subfascial position will experience less animation compared to subpectoral.[21,23,24]

The mechanism of animation is important to understand. The unaltered pectoralis major muscle originates superiorly from the clavicle, medially from the sternal border, and inferiorly from the costal margin. It inserts on the humerus and serves to adduct and flex the humerus with contraction. When the inferior origin of the muscle is divided, contraction will result in foreshortening of the muscle in the vertical orientation. When an implant is placed under the pectoralis major, the resulting scar or capsule will essentially anchor the implant to the pectoralis muscle. When the muscle contracts and vertically foreshortens, it will pull the capsule and implant with it, resulting in the animation deformity. The degree of animation will vary from patient to patient based on the density of the scar or capsule, the amount of laxity within the periprosthetic space, the amount of breast parenchyma overlying the pectoralis major, and the strength of the pectoralis major.

The optimal management for problematic animation deformity is to convert the subpectoral implant to a subglandular or subfascial position. Lesavoy et al reviewed 36 patients who had animation deformity and demonstrated complete correction with removal of the subpectoral implant, resuspending the pectoralis to the chest wall, and insertion of a new implant in the subglandular space.[27] The basis for this is that the forces generated by muscle contraction on the implant are eliminated as the muscle is replaced to its anatomical position. The subpectoral pocket is also compressed by the newly placed subglandular implant, which eliminates the potential risk of implant movement back into the old pocket and fluid collection in the pocket. This technique is effective for patients with malposition, capsular contracture, and symmastia as well.

5.6.3 Parenchymal Atrophy

Parenchymal atrophy associated with primary breast augmentation has been another topic of discussion and controversy. Handel stated, "The long-term presence of implants typically results in changes in breast anatomy and physiology, including parenchymal atrophy, tissue thinning, and diminished skin blood supply."[34] Tebbetts and Teitelbaum have stated, "The weight and pressure of high- and extra-high-projection implants potentially causes more stretching and thinning of the breast envelope (skin and subcutaneous tissue) and more parenchymal atrophy compared with smaller or less projecting implants"[35] Thus, the long-term changes associated with breast implants can have significant ramifications on the parenchyma, pectoralis major muscle, and chest wall.

Parenchymal and pectoral major atrophy as a function of subglandular and subpectoral placement has been evaluated. Prior studies have demonstrated that, compared with subglandular augmentation mammaplasty, submuscular augmentation reduces contour deformities and decreases implant edge visibility, rippling, and capsular contracture; however, subpectoral augmentation has a higher risk of implant malposition and breast asymmetry.[27,35] The consequences of pressure placed on soft tissues have been studied and demonstrated that muscle is the most susceptible to damage due to ischemia and deformation.[36,37]

In a randomized prospective study by Roxo et al, the authors studied 58 patients of whom 24 were randomized into the subglandular cohort and 24 into the subpectoral cohort, with 10 serving as unoperated controls.[38,39] Comparisons between the subglandular and subpectoral cohorts were made relative to the unoperated controls at various time points that included 0, 6, and 12 months. Patient and implant characteristics were similar between all cohorts. Magnetic resonance imaging (MRI) analysis of parenchymal volume demonstrated a significant reduction in volume comparing the subglandular and subpectoral cohorts at 6 months (27.7% versus 23.08%, respectively). When implants were placed in the subpectoral position, there was a significant reduction in the volume of the pectoralis major muscle at 6 and 12 months (46.38% versus 49.8%, respectively). The conclusions of the study were that parenchymal volume was significantly decreased 6 months after surgery in both cohorts but that the volume was 16.6% lower in the submuscular group than in the subglandular group. In addition, there was a significant regain in parenchymal volume in both cohorts at 12-month follow-up; however, the significant volume loss remained in the subglandular cohort ($p < 0.001$). There was no significant parenchymal volume loss in the submuscular group at 12 months following augmentation. Finally, the pectoralis major muscle was demonstrated to be susceptible to pressure-related compression that did not improve during the time interval studied.

Other studies have demonstrated similar finding to the Roxo study. Kovacs et al measured 3D surface area in 17 patients (34 breasts) following subpectoral breast augmentation with round implants and in 10 patients (20 breasts) following placement of anatomic implants via an axillary or inframammary approach.[40] Measurements were obtained before and 6 months postoperatively. The breast projection increase was 22% less than expected for round implants and 25% less than expected for anatomic implants based on the manufacturer implant parameters ($p < 0.01$), without essential differences regarding the surgical incision. It was demonstrated that breast projection was 20% less than expected 6 months after surgery following subpectoral augmentation with round implants. Tepper et al also used 3D breast volume measurements in 14 patients (28 breasts) following breast augmentation and demonstrated breast projection was 20.9% less than expected 6 months after surgery.[41] Three-dimensional imaging scans demonstrated actual changes that occurred following breast augmentation that included the breast volume, the increase in the internal angle of the breast projection, and the sternal notch–to-nipple distance. The authors also found that breast augmentation resulted in less than expected anterior–posterior projection, possibly due to tissue attenuation occurring anterior to the implant.

In addition to implant location, other factors such as implant volume and projection can also affect the soft tissue characteristics of the breast following augmentation. Tebbetts and Teitelbaum have opined that the weight and pressure associated with high-projection implants can result in more stretching and thinning of the skin and subcutaneous tissues of the breast and more parenchymal atrophy compared with smaller or less-projecting implants.[35] Although sometimes true, this is dependent on other factors, such as the ratio between implant volume and parenchymal volume, as well as soft tissue compliance. Previous studies have demonstrated that when an implant is inserted, the forces applied to the breast and the surrounding tissues will result in some degree of remodeling to resist the effects of that force.[38,39,40,41] The short-term effects will be related to creep and stress relaxation. If the surrounding tissues do not adequately compensate, long-term and potentially irreversible effects may ensue. These include parenchymal atrophy, dermal thinning, and osseous (rib cage) deformation. The question is whether these changes are related to implant contour (high profile) or implant volume. Nahabedian has stated, "[T]he tipping point is not based solely on the projection of the device, but also on the relationship among implant volume, soft-tissue compliance, and parenchymal volume because deformational changes can occur with any breast implant, regardless of projection."[42] Slavin has stated, "Drs. Tebbetts-and Teitelbaum are correct in their assertion that increasing the projection of implants is likely to be harmful to breast tissues, but low- and moderate-profile implants have not proven to be a panacea."[43]

5.6.4 Sensory Changes

Alterations to the sensation of the breast following subglandular, subfascial, and subpectoral breast augmentation have been described. It is commonly stated that up to 50% of patients may have a transient alteration in sensation to the breast and NAC and that up to 16% may experience permanent sensory changes.[44] It has been proposed that subpectoral breast augmentation may result in less sensory disturbance than subglandular and subfascial because of less disruption of the neural pathways.

Anatomic studies have demonstrated that sensation to the NAC is through the medial and lateral cutaneous branches of the third to the sixth intercostal nerves.[5] The fourth lateral cutaneous nerve is the dominant sensory nerve in 79% of patients and courses within and pierces the pectoral fascia at the midaxillary line before entering the parenchyma at the midclavicular line and finally arriving at the NAC in 93% of breasts.[5]

In a systematic review of 36 studies, Ducic et al determined that the risk of any nerve injury after breast augmentation ranged from 13.57% to 15.44%.[44] The most commonly injured nerves included the intercostal cutaneous nerves, with a risk that ranged from 8.86% to 10.01%, followed by the T3–T5 intercostal cutaneous nerves to the NAC, with a risk that ranged from 4.64% to 5.43%; the intercostobrachial nerve (0.05%); and the long thoracic nerve (0.01%). In that review, the authors examined whether implant placement in the subpectoral or subglandular plane made a difference. In one study, submuscular placement was associated with sensation changes, whereas in another study, subglandular placement was implicated. Overall, however, the meta-analysis demonstrated no difference in breast sensory changes between subpectoral and subglandular placement ($p = 0.2613$).

Individual studies have had mixed outcomes with regard to postoperative sensation following augmentation mammaplasty. Banbury and coworkers evaluated sensation of the breast in 47 patients following subpectoral augmentation that included the NAC and the four peripheral quadrants.[17] They demonstrated a significant difference in vibratory sensation at 3 and 6 months postoperatively, whereas pressure demonstrated a significant alteration at the 3-month but not at the 6-month period. Courtiss and Goldwyn evaluated breast sensation in 249 breasts following subglandular augmentation and demonstrated a 15% reduction in sensation of the NAC 2 years postoperatively.[45] Brown et al evaluated 162 women following subfascial augmentation for sensory changes before and following surgery at 2, 6, and 12 weeks.[46] There was a statistical decrease in sensation in all areas of the breast 2 weeks following surgery ($p < 0.01$). Most women (92.5%) regained preoperative levels of sensation by 12 weeks in all areas of the breast except for the lower-outer quadrants. There was a failure to return to normal sensation in 4% of NACs and 16.15% of lower outer quadrants by 12 weeks after surgery.

5.6.5 Symmastia

Symmastia is an uncommon occurrence with breast augmentation and can occur with subglandular and subpectoral implant placement.[47] With subglandular, it is usually due to medial overdissection or the placement of a breast implant that is too large. With subpectoral, it is usually associated with detachment of the medial origin of the pectoralis major muscle. In both situations, the implants may be in direct contact or close proximity.

A variety of techniques have been described for the correction of symmastia.[47] When the original device was subglandular, creation of a subpectoral pocket will usually correct the problem. When the original device was subpectoral, several options are available that include the creation of a neosubpectoral pocket, medial capsulorrhaphy, and the use of capsular flaps with or without reinforcement with synthetic or biologic materials. Spear et al have described the role of neo-pocket creation in 23 patients with symmastia, demonstrating no recurrence at an average follow-up of 22 months.[47]

5.6.6 Breast Cancer, Imaging, and Surveillance

The relationship of breast neoplasms to prosthetic devices has always been a concern. Over the years, several epidemiologic studies have essentially demonstrated no association between the two.[48,49] The incidence of breast cancer following augmentation generally parallels that of women who have not had breast augmentation. Most of these cancers will generally involve the parenchymal tissues of the breast; however, some can involve the chest wall or capsular tissues. Diagnosis of these tumors has been reported to be complicated in the presence of breast implants, with studies demonstrating that breast imaging can be obscured in approximately 30% of women.[50,51] Fortunately, there are a variety of specialized techniques that can facilitate diagnosis, including implant displacement techniques during mammography and MRI scans.[52]

The location of the implant in the subpectoral or subglandular position has been presumed to affect the accuracy of breast cancer detection and imaging. Spear et al previously demonstrated that women with subpectoral implants were more likely to detect breast cancer by palpation (75%) compared to women with subglandular implants (43.8%).[53] It has also been assumed that women with subglandular or subfascial implants will be more difficult to assess via mammography alone because the pectoral–parenchymal interface may be obscured, whereas it is more easily identified in women with subpectoral implants.[15]

In a recent case-control study comparing 48 previously augmented women who developed breast cancer and 302 controls with breast cancer but without a history of breast augmentation, associations between subglandular and subglandular implant placement were studied.[49] Demographic evaluation demonstrated that more women had subpectoral implants (68.9%) than subglandular implants (31.1%). Whether the implants were subpectoral or subglandular demonstrated no clinically relevant differences in method of cancer detection, biopsy technique, stage at diagnosis, and surgical intervention. In addition, there were no differences in tumor size, lymph node spread, or metastasis between subpectoral and subglandular augmentation. Other findings of interest included comparability in the identification of a palpable mass and in mammographic diagnosis. In contrast to the findings by Spear, the Sosin study found that a palpable mass was identified in 57.1% of patients with subglandular implants and in 54.8% patients with subpectoral implants.[49] Breast lesions were seen on mammography at comparable rates in both cohorts, 78.6% for subglandular and 71% in the subpectoral. The subglandular cohort had a lower false-negative rate (14.3%) versus 25.8% for the subpectoral cohort. Mean Breast Imaging, Reporting, and Data System (BIRADS) scores were nearly identical, at 4.0 for subglandular and 3.95 for subpectoral. Mammography was found to be 1.5-fold more sensitive in detecting breast cancer in patients with subpectoral implants (41.9%) than in those with subglandular implants (28.6%). Interestingly, screening MRI in women with subglandular implants was performed more often (14.3%) compared to the subpectoral group (3.2%). This may be partly due to the finding that more patients with subglandular implants were *BRCA* gene mutation carriers and not ideal candidates for mammography.

In the event of a breast cancer diagnosis following breast augmentation, all oncologic options remain available and include breast conservation and mastectomy. The mastectomy can be skin- or nipple-sparing, and the reconstruction can include prosthetic devices or autologous flaps. Prosthetic reconstruction following mastectomy in a previously augmented patient can be accomplished using tissue expanders or implants.[54] If the previous device was subglandular, then prosthetic reconstruction can be performed by placing the device in the prepectoral or the subpectoral space. If the previous device was subpectoral, then the same subpectoral pocket is usually used; however, a prepectoral repositioning can be considered. These reconstructions can be performed in one or two stages using tissue expanders or implants. If a flap is chosen, the pectoralis major muscle is always placed back on the chest wall and the flap is placed above the pectoralis major muscle.

5.7 Conclusion

Breast augmentation can be safely performed in the subglandular, subfascial, and subpectoral positions. Subglandular placement offers enhanced projection but higher rates of capsular contracture. Subpectoral placement offers reduced capsular contracture but increased breast animation. Subfascial placement offers reduced capsular contracture but a very thin layer between the muscle and parenchyma.

Key Points

- Decision making often depends on the size of the natural breast, the patient's degree of physical activity, and an appreciation of patient expectations.
- In general, the subpectoral position is typically recommended in patients with a thin body habitus and an upper pole pinch test < 2 cm, whereas the subglandular or subfascial plane can be considered in patients with an upper pole pinch thickness > 2 cm.
- The most common pocket locations are the partial submuscular or dual-plane (79.5%), complete submuscular (12.7%), subglandular (5.4%), and subfascial (2.4%).[19] These percentages vary globally, as subfascial placement is more common in Europe and South America.
- Subglandular placement offers enhanced projection but higher rates of capsular contracture.
- Subpectoral placement offers reduced capsular contracture but increased breast animation.
- Subfascial placement offers reduced capsular contracture but a very thin layer between the muscle and parenchyma.

References

[1] Larson DL, Basir Z, Bruce T. Is oncologic safety compatible with a predictably viable mastectomy skin flap? Plast Reconstr Surg. 2011; 127(1):27–33

[2] van Deventer PV, Graewe FR. The blood supply of the breast revisited. Plast Reconstr Surg. 2016; 137(5):1388–1397

[3] Michelle le Roux C, Kiil BJ, Pan WR, Rozen WM, Ashton MW. Preserving the neurovascular supply in the Hall-Findlay superomedial pedicle breast reduction: an anatomical study. J Plast Reconstr Aesthet Surg. 2010; 63(4):655–662

[4] Wueringer E, Tschabitscher M. New aspects of the topographical anatomy of the mammary gland regarding its neurovascular supply along a regular ligamentous suspension. Eur J Morphol. 2002; 40(3):181–189

[5] Schlenz I, Kuzbari R, Gruber H, Holle J. The sensitivity of the nipple-areola complex: an anatomic study. Plast Reconstr Surg. 2000; 105(3):905–909

[6] Jaspars JJ, Posma AN, van Immerseel AA, Gittenberger-de Groot AC. The cutaneous innervation of the female breast and nipple-areola complex: implications for surgery. Br J Plast Surg. 1997; 50(4):249–259

[7] Prakash KG, Saniya K. Anatomical study of pectoral nerves and its implications in surgery. J Clin Diagn Res. 2014; 8(7):AC01–AC05

[8] Gil YC, Lee KW, Chang DY, Park SH, Kim HJ, Kim HM. Positional relationship between the pectoralis major and external abdominal oblique muscles for consideration during dual-plane breast augmentation. Clin Anat. 2018; 31(3): 339–346

[9] Lin J, Song J, Chen X, et al. Anatomy and clinical significance of pectoral fascia. Plast Reconstr Surg. 2006; 118(7):1557–1560

[10] Tebbetts JB. Does fascia provide additional, meaningful coverage over a breast implant? Plast Reconstr Surg. 2004; 113(2):777–779, author reply 779--780

[11] Graf RM, Bernardes A, Rippel R, Araujo LR, Damasio RC, Auersvald A. Subfascial breast implant: a new procedure. Plast Reconstr Surg. 2003; 111(2):904–908

[12] Hidalgo DA, Spector JA. Breast augmentation. Plast Reconstr Surg. 2014; 133 (4):567e–583e

[13] Strasser EJ. Results of subglandular versus subpectoral augmentation over time: one surgeon's observations. Aesthet Surg J. 2006; 26(1):45–50

[14] Stevens WG, Nahabedian MY, Calobrace MB, et al. Risk factor analysis for capsular contracture: a 5-year Sientra study analysis using round, smooth, and textured implants for breast augmentation. Plast Reconstr Surg. 2013; 132 (5):1115–1123

[15] Silverstein MJ, Handel N, Gamagami P. The effect of silicone-gel-filled implants on mammography. Cancer. 1991; 68(5) Suppl:1159–1163

[16] Spear SL, Schwartz J, Dayan JH, Clemens MW. Outcome assessment of breast distortion following submuscular breast augmentation. Aesthetic Plast Surg. 2009; 33(1):44–48

[17] Banbury J, Yetman R, Lucas A, Papay F, Graves K, Zins JE. Prospective analysis of the outcome of subpectoral breast augmentation: sensory changes, muscle function, and body image. Plast Reconstr Surg. 2004; 113(2):701–707, discussion 708–711

[18] Stoff-Khalili MA, Scholze R, Morgan WR, Metcalf JD. Subfascial periareolar augmentation mammaplasty. Plast Reconstr Surg. 2004; 114(5):1280–1288, discussion 1289–1291

[19] Hidalgo DA, Sinno S. Current trends and controversies in breast augmentation. Plast Reconstr Surg. 2016; 137(4):1142–1150

[20] Cronin TD, Gerow FJ. Augmentation mammaplasty: a new "natural feel" prosthesis. In: Transactions of the Third International Congress of Plastic Surgery. Amsterdam: Excerpta Medica Foundation; 1964:41–49

[21] Hunstad JP, Webb LS. Subfascial breast augmentation: a comprehensive experience. Aesthetic Plast Surg. 2010; 34(3):365–373
[22] Góes JCS, Landecker A. Optimizing outcomes in breast augmentation: seven years of experience with the subfascial plane. Aesthetic Plast Surg. 2003; 27 (3):178–184
[23] Brown T. Subfascial breast augmentation: is there any advantage over the submammary plane? Aesthetic Plast Surg. 2012; 36(3):566–569
[24] Graf RM, Ono MCC, Tolazzi ARD. Subfascial breast augmentation. In: Spear SL, Willey SC, Robb GL, Hammond DC, Nahabedian MY, eds. Surgery of the Breast: Principles and Art. 3rd ed. Philadelphia, PA: Lippincott Williams & Wilkins; 2011:1283–1289
[25] Dempsey WC, Latham WD. Subpectoral implants in augmentation mammaplasty. Preliminary report. Plast Reconstr Surg. 1968; 42(6):515–521
[26] Tebbetts JB. Dual plane breast augmentation: optimizing implant-soft-tissue relationships in a wide range of breast types. Plast Reconstr Surg. 2001; 107 (5):1255–1272
[27] Lesavoy MA, Trussler AP, Dickinson BP. Difficulties with subpectoral augmentation mammaplasty and its correction: the role of subglandular site change in revision aesthetic breast surgery. Plast Reconstr Surg. 2010; 125(1):363–371
[28] Adams WP, Jr, Mallucci P. Breast augmentation. Plast Reconstr Surg. 2012; 130(4):597e–611e
[29] Headon H, Kasem A, Mokbel K. Capsular Contracture after Breast Augmentation: An Update for Clinical Practice. Arch Plast Surg. 2015; 42(5):532–543
[30] Codner MA, Mejia JD, Locke MB, et al. A 15-year experience with primary breast augmentation. Plast Reconstr Surg. 2011; 127(3):1300–1310
[31] Tebbetts J. Discussion: subfascial periareolar augmentation mammaplasty. Plast Reconstr Surg. 2004; 114(5):1289
[32] Mofid MM, Singh NK. Pocket conversion made easy: a simple technique using alloderm to convert subglandular breast implants to the dual-plane position. Aesthet Surg J. 2009; 29(1):12–18
[33] Spear SL, Carter ME, Ganz JC. The correction of capsular contracture by conversion to "dual-plane" positioning: technique and outcomes. Plast Reconstr Surg. 2003; 112(2):456–466
[34] Handel N. Secondary mastopexy in the augmented patient: a recipe for disaster. Plast Reconstr Surg. 2006; 118(7) Suppl:152S–163S, discussion 164S–165S, 166S––167S
[35] Tebbetts JB, Teitelbaum S. High- and extra-high-projection breast implants: potential consequences for patients. Plast Reconstr Surg. 2010; 126(6):2150–2159
[36] Siu PM, Tam EW, Teng BT, et al. Muscle apoptosis is induced in pressure-induced deep tissue injury. J Appl Physiol (1985). 2009; 107(4):1266–1275
[37] Gawlitta D, Li W, Oomens CW, Baaijens FP, Bader DL, Bouten CV. The relative contributions of compression and hypoxia to development of muscle tissue damage: an in vitro study. Ann Biomed Eng. 2007; 35(2):273–284
[38] Roxo ACW, Nahas FX, Salin R, de Castro CC, Aboudib JH, Marques RG. Volumetric evaluation of the mammary gland and pectoralis major muscle following subglandular and submuscular breast augmentation. Plast Reconstr Surg. 2016; 137(1):62–69
[39] Roxo ACW, Nahas FX, Bazi F, de Castro CC, Aboudib JH, Marques RG. Evaluation of the effects of silicone implants on the breast parenchyma. Aesthet Surg J. 2015; 35(8):929–935
[40] Kovacs L, Eder M, Zimmermann A, et al. Three-dimensional evaluation of breast augmentation and the influence of anatomic and round implants on operative breast shape changes. Aesthetic Plast Surg. 2012; 36(4):879–887
[41] Tepper OM, Small KH, Unger JG, et al. 3D analysis of breast augmentation defines operative changes and their relationship to implant dimensions. Ann Plast Surg. 2009; 62(5):570–575
[42] Nahabedian MY. Discussion: High- and extra-high-projection breast implants: potential consequences for patients. Plast Reconstr Surg. 2010; 126 (6):2165–2167
[43] Slavin SA. Discussion: High- and extra-high-projection breast implants: potential consequences for patients. Plast Reconstr Surg. 2010; 126(6):2163–2164
[44] Ducic I, Zakaria HM, Felder JM, III, Fantus S. Nerve injuries in aesthetic breast surgery: systematic review and treatment options. Aesthet Surg J. 2014; 34 (6):841–856
[45] Courtiss EH, Goldwyn RM. Breast sensation before and after plastic surgery. Plast Reconstr Surg. 1976; 58(1):1–13
[46] Brown T. Objective sensory changes following subfascial breast augmentation. Aesthet Surg J. 2016; 36(7):784–789
[47] Spear SL, Dayan JH, Bogue D, et al. The "neosubpectoral" pocket for the correction of symmastia. Plast Reconstr Surg. 2009; 124(3):695–703
[48] Deapen D. Breast implants and breast cancer: a review of incidence, detection, mortality, and survival. Plast Reconstr Surg. 2007; 120(7) Suppl 1:70S–80S
[49] Sosin M, Devulapalli C, Fehring C, et al. Breast cancer following augmentation mammaplasty: a case-control study. Plast Reconstr Surg. 2018; 141(4):833–840
[50] Handel N, Silverstein MJ. Breast cancer diagnosis and prognosis in augmented women. Plast Reconstr Surg. 2006; 118(3):587–593, discussion 594––596
[51] Miglioretti DL, Rutter CM, Geller BM, et al. Effect of breast augmentation on the accuracy of mammography and cancer characteristics. JAMA. 2004; 291 (4):442–450
[52] Eklund GW, Busby RC, Miller SH, Job JS. Improved imaging of the augmented breast. AJR Am J Roentgenol. 1988; 151(3):469–473
[53] Spear SL, Clemens MW, Dayan JH. Considerations of previous augmentation in subsequent breast reconstruction. Aesthet Surg J. 2008; 28(3):285–293
[54] Nahabedian MY, Patel K. Management of common and uncommon problems after primary breast augmentation. Clin Plast Surg. 2009; 36(1):127–138, vii

6 Fat Grafting for Primary Augmentation

Ash Patel, Kristen Rezak, and Emily Van Kouwenberg

Summary

This chapter will focus on fat grafting for primary breast augmentation. Patient selection, process of graft survival, techniques of fat grafting, outcomes and complications, oncologic considerations, and postoperative breast screening will be discussed. Although some controversies still exist regarding primary augmentation with fat grafting, this technique continues to gain popularity among plastic surgeons. Patients should undergo extensive counseling before proceeding with fat grafting to the breast, including potential risks, complications, and effects on future cancer screening.

Keywords: fat grafting, primary breast augmentation, stromal vascular fraction, adipose-derived stem cells, fat injection, fat graft survival, fat necrosis

6.1 Introduction

Fat transplantation was first described by Gustav Adolf Neuber in 1893 for reconstruction of facial scars.[1] Autologous fat transfer to the breast was later described by Vincenz Czerny in 1895, after he successfully transferred a back lipoma to fill a breast defect.[2] Fat transfer procedures continued to develop until the mid-1900s, when fat grafting lost popularity because of high reported resorption rates. A 1950 study by Peer reported fat loss averaging 45% 1 year after transfer.[3] Fat grafting had a resurgence in the 1980s, when liposuction became available as a minimally invasive technique for harvest. In 1987, Bircoll reported a case of successful and long-lasting fat transfer to the breast using liposuction.[4] Later that same year, fat transplant to the breast was denounced by the American Society of Plastic and Reconstructive Surgeons (ASPRS, as the American Society of Plastic Surgeons [ASPS] was then named) Ad-Hoc Committee on New Procedures for potential interference with breast cancer detection.[5]

In 2007, the ASPS Fat Graft Task Force was created to evaluate the efficacy and safety of fat grafting to the breast. A report was released by the group in 2009 suggesting a potential role for fat grafting to the breast and other sites, but inadequate data was available to make specific recommendations. Their review of the literature included reports of fat grafting to the breast to treat micromastia, postaugmentation deformities, congenital deformities such as Poland syndrome and tuberous breast deformity, and defects after surgical resection for breast cancer. No evidence of delayed detection of breast cancer after fat grafting was found, and complication rates appeared appropriate, with only rare cases of severe complications and death; the primary cause of poor results was found to be graft volume loss. The task force reported that fat grafting "can be considered a safe method of augmentation and correction of defects associated with various medical conditions." The study concluded that although fat grafting to the breast and other sites can be considered, outcomes are surgeon- and technique-dependent.[6] Since that time, there has been a resurgence of fat grafting to the breast, with new innovations aimed to enhance fat retention rates.

6.2 Patient Selection and Preoperative Assessment

There are multiple potential uses for fat grafting in the breast, including primary breast reconstruction after mastectomy or lumpectomy, revision reconstruction, correction of congenital deformities such as Poland syndrome or tuberous breast deformity, and primary or secondary breast augmentation. Advantageous qualities of autologous fat include accessibility, simplicity of harvest, and most importantly, lack of immunogenic response. Patients should undergo extensive counseling before proceeding with fat grafting to the breast, including potential risks, complications, and effects on future cancer screening. Patients must understand the likelihood of partial graft resorption, the possible need for multiple procedures, and the possibility of unfavorable or inadequate results. Patients must also be counseled on the controversies of fat grafting.

A good candidate for fat grafting breast augmentation is a patient with appropriate expectations, desire for modest augmentation, adequate donor site adiposity, stable weight, and nonptotic breasts. Patients desiring more pronounced breast enlargement with substantial projection may be better suited for implant augmentation. Although the optimal candidate would have ample donor adiposity, low body mass index (BMI) is not an absolute contraindication. Studies have shown that satisfactory augmentation can be achieved in underweight patients (BMI ≤ 18.5).[7] Preoperative weight stability will contribute to a more predictable result, as significant weight loss or gain after fat grafting will result in similar effects at the recipient site. Breast ptosis should be addressed with mastopexy prior to fat grafting augmentation; combining these into a single procedure may decrease fat survival as a result of temporary decreased perfusion to the breast. Fat grafting alone will not address ptosis, and failure to correct ptosis will result in suboptimal outcomes.

Careful consideration is needed in patients at increased risk for breast cancer, such as those with family history, personal history, or relevant genetic mutation. Currently there are no studies that prove delayed detection of breast cancer or increased risk for breast cancer after autologous fat transfer to the breast, but these topics are still controversial. In light of these controversies, however, the ASPS has declared that fat grafting to the breast should no longer be considered an experimental practice and should instead be considered part of reconstructive surgery in patients with breast cancer.[8] Although there is not an absolute contraindication in these patients, extensive counseling is required. Patients must understand that postoperative changes to the breast could potentially lead to radiographic changes and increased likelihood of a need for biopsy.

Prior to surgery, photographs should be taken and the specific areas requiring augmentation identified. Communication with the patient is important to determine expectations and goals, including volume of augmentation; depending on the volume desired, the likelihood of multiple sessions should be reemphasized. Donor sites should be chosen preoperatively based on areas of available adiposity and patient preference. Preoperative mammograms should be performed, and the patient should be agreeable to repeat mammograms with the same radiologist 1 year after surgery to establish a new baseline.

Patients should be generally healthy with optimization of preexisting medical conditions. Preoperative risk stratification should be performed, including risk for perioperative venous thromboembolism (VTE); patients at increased risk for VTE should receive appropriate preventative measures. A full abdominal exam should be performed to rule out hernia prior to abdominal liposuction.

6.3 Process of Graft Survival

Survival of transplanted fat initially depends on diffusion of nutrients from surrounding plasma until neovascularization begins, usually within 48 hours.[9] As a result, ideal fat for transplantation has a high surface area–to-volume ratio to optimize absorption of nutrients from surrounding tissues for graft survival. Although fat deposits must be large enough to preserve cellular composition, excessively large deposits have a higher likelihood of central necrosis. Fat can ultimately be lost as a result of ischemia, apoptosis, or adipocyte dedifferentiation. Even distribution of fat during transfer is also important to maximize resorption of graft that does not survive.

In addition to adipocytes, harvested fat contains stromal cells in a portion termed the stromal vascular fraction (SVF). The SVF contains a high ratio of adipose-derived stem cells (ADSCs), which can differentiate into adipocytes or epithelial cells required for angiogenesis; these cells also secrete growth factors that promote angiogenesis and graft survival. Studies suggest that there are different zones of survival within nonvascularized transplanted fat. The peripheral zone has the highest survival of transplanted adipocytes, while the central zone has the greatest loss of both adipocytes and stromal cells. Between these layers is an intermediate zone where there is low survival of adipocytes but retention of viable adipose-derived stromal cells. This layer is thought to be the regenerating zone, with eventual replacement of lost adipocytes with new adipocytes as a result of the preserved stromal cells. This theory highlights the importance of stromal cell viability for ultimate graft retention volume.[10] The dead adipocytes undergo slow absorption and act to reserve space for eventual replacement with new adipocytes; adipogenesis is typically completed by 12 weeks. If dead adipocytes are inadequately removed by macrophages, then oil cysts, fibrosis, and calcifications can result.[11]

Fat graft survival can be optimized with atraumatic methods of harvesting, processing, and injection, although such techniques are yet to be standardized.[12] Atraumatic technique maximizes the ratio of viable adipocytes and stromal cells that are critical for graft retention. Capacity for adipocyte revascularization differs among different patients; although not completely understood, older age may negatively affect this process.

6.4 Technique

6.4.1 Preparation and Anesthesia

Antiseptic skin cleanser is used at home for 3 days prior to surgery. The patient should be marked while standing in the preoperative holding area. Markings should include anatomic breast boundaries, areas of desired augmentation, and any contour irregularities to be corrected. Donor sites for fat harvest should be marked, as well as areas where liposuction should be avoided (e.g., zones of adherence).

Although fat grafting breast augmentation is typically performed under general anesthesia, it can also be performed using local anesthetic and sedation in accredited surgical facilities. Initial patient positioning depends on the site of harvest. Supine positioning may be adequate for liposuction of the abdomen, flanks, lateral and medial thighs, and knees, but harvest from the back or buttocks may require prone positioning with subsequent repositioning for injection. Sequential compression devices should be placed whenever possible to prevent VTE. All pressure points should be adequately padded. Unless contraindicated, chlorhexidine is used for sterile preparation.

Perioperative antibiotics are typically administered before the procedure. Careful volume monitoring is performed to avoid under- or overresuscitation, and fluid is administered depending on vital signs and urine output.[13,14]

6.4.2 Fat Harvest

Donor sites for fat harvest should be chosen based on patient morphology; options include the abdomen, flanks, back, hips, thighs, and buttocks. Based on current studies, fat harvests from various sites lead to comparable results, and there is not a preferred site for harvest.[15,16,17,18] Entrance incisions should be made asymmetrically within or parallel to relaxed skin tension lines or previous scars. A superwet technique is commonly employed, using tumescent solutions with epinephrine and lidocaine or with epinephrine alone to reduce blood loss. When lidocaine is included, a serum concentration of 35 mg/kg is widely considered to be safe. Patients typically reach peak serum concentration of lidocaine with its active metabolite, monoethylglycinexylidide, 8 to 28 hours after infiltration.[19] Marcaine should be avoided in wetting solutions, given its longer duration of action and increased systemic risk. Current studies show similar adipocyte viability after harvest with wet or dry liposuction techniques.[20,21] Exposure to lidocaine with epinephrine has not been shown to affect adipocyte viability or retention when there is adequate washing prior to injection, but inadequate removal of local anesthetic can negatively impact adipocyte function.[16,17,22,23]

Studies suggest that use of smaller harvest cannulas, such as 2- to 4-mm cannulas, may result in less graft retention compared to larger cannulas, despite eventual use of small injection cannulas.[24,25] Larger harvest cannulas are thought to result in less damage to harvested fat, in part due to less shear stress.[26] Data evaluating cannula size is limited in the setting of tumescent infiltration techniques, and it is unclear whether use of wetting solutions can decrease the shear stress associated with smaller cannulas.[16] Larger cannulas, however, harvest larger fat fragments that may lead to accidental bolus injection when

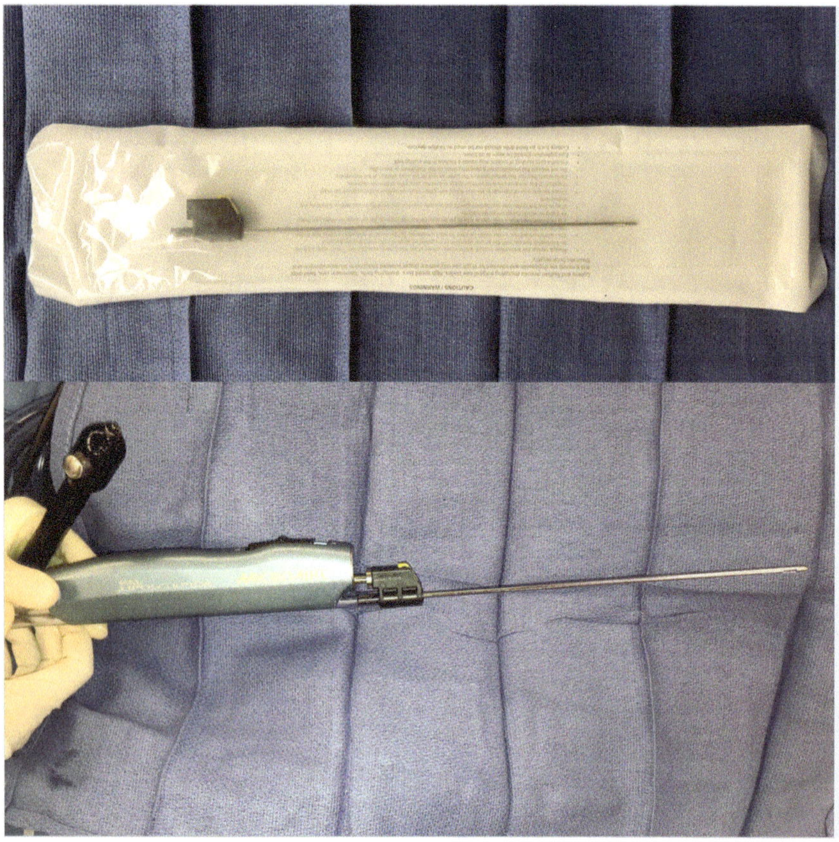

Fig. 6.1 Disposable 3-mm liposuction cannulas.

using smaller injection cannulas. As a result, a 3-mm cannula with multiple holes is typically used. Disposable cannulas should be used when harvesting for fat transfer (▶ Fig. 6.1).

Fat is most commonly harvested by traditional suction-assisted or power-assisted liposuction. Higher negative pressures should be avoided, as this can potentially decrease the final number of viable adipocytes and stromal vascular fraction cells.[27,28] Careful attention should be paid to preserve the superficial layer of adipose tissue and to avoid creation of contour irregularities; smaller cannulas should be used in more superficial or critical areas.

Manual fat harvest is another commonly performed technique, using a 10-mL syringe connected to a blunt liposuction cannula; the plunger is held in a partially-pulled-back position to achieve negative pressure.[29] Some authors feel that this technique minimizes damage to adipocytes compared to mechanical suction, however, currently there is no evidence that either method leads to superior results.[17,29,30,31,32] Although some studies have shown greater counts of viable adipocytes or greater enzymatic activity with fat harvested from a manual technique compared to mechanical techniques, other studies have shown that fat harvested by suction-assisted or ultrasound-assisted liposuction has similar adipocyte and ADSC viability and function.[16,32,33,34,35] In contrast, laser-assisted liposuction has been linked to decreased viability and function of stromal cells and should thus be avoided.[36] A newer method of water jet–assisted liposuction has promising potential applications in fat grafting, with studies showing greater retention of adipocytes with this method than with manual harvest.[37,38]

Adequate fat should be harvested to account for fat lost during processing and to allow for overcorrection during fat injection. Entrance sites are closed with rapidly absorbed simple sutures.

6.4.3 Fat Processing

The most common method of fat processing over time has been centrifugation.[15] Centrifugation separates lipoaspirate into three layers: a top oily layer containing chylomicrons and triglycerides, a middle layer of fat optimal for grafting, and a bottom layer containing blood products, serum, and infiltration fluid. The bottom layer can be drained by removing the cap from the bottom of the syringe, and the top layer can be poured off, leaving behind purified fat.[30] Separation of fat by centrifugation increases the concentration of adipocytes in the graft and removes lipases, proteases, and other enzymes that lead to fat degradation. Nonviable cells are also removed, decreasing the postoperative inflammatory response. Although there is no standardized duration or revolutions per minute (rpm), Emmanuel Delay reports processing for 3 minutes at 3,200 rpm, while Sydney Coleman recommends 3 minutes at 3,000 rpm.[29,30,39] Studies show that excessive centrifugation forces can lead to increased damage to adipocytes and ADSCs in fat harvested by mechanical liposuction.[16,40,41,42] In contrast, lower centrifugation forces are likely to leave residual debris. Son et al found force under 4,000 rpm to be safe without affecting adipocyte or stromal cell viability.[43]

Another option is decantation, in which the adipose tissue and associated fluid are separated by gravity. This is typically

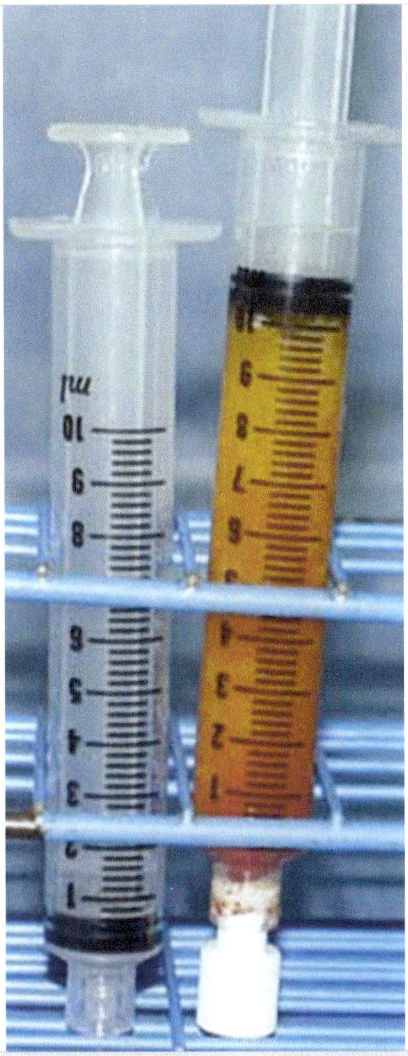

Fig. 6.2 Fat separation by decantation. (Reproduced from Herman CK, Strauch B. Encyclopedia of Aesthetic Rejuvenation through Volume Enhancement. New York, NY: Thieme Medical Publishers; 2014.)

performed directly in syringes, although commercial devices also exist (▶ Fig. 6.2). Decantation is an inexpensive and easy approach to fat processing, however, it often results in inadequate removal of fluid. Remaining infiltration fluid and adipose-secreted cytokines and enzymes can lead to decreased adipocyte viability and increased resorption.[44] Separation by cotton gauze rolling is another inexpensive approach, in which the fat is gently rolled over nonadherent gauze to remove fluid. Although this is a viable option for small-volume fat grafting, it is not practical for processing large quantities of lipoaspirate.

In filtering techniques, lipoaspirate is passed through a filter to preserve larger particles while ridding it of fluid and smaller particles. Many commercial filter devices have added washing steps to help remove infiltration fluid and inflammatory molecules to improve graft survival.[18] The authors recommend using washing and filtering techniques for effective and efficient processing of lipoaspirate, using a closed system to decrease fat desiccation and contamination (▶ Fig. 6.3).

Although many studies have compared these methods, results are conflicting and no technique has been proven to provide superior results.[16,17,45,46] Some authors have attempted to increase retention of fat grafts by supplementation with various biologic products including insulin, vascular endothelial growth factor (VEGF), or platelet-rich plasma (PRP).[4,29,47,48,49,50,51] In other countries, cell-assisted lipotransfer (CAL) is gaining traction, using techniques of autologous stem cell enrichment to improve graft survival.[52]

6.4.4 Fat Injection

The technique of fat injection is the most critical factor affecting fat retention and patient outcomes.[29] Fat is prepared into small syringes with small-diameter cannulas; 5-mL or 10-mL syringes and 2-mm blunt cannulas are used (▶ Fig. 6.4). Blunt cannulas minimize risk for intravascular injection and allow better dispersion of the fat into small aliquots.[54] Entrance sites for fat injection into the breast are placed with a 16-gauge needle, using previous scars whenever possible and avoiding the sternum to prevent hypertrophic scarring. Several entrance sites may be required to allow transfer along multiple directions and planes. To minimize risk for pneumothorax, the cannula is inserted with a slight anterior inclination of the cannula tip to avoid deep penetration into the chest wall. Furthermore, the cannula is inserted gently, without forced entry against resistance.

Multiple tunnels are first created with the cannula, and then injection is performed during cannula withdrawal; small amounts of fat, approximately 0.2 mL, are injected with each pass. Bolus injection is avoided because it is associated with increased rates of fat necrosis, liponecrotic cysts, and surgical site infection.[29] Slow injection speeds are preferred to prevent graft damage by shear stress.[54] Although the authors inject manually, automated injection devices exist to aid in controlled delivery of small fat volumes with minimal shear stress.[55,56] Fat is transferred from multiple directions and in multiple planes, building from deep to superficial to create a honeycomb distribution of fat.

Most surgeons recommend distributing the fat into the subcutaneous, retroglandular, or perimuscular spaces, while avoiding injection into the glandular tissue.[15,17] Avoiding breast parenchyma allows easier injection and theoretically decreases risk for infection. Although the effect of ADSCs on malignant and premalignant cells in the breast remains unclear, avoiding injection into breast tissue also minimizes any potential interactive effects.[17,57] Intramuscular injection is generally avoided because fat retention is less than in other planes, despite excellent perfusion of the muscle; this may be due to displacement of the graft during pectoralis contraction.[58] For these reasons, the authors primarily inject fat into the subcutaneous and retroglandular spaces.

The amount of fat injected is often limited by what the recipient site is able to accommodate based on skin envelope pliability and vascularity. If possible, overcorrection by 40% should be attempted to account for resorption. At the same time, grafting should be conservative so as not to exceed what the recipient site can accommodate. Excessive graft placement will result in increased interstitial pressure and graft ischemia, which will lead to increased resorption and risk for fat necrosis. The surgeon must use careful judgment when balancing these considerations. Pre-expansion devices can be considered preopera-

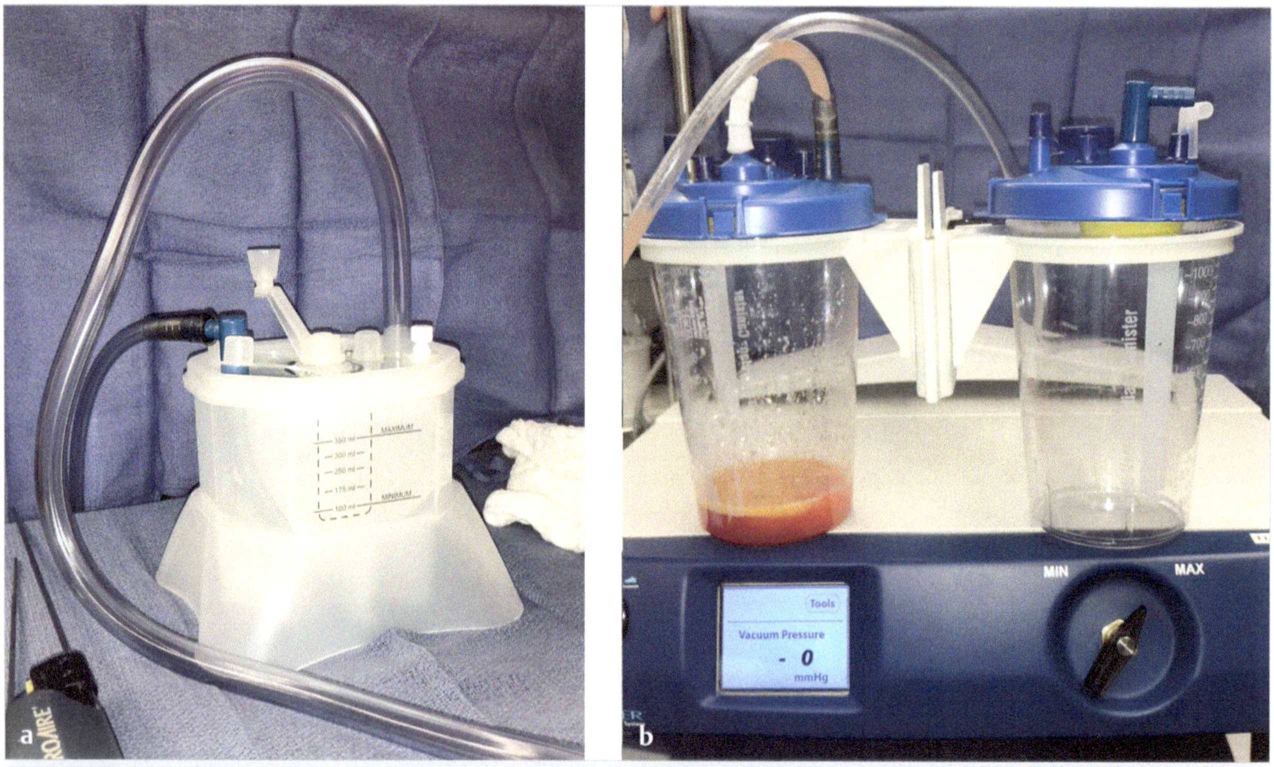

Fig. 6.3 **(a,b)** Disposable, closed-system device for washing and filtering of harvested fat (Revolve System, Allergan PLC, Dublin, Ireland).

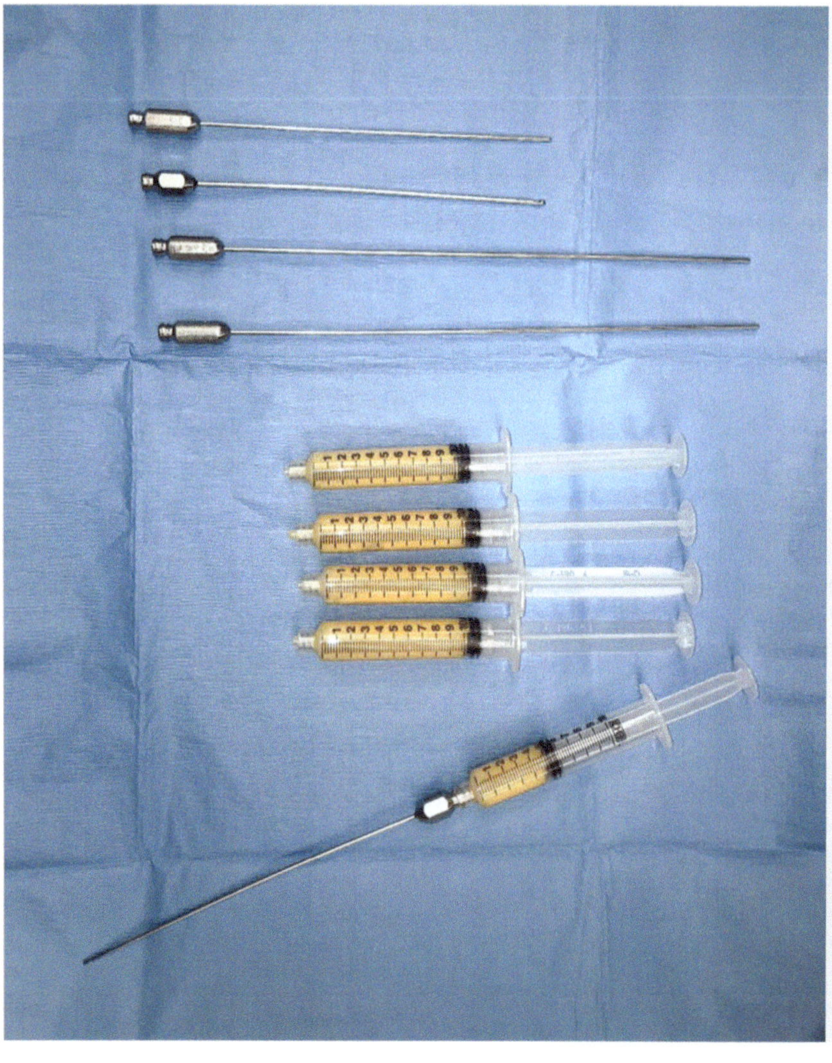

Fig. 6.4 Syringes and blunt injection cannulas.

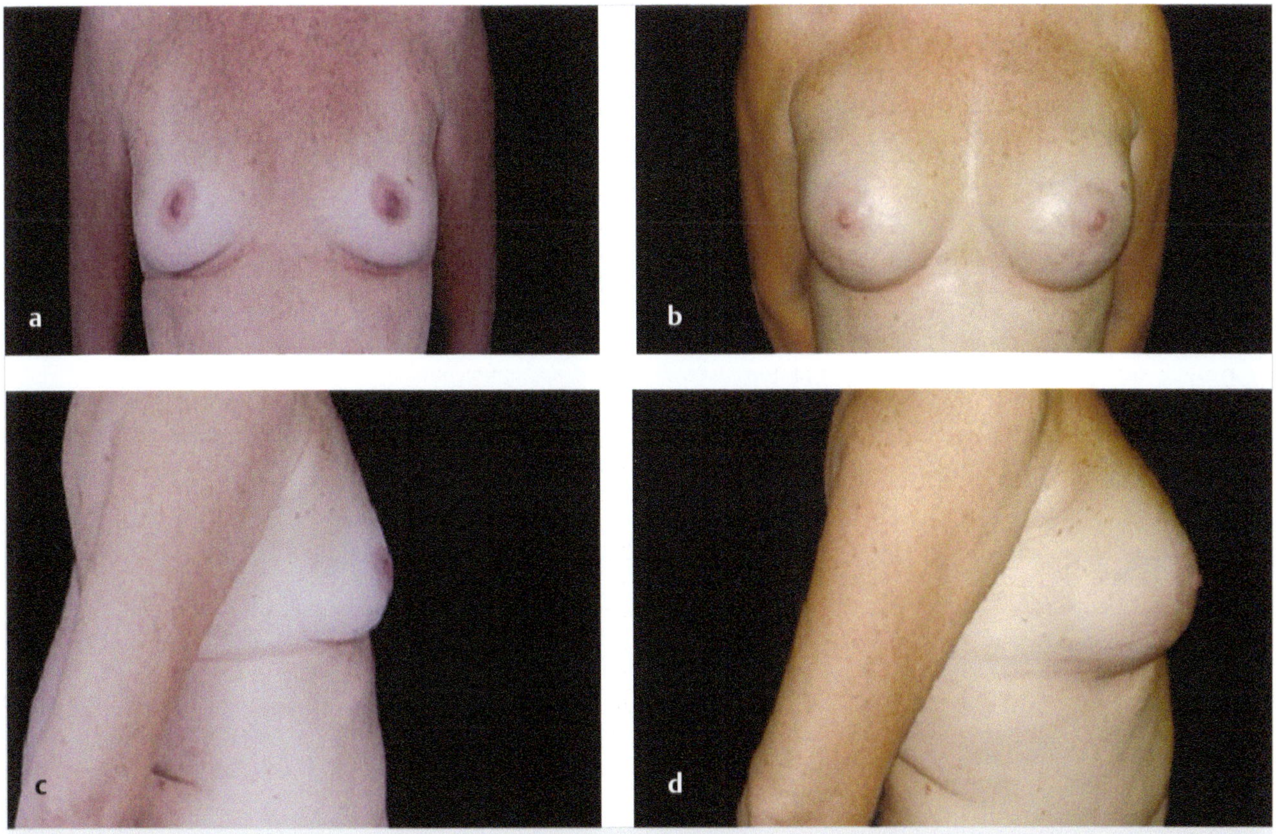

Fig. 6.5 (a,c) Pre- and **(b,d)** postoperative photographs after three sessions of fat grafting breast augmentation. A total of 253 mL was injected into the right breast and 249 mL into the left breast. (Reproduced from Herman CK, Strauch B. Encyclopedia of Aesthetic Rejuvenation through Volume Enhancement. New York, NY: Thieme Medical Publishers; 2014.)

tively in patients with tight skin envelopes to prepare the recipient site to accept larger graft volumes.[59] Upon completion, entrance sites are closed with rapidly absorbed simple sutures. Studies report injecting 50–600 mL per breast each session, for a total of one to five sessions.[15] The authors typically inject 200–250 mL per breast in most women; however, larger-breasted women can often accommodate more.

The Coleman technique can also be used and has been found to be associated with favorable and long-lasting results in a systematic review.[29] This technique includes manual suction with a 10-mL syringe and a two-hole cannula, followed by processing by centrifugation. The fat is then transferred to 3-mL syringes and injected using blunt infiltration cannulas. The fat is primarily injected into the pectoralis major muscle and the perimuscular spaces, while injection into the parenchyma is limited. Breast shaping is achieved with subcutaneous injection. Arguably the most important technical point of this method is injection in small aliquots and from multiple directions.[54]

6.5 Postoperative Management

Compression garments are worn over donor sites for at least 2 weeks. When small-volume liposuction is performed, patients can typically return to light duty work in 5 days, whereas patients requiring larger-volume liposuction are out of work for 7 to 10 days. Pressure to the breasts is avoided for 6 weeks, and mammograms are deferred for 6 months. Patients can generally return to exercise and regular activities 4 weeks after surgery.

The majority of postoperative edema resolves after the first month; however, patients should be counseled that the overall volume of the breast will continue to decrease over the following months as a result of fat resorption. In a patient with stable weight, the volume typically stabilizes after 3 to 6 months postoperatively.[30] Publications vary, reporting one to five sessions of fat grafting needed to achieve desired augmentation (▶ Fig. 6.5).[15,49] Repeat fat grafting can be performed 6 months after surgery.

6.6 Outcomes

Outcomes are largely dependent on surgeon technique, which is not yet standardized. Typically 30–40% of fat is lost by resorption over 3 to 6 months; this percentage can be higher with resorption over a longer period of time when fat is inadequately purified for transfer.[30,53] Fat resorption is often less after subsequent sessions of fat grafting.[30] After initial resorption, volume usually remains stable in the long term, confirmed by studies using three-dimensional (3D) imaging technology.[30] One caveat is that grafted fat is affected by patient weight fluctuation, with increase or decrease in size corresponding to weight gain or loss, respectively.

Augmentation with fat grafting is often modest and limited to one cup size increase per session. Multiple procedures are often required to achieve adequate augmentation, in contrast to implant-based augmentation, which offers reproducible results in a single-stage procedure. Given that fat grafting is autologous, however, complications associated with foreign body are avoided, including implant infection, extrusion, malposition, rupture, capsular contracture, and potential need for replacement. Risk for breast implant–associated anaplastic large cell lymphoma (BIA-ALCL) can also be avoided. Fat grafting has additional benefits, including decreased scar burden, potential to improve skin quality and stretch marks, and a more natural appearance.

A prospective study conducted by Spear et al found disproportionately high patient satisfaction after fat grafting to the breasts, despite only modest augmentation. Patients reported "feeling more attractive, sexually confident, and at ease during sexual activity."[60]

6.7 Complications

Early complications after autologous fat grafting most commonly include surgical site infection, contour irregularities, and inadequate augmentation; rarer complications include sepsis, pneumothorax from cannula penetration, or fat embolism from intravascular injection. Late complications are usually the result of fat necrosis and include fat resorption, liponecrotic cysts, and formation of calcifications. Changes in nipple sensation or lactation are not expected with fat grafting augmentation. Both early and late complications are highly associated with surgeon technique, as demonstrated by the wide variation of complication rates reported in the literature.

Localized infection can occur at the donor or recipient site and can typically be treated with suture removal, wound care, and antibiotics. Contour irregularities and inadequate augmentation can be addressed with additional rounds of fat grafting after the site has been given adequate time to heal and stabilize.

Although occurrence of pneumothorax is rare, this risk should not be overlooked, and precautions should be taken. If a pneumothorax does occur, it typically presents as respiratory compromise with oxygen desaturation, warranting an emergent chest X-ray. Pneumothorax should be treated with needle decompression, chest tube, or vascular interventional radiology (VIR) image-guided pigtail drain depending on patient stability. Typically, patients recover completely without long-term sequelae.

There is also a risk of fat embolism if fat is injected into a large vessel, classically presenting as a triad with altered mental status, respiratory compromise, and petechial rash. To minimize risk, blunt cannulas are used, and fat is injected during rapid withdrawal of the cannula while avoiding bolus injection. Studies evaluating fat embolism after gluteal fat grafting have suggested increased risk with intramuscular injection; for this reason, injection into the pectoralis major where large perforators are located is generally avoided.[61,62] Risk can be higher in patients with chest wall deformities, such as those with Poland syndrome who have inferiorly displaced subclavian vessels. Patients are treated with supportive care.

Clinically apparent fat necrosis occurs in about 3% of cases performed by experienced surgeons, but rates can be significantly higher depending on technique employed.[15,30] Fat necrosis is more likely to occur when fat is injected in large aliquots or when excessive fat is injected into the recipient site. Fat necrosis presents as a firm lump that is slightly tender to the touch. Although fat necrosis can usually be recognized on physical exam, imaging is occasionally required. Mammography should be avoided the first 6 months after surgery, and any concerning masses identified in the early postoperative period should be evaluated with ultrasound or magnetic resonance imaging (MRI).

Donor site complications can also occur, and they mirror those of general liposuction. Most commonly, contour irregularities can occur at the donor site if careful attention is not paid to liposuction technique. Other aesthetic complications include hypertrophic scarring of the entrance sites or obliteration of zones of adherence. Infection at the donor site, although rare, can occur and occasionally progress to abscess formation requiring drainage, or even more rarely, to sepsis.

A recent meta-analysis found a 12.6% complication rate for breast augmentation by fat transfer, including < 3% rate of cytosteatonecrotic lesions; most complications were acute or subacute, with very few long-term complications reported.[15] In this study, only 16 of 2,203 patients required reoperation for complication. In comparison, Hidalgo et al reported that up to 36% of patients with implant augmentation required secondary surgery over 10 years to address complications such as capsular contracture, implant malposition, and implant failure.[61]

6.8 Postoperative Breast Screening

Postsurgical changes can be seen on mammogram or other imaging after any breast surgery and can lead to architectural distortion. Mammographic findings after autologous fat grafting are typically due to fat necrosis, which can appear as oil cysts, microcalcifications, coarse calcifications, focal masses, or spiculated areas of increased opacity.[62] Oil cysts are more common after bolus injection and can be identified as radiolucent round or ellipsoid lesions surrounded by a thin, smooth, calcified "egg-shell" rim. A meta-analysis found radiologic changes in 75.7% of patients after fat grafting to the breast, most commonly including benign calcifications or liponecrotic cysts.[15] Ten studies included in the meta-analysis focused exclusively on radiologic assessment after fat grafting, and none of these studies showed interference with breast cancer screening as a result of such changes.[15]

A 2008 study evaluated the occurrence and character of such changes in 20 patients with history of autologous fat grafting; all mammograms evaluated were performed at least 6 months after surgery.[63] The most common finding was bilateral scattered microcalcifications, followed by oil cysts with or without associated microcalcifications. Another common finding was heterogeneity of pectoral muscle density, sometimes with microcalcifications. 85% of patients were classified as Breast Imaging Reporting and Data System (BI-RADS) 2 ("benign finding"), while 15% of patients were found to have microcalcifications in clusters, resulting in an initial BI-RADS 3 classification ("probably benign finding" with short-interval mammographic follow-up recommended). All of the BI-RADS 3 patients were reclassified to BI-RADS 2 after follow-up mammography.

Another study by Rubin et al compared mammographic changes 1 year after fat transfer breast augmentation to those after breast reduction; all patients had normal preoperative mammograms. Postoperative mammograms performed 1 year after surgery were reviewed in a blinded fashion by breast imaging radiologists. The study found significantly fewer radiographic abnormalities, significantly lower BI-RADS scores, and fewer recommendations for biopsy in the lipotransfer group compared to the reduction mammoplasty group.[63]

With trained breast radiologists, cancer screening after fat grafting breast augmentation should not be problematic.[64] Mammograms can be performed prior to surgery and 1 year after surgery to establish baseline imaging. Patients who do not have any postoperative concerns are then instructed to undergo the same breast screening as the general population.

6.9 Oncologic Safety

Concern that fat grafting can potentially increase breast cancer risk stems from the theory that adipocytes and ADSCs can promote neoplastic cell production. Proposed mechanisms include increased local estrogen production as a result of adipose-derived aromatase and increased angiogenesis as a result of ADSCs.

In a 2003 murine study evaluating effects of adipocytes on tumor cells, adipocyte-secreted cytokines were shown to promote tumorigenesis in the presence of malignant breast ductal epithelial cells.[65] The cytokines were found to induce transcription factors that increased angiogenesis as well as cell survival, proliferation, and invasive potential. Adipocyte-secreted factors were also found to stabilize pro-oncogenic factors by decreased expression of inhibitors. Another 2003 study using a rat model found promotion of estrogen receptor (ER)-positive tumor cells by mature adipocytes, hypothetically related to adipocyte-produced estrogen.[66] In contrast to mature adipocytes, premature adipocytes did not promote tumorigenesis and were associated with increased expression of tumor inhibitors.

Multiple studies have also been done to evaluate the interaction between ADSCs and breast cancer cells. While one 2009 mouse study found promotion of human breast cancer cell proliferation in the presence of human ADSCs,[67] another mouse model study reported a protective effect of stem cells against breast cancer.[68] The latter study showed an inhibition of tumor growth and metastasis when adipose-derived mesenchymal stromal cells were injected into mouse mammary tissue that had also been injected with breast cancer cells. Although multiple studies have shown an antitumor effect of stromal cells, other studies suggest no effect or the opposite effect, with variation depending on the type of stromal cells and tumor cells used.[68]

As described, current studies show contradictory evidence regarding the interaction of adipocytes and ADSCs with breast cancer cells and the resulting effect on tumorigenesis. In a recent meta-analysis including 2,023 patients who underwent fat grafting augmentation with a mean follow-up of 22 months, only two (0.09%) patients were diagnosed with breast cancer during their follow-up period; no study devoted to evaluation of oncological risk after fat grafting to the breast was identified in the study.[15] A clinical study with 10-year follow-up after fat grafting to the breast for reconstruction or aesthetic augmentation found no increased risk of breast cancer recurrence or new breast cancers in fat-grafted patients.[30] Studies have also been conducted to evaluate effects of fat grafting specifically in patients with known breast cancer history. A multicenter case-cohort study by Myckatyn et al including 1,197 patients did not find a higher recurrence rate among patients who underwent fat grafting as part of their immediate reconstruction after mastectomy.[69] Similarly, a matched case-control study by Petit et al evaluating 644 patients who underwent breast conservation therapy did not find higher rates of recurrence or other primary breast cancers among those who underwent fat grafting.[70] A prior study by the same author group found increased rates of local recurrence after fat grafting in the setting of carcinoma in situ, with potentially increased risk with younger age (< 50 years old), high-grade cancer, positive Ki-67, and quadrantectomy procedures; the study also suggested higher risk with shorter periods of time between surgical resection and fat grafting reconstruction.[71] In their follow-up study, however, the authors reported that additional analysis of the same patient series after a longer period of follow-up did not show any statistically significant differences in recurrence rates between patients who had undergone fat grafting and patients who had not.[70,71] Although animal studies have shown potential for increased cancer risk in the presence of adipocytes and ADSCs, this is yet to be seen in human studies.[72,73]

Further studies are needed to clarify the controversies that surround fat grafting, including large, prospective, controlled studies. Currently a phase III randomized multicenter trial titled Adipose Tissue Transfer for Moderate Breast Cancer Conservative Treatment Sequela (GRATSEC) is underway in France to evaluate effects of fat transfer on breast cancer surveillance and recurrence.[15] The Plastic Surgery Foundation has also initiated a General Registry of Autologous Fat Transfer (GRAFT) project to obtain national data in the United States. Recommendations vary among societies, but most agree that fat grafting augmentation should be avoided in patients at high risk for breast cancer and that all patients should undergo preoperative radiologic evaluation and regular postoperative screening.[15] In the United States, patients with history of fat grafting to the breast generally undergo the same screening regimen as those who have not.

6.10 Other Indications

There are many indications for fat grafting to the breast beyond cosmetic augmentation, including breast reconstruction of oncologic defects or congenital malformations. Fat grafting can be used for primary reconstruction after lumpectomy or mastectomy, as well as for revision breast reconstruction to achieve augmentation or correction of contour deformities (▶ Fig. 6.6). Fat grafting can also be used to improve skin quality of the irradiated breast, although more conservative volumes should be injected in this setting given decreased vascularity.

Various breast malformations can be addressed with autologous fat transfer, such as sternocostal hollowing associated with pectus excavatum. Focused fat transfer can be delivered to sites of deficiency in these patients, either alone or in combination with a customized implant, to improve breast appearance

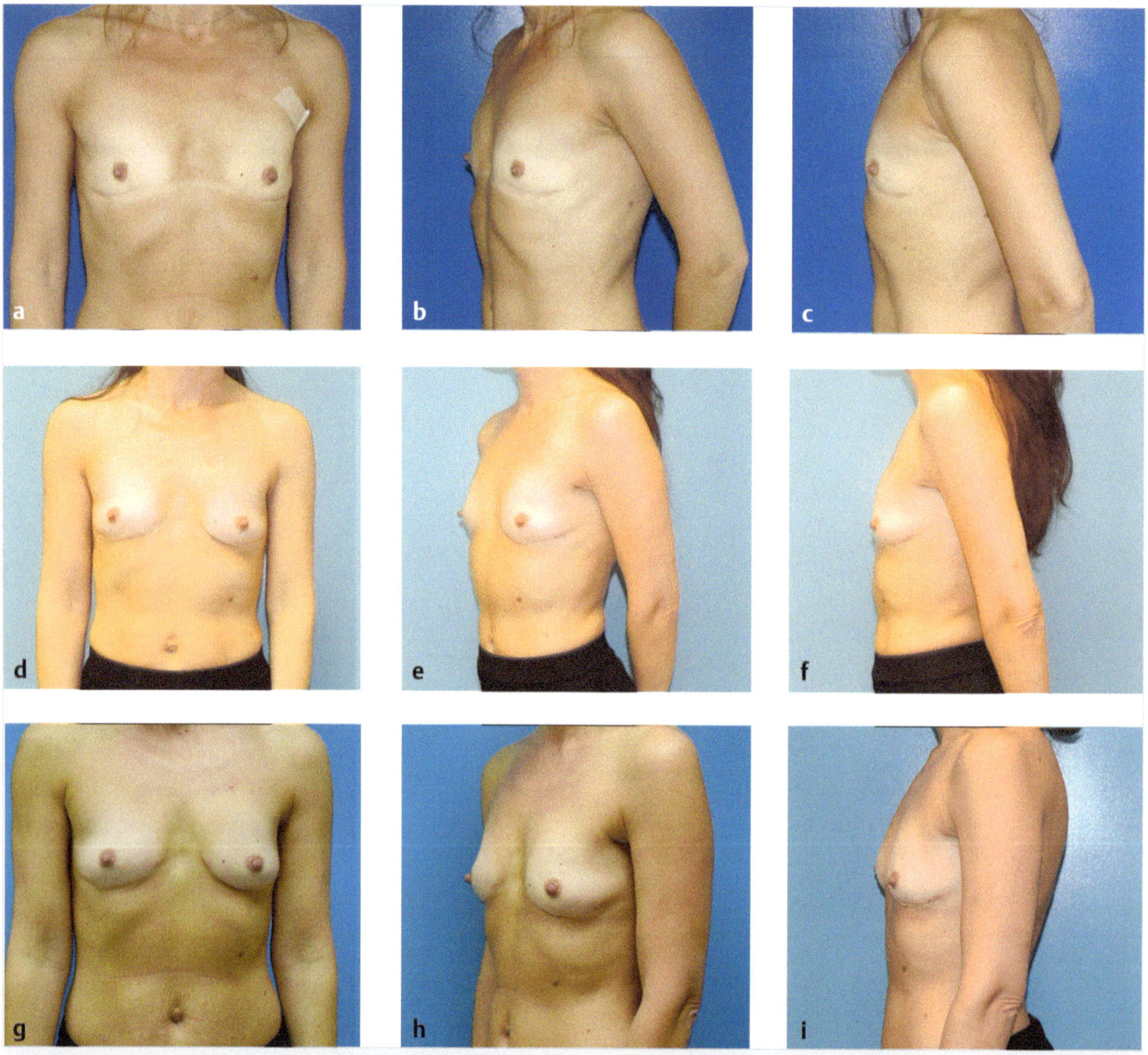

Fig. 6.6 Pre- and postoperative photographs after bilateral breast reconstruction with two sessions of fat grafting. Patient had prior history of multiple breast operations after bilateral silicone implant ruptures, with eventual removal of implants and excision of a left breast benign mass. As a result, the patient had minimal residual breast tissue and contour abnormalities warranting reconstruction. **(a–c)** Preoperative. **(d–f)** Four months after first session (100 mL into each breast). **(g–i)** Two months after second session of fat grafting (100 mL into each breast).

significantly. Tuberous breast deformity can be addressed with directed fat transfer to improve contour, superior pole fullness, and general volume, and to increase breast base width (▸ Fig. 6.7). Although this is an option for mild cases, Brault et al found greater satisfaction among tuberous breast patients treated with implant augmentation compared to fat grafting.[74] Fat grafting can also be employed in cases of breast asymmetry, in which augmentation with fat will achieve a more natural appearance to match the contralateral breast than could be achieved with an implant. In such circumstances of malformation, fat transfer is advantageous over breast implant augmentation because of its ability to deliver localized augmentation to specific sites.

Fat grafting can also be utilized for primary or revision implant-based augmentation. Primary composite breast augmentation with both implant and fat grafting is a good option for patients who desire greater volume than can be achieved with fat grafting alone, but also a more natural appearance than can be achieved with implants alone. The addition of fat grafting can provide a softer transition between the superior pole and the chest, a more natural cleavage, and enhanced soft tissue coverage of the implant, all of which are particularly useful in thin patients. Camouflaging the implant with fat grafting also allows subfascial or prepectoral implant placement in patients who would not otherwise be candidates, reducing risk for persistent pain and animation deformity.[75] Furthermore, natural shape can be achieved without use of anatomic implants, eliminating risk for malrotation.[76]

There are also indications for fat grafting in secondary procedures after implant-based augmentation, including correction

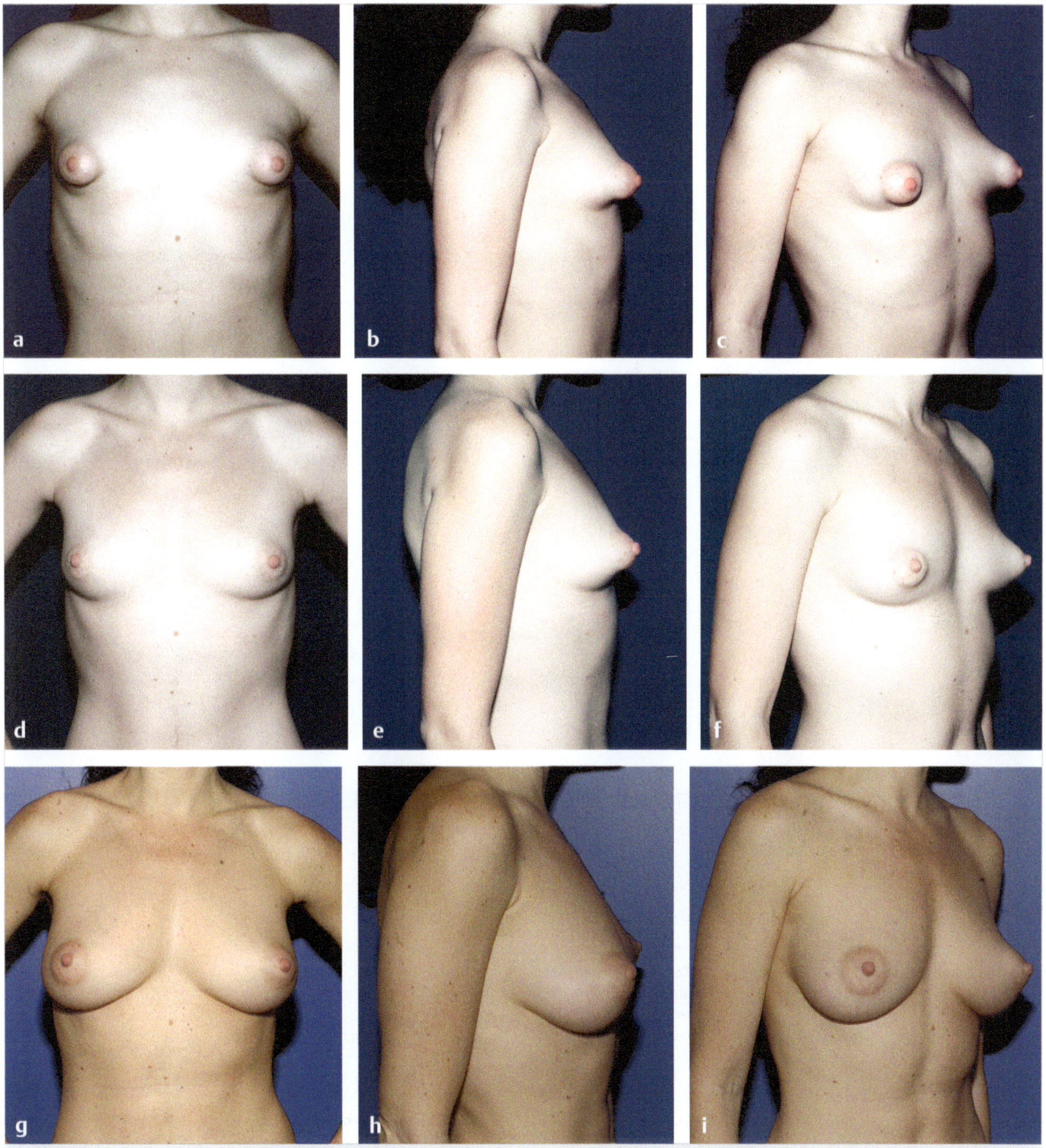

Fig. 6.7 Pre- and postoperative photographs after reconstruction of tuberous breast deformity with fat grafting augmentation. **(a–c)** Preoperative. **(d–f)** Eight months after first session of fat grafting (380 mL into right breast, 370 mL into left breast). **(g–i)** Almost five years after second session of fat grafting (340 mL into right breast, 300 mL into left breast). (Reproduced from Coleman SR, Mazzola RF, Pu LLQ. Fat Injection: from Filling to Regeneration. 2nd Edition. New York, NY: Thieme Medical Publishers; 2018.)

of small or large contour deformities (▶ Fig. 6.8). Fat grafting can be used to reduce intermammary distance in patients who complain of a wide space between the breasts; this is otherwise difficult to address, as the anatomic footprint should be preserved during surgical dissection.[77] Wide intermammary distance is a common challenge in transgender patients undergoing breast augmentation, and fat grafting can be utilized in these patients to achieve a more feminine appearance. Successful treatment of capsular contracture and double-bubble deformity with fat grafting alone have also both been reported.[53,78]

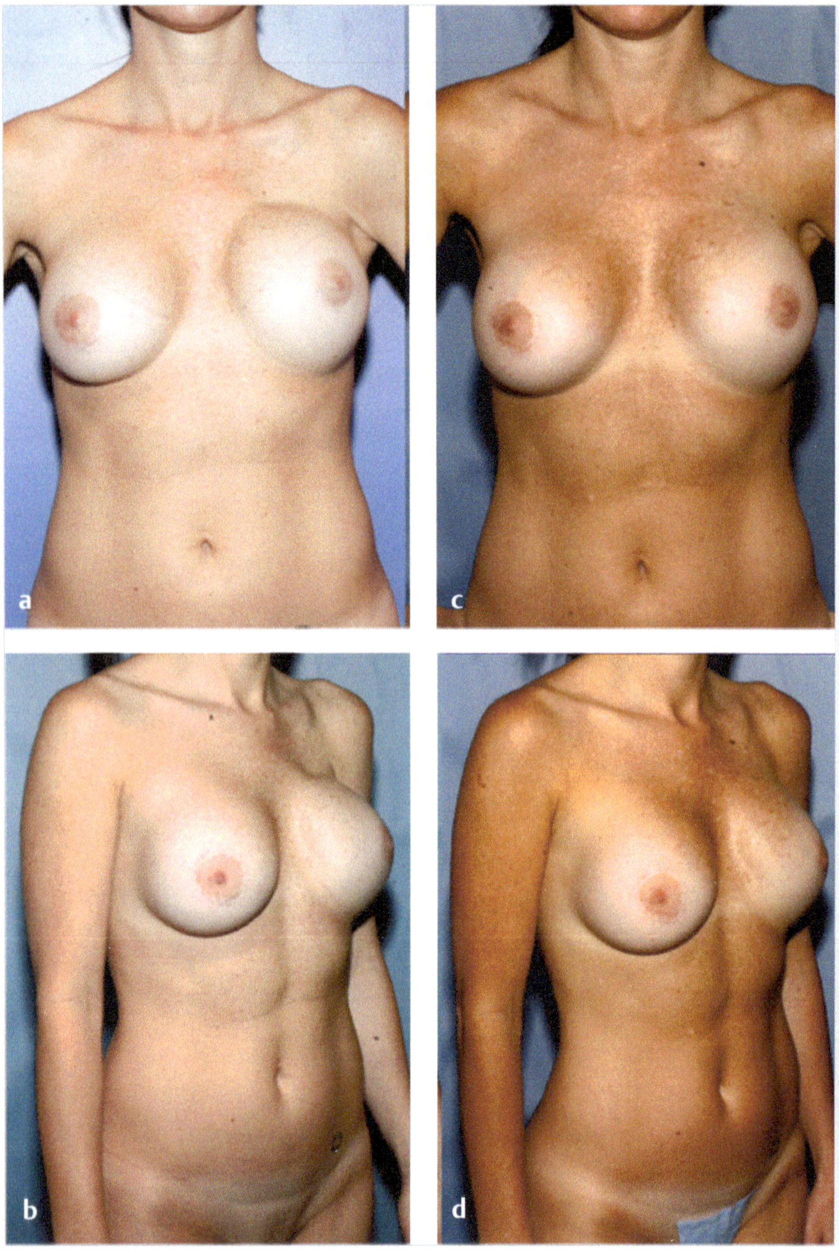

Fig. 6.8 (a,b) Preoperative and **(c,d)** 7-month postoperative photographs of left breast revision reconstruction with fat grafting to soften the superior pole and axilla with improved postoperative appearance and decreased implant discomfort. Patient had undergone right mastopexy and bilateral saline implants 17 years previously for reconstruction of left breast and chest deformities associated with Poland syndrome. In the revision, 177.5 mL was injected into the upper pole of the left breast and 30 mL into the axilla. (Reproduced from Herman CK, Strauch B. Encyclopedia of Aesthetic Rejuvenation through Volume Enhancement. New York, NY: Thieme Medical Publishers; 2014.)

6.11 Innovations

Multiple innovations have been made in an attempt to increase graft retention. Probably the most controversial is supplementation with adipose-derived regenerative cells (ADRCs), such as ADSCs. In 2006 Matsumoto described cell-assisted lipotransfer (CAL) as a technique in which ADSCs isolated from lipoaspirate were added to fat prior to injection; in this animal model study, CAL was found to have a 35% greater fat retention with improved neovascularization.[52] Studies suggest that supplementation can increase neovascularization, adipocyte differentiation, and, ultimately, long-term graft retention while preventing apoptosis, especially in hypoxic conditions.[50,51,79,80] This may be the result of multiple growth factors expressed by ADSCs, such as VEGF and IGF-1.[79,80] ADSCs have also been found to have an immunosuppressive effect, which can decrease inflammation leading to graft loss.[81] Stromal vascular fraction with ADSCs can be obtained from harvested fat by digestion of fat with collagenase and separation by centrifugation; SVF cells can then be expanded by culture or used immediately.[52,82,83] SVF can also be obtained from the lipoaspirate fluid, although this method results in a smaller percentage of ADSCs.[84,85]

Although some studies show promising data, many other studies, including a recent meta-analysis, have not found superior graft take and volume gain with this technique.[15,84,86] Furthermore, CAL requires greater volume of fat harvest, more operative time, and a laboratory for fat processing. Given varied reports, additional time and cost, and potential neoplastic concerns, CAL should not be routinely used, although it may have potential application in suboptimal recipient sites such as the irradiated breast. Currently, no clinical studies have shown increased recurrence when applied to breast cancer patients, although the oncologic risks of this method are still poorly understood.[87,88]

Optimization of the recipient site is another drive for innovation. Pre-expansion devices such as the Brava device can be used preoperatively to prepare the recipient site.[59] The goal of pre-expansion is to increase the interstitial space and thereby increase the volume of fat that the recipient site can safely accept. The device works by applying negative pressure to the breasts to cause an inflow of fluid and, as a result, transient breast enlargement. The negative pressure has an added benefit of increased angiogenesis, further optimizing the recipient site. When worn nightly, the Brava can increase breast size one cup over 4 to 6 weeks; Khouri recommends pre-expansion beyond the final volume goal prior to grafting. Postoperative use of Brava is also advocated to immobilize the fat graft and further promote angiogenesis.[59] Brava has been associated with larger fat injection volumes and higher graft survival rates, reportedly reaching 82% average retention (▸ Fig. 6.9).[89,90,91] Brava comes with added costs and requires patient compliance.

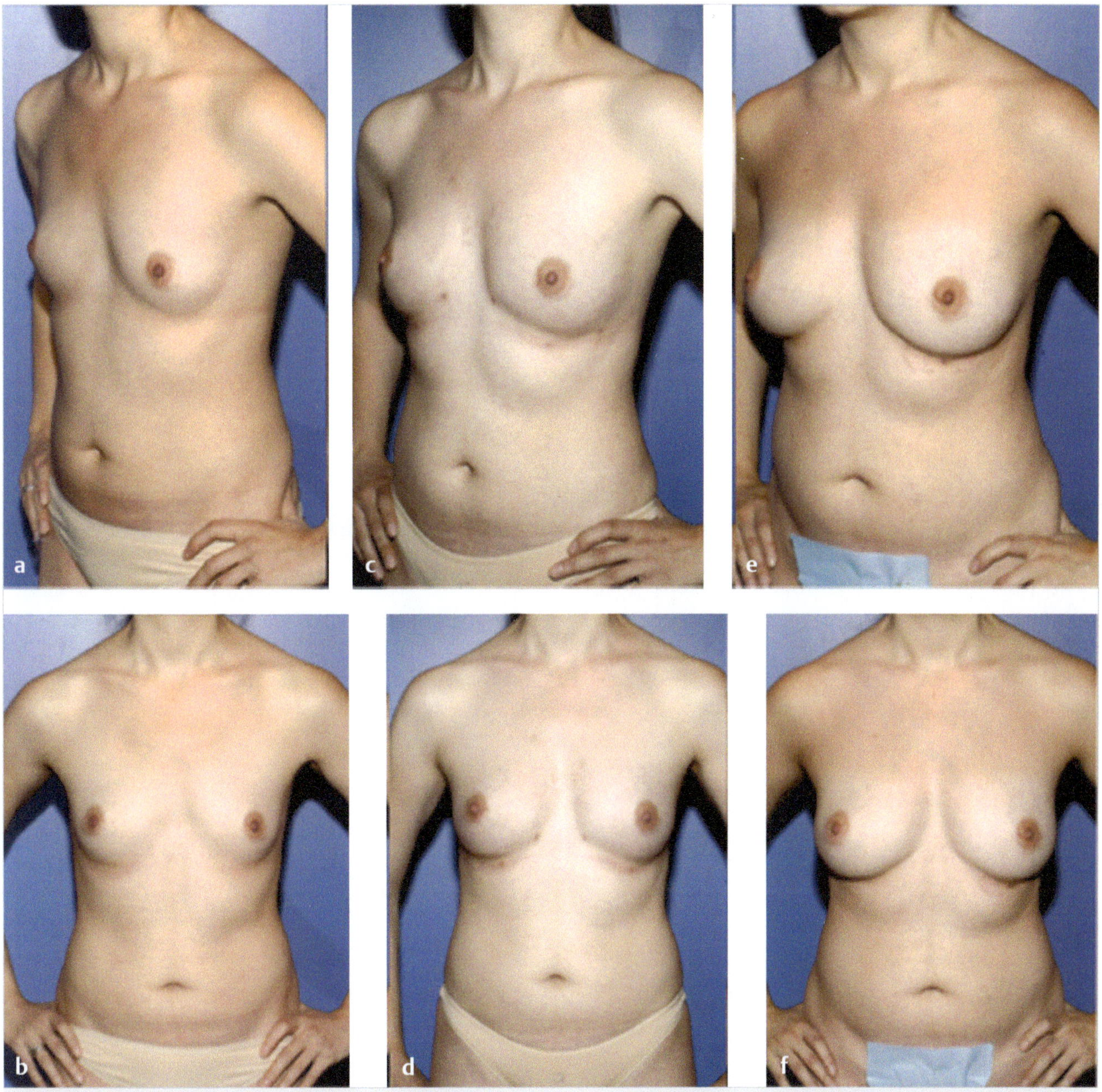

Fig. 6.9 Fat grafting augmentation using preoperative Brava expansion (Brava, LLC, Miami, FL). **(a,b)** Preoperative. **(c,d)** Three months after first session (232.5 mL into right breast, 230 mL into left breast). **(e,f)** Twenty-one months after second session of fat grafting (237.5 mL into right breast, 287.5 mL into right breast). (Reproduced from Herman CK, Strauch B. Encyclopedia of Aesthetic Rejuvenation through Volume Enhancement. New York, NY: Thieme Medical Publishers; 2014.)

6.12 Conclusion

Breast augmentation by autologous fat transfer can be considered in select patients after thorough counseling. Favorable, long-lasting, and reproducible results are possible with refined technique and surgeon experience. Patients should undergo extensive counseling before proceeding with fat grafting to the breast, including potential risks, complications, and effects on future cancer screening. Patients must understand the likelihood of partial graft resorption, possible need for multiple procedures, and possibility of unfavorable or inadequate results. Patients must also be informed about the controversies of fat grafting.

Key Points

- Advantageous qualities of autologous fat include lack of immunogenic response, accessibility, simplicity of harvest, decreased scar burden, potential to improve skin quality and stretch marks, and natural appearance. Complications associated with foreign body are avoided with autologous fat, such as implant infection, extrusion, malposition, rupture, capsular contracture, and potential need for replacement.
- Patients should undergo extensive counseling prior to fat grafting to the breast, including likelihood of partial graft resorption, possible need for multiple procedures, potential risks and complications, effects on future cancer screening, and the controversies of fat grafting. Careful consideration is needed in patients at high risk for breast cancer.
- Optimal candidates for fat grafting breast augmentation are those with appropriate expectations, desire for modest augmentation, adequate donor site adiposity, stable weight, and nonptotic breasts.
- Outcomes after fat grafting breast augmentation are largely dependent on surgeon technique, which is yet to be standardized.
- Atraumatic fat harvest, processing, and injection are needed to maximize the ratio of viable adipocytes and stromal cells, which are critical for graft retention; the technique of fat injection is the most critical factor affecting outcomes.
- Postsurgical changes can be seen on breast imaging after fat grafting and can lead to architectural distortion. Although these changes have potential to increase biopsy rates, this can typically be avoided when imaging is read by trained breast radiologists. In the United States, patients who have a history of fat grafting to the breast generally undergo the same screening regimen as those who do not.
- Current animal studies show contradictory evidence regarding the interaction of adipocytes and ADSCs with breast cancer cells, and the resulting effect on tumorigenesis. Numerous human studies, however, are yet to show increased cancer risk after fat grafting to the breast. Further studies are needed to clarify the controversies that surround fat grafting, including large, prospective, controlled studies.

References

[1] Neuber GA. Fat transplantation [in German]. Chir Kong Verhandl. 1893; 22:66–68

[2] Czerny V. Plastic replacement of the breast with a lipoma [in German]. Chir Kong Verhandl. 1895; 24:216–217

[3] Peer LA. Loss of weight and volume in human fat grafts: with postulation of a "cell survival theory.". Plast Reconstr Surg. 1950; 5:217–230

[4] Bircoll M, Novack BH. Autologous fat transplantation employing liposuction techniques. Ann Plast Surg. 1987; 18(4):327–329

[5] ASPRS Ad-Hoc Committee on New Procedures.. Report on autologous fat transplantation. Plast Surg Nurs. 1987; 7(4):140–141

[6] Gutowski KA, ASPS Fat Graft Task Force. Current applications and safety of autologous fat grafts: a report of the ASPS Fat Graft Task Force. Plast Reconstr Surg. 2009; 124(1):272–280

[7] Chiu CH. Autologous fat grafting for breast augmentation in underweight women. Aesthet Surg J. 2014; 34(7):1066–1082

[8] American Society of Plastic Surgeons. ASPS Recommended Insurance Coverage Criteria: Autologous Fat Grafting to the Breast. Arlington Heights, IL: ASPS; 2015. URL: https://www.plasticsurgery.org/Documents/Health-Policy/Reimbursement/insurance-2015-autologous-fat-grafting-breast.pdf (Accessed July 10, 2019)

[9] Mizuno H, Hyakusoku H. Fat grafting to the breast and adipose-derived stem cells: recent scientific consensus and controversy. Aesthet Surg J. 2010; 30 (3):381–387

[10] Eto H, Kato H, Suga H, et al. The fate of adipocytes after nonvascularized fat grafting: evidence of early death and replacement of adipocytes. Plast Reconstr Surg. 2012; 129(5):1081–1092

[11] Kato H, Mineda K, Eto H, et al. Degeneration, regeneration, and cicatrization after fat grafting: dynamic total tissue remodeling during the first 3 months. Plast Reconstr Surg. 2014; 133(3):303e–313e

[12] Longaker MT, Aston SJ, Baker DC, Rohrich RJ. Fat transfer in 2014: what we do not know. Plast Reconstr Surg. 2014; 133(5):1305–1307

[13] Rohrich RJ, Leedy JE, Swamy R, Brown SA, Coleman J. Fluid resuscitation in liposuction: a retrospective review of 89 consecutive patients. Plast Reconstr Surg. 2006; 117(2):431–435

[14] Tabbal GN, Ahmad J, Lista F, Rohrich RJ. Advances in liposuction: five key principles with emphasis on patient safety and outcomes. Plast Reconstr Surg Glob Open. 2013; 1(8):e75

[15] Voglimacci M, Garrido I, Mojallal A, et al. Autologous fat grafting for cosmetic breast augmentation: a systematic review. Aesthet Surg J. 2015; 35(4):378–393

[16] Strong AL, Cederna PS, Rubin JP, Coleman SR, Levi B. The current state of fat grafting: a review of harvesting, processing, and injection techniques. Plast Reconstr Surg. 2015; 136(4):897–912

[17] Largo RD, Tchang LA, Mele V, et al. Efficacy, safety and complications of autologous fat grafting to healthy breast tissue: a systematic review. J Plast Reconstr Aesthet Surg. 2014; 67(4):437–448

[18] Hivernaud V, Lefourn B, Guicheux J, et al. Autologous fat grafting in the breast: critical points and technique improvements. Aesthetic Plast Surg. 2015; 39(4):547–561

[19] Kenkel JM, Lipschitz AH, Shepherd G, et al. Pharmacokinetics and safety of lidocaine and monoethylglycinexylidide in liposuction: a microdialysis study. Plast Reconstr Surg. 2004; 114(2):516–524, discussion 525–526

[20] Agostini T, Lazzeri D, Pini A, et al. Wet and dry techniques for structural fat graft harvesting: histomorphometric and cell viability assessments of lipoaspirated samples. Plast Reconstr Surg. 2012; 130(2):331e–339e

[21] Agostini T, Spinelli G, Perello R, Bani D, Boccalini G. Analysis of lipoaspirated following centrifugation: wet versus dry harvesting technique. J Craniofac Surg. 2016; 27(6):1489–1493

[22] Zielins ER, Brett EA, Longaker MT, Wan DC. Autologous fat grafting: the science behind the surgery. Aesthet Surg J. 2016; 36(4):488–496

[23] Moore JH, Jr, Kolaczynski JW, Morales LM, et al. Viability of fat obtained by syringe suction lipectomy: effects of local anesthesia with lidocaine. Aesthetic Plast Surg. 1995; 19(4):335–339

[24] Kirkham JC, Lee JH, Medina MA, III, McCormack MC, Randolph MA, Austen WG, Jr. The impact of liposuction cannula size on adipocyte viability. Ann Plast Surg. 2012; 69(4):479–481

[25] Erdim M, Tezel E, Numanoglu A, Sav A. The effects of the size of liposuction cannula on adipocyte survival and the optimum temperature for fat graft storage: an experimental study. J Plast Reconstr Aesthet Surg. 2009; 62(9): 1210–1214

[26] Tambasco D, Arena V, Finocchi V, Grussu F, Cervelli D. The impact of liposuction cannula size on adipocyte viability. Ann Plast Surg. 2014; 73(2):249–251

[27] Cheriyan T, Kao HK, Qiao X, Guo L. Low harvest pressure enhances autologous fat graft viability. Plast Reconstr Surg. 2014; 133(6):1365–1368

[28] Mojallal A, Auxenfans C, Lequeux C, Braye F, Damour O. Influence of negative pressure when harvesting adipose tissue on cell yield of the stromal-vascular fraction. Biomed Mater Eng. 2008; 18(4–5):193–197

[29] Rosing JH, Wong G, Wong MS, Sahar D, Stevenson TR, Pu LL. Autologous fat grafting for primary breast augmentation: a systematic review. Aesthetic Plast Surg. 2011; 35(5):882–890
[30] Delay E, Garson S, Tousson G, Sinna R. Fat injection to the breast: technique, results, and indications based on 880 procedures over 10 years. Aesthet Surg J. 2009; 29(5):360–376
[31] Smith P, Adams WP, Jr, Lipschitz AH, et al. Autologous human fat grafting: effect of harvesting and preparation techniques on adipocyte graft survival. Plast Reconstr Surg. 2006; 117(6):1836–1844
[32] Pu LL, Coleman SR, Cui X, Ferguson RE, Jr, Vasconez HC. Autologous fat grafts harvested and refined by the Coleman technique: a comparative study. Plast Reconstr Surg. 2008; 122(3):932–937
[33] Keck M, Kober J, Riedl O, et al. Power assisted liposuction to obtain adipose-derived stem cells: impact on viability and differentiation to adipocytes in comparison to manual aspiration. J Plast Reconstr Aesthet Surg. 2014; 67(1): e1–e8
[34] Pu LL, Cui X, Fink BF, Cibull ML, Gao D. The viability of fatty tissues within adipose aspirates after conventional liposuction: a comprehensive study. Ann Plast Surg. 2005; 54(3):288–292, discussion 292
[35] Schafer ME, Hicok KC, Mills DC, Cohen SR, Chao JJ. Acute adipocyte viability after third-generation ultrasound-assisted liposuction. Aesthet Surg J. 2013; 33(5):698–704
[36] Chung MT, Zimmermann AS, Paik KJ, et al. Isolation of human adipose-derived stromal cells using laser-assisted liposuction and their therapeutic potential in regenerative medicine. Stem Cells Transl Med. 2013; 2(10):808–817
[37] Yin S, Luan J, Fu S, Wang Q, Zhuang Q. Does water-jet force make a difference in fat grafting? In vitro and in vivo evidence of improved lipoaspirate viability and fat graft survival. Plast Reconstr Surg. 2015; 135(1):127–138
[38] Meyer J, Salamon A, Herzmann N, et al. Isolation and differentiation potential of human mesenchymal stem cells from adipose tissue harvested by water jet-assisted liposuction. Aesthet Surg J. 2015; 35(8):1030–1039
[39] Coleman SR, Saboeiro AP. Lipoaugmentation. 3rd ed. Philadelphia, PA: Lippincott Williams & Wilkins; 2011
[40] Ferraro GA, De Francesco F, Tirino V, et al. Effects of a new centrifugation method on adipose cell viability for autologous fat grafting. Aesthetic Plast Surg. 2011; 35(3):341–348
[41] Pulsfort AK, Wolter TP, Pallua N. The effect of centrifugal forces on viability of adipocytes in centrifuged lipoaspirates. Ann Plast Surg. 2011; 66(3):292–295
[42] Kurita M, Matsumoto D, Shigeura T, et al. Influences of centrifugation on cells and tissues in liposuction aspirates: optimized centrifugation for lipotransfer and cell isolation. Plast Reconstr Surg. 2008; 121(3):1033–1041, discussion 1042--1043
[43] Son D, Choi T, Yeo H, Kim J, Han K. The effect of centrifugation condition on mature adipocytes and adipose stem cell viability. Ann Plast Surg. 2014; 72 (5):589–593
[44] Hoareau L, Bencharif K, Girard AC, et al. Effect of centrifugation and washing on adipose graft viability: a new method to improve graft efficiency. J Plast Reconstr Aesthet Surg. 2013; 66(5):712–719
[45] Gupta R, Brace M, Taylor SM, Bezuhly M, Hong P. In search of the optimal processing technique for fat grafting. J Craniofac Surg. 2015; 26(1):94–99
[46] Minn KW, Min KH, Chang H, Kim S, Heo EJ. Effects of fat preparation methods on the viabilities of autologous fat grafts. Aesthetic Plast Surg. 2010; 34(5): 626–631
[47] Mu D-L, Luan J, Mu L, Xin MQ. Breast augmentation by autologous fat injection grafting: management and clinical analysis of complications. Ann Plast Surg. 2009; 63(2):124–127
[48] Yi CG, Xia W, Zhang LX, et al. VEGF gene therapy for the survival of transplanted fat tissue in nude mice. J Plast Reconstr Aesthet Surg. 2007; 60(3): 272–278
[49] Fulton JE. Breast contouring with "gelled" autologous fat: a 10 year update. Int J Cosmet Surg Aesthetic Dermatol. 2003; 5:155–163
[50] Gentile P, Orlandi A, Scioli MG, et al. A comparative translational study: the combined use of enhanced stromal vascular fraction and platelet-rich plasma improves fat grafting maintenance in breast reconstruction. Stem Cells Transl Med. 2012; 1(4):341–351
[51] Lucarelli E, Beccheroni A, Donati D, et al. Platelet-derived growth factors enhance proliferation of human stromal stem cells. Biomaterials. 2003; 24(18): 3095–3100
[52] Matsumoto D, Sato K, Gonda K, et al. Cell-assisted lipotransfer: supportive use of human adipose-derived cells for soft tissue augmentation with lipoinjection. Tissue Eng. 2006; 12(12):3375–3382
[53] Coleman SR, Saboeiro AP. Fat grafting to the breast revisited: safety and efficacy. Plast Reconstr Surg. 2007; 119(3):775–785, discussion 786--787
[54] Lee JH, Kirkham JC, McCormack MC, Nicholls AM, Randolph MA, Austen WG, Jr. The effect of pressure and shear on autologous fat grafting. Plast Reconstr Surg. 2013; 131(5):1125–1136
[55] Atashroo D, Raphel J, Chung MT, et al. Studies in fat grafting: Part II. Effects of injection mechanics on material properties of fat. Plast Reconstr Surg. 2014; 134(1):39–46
[56] Chung MT, Paik KJ, Atashroo DA, et al. Studies in fat grafting: Part I. Effects of injection technique on in vitro fat viability and in vivo volume retention. Plast Reconstr Surg. 2014; 134(1):29–38
[57] Parrish JN, Metzinger SE. Autogenous fat grafting and breast augmentation: a review of the literature. Aesthet Surg J. 2010; 30(4):549–556
[58] Herold C, Ueberreiter K, Cromme F, Grimme M, Vogt PM. Is there a need for intrapectoral injection in autologous fat transplantation to the breast? An MRI volumetric study [in German]. Handchir Mikrochir Plast Chir. 2011; 43 (2):119–124
[59] Khouri R, Del Vecchio D. Breast reconstruction and augmentation using pre-expansion and autologous fat transplantation. Clin Plast Surg. 2009; 36(2): 269–280, viii
[60] Spear SL, Pittman T. A prospective study on lipoaugmentation of the breast. Aesthet Surg J. 2014; 34(3):400–408
[61] Hidalgo DA, Spector JA. Breast augmentation. Plast Reconstr Surg. 2014; 133 (4):567e–583e
[62] Carvajal J, Patiño JH. Mammographic findings after breast augmentation with autologous fat injection. Aesthet Surg J. 2008; 28(2):153–162
[63] Rubin JP, Coon D, Zuley M, et al. Mammographic changes after fat transfer to the breast compared with changes after breast reduction: a blinded study. Plast Reconstr Surg. 2012; 129(5):1029–1038
[64] Veber M, Tourasse C, Toussoun G, Moutran M, Mojallal A, Delay E. Radiographic findings after breast augmentation by autologous fat transfer. Plast Reconstr Surg. 2011; 127(3):1289–1299
[65] Iyengar P, Combs TP, Shah SJ, et al. Adipocyte-secreted factors synergistically promote mammary tumorigenesis through induction of anti-apoptotic transcriptional programs and proto-oncogene stabilization. Oncogene. 2003; 22 (41):6408–6423
[66] Manabe Y, Toda S, Miyazaki K, Sugihara H. Mature adipocytes, but not preadipocytes, promote the growth of breast carcinoma cells in collagen gel matrix culture through cancer-stromal cell interactions. J Pathol. 2003; 201(2):221–228
[67] Muehlberg FL, Song YH, Krohn A, et al. Tissue-resident stem cells promote breast cancer growth and metastasis. Carcinogenesis. 2009; 30(4):589–597
[68] Sun B, Roh KH, Park JR, et al. Therapeutic potential of mesenchymal stromal cells in a mouse breast cancer metastasis model. Cytotherapy. 2009; 11(3): 289–298, 1, 298
[69] Myckatyn TM, Wagner IJ, Mehrara BJ, et al. Cancer risk after fat transfer: a multicenter case-cohort study. Plast Reconstr Surg. 2017; 139(1):11–18
[70] Petit JY, Maisonneuve P, Rotmensz N, Bertolini F, Rietjens M. Fat grafting after invasive breast cancer: a matched case-control study. Plast Reconstr Surg. 2017; 139(6):1292–1296
[71] Petit JY, Rietjens M, Botteri E, et al. Evaluation of fat grafting safety in patients with intraepithelial neoplasia: a matched-cohort study. Ann Oncol. 2013; 24 (6):1479–1484
[72] Krastev TK, Jonasse Y, Kon M. Oncological safety of autologous lipoaspirate grafting in breast cancer patients: a systematic review. Ann Surg Oncol. 2013; 20(1):111–119
[73] Agha RA, Fowler AJ, Herlin C, Goodacre TE, Orgill DP. Use of autologous fat grafting for breast reconstruction: a systematic review with meta-analysis of oncological outcomes. J Plast Reconstr Aesthet Surg. 2015; 68(2):143–161
[74] Brault N, Stivala A, Guillier D, et al. Correction of tuberous breast deformity: a retrospective study comparing lipofilling versus breast implant augmentation. J Plast Reconstr Aesthet Surg. 2017; 70(5):585–595
[75] Auclair E, Blondeel P, Del Vecchio DA. Composite breast augmentation: soft-tissue planning using implants and fat. Plast Reconstr Surg. 2013; 132(3): 558–568
[76] Kerfant N, Henry AS, Hu W, Marchac A, Auclair E. Subfascial primary breast sugmentation with fat grafting: a review of 156 cases. Plast Reconstr Surg. 2017; 139(5):1080e–1085e
[77] Serra-Mestre JM, Fernandez Peñuela R, Foti V, D'Andrea F, Serra-Renom JM. Breast cleavage remodeling with fat grafting: a safe way to optimize symmetry and reduce intermammary distance. Plast Reconstr Surg. 2017; 140(5): 665e–672e
[78] Bresnick SD. Management of a common breast augmentation complication: treatment of te double-bubble deformity with fat grafting. Ann Plast Surg. 2016; 76(1):18–22

[79] Zhu M, Zhou Z, Chen Y, et al. Supplementation of fat grafts with adipose-derived regenerative cells improves long-term graft retention. Ann Plast Surg. 2010; 64(2):222–228

[80] Rehman J, Traktuev D, Li J, et al. Secretion of angiogenic and antiapoptotic factors by human adipose stromal cells. Circulation. 2004; 109(10):1292–1298

[81] Puissant B, Barreau C, Bourin P, et al. Immunomodulatory effect of human adipose tissue-derived adult stem cells: comparison with bone marrow mesenchymal stem cells. Br J Haematol. 2005; 129(1):118–129

[82] Zuk PA, Zhu M, Mizuno H, et al. Multilineage cells from human adipose tissue: implications for cell-based therapies. Tissue Eng. 2001; 7(2):211–228

[83] Zuk PA, Zhu M, Ashjian P, et al. Human adipose tissue is a source of multipotent stem cells. Mol Biol Cell. 2002; 13(12):4279–4295

[84] Wang L, Luo X, Lu Y, Fan ZH, Hu X. Is the resorption of grafted fat reduced in cell-assisted lipotransfer for breast augmentation? Ann Plast Surg. 2015; 75 (2):128–134

[85] Kamakura T, Ito K. Autologous cell-enriched fat grafting for breast augmentation. Aesthetic Plast Surg. 2011; 35(6):1022–1030

[86] Jung HK, Kim CH, Song SY. Prospective 1-year follow-up study of breast augmentation by cell-assisted lipotransfer. Aesthet Surg J. 2016; 36(2):179–190

[87] Alperovich M, Lee ZH, Friedlander PL, Rowan BG, Gimble JM, Chiu ES. Adipose stem cell therapy in cancer reconstruction: a critical review. Ann Plast Surg. 2014; 73 Suppl 1:S104–S107

[88] Pérez-Cano R, Vranckx JJ, Lasso JM, et al. Prospective trial of adipose-derived regenerative cell (ADRC)-enriched fat grafting for partial mastectomy defects: the RESTORE-2 trial. Eur J Surg Oncol. 2012; 38(5):382–389

[89] Khouri RK, Eisenmann-Klein M, Cardoso E, et al. Brava and autologous fat transfer is a safe and effective breast augmentation alternative: results of a 6-year, 81-patient, prospective multicenter study. Plast Reconstr Surg. 2012; 129(5):1173–1187

[90] Khouri RK, Khouri RK, Jr, Rigotti G, et al. Aesthetic applications of Brava-assisted megavolume fat grafting to the breasts: a 9-year, 476-patient, multicenter experience. Plast Reconstr Surg. 2014; 133(4):796–807, discussion 808–809

[91] Del Vecchio DA, Bucky LP. Breast augmentation using preexpansion and autologous fat transplantation: a clinical radiographic study. Plast Reconstr Surg. 2011; 127(6):2441–2450

Part III

Management of the Ptotic Breast

III

7 Preoperative Evaluation of Patients with Macromastia and Ptosis

Katherine H. Carruthers, Pankaj Tiwari, and Ergun Kocak

Summary

The preoperative evaluation of patients with macromastia and ptosis is a complex topic, as the definition of macromastia is not always clear. It is generally accepted that reduction mammaplasty can be a therapeutic rather than purely cosmetic procedure. However, regardless of whether the breast reduction surgery is motivated by cosmetic or therapeutic goals, the essence of the procedure remains the same. The goals of surgery are to reduce breast weight and volume, improve shape and asymmetry, remove excess skin, and reposition the nipple areola complex (NAC). The realization of these goals results in the regaining of a more youthful appearance. A thorough history and physical exam are an essential part of the preoperative assessment and enable the physician to recognize modifiable risk factors. However, surgeons should not limit patient access to this therapeutic procedure based on isolated comorbidities. It has been widely published that reduction mammaplasty surgery has one of the highest satisfaction rates of all plastic surgical procedures, and postoperative outcomes have repeatedly been shown to improve quality of life and provide positive emotional and aesthetic results that are long-lasting.

Keywords: macromastia, ptosis, breast reduction, reduction mammoplasty, preoperative planning

7.1 Introduction

Breast reduction surgery is one of the most common plastic surgical procedures, with over 60,000 operations performed annually.[1,2] It is generally accepted that reduction mammaplasty can be a therapeutic rather than purely cosmetic procedure. However, regardless of whether the breast reduction surgery is motivated by cosmetic or therapeutic goals, the essence of the procedure remains the same. The goals of surgery are to reduce breast weight and volume, improve shape and asymmetry, remove excess skin, and reposition the nipple areola complex (NAC).[3] The realization of these goals results in the regaining of a more youthful appearance. It has been widely published that reduction mammaplasty surgery has one of the highest satisfaction rates of all plastic surgical procedures.[4] In cases where patients present with symptomatic macromastia, more than 90% report improvement or resolution in symptoms after surgical intervention.[5,6] Postoperative outcomes have repeatedly been shown to improve quality of life and provide positive emotional and aesthetic results that are long-lasting.[5,7]

7.1.1 Definition of Macromastia

The definition of macromastia is not always clear, and therefore, the preoperative management of patients with breast hypertrophy is a complex topic. However, there are a few minimum criteria that must be met in order to classify a patient as having symptomatic macromastia. History and physical examination are an essential part of the preoperative evaluation, and certain topics, as described in the following sections, must be addressed to support the diagnosis adequately. It has been argued that symptomatic macromastia is better defined by a complex combination of physical and emotional complaints than simply by breast volume and the amount of tissue to be removed.[8]

7.2 Preoperative Consultation

The goals for the initial preoperative consultation are to understand the patient's current complaints; to establish whether the patient's goals for surgery are cosmetic, therapeutic, or both; and to determine the risks and benefits of surgical intervention. Documentation is one of the simplest things a physician can do preoperatively to ensure that the elective breast surgery is successful. At a minimum, photographs illustrating severe breast hypertrophy are necessary, but other reports of associated symptoms can also be useful, especially if the patient is seeking insurance coverage for the surgery. The components of a thorough preoperative evaluation are discussed in detail in this and the following sections.

7.2.1 Presenting Symptoms

If it is established that the motivation for surgery is therapeutic rather than cosmetic, most insurance companies require patients to obtain preauthorization for surgical procedures. It is essential that the physician be aware of the required information and documentation at the preoperative appointment, since preauthorization is based heavily on subjective information and symptom duration that may not surface unless the appropriate questions are asked (Box 7.1 (p. 88), Box 7.2 (p. 89)).[6]

Box 7.1 Key Elements of History to Assess for Risk of Breast Reduction Complications

- Patient symptoms and expectations
- Comorbidities (including diabetes, hypertension, coagulopathy, connective tissue disorders, obesity)
- Previous hypertrophic scarring
- Smoking habits
- Obstetric history
- Medications
- Mammogram status

Box 7.2 Key Elements of Physical Examination to Assess for Risk of Breast Reduction Complications

- Shape
- Symmetry
- Contours
- Scar location
- Skin quality and elasticity
- Nipple areola complex (NAC) shape
- NAC position relative to inframammary fold (IMF)
- NAC position relative to the volume of the breast
- Volume distribution of both skin and parenchyma
- Specific measurements (suprasternal notch–to-nipple distance, breast base width, nipple-to-IMF distance, nipple-to-midline distance)
- Estimated volume of resection

A subjective history of neck pain, shoulder pain, lower back pain, and mastodynia is the most common combination of presenting symptoms of patients with macromastia.[5] These symptoms must be causing significant pain for greater than 1 year in order for the condition to be acknowledged by insurers.[3,9,10] Typically, the natural history involves the onset of pain during late adolescence with slow progression of symptoms as the breasts fully develop over time. Breast hypertrophy may eventually cause a change in posture resulting in progressive kyphosis, which could possibly be a subconscious attempt to hide the macromastia or the inevitable result of excess weight on the anterior chest wall.[7,11] When present, kyphosis should be documented through plain film X-rays of the cervical and thoracic spine, and any patients with chronic back pain should be evaluated by a qualified spine surgeon to rule out neurologic pathology.[11]

Patients may attempt to offset the added weight of their breast hypertrophy with use of wide-strap support bras or even multiple sports bras; however, this often fails to improve the pain and may actually cause new-onset shoulder pain and shoulder grooving due to the pressure of the bra straps. The use of multiple support or compression garments naturally leads to the onset of intertrigo. Baby powder or antiperspirant may improve the symptoms temporarily; however, chronic skin irritation will ultimately occur and lead to superficial bacterial or fungal infections and tissue maceration with skin breakdown.[9,10] Additionally, the long-term result of macromastia is ultimately breast ptosis. The weight of the excess breast volume will pull the tissues caudally, necessitating the use of constant support bras, which further exacerbates the issue of intertrigo, as just mentioned.

Other serious complaints often associated with macromastia include respiratory difficulty, which can lead to inability to exercise and, ultimately, decreased functional capacity.[3] In extreme cases, this debilitation can prevent patients from performing physically demanding jobs and cause lifelong disability.[3] Less common presenting complaints include neurologic symptoms such as ulnar paresthesias and chronic occipital headaches.[4] Since patients may not be aware of the association between breast hypertrophy and these complaints, they may not mention them unless specifically asked by the physician.

It is generally recommended that conservative treatments be attempted prior to proceeding with reduction surgery. Insurance companies may ask for documentation showing that the patient has failed conservative measures for at least 3 months prior to seeking approval for a therapeutic reduction mammaplasty.[9,10] Nonsurgical treatment options include trials of nonsteroidal anti-inflammatory medications, dermatologic intervention for skin concerns, and use of specialized support bras. Even physical therapy and chiropractic manipulation are encouraged before surgical intervention is considered indicated. However, these nonoperative interventions have been shown to be only rarely successful in improving symptoms in the long term.[12]

In addition to the physical manifestations that can cause a patient to present for evaluation for possible reduction mammaplasty, the psychologic manifestations can also be profound. Specifically in younger patient populations, macromastia can lead to a decrease in self-confidence, particularly in social situations where sexual attention may occur and in athletic settings where the individual is required to wear activewear or swimwear. This is more than just a cosmetic concern; it has the potential to lead to an actual impediment to emotional development in adolescents. Despite this, some insurers will not cover breast reduction surgery in patients under the age of 18 years old.[4,6] Elective breast surgery in this adolescent population is discussed in detail in Section 7.2.5.

It is important to note that with all of the presenting complaints outlined here, the severity of symptoms does not always correlate with degree of breast hypertrophy.[13] Thus, physicians should not discourage patients with relatively mild macromastia from proceeding with surgery if it has been determined that the patient's complaints are truly due to her breast hypertrophy and not other somatic or psychological pathology.

7.2.2 Medical and Surgical History

Once the chief complaint has been thoroughly addressed, it is important to obtain a complete medical and surgical history, as this can identify early risk factors for surgical complications and initiate the process for surgical optimization. Medications must be reviewed, specifically identifying any current or prolonged history of steroid use, which can negatively impact wound healing; any anticoagulation medications, which can lead to increased risk of intraoperative and postoperative bleeding and hematoma formation; and the use of hormonal birth control or oral estrogens, which can dramatically increase the likelihood of postoperative deep venous thrombosis (DVT) or pulmonary embolus (PE). In cases where these medications are identified, surgeons must work with the primary care and specialty care physicians to determine whether it is safe to discontinue their use temporarily for surgery or whether the risk of doing so outweighs the benefits of this elective procedure.

Several other topics are important factors in the preoperative planning of any breast-related surgery. One is the patient's individual weight history, including any major weight loss such as in the postbariatric setting, which can have profound impact on the reduction technique employed and the surgical outcome. Additionally, a history of prior soft tissue infections, especially methicillin-resistant *Staphylococcus aureus* (MRSA) infections, should be identified, as these can increase the risk of future infections, and any intraoperative antibiotic therapy may need to be adjusted accordingly. Finally, a personal or family history of keloids or unfavorable scars should be reviewed. Since reduction mammaplasty requires long incisions and, therefore, results in extensive scars, the risk of scar hypertrophy, hyperpigmentation, or keloid formation should be discussed in the preoperative setting.

7.2.3 Breast History

A detailed breast history is absolutely essential to providing appropriate patient care and preventing potentially unfavorable postoperative complications. Any current or past breast masses should be thoroughly investigated to ensure that malignancy is ruled out. Additionally, any previous breast biopsies, whether benign or malignant; any personal history of breast cancer, with or without surgical treatment; and any family history of breast cancer need to be outlined. The date of the patient's last mammogram should also be noted, along with the results and any secondary testing performed. In patients who are identified preoperatively as being high-risk for future breast malignancy, it is prudent to discuss with the patient the surgical plan if an occult malignancy is encountered intraoperatively.

Outside of breast cancer, A few other aspects of breast history should be discussed because they can have an impact on surgical planning. Any previous breast surgery, such as a prior augmentation, reduction, or mastopexy, needs to be identified. Additionally, any future plans for pregnancy should be explored, as this can dramatically change the breast volume and degree of ptosis. As such, some physicians recommend that elective breast surgery be deferred until no further childbearing is planned. Deferring surgery also alleviates concerns regarding the ability to breastfeed postoperatively, which is discussed in more detail in Section 7.5.1, Possible Complications.

7.2.4 Comorbidities

After thoroughly evaluating the physical and emotional symptoms and establishing an accurate diagnosis of symptomatic macromastia, the discussion should turn to the topic of comorbidities. Since the only true method for correcting the symptoms associated with breast hypertrophy and ptosis is surgery, which is discussed in detail in Chapter 8, Mastopexy Techniques—Basic Principles, identifying comorbid conditions that could threaten the success of a surgical intervention is essential.

Use of Tobacco Products

Regardless of whether a reduction mammaplasty or an isolated mastopexy is planned, a vascular pedicle to the nipple must be isolated, and tobacco use can have a major impact on wound healing or blood flow with nipple translocation. It has been reported that smoking can double or even triple the risk of major postoperative complications, specifically fat necrosis and other wound complications leading to reoperation.[2,14,15,16] If the patient is a current tobacco user, cessation of all tobacco products must be achieved for a minimum of 3 to 4 weeks before surgery. Even passive or secondhand smoke can have clinically significant negative effects on vascular perfusion and wound healing. This abstinence from nicotine products should, if at all possible, be continued for another 3 to 4 weeks after surgery as well, to facilitate wound healing.[16,17] There has been a recent trend toward preoperatively screening patients for tobacco exposure with urine cotinine tests. Most in-office tests can detect direct or passive exposure over the past 4 days and are an excellent way for nicotine abstinence to be verified in an economic and convenient manner. If, for whatever reason, complete abstinence is not achieved but surgery proceeds, the physician should limit the distance the nipple is translocated and perform a far less aggressive dissection in hopes of maintaining blood flow to the skin.

Obesity

Any patient with a body mass index (BMI) greater than or equal to 30 is considered obese.[11] A high BMI has been shown to be associated with wound healing complications, such as skin and fat necrosis, and a greatly increased risk of infection.[18,19,20] In one study in which patients were grouped based on the degree of obesity, those considered moderately obese (BMI 30–35) had a relative risk (RR) for major complications after reduction mammaplasty of 1.45 compared to the general population, and those considered severely obese (BMI 35–40) had an RR of 1.71 for major complications compared to the general population.[20] Additionally, obese patients have increased anesthesia risks.

Although it is certainly reasonable for the surgeon to calculate a patient's BMI at the preoperative visit, the individual patient's surgical risk stratification should be determined in collaboration with a primary care physician (PCP). Additionally, obese patients should be screened for diabetes, as this is a separate risk factor from obesity for postoperative complications and causes a significantly higher risk of nipple necrosis.[21] In cases where a reduction mammaplasty is being performed on an obese diabetic patient, the surgeon may need to accept a smaller volume reduction in order to prevent complications related to metabolic syndrome.

Since an increased BMI is considered a modifiable risk-factor, the option of preoperative weight loss should be encouraged in all overweight and obese patients if possible. In patients with a BMI over 30, this may even be required by some insurance agencies as a prerequisite for insurance coverage of the proposed breast reduction surgery.[4,6] However, some argue that weight loss may be difficult to achieve in patients with symptomatic macromastia due to the reduced functional capacity outlined in Section 7.2.1 and that surgery may promote additional weight loss after recovery.[22] It has been shown that obese patients lose an average of almost 9 lb (4 kg) after breast reduction surgery, which is far more than the weight lost through the surgical resection of breast tissue.[13] A large multicenter prospective trial called the Breast Reduction Assessment: Value and Outcomes (BRAVO) study showed that obesity did not change the benefits of reduction mammaplasty surgery and that, despite pressure from insurance companies, physicians should not use obesity as a justification for not surgically treating symptomatic macromastia.[12] However, patients should be informed of the effects of significant weight gain or loss after surgery, as this can permanently distort previously acceptable aesthetic results.

7.2.5 Age

Although most patients who present for evaluation of symptomatic macromastia are 30–40 years of age, there is a small proportion of patients who present well before or after this age seeking surgical intervention for their breast hypertrophy or ptosis.[3] Additional time should be spent in the preoperative setting when considering treatment of macromastia in such younger or older patients, as special consideration needs to be given to ensure proper management.

Adolescent Patients

The adolescent female patient population is usually defined as girls 11–17 years of age. In the past, there has been a general reluctance to treat these patients surgically, as it was felt that intervention for cosmetic reasons should be deferred until adulthood. However, recently, there has been a slowly growing trend to intervene at an earlier age, since multiple studies demonstrate the significant emotional sequelae that can occur if macromastia is left untreated.[23] For example, macromastia in the adolescent can cause social issues and stressors, leading the adolescent patient to avoid social situations where there is chance for ridicule or other undesirable peer responses. This reluctance to be involved in the social setting can ultimately impede emotional growth.[14] As such, increasing numbers of young patients are being referred by their pediatrician, PCP, or gynecologist for plastic surgical evaluation and possible treatment of their breast hypertrophy.[23] In these cases, physicians should encourage parental involvement and education, as patients who are under the age of 18 are considered a venerable population and will need parent or guardian consent for any surgical intervention. Additionally, it is important to note that adolescent patients tend to be more motivated by cosmetic concerns than the adult patient population is. Therefore, before proceeding with breast reduction surgery, the treating physician needs to be sure that the patient and her parents understand that they will be trading breast size for extensive permanent scars.

There is a general consensus among physicians that, regardless of age, it is better to wait for surgery until after complete breast development. However, in cases as just described where emotional disturbances are present because of the macromastia, surgery can reasonably be performed as early as after 1 to 2 years of stable breast size. This precaution is in place to decrease or prevent the risk of postoperative recurrence of excess breast tissue.

Additionally, in order to ensure proper treatment, it is important to identify the type of macromastia present in each patient, as certain types have a higher chance of recurrence and should be managed accordingly. Usually, adolescent patients have what is known as adolescent macromastia. In these cases, a reduction mammaplasty is a reasonable option once breast size has plateaued. However, there is a growing proportion of patients with BMI over 30 who have obesity-related breast hypertrophy. In these cases, patients should be strongly encouraged to lose weight, as doing so can often dramatically reduce breast size, which is not necessarily the case for other types of macromastia. Rarely, patients with juvenile gigantomastia will present for surgical evaluation. These patients have extreme cases of breast hypertrophy at a very young age and, due to the high rate of symptom recurrence, should be counseled on the increased likelihood of needing repeat reduction surgery.[8,23,24]

Elderly Patients

Patients over the age of 65 occasionally present for breast reduction consultation; however, their issue is often more with breast ptosis than with actual macromastia. Additionally, they tend to be more motivated by symptom control than by aesthetic concerns.[1] In forming an operative plan in accordance with this, the physician must recall that the elderly patient population has significantly more comorbidities and, therefore, is at increased surgical risk. This risk includes not just wound healing but also increased risk with general anesthesia. As such, the preoperative evaluation of these patients should be coordinated with a PCP or medical specialist to order and review any necessary electrocardiograms (EKG), chest X-rays, or other screening exams. Approval from these consulting physicians should also be obtained in writing prior to scheduling of any elective surgery.

Patients need to be counseled on their individual risk of surgical complication to decide whether this outweighs the benefits of the procedure. Despite the need for this extended workup, physicians should remember that reduction mammaplasty and mastopexy can be safely performed in older patients with appropriate patient selection and collaboration from consulting physicians.[1] Elective breast surgery is, overall, considered a low-risk procedure with small chance for significant blood loss, and the elderly population should not be excluded from the documented benefits of surgery based on age alone.[1]

7.2.6 Postradiation

Evaluating the postradiation patient for elective breast surgery can be a daunting task, since there is a reported complication rate of between 50 and 60% in this population.[25,26] It has been shown that the amount of radiation is directly proportional to risk for surgical complications such as delayed wound healing, nipple necrosis, and prolonged erythema.[27] Therefore, if surgery is attempted, it is important for the surgeon to be cautious intraoperatively; design flaps with shorter, wider pedicles; and avoid excessive undermining of flaps to give the tissue the best chance for survival. Additionally, the choice of pedicle may need to be based on the previous lumpectomy location, with the understanding that past surgery may have disrupted the normal blood flow, and therefore the lumpectomy site should, if possible, not be included in the pedicle.[27] In the event that a wound complication is encountered in the postoperative setting, physicians may consider ordering hyperbaric oxygen therapy, which has been shown to improve delayed wound healing in the irradiated patient.[28] Overall, as long as patients are educated on the risks of surgery on irradiated tissue, they should not be discouraged from undergoing reduction mammaplasty for symmetry or other cosmetic concerns.

Alternatively, as a way of avoiding additional surgery on irradiated tissue, some patients with a known existing breast malignancy who are undergoing lumpectomy may be offered the option of a simultaneous oncoplastic reduction at the time of mass resection.[29] Not only does this reduce the total number of operations, but it allows the reduction to be performed before any radiation treatment is begun, dramatically reducing the rate of wound healing complications.[30]

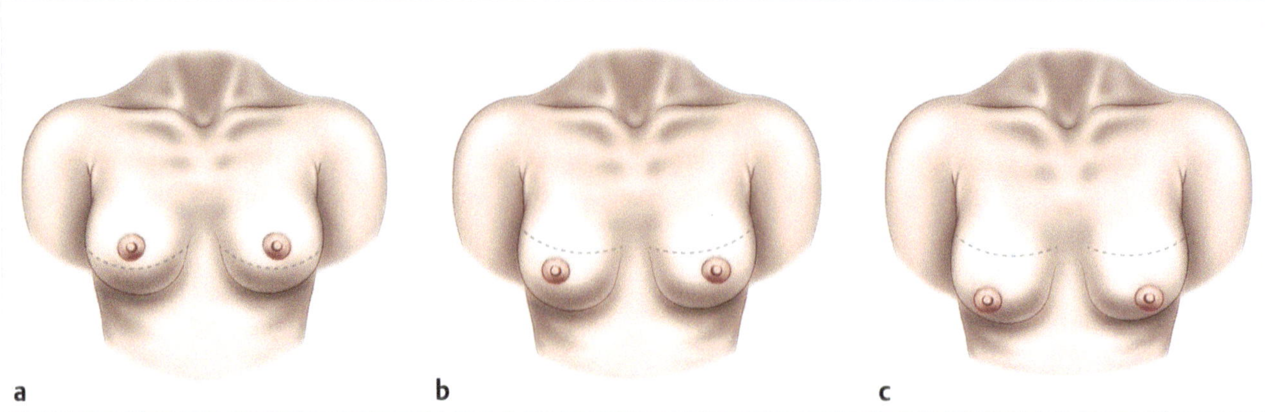

Fig. 7.1 Regnault's breast ptosis classification system. (a) First-degree/minor ptosis: the nipple lies at the level of the submammary fold, above the lower contour of the gland and skin brassiere. (b) Second-degree/moderate ptosis: the nipple lies below the level of the fold but remains above the lower contour of the breast and skin brassiere. (c) Third-degree/major ptosis: the nipple lies below the fold level and at the lower contour of the breast and skin brassiere. (Adapted from Regnault P. Breast ptosis. Definition and treatment. Clin Plast Surg 1976;3(2):193–203.)

7.2.7 Psychosocial Factors

Approximately 30% of patients who seek breast reduction surgery have a history of a psychiatric disorder that required some form of treatment.[31] Although most disorders are mild forms of anxiety or depression, identifying patients with a psychiatric history is important because patients with depression generally have unrealistic expectations and perceive their surgical outcomes as worse compared to the general population.[5] Even when patients do not have a diagnosed condition, those with poor coping mechanisms or poor support systems may not be good candidates for elective surgery. In these cases, surgery may not resolve their emotional distress, and an individual's dissatisfaction about her breasts may just shift to another part of her body after surgery.[32]

When assessing patients at their initial preoperative appointment, physicians should consider a complex psychiatric history or a history of multiple cosmetic procedures as indicators of a more complex emotional or psychological situation. However, in select cases, studies have shown that reduction mammaplasty may be considered as a possible way to significantly improve depression, anxiety, and low self-esteem in patients whose large breasts are the true source of their emotional distress.[31,32] In these patients, positive emotional results have shown to last for up to 5 years after surgery.[5]

7.2.8 Physical Examination

It is important to have a complete understanding of the patient's preoperative breast aesthetics in order to plan for possible surgical intervention. Elements of the breast that should be examined include the preoperative breast size, the areolar diameter, the NAC position, and degree of nipple ptosis. Breast and nipple ptosis can be assessed by analyzing the NAC in relation to the inframammary fold (IMF). This technique was discussed in an early paper by Regnault in which breast ptosis was grouped into three broad categories.[33] He describes first-degree, or minor, ptosis as when "the nipple lies at the level of the submammary fold, above the lower contour of the gland and skin brassiere." Second-degree, or moderate, ptosis occurs when "the nipple lies below the level of the fold but remains above the lower contour of the breast and skin brassiere." Finally, third-degree, or major, ptosis is found when "the nipple lies below the fold level and at the lower contour of the breast and skin brassiere" (▶ Fig. 7.1).[33,34] Additionally, the physician should mention any preexisting asymmetry, for example, differences in shape, volume, or anatomy such as a constricted pole. Assessment of the breast skin should also be completed as part of the physical exam. The skin quality, the amount of skin excess, and the presence of scars that would interfere with pedicle design should all be noted. This is of particular importance for postbariatric patients, who typically have excessive skin laxity and deflated tissue (see Chapter 10). Additionally, the physician must palpate the entirety of the breast for any masses.[14] Finally, photographs of the patient in the anteroposterior (AP), oblique, and lateral views should be obtained. These images can then be used for the patient's medical record, for preoperative planning, and for any required insurance documentation.

Some physicians advocate for recording specific breast surface measurements at the time of the preoperative appointment. Standard measurements that are often recorded include the sternal notch–to-nipple distance, the IMF-to-nipple distance, intermammary distance, and chest circumference. Additional measurements that have been proposed include orthogonal surface breast measurement (▶ Fig. 7.2). The horizontal breast distance is measured from the lateralmost aspect of the breast mound on the chest wall, over the nipple, to the medialmost aspect of the breast mound on the sternum. The vertical breast distance is recorded by measuring from the most cephalad point of the palpable breast tissue, over the nipple, to the IMF (▶ Fig. 7.3).[35] These measurements can be recorded not just for determination of the preoperative breast size and ptosis, but also to predict reduction mammaplasty resection weights, as discussed in Section 7.4, Preoperative Planning: Resection Weight and Size Goals.[35]

7.3 Preoperative Workup

The preoperative evaluation does not end with the initial consultation. Surgeons should work with primary care physicians

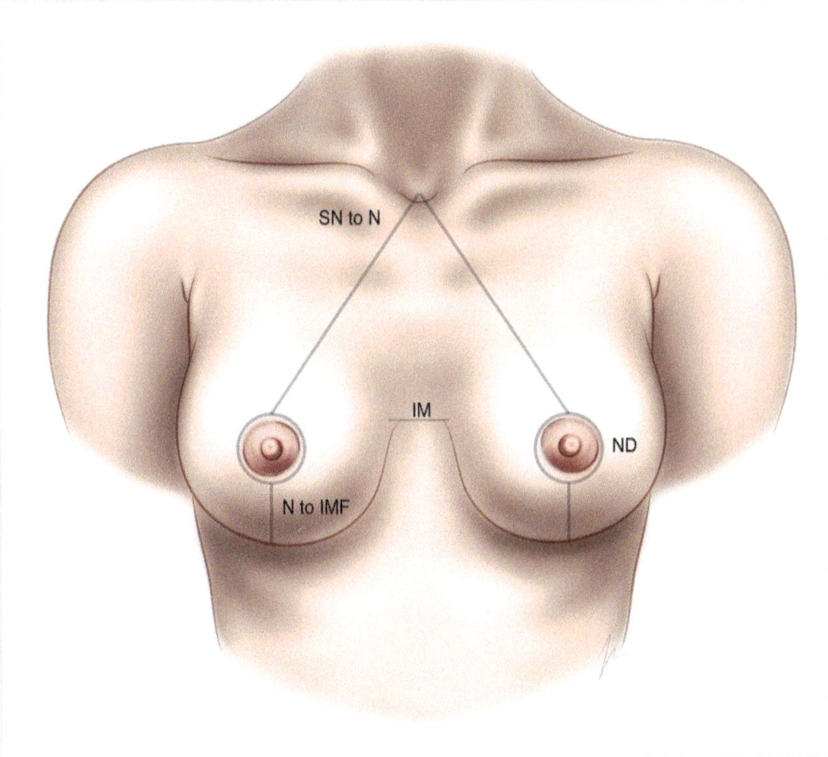

Fig. 7.2 Surface measurements of the breast. SS to N: sternal notch to nipple; IM: intermammary; N to IMF: nipple to inframammary fold; ND: nipple diameter.

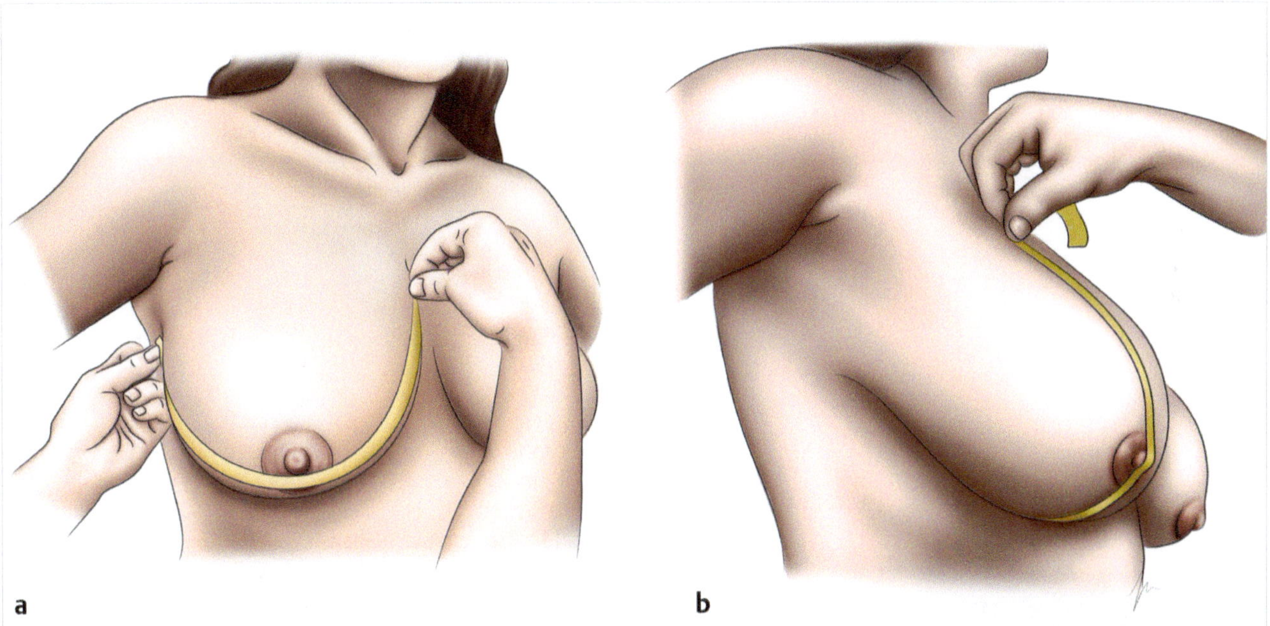

Fig. 7.3 **(a)** The horizontal measurement begins on the lateral aspect of the breast at the level of the lateral inframammary fold (IMF) and proceeds inferiorly, ending at the medial extent of the IMF where it approaches the sternum. **(b)** The vertical dimension is measured from the center of the IMF, over the breast meridian, to the superiormost aspect of the breast. (Adapted from Kocak E, Carruthers KH, McMahan JD. A reliable method for the preoperative estimation of tissue to be removed during reduction mammaplasty. Plast Reconstr Surg 2011;127(3):1059–1064.)

to optimize the patient's general health status prior to surgery. This includes eliminating or improving any modifiable risk factors or comorbidities, as just outlined. Although patients are often eager to proceed with surgical intervention, physicians must remember that reduction mammaplasty and mastopexy are elective surgeries and should be postponed until the patient is appropriately optimized.

7.3.1 Laboratory Studies

Preoperative blood work is a valuable tool for assessing a patient's overall health status prior to surgery. A complete blood count (CBC), complete metabolic panel (CMP), and coagulation studies, such as prothrombin time (PT), activated partial thromboplastin time (aPTT), and international normalized ratio (INR), are all basic studies that can provide a good general picture of a patient's health. Specific nutrition labs, such as albumin and prealbumin, should always be considered in addition to the basic labs if there is any concern for malnutrition, as this can greatly impact postoperative healing. It should be noted that even obese patients can be malnourished and should be screened for hypoalbuminemia regardless of BMI. It is reasonable to consider protein supplementation when testing indicates an albumin level of less than or equal to 3.0 g/dL.[36] Once initiated, these supplements should be continued through the early postoperative period to facilitate the initial wound healing.

7.3.2 Imaging Studies

Although there is little disadvantage to recommending a screening mammography prior to elective breast surgery, the American College of Surgeons (ACS) has issued no formal recommendations in regard to preoperative or postoperative imaging. Therefore, at a minimum, physicians should recommend that their patients follow the same guidelines as any nonoperative, asymptomatic patient in the general population. These guidelines advise any patients over 45 years old or any patients with a past personal history of breast cancer to undergo an annual mammogram.[37] In select cases, patients over 25 years of age may undergo screening if there is a strong family history of breast cancer. Mammograms are not typically recommended for patients less than 25 years old, as they are less sensitive in the dense breast tissue of younger patients. Ultrasound is the imaging modality of choice in the rare instances where young patients require breast imaging studies. Most surgeons require a mammogram within the last 12–24 months prior to surgery.[17] In some cases, a normal mammogram within this time period is also an insurance requirement.[9] No more advanced imaging is warranted in the preoperative setting if the screening mammography is normal.

Nationally, 11% of all mammograms performed warrant further evaluation and subsequent testing.[38] It should be noted that the rate of false positives is higher in patients with BMI > 30. Despite this, all suspicious masses should be thoroughly worked up regardless of the patient's BMI. It has been reported that malignancy is found in approximately 1.5% of all breast reduction specimens, and this discovery can dramatically complicate the clinical picture.[38] By requiring patients to have a recent, normal mammogram or to have a thorough malignancy workup when appropriate, it is hoped that this number will decline over time.

Because reduction mammaplasty and mastopexy will cause changes, including fat necrosis, fibrosis, and scar formation, that are visible on all subsequent postoperative breast imaging, some physicians recommend obtaining a new baseline mammogram 6 to 12 months postoperatively (▶ Fig. 7.4).[39,40] Although somewhat controversial, it is argued that establishing a new baseline will decrease the difficulty in detecting malignancy in future imaging studies.

7.4 Preoperative Planning: Resection Weight and Size Goals

When discussing current breast size and postoperative size goals, most patients feel comfortable discussing in terms of cup sizes and chest circumference measurements. However, often they are not aware that this sizing system is not standardized across companies or bra styles and is not an ideal way to quantify breast size (see also Chapter 2).[41] As such, photographs can be useful tools to help illustrate realistic postoperative sizing options and understand patient goals in regard to the amount of breast tissue that needs to be resected at the time of surgery. However, patients need to be informed of what postoperative size goals are realistic given their preoperative breast size. Extensive resection of tissue from the pedicle and thinning of the skin flaps can lead to serious complications. Thus, very large volume reductions are not always possible.

Prediction of breast tissue resection weights is an essential part of preoperative planning and is often required for insurance preauthorization. Insurance companies will use this information to determine whether they believe that surgery will result in a medical benefit for the patient.[7] Typically, for patients with an average body surface area (BSA), at least 400–500 mL of breast tissue per side is required for insurance approval.[11] In cases where less than 400 mL of breast tissue is to be removed but there is an excess in breast skin, a cosmetic mastopexy may be more appropriate.[17] For patients with 1 kg or more of excess breast tissue, regardless of BSA, a therapeutic reduction mammaplasty is usually covered.[9] Additionally, patients with greater than one cup size in asymmetry between breasts may qualify for insurance coverage regardless of the predicted resection weights.

Most insurance companies have adopted the Schnur Sliding Scale as a tool for further identifying patients who would experience medical benefit from breast reduction surgery. In 1991, Schnur published his technique which was based on the patient's individual BSA, calculated using height and weight measurements and the Mosteller formula, to predict the resection weight per breast.[9,10,42] If, when entered into Schnur's table, the patient's body surface area resulted in a resection weight that fell below the 22nd percentile, then the surgery would be deemed cosmetic and not medically necessary. However, since the time of this initial publication, Schnur and others have reported that this table is, in fact, not a useful tool for predicting improvement in symptoms.[12,43] Not only does the technique not account for patients with smaller skeletal frames, but the accuracy, reliability, and utility of predicting medical benefit based on a resection weight is highly controversial.

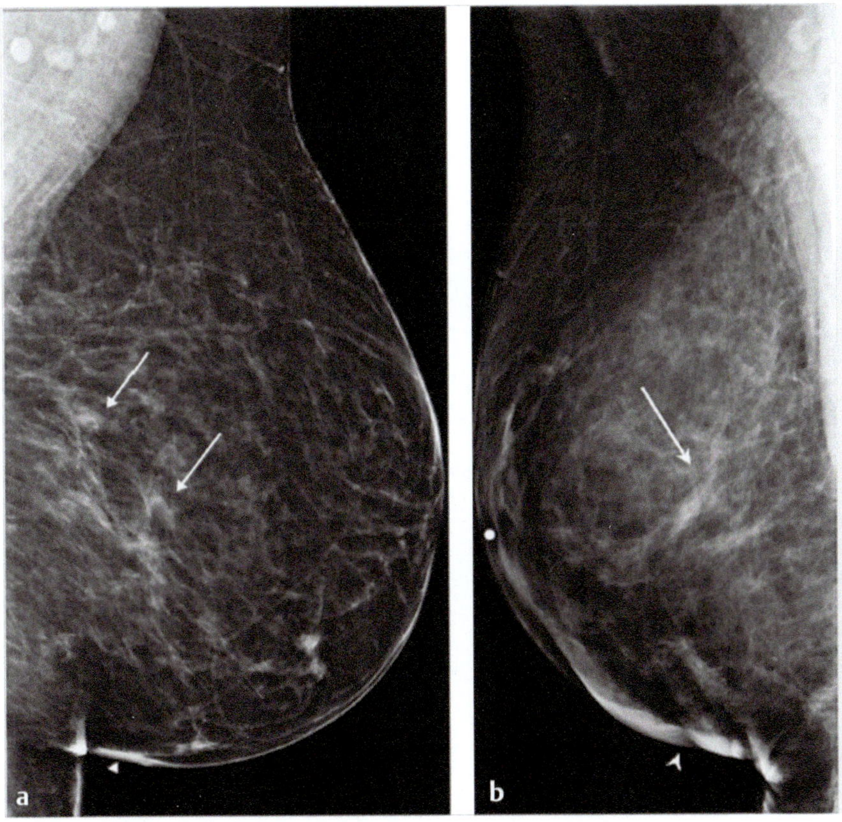

Fig. 7.4 **(a)** Medial lateral oblique mammographic view shows a band of mildly distorted tissue *(long arrows)* obliquely oriented in the breast, unusual in distribution for normal breast parenchyma but typical for postreduction change. Note skin thinkening in inframammary fold region *(arrowhead)*, also a common postreduction change. **(b)** Medial lateral oblique view in another patient showing the characteristic postreduction band of scar tissue *(long arrow)* and significant skin thickening *(arrowhead)* extended from nipple inferiorly to the inframammary fold. Note how high the nipple is situated on the breast *(marker ball)*.

In the past, multiple published studies have shown no significant correlation between resection weight and symptom improvement.[12,44,45]

Most practicing physicians would argue that it is more important for breast size to be proportional to body frame than for specific resection weights to be met. As such, publications have begun to emerge that advocate for anthropometric chest and breast measurements to be employed, rather than BSA or BMI calculations, when predicting breast tissue resection weights. This better accounts for variability in chest wall size and relies less on overall body volume. Chest circumference, sternal notch–to-nipple distance, nipple-to-IMF distance, and surface-based horizontal and vertical breast measurements have all been proposed.[35,46] The precise technique for obtaining these measurements was outlined previously. In one published study, it was shown that horizontal and vertical breast surface measurements alone could be used to estimate resection weights accurately.[35] Therefore, if insurance companies continue to require a preoperative approximate resection weight, regardless of data that shows that this is not a useful way to predict improvement in symptomatic macromastia, physicians should consider using surface measurements to provide an estimate that is more reflective of skeletal frame and body proportion.

7.5 Patient Education

It is very important that patients understand the risks and benefits of surgery before they agree to proceed with any surgical intervention. Educating patients on the possible complications as well as the expected outcomes after surgery is essential for the patient to perceive their surgery as successful. According to the BRAVO study, complications are higher with greater resection weights.[3,17,47] However, regardless of resected volume, overall surgical complication risk is approximately 5%.[48] From a medicolegal standpoint, the patient must be fully informed of this information prior to signing any surgical consent forms.[17]

7.5.1 Possible Complications

The most common complication after a reduction mammaplasty is delayed wound healing.[17,47] Additional complications include breast asymmetry, bottoming-out, and loss of sensation.[37] Occasionally, patients may encounter fat necrosis, leading to wound drainage, hematoma or seroma formation, infection, or even NAC necrosis, which is typically associated with larger resection weights and longer pedicle length.[7,17,18]

Loss of ability to breastfeed is another major concern. It has been documented that there is an approximately 50% chance of having an inability to breastfeed after reduction mammaplasty regardless of the surgical technique employed.[49] Therefore, the physician must determine whether the patient is currently able to breastfeed and how strong her desire is to breastfeed in the future. If she is adamant about maintaining this ability postoperatively, it is yet another reason to postpone surgery until after the patient has finished having children.

One of the points that patients must always understand is that they are trading a reduction in breast size for permanent breast scarring.[17] Hypertrophic scars, keloids, and painful scars may develop after surgery, but it is common to wait 6 months to 1 year before considering scar revision.[14,37] Since the scars associated with either reduction mammaplasty or mastopexy can be extensive, they can lead to patient dissatisfaction if not discussed preoperatively.[7,50]

7.5.2 Expected Outcomes

Despite the possible complications just outlined, studies have shown that the vast majority of patients are satisfied with their reduction mammaplasty, with approximately 75% indicating that they were "extremely satisfied" with outcome even if only a moderate amount of tissue was resected.[3,5] Moreover, 97% of patients would have the operation again and indicate a significantly improved quality of life postoperatively.[7,32,51] Shoulder pain and breast pain are the symptoms most constantly improved by surgery, but there have been published reports indicating that surgery also improves posture and results in at least partial correction of some preoperative spinal malalignment.[13,52] Another study showed that breast surgery can result in improved functionality, with approximately 75% of patients with a preoperative working disability returning to their jobs after reduction mammaplasty.[53] There are also reports of patients with a postoperative increase in ability to exercise, increased sociability and emotional stability, and improved sexual functioning.[5,7,11,13,31,32] Studies have even shown that an improved self-image persists at least to the 3- and 6-month follow-up appointments.[4,50]

7.6 Conclusions

Elective breast surgeries, including reduction mammaplasty and mastopexy, are considered to be some of the most successful surgeries performed in the field of plastic surgery.[5] When performing the preoperative assessment, a thorough history and physical examination is essential and enables the physician to identify each individual patient's motivation for surgery. Physicians who perform these procedures must understand the insurance criteria for coverage of breast reduction surgery. However, surgeons should not limit patient access to reduction mammoplasty based on a strict definition of symptomatic macromastia. Regardless of breast tissue resection weights, most patients consistently gain a more youthful appearance and experience a long-lasting improvement in quality of life after breast reduction surgery.[50]

Key Points

- The goals of reduction mammaplasty surgery are to reduce breast weight and volume, improve shape and asymmetry, and reposition the nipple areola complex (NAC).
- Patients present for consultation with complaints including a history of neck pain, shoulder grooving from bra straps, and intertrigo.
- Elements of the breast that should be examined include the preoperative breast size, the areolar diameter, the NAC position, and the degree of nipple ptosis.
- The scars associated with breast reduction surgery can be extensive, and each patient's individual risk of scar hypertrophy, hyperpigmentation, or keloid formation should be acknowledged.
- The potential loss of ability to breastfeed must be considered when deciding whether a reduction mammaplasty is appropriate for a specific patient at a given time.

References

[1] Nelson JA, Fischer JP, Wink JD, Kovach SJ, III. A population-level analysis of bilateral breast reduction: does age affect early complications? Aesthet Surg J. 2014; 34(3):409–416

[2] Karamanos E, Wei B, Siddiqui A, Rubinfeld I. Tobacco use and body mass index as predictors of outcomes in patients undergoing breast reduction mammoplasty. Ann Plast Surg. 2015; 75(4):383–387

[3] Brown DM, Young VL. Reduction mammoplasty for macromastia. Aesthetic Plast Surg. 1993; 17(3):211–223

[4] Ducic I, Iorio ML, Al-Attar A. Chronic headaches/migraines: extending indications for breast reduction. Plast Reconstr Surg. 2010; 125(1):44–49

[5] Valtonen JPSL, Setälä LP, Mustonen PK, Blom M. Can the efficacy of reduction mammoplasty be predicted? The applicability and predictive value of Breast-Related Symptoms Questionnaire in measuring breast-related symptoms pre- and postoperatively. J Plast Reconstr Aesthet Surg. 2014; 67(5):676–681

[6] Seitchik MW. Reduction mammaplasty: criteria for insurance coverage. Plast Reconstr Surg. 1995; 95(6):1029–1032

[7] Brühlmann Y, Tschopp H. Breast reduction improves symptoms of macromastia and has a long-lasting effect. Ann Plast Surg. 1998; 41(3):240–245

[8] Netscher DT, Mosharrafa AM, Laucirica R. Massive asymmetric virginal breast hypertrophy. South Med J. 1996; 89(4):434–437

[9] Aetna. Breast Reduction Surgery and Gynecomastia Surgery. URL: http://www.aetna.com/cpb/medical/data/1_99/0017.html. Last reviewed May 22, 2019. Accessed July 12, 2019

[10] Bridgespan. Medical Policy Manual: Reduction Mammaplasty. URL: https://www.policy.bridgespanhealth.com/surgery/sur60.pdf. Effective: December 17, 2018. Accessed July 12, 2019

[11] Aydin D, Hansen LB, Ikander P, Drejøe JB, Lambaa S, Hölmich LR. Poor adherence to clinical guidelines for women undergoing breast reduction. Dan Med J. 2016; 63(1):A5179

[12] Nguyen JT, Wheatley MJ, Schnur PL, Nguyen TA, Winn SR. Reduction mammaplasty: a review of managed care medical policy coverage criteria. Plast Reconstr Surg. 2008; 121(4):1092–1100

[13] Miller AP, Zacher JB, Berggren RB, Falcone RE, Monk J. Breast reduction for symptomatic macromastia: can objective predictors for operative success be identified? Plast Reconstr Surg. 1995; 95(1):77–83

[14] Hammond DC, Loffredo M. Breast reduction. Plast Reconstr Surg. 2012; 129 (5):829e–839e

[15] Schumacher HH. Breast reduction and smoking. Ann Plast Surg. 2005; 54(2): 117–119

[16] Bartsch RH, Weiss G, Kästenbauer T, et al. Crucial aspects of smoking in wound healing after breast reduction surgery. J Plast Reconstr Aesthet Surg. 2007; 60(9):1045–1049

[17] Shestak KC, Davidson EH. Assessing risk and avoiding complications in breast reduction. Clin Plast Surg. 2016; 43(2):323–331

[18] Henry SL, Crawford JL, Puckett CL. Risk factors and complications in reduction mammaplasty: novel associations and preoperative assessment. Plast Reconstr Surg. 2009; 124(4):1040–1046

[19] Nelson JA, Fischer JP, Chung CU, et al. Obesity and early complications following reduction mammaplasty: an analysis of 4545 patients from the 2005–2011 NSQIP datasets. J Plast Surg Hand Surg. 2014; 48(5):334–339

[20] Myung Y, Heo CY. Relationship between obesity and surgical complications after reduction mammaplasty: a systematic literature review and meta-analysis. Aesthet Surg J. 2016

[21] Lewin R, Göransson M, Elander A, Thorarinsson A, Lundberg J, Lidén M. Risk factors for complications after breast reduction surgery. J Plast Surg Hand Surg. 2014; 48(1):10–14

[22] Sarıcı M, Demirseren ME, Durgun M, Ceran C, Yenidunya MO. Effects of reduction mammoplasty on metabolic profile and body weight. Aesthetic Plast Surg. 2011; 35(6):995–999

[23] Xue AS, Wolfswinkel EM, Weathers WM, Chike-Obi C, Heller L. Breast reduction in adolescents: indication, timing, and a review of the literature. J Pediatr Adolesc Gynecol. 2013; 26(4):228–233

[24] Rohrich RJ, Thornton JF, Sorokin ES. Recurrent mammary hyperplasia: current concepts. Plast Reconstr Surg. 2003; 111(1):387–393, quiz 394

[25] Patel KM, Hannan CM, Gatti ME, Nahabedian MY. A head-to-head comparison of quality of life and aesthetic outcomes following immediate, staged-immediate, and delayed oncoplastic reduction mammaplasty. Plast Reconstr Surg. 2011; 127(6):2167–2175

[26] Kronowitz SJ, Hunt KK, Kuerer HM, et al. Practical guidelines for repair of partial mastectomy defects using the breast reduction technique in patients undergoing breast conservation therapy. Plast Reconstr Surg. 2007; 120(7): 1755–1768

[27] Spear SL, Rao SS, Patel KM, Nahabedian MY. Reduction mammaplasty and mastopexy in previously irradiated breasts. Aesthet Surg J. 2014; 34(1):74–78

[28] Korpinar S, Cimsit M, Cimsit B, Bugra D, Buyukbabani N. Adjunctive hyperbaric oxygen therapy in radiation-induced non-healing wound. J Dermatol. 2006; 33(7):496–497

[29] Emiroglu M, Salimoglu S, Karaali C, et al. Oncoplastic reduction mammoplasty for breast cancer in women with macromastia: oncological long-term outcomes. Asian J Surg. 2017; 40(1):41–47

[30] Kronowitz SJ, Kuerer HM, Buchholz TA, Valero V, Hunt KK. A management algorithm and practical oncoplastic surgical techniques for repairing partial mastectomy defects. Plast Reconstr Surg. 2008; 122(6):1631–1647

[31] Cerovac S, Ali FS, Blizard R, Lloyd G, Butler PE. Psychosexual function in women who have undergone reduction mammaplasty. Plast Reconstr Surg. 2005; 116(5):1306–1313

[32] Faria FS, Guthrie E, Bradbury E, Brain AN. Psychosocial outcome and patient satisfaction following breast reduction surgery. Br J Plast Surg. 1999; 52(6):448–452

[33] Regnault P. Breast ptosis. Definition and treatment. Clin Plast Surg. 1976; 3 (2):193–203

[34] Kirwan L. A classification and algorithm for treatment of breast ptosis. Aesthet Surg J. 2002; 22(4):355–363

[35] Kocak E, Carruthers KH, McMahan JD. A reliable method for the preoperative estimation of tissue to be removed during reduction mammaplasty. Plast Reconstr Surg. 2011; 127(3):1059–1064

[36] Leung JSSJ, Seto A, Li GK. Association between preoperative nutritional status and postoperative outcome in head and neck cancer patients. Nutr Cancer. 2017; 69(3):464–469

[37] Hall-Findlay EJ, Shestak KC. Breast reduction. Plast Reconstr Surg. 2015; 136 (4):531e–544e

[38] Campbell MJ, Clark CJ, Paige KT. The role of preoperative mammography in women considering reduction mammoplasty: a single institution review of 207 patients. Am J Surg. 2010; 199(5):636–640

[39] Ortiz-Pomales YT, Priyanka Handa, Newell MS, Losken A. Reduction mammaplasty and breast cancer screening. Clin Plast Surg. 2016; 43(2):333–339

[40] Cathcart RS, III, Hagerty RC. Preoperative and postoperative considerations in elective breast operations. Ann Plast Surg. 1989; 22(6):533–538

[41] Bengtson BP, Glicksman CA. The standardization of bra cup measurements: redefining bra sizing language. Clin Plast Surg. 2015; 42(4):405–411

[42] Schnur PL, Hoehn JG, Ilstrup DM, Cahoy MJ, Chu CP. Reduction mammaplasty: cosmetic or reconstructive procedure? Ann Plast Surg. 1991; 27(3):232–237

[43] Strong B, Hall-Findlay EJ. How does volume of resection relate to symptom relief for reduction mammaplasty patients? Ann Plast Surg. 2015; 75(4):376–382

[44] Spector JA, Singh SP, Karp NS. Outcomes after breast reduction: does size really matter? Ann Plast Surg. 2008; 60(5):505–509

[45] Radosa JC, Radosa MP, Baum S, Mavrova R, Camara O. Reduction mammaplasty for symptomatic macromastia: which factors influence the post-operative outcome? Arch Gynecol Obstet. 2013; 287(4):715–722

[46] Kececi Y, Sir E. Prediction of resection weight in reduction mammaplasty based on anthropometric measurements. Breast Care (Basel). 2014; 9(1):41–45

[47] Cunningham BL, Gear AJ, Kerrigan CL, Collins ED. Analysis of breast reduction complications derived from the BRAVO study. Plast Reconstr Surg. 2005; 115 (6):1597–1604

[48] Fischer JP, Cleveland EC, Shang EK, Nelson JA, Serletti JM. Complications following reduction mammaplasty: a review of 3538 cases from the 2005–2010 NSQIP data sets. Aesthet Surg J. 2014; 34(1):66–73

[49] Kakagia D, Tripsiannis G, Tsoutsos D. Breastfeeding after reduction mammaplasty: a comparison of 3 techniques. Ann Plast Surg. 2005; 55(4):343–345

[50] Shakespeare V, Cole RP. Measuring patient-based outcomes in a plastic surgery service: breast reduction surgical patients. Br J Plast Surg. 1997; 50(4): 242–248

[51] Hermans BJ, Boeckx WD, De Lorenzi F, van der Hulst RR. Quality of life after breast reduction. Ann Plast Surg. 2005; 55(3):227–231

[52] Karabekmez FEGA, Gokkaya A, Isik C, Saglam I, Efeoglu FB, Gorgu M. Does reduction mammaplasty revert skeletal disturbances in the vertebral column of patients with macromastia? A preliminary study. Aesthetic Plast Surg. 2014; 38(1):104–112

[53] Atterhem H, Holmner S, Janson PE. Reduction mammaplasty: symptoms, complications, and late results. A retrospective study on 242 patients. Scand J Plast Reconstr Surg Hand Surg. 1998; 32(3):281–286

8 Mastopexy Techniques—Basic Principles

Elizabeth J. Hall-Findlay

Summary

Numerous techniques have been described to perform a mastopexy. This chapter reviews key concepts in understanding the footprint and how to get good, consistent, predictable results. Assessment of ptosis is re-evaluated to make surgical planning easier. The concept of parenchymal rearrangement is emphasized versus the failure of the skin as a brassiere. Different methods are reviewed, and emphasis is placed on the inferior flap of Ribeiro as being the most effective.

Keywords: mastopexy, ptosis, nipple ptosis, glandular ptosis, breast footprint, upper breast border, inferior flap mastopexy, parenchymal rearrangement, skin brassiere

8.1 Introduction

The most common complication after mastopexy is recurrent ptosis. This problem results from a lack of understanding of the principles of aesthetic breast surgery. Most patients who are candidates for mastopexy have already proven that their skin has functioned poorly as a brassiere. Trying to tighten up the skin envelope and then expecting the skin to hold the shape against gravity is doomed to failure.

The key to achieving good consistent results in mastopexy surgery is first to understand the role of the breast footprint. The surgeon then needs to understand the difference between nipple ptosis and glandular ptosis and then to plan accordingly. Correcting nipple ptosis is the easy part. Correcting glandular ptosis entails an understanding of what true ptosis is and how important parenchymal reshaping is to the final outcome.

We have been taught over the years that the inframammary fold (IMF) is the best landmark for determining ptosis.[1] Unfortunately, this classification is misleading because it relates only to nipple ptosis and does not take into account glandular ptosis. The upper breast border is a better landmark than the IMF for planning a mastopexy.

8.2 Key Concepts

8.2.1 Breast Footprint

The actual attachment of the breast to the chest wall (footprint or base[2,3]) varies significantly from patient to patient, and the breast borders can be only minimally changed with surgery. Some patients are "high-breasted" and some patients are "low-breasted." It is important to understand that the breast borders can be altered only by adding or removing volume. The upper breast border can be elevated only with an implant (or fat injections), and the lower breast border (IMF) can be elevated when weight is removed, but it descends when weight is added. The medial and lateral breast borders are adjusted by adding volume (implant) or removing volume (liposuction). It is less about the skin than it is about the volume and weight (▶ Fig. 8.1, ▶ Fig. 8.2).[4,5,6,7,8]

8.2.2 Nipple Ptosis

The nipple needs to be "centralized" on the breast mound. The surgeon needs to understand not only the footprint but what can and cannot be achieved with manipulating the breast mound in order to determine the ideal nipple position. On an average "C-cup" breast on an average woman, the ideal nipple position is about 8–10 cm below the upper breast border and about 8–10 cm from the chest midline (drawn as a straight line, not curved around the breast).[9] Although some surgeons state that breasts look best with the nipple at 55% up from the bottom of the breast just above the horizontal meridian,[10] this could lead to patient dissatisfaction. Over time, breasts tend to bottom out, and high nipples are very difficult for patients to hide in clothing and bathing suits without suffering "nipple slip." The high nipple might look good in magazines with the back arched and the arms elevated to reduce glandular ptosis, but the high nipple can be a problem in clothing (▶ Fig. 8.3).

8.2.3 Glandular Ptosis

The surgeon needs to determine how much of the gland is sagging, or ptotic, and correct it. Ptotic gland tissue can be either removed (breast reduction) or moved (mastopexy). Although nipple ptosis can be easily corrected by repositioning, the breast mound needs to be corrected with parenchymal reshaping. Adjusting the skin brassiere will not correct glandular ptosis. The location of the IMF is less important than the actual amount of ptotic gland (▶ Fig. 8.4).

It is clear from the above that the Regnault[1] classification of breast ptosis (nipple position in relation to the IMF) can be misleading. What is important is an assessment of the breast mound—both the amount of glandular ptosis and the degree of nipple ptosis. The position of the IMF can be misleading in planning. It is important, however, for the surgeon to understand that the upper portion of the footprint will not change. The upper breast border is a better landmark for decision making (Spear S; personal communication).

8.2.4 Skin Brassiere versus Parenchymal Reshaping

Gravity wins. Skin is not a particularly good brassiere, especially when it has already shown that it is not good at holding the breast up, as occurs with most patients presenting for a mastopexy (▶ Fig. 8.5).

8.2.5 The Wise Pattern

The Wise pattern (not just the keyhole opening) is important for the surgeon to use as a template for the parenchyma (and not the skin)—for what should be left behind. Dr Robert Wise developed the pattern from a deconstructed brassiere.[11] Note that when the pattern is closed, it results in a nice coned breast shape. He used it for a skin pattern, but it is better used for the parenchymal pattern (▶ Fig. 8.6a,b).

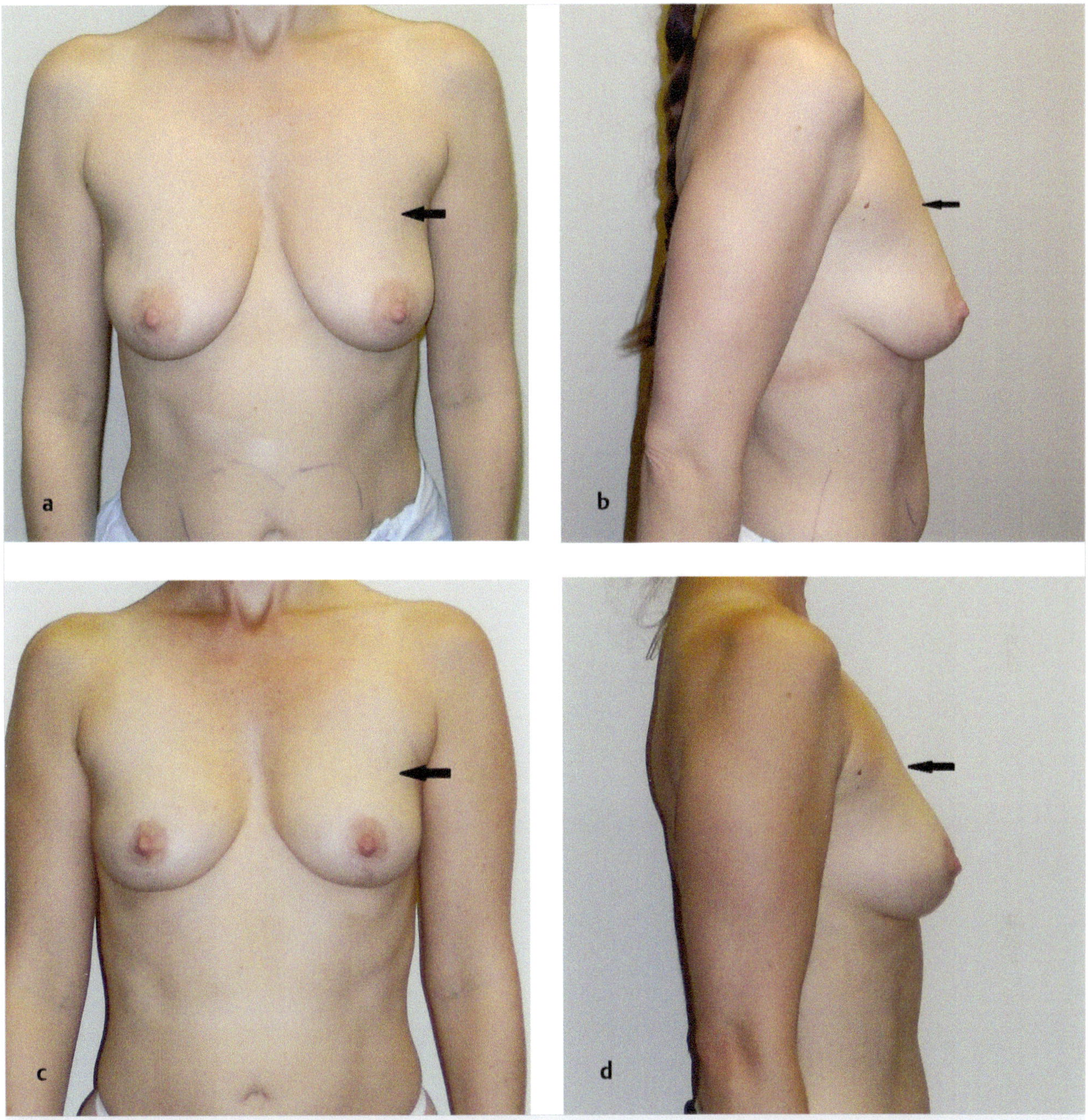

Fig. 8.1 Mastopexy in patient with high footprint. **(a,b)** Patient aged 41 at presentation. The black arrow marks the higher upper breast border, which does not change after a mastopexy. She was 5 ft 2 in (157 cm) tall, weighed 110 lb (50 kg), and had skin only removed from both breasts. **(c,d)** Patient at 15 months after surgery, which involved "moving" the glandular ptosis via an inferior flap; in her case, the inferior flap was held up under a pectoralis sling. Although the sling can be powerful, the flap sometimes remains as a bump, and it is better to let both the flap and the breast parenchyma settle as a unit.

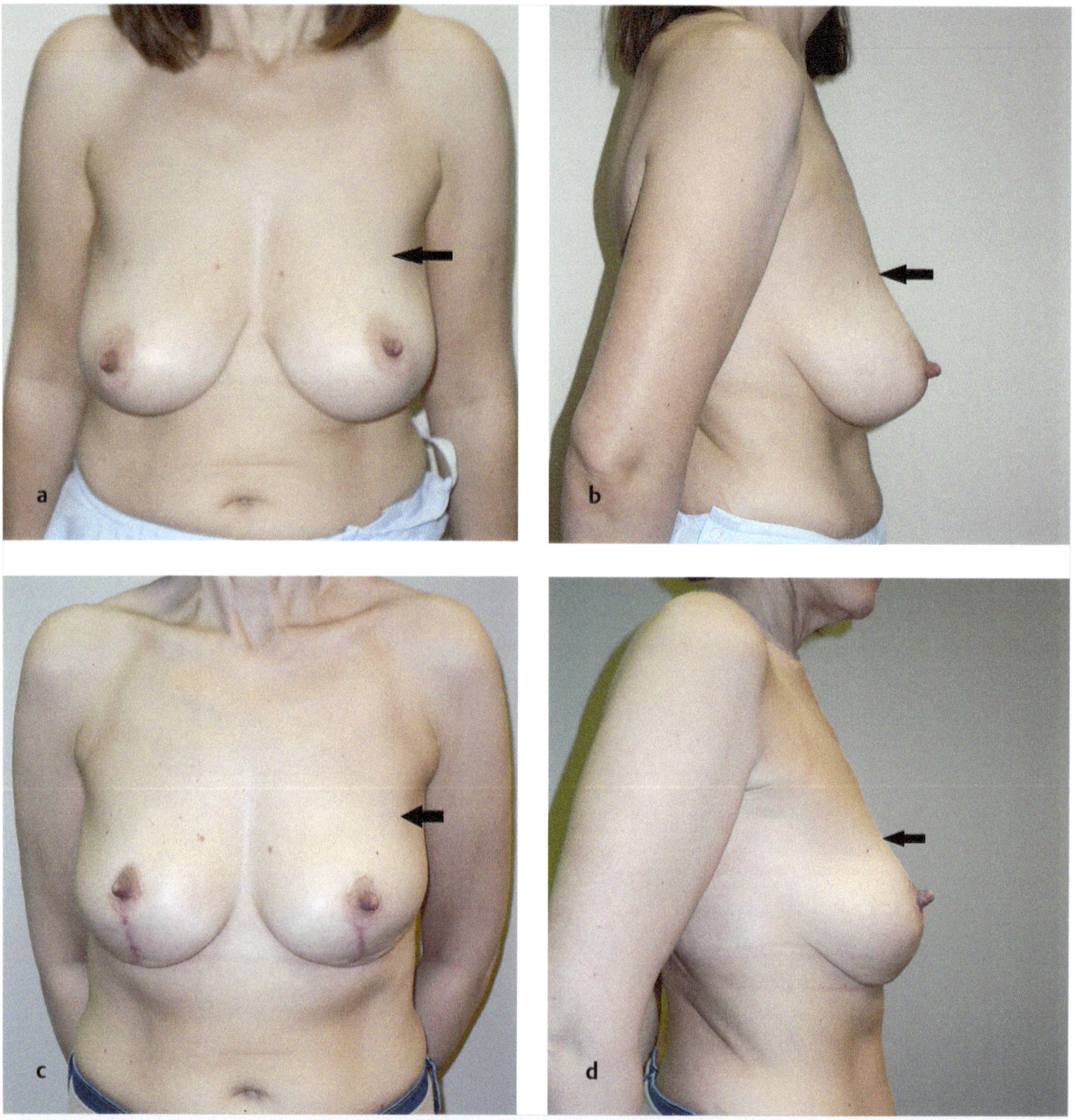

Fig. 8.2 Mastopexy in patient with low footprint. **(a,b)** Patient aged 46 at presentation. The black arrow marks the relatively low upper breast border, which does not change after a mastopexy or a breast reduction. She was 5 ft 3 in (160 cm) tall, weighed 122 lb (55 kg), and had 64 grams removed from the right breast and 181 grams from the left breast along with 250 mL of liposuction. **(c,d)** Patient at 9 months after surgery, which involved removing the glandular ptosis.[8] Note also how the upper breast border *(large arrows)* has not changed postoperatively.

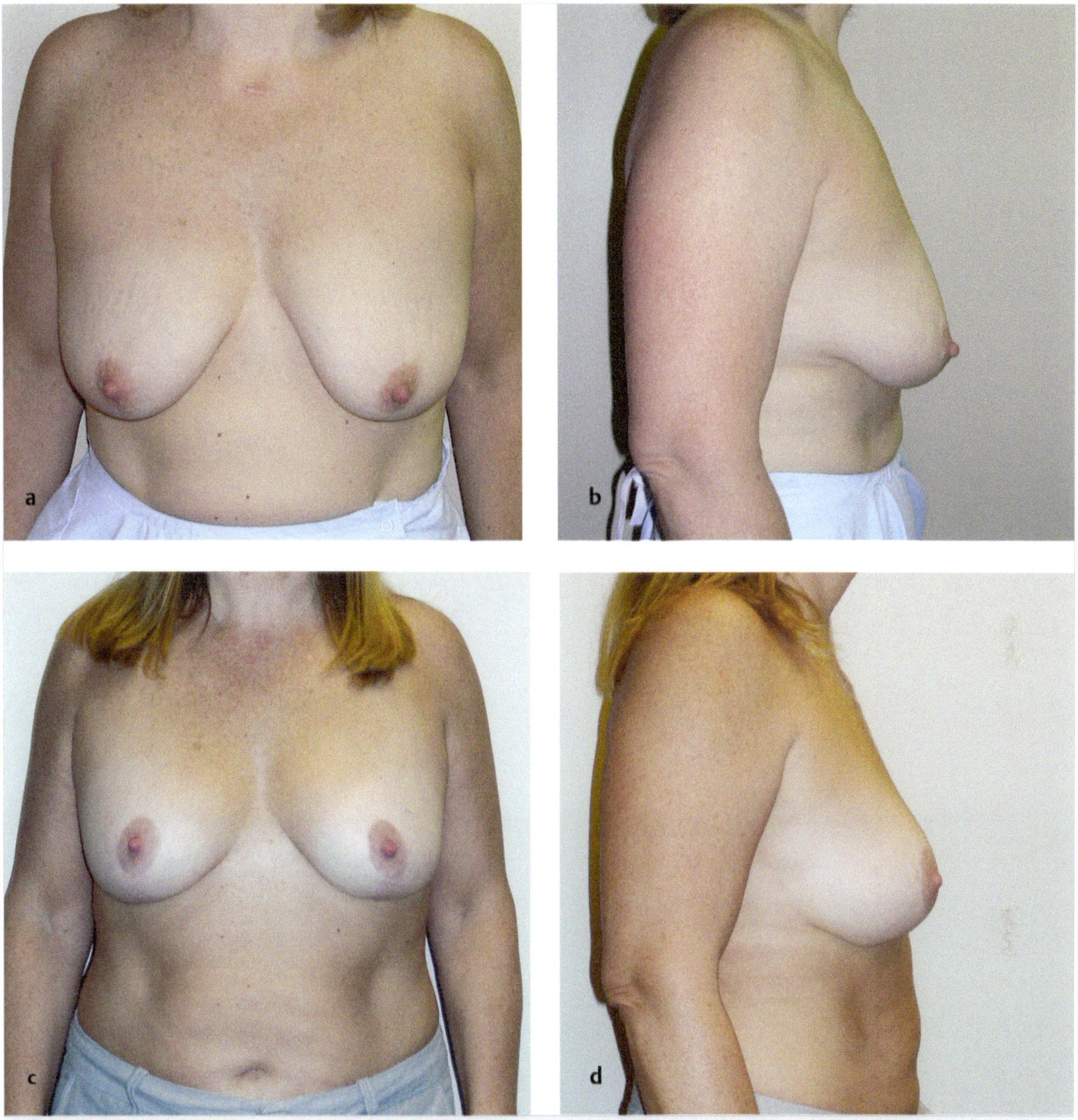

Fig. 8.3 Nipple ptosis. **(a,b)** Patient aged 23 at presentation with nipple ptosis and only a small amount of glandular ptosis. She was 5 ft 5 in (165 cm) tall, weighed 164 lb (74 kg), and had skin only removed from both breasts. **(c,d)** Patient at 6 years after surgery, which involved some glandular ptosis correction but mainly nipple ptosis correction. She did have an inferior flap held up with a pectoralis sling (which was probably not necessary).

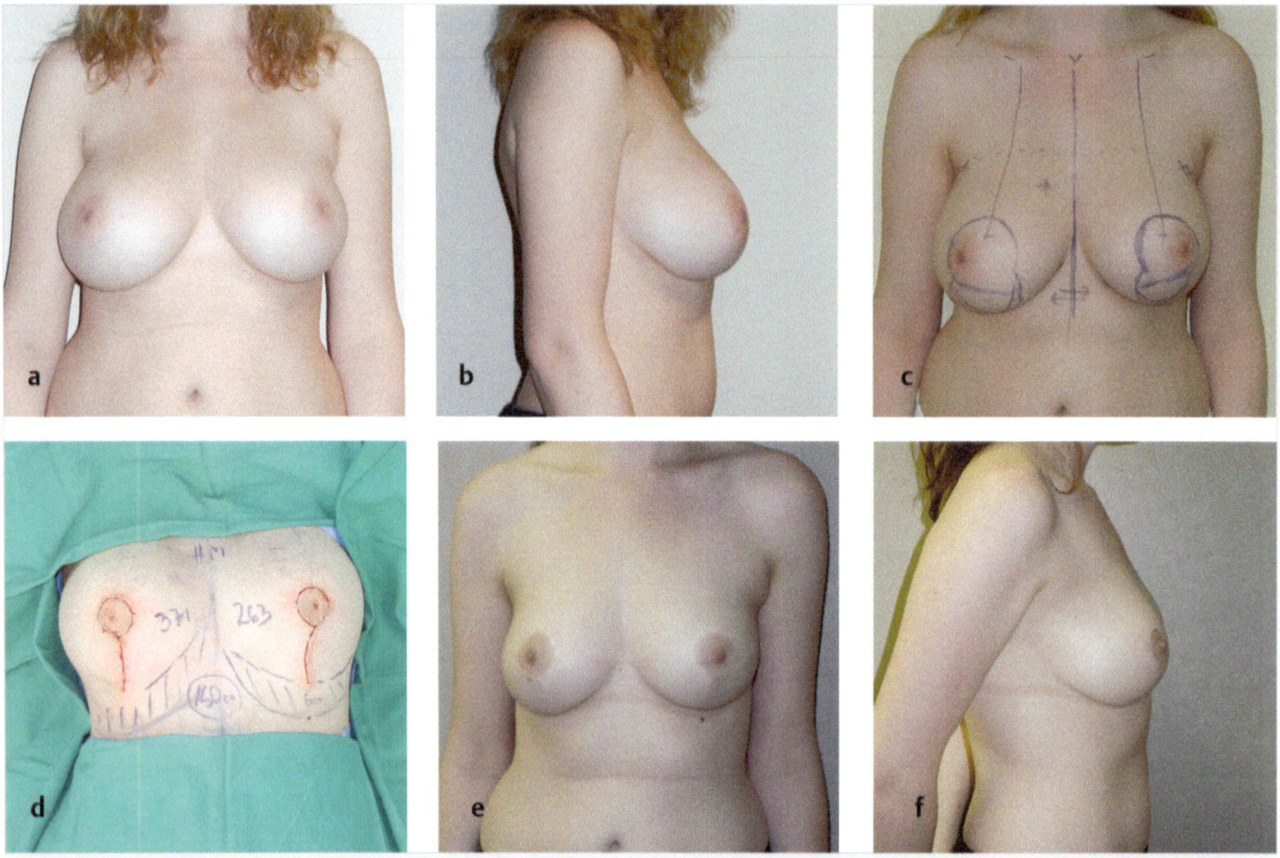

Fig. 8.4 Glandular ptosis. **(a,b)** Patient aged 18 at presentation with glandular ptosis but without nipple ptosis, so the position of the nipple in relation to the inframammary fold (IMF) is irrelevant. She was 5 ft 8 in (173 cm) tall and weighed 153 lb (69 kg). **(c,d)** Correction of glandular ptosis by removal of 371 grams from the right breast and 263 grams from the left breast. She had another 150 mL of fat removed with liposuction. The nipples were, however, too lateral, and they needed to be moved to the ideal breast meridian. **(e,f)** Patient at 2 years after her breast reduction. Her IMF was raised 2 cm by removing the tissue just above the fold. This removed weight, which then allowed the fold to rise.

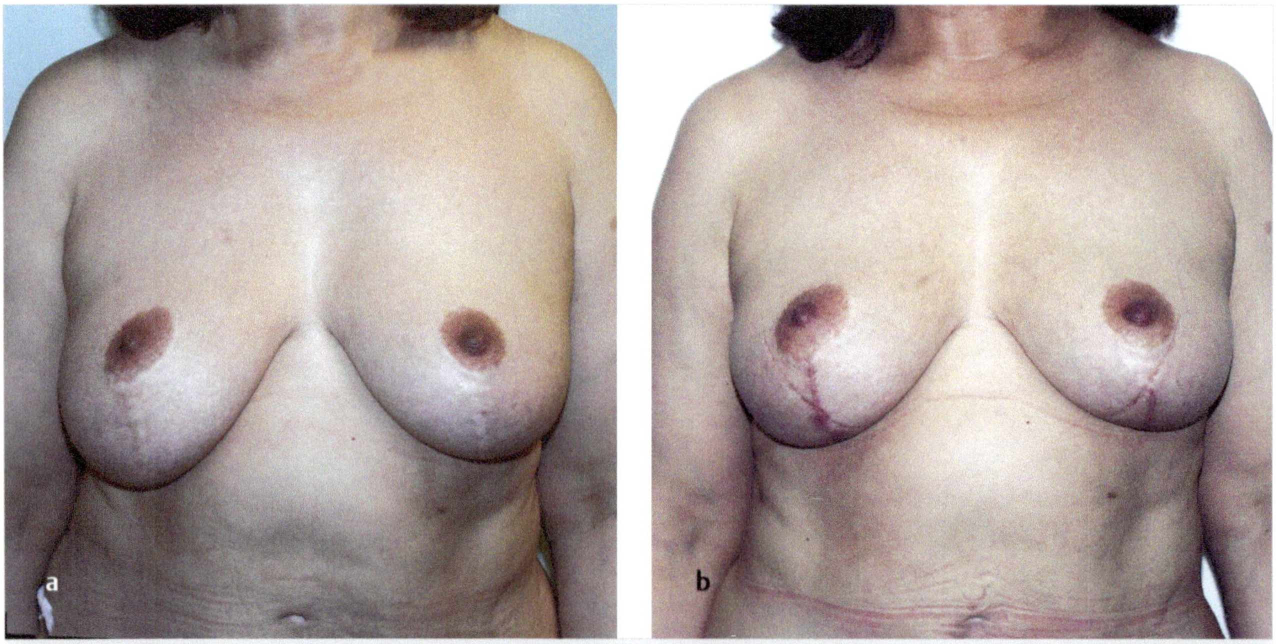

Fig. 8.5 Principles of mastopexy. **(a)** This patient underwent a breast reduction with removal of glandular ptosis on her left breast and a mastopexy only on her right breast using overlapping dermal flaps. She is shown at 6 years after surgery. Her nipple ptosis has been corrected, but she still has glandular ptosis on the right. This result shows that dermal flaps are not successful in the long term at correcting glandular ptosis. We know that skin stretches with tension (skin expansion), and unless the parenchyma is corrected, the skin will not act as a good brassiere. The parenchyma either needs to be "removed." as in a reduction (left breast), or "moved," as should have been performed on the right breast. **(b)** Patient had 150 g of ptotic gland removed from the right breast later during the subsequent correction.

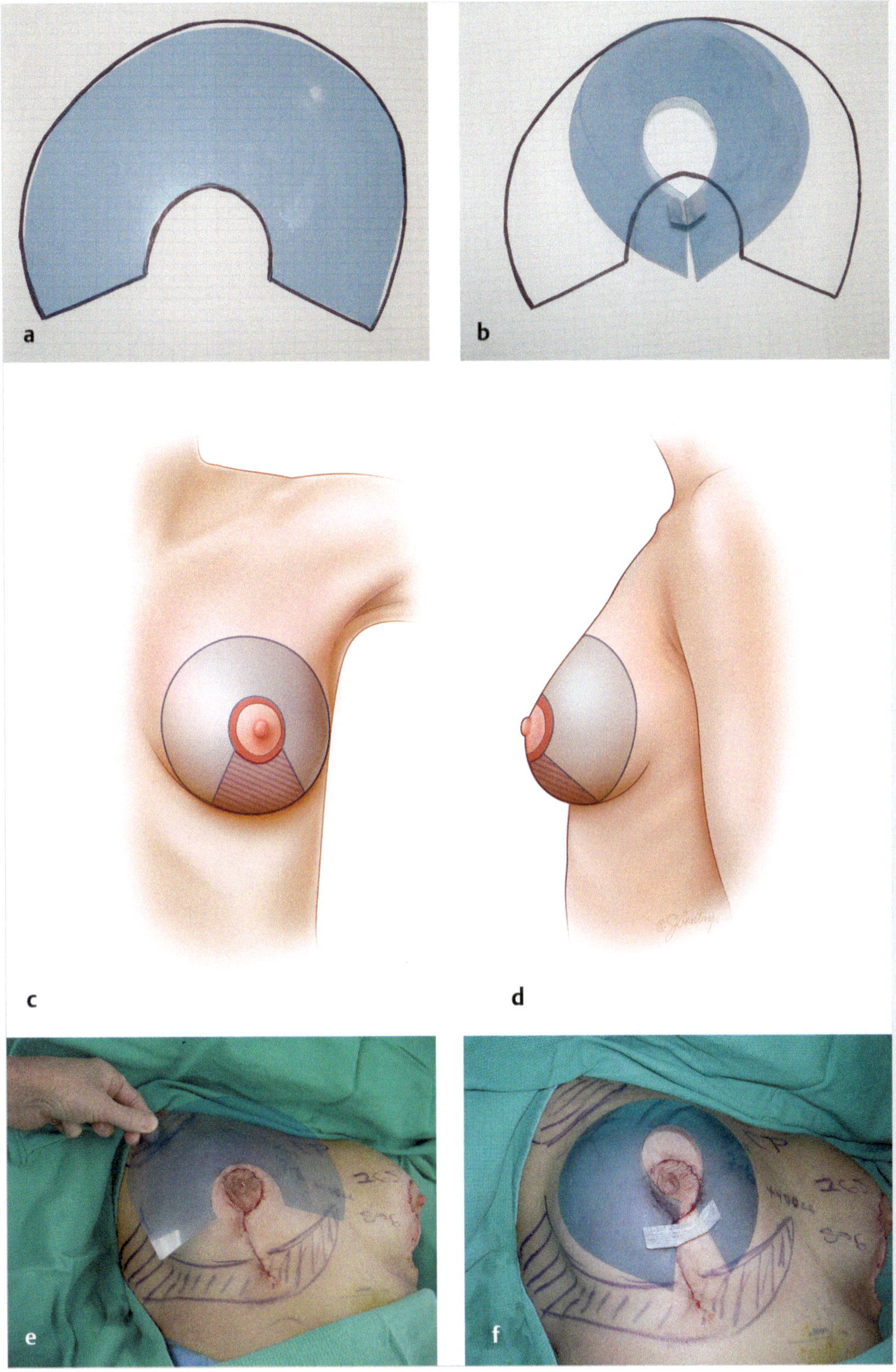

Fig. 8.6 Wise pattern. **(a,b)** The original Wise pattern was developed by Robert Wise from a brassiere design. He used it for the skin pattern, but it is actually better as a pattern for the parenchyma that is left behind. The pattern, when closed, gives a good cone shape to the breast. **(c,d)** The pattern concept is shown. Parenchyma beyond the limits of the Wise pattern is removed by direct excision and tailored out (cross-hatched areas) by liposuction. (Reproduced from Hall-Findlay EJ. Aesthetic Breast Surgery: Concepts & Techniques. New York, NY: Thieme Medical Publishers; 2011.) **(e,f)** The Wise pattern design shown on the breasts. An inferior vertical wedge of skin and breast tissue is removed, and when the pattern is brought together, it results in a nicely projected breast shape.

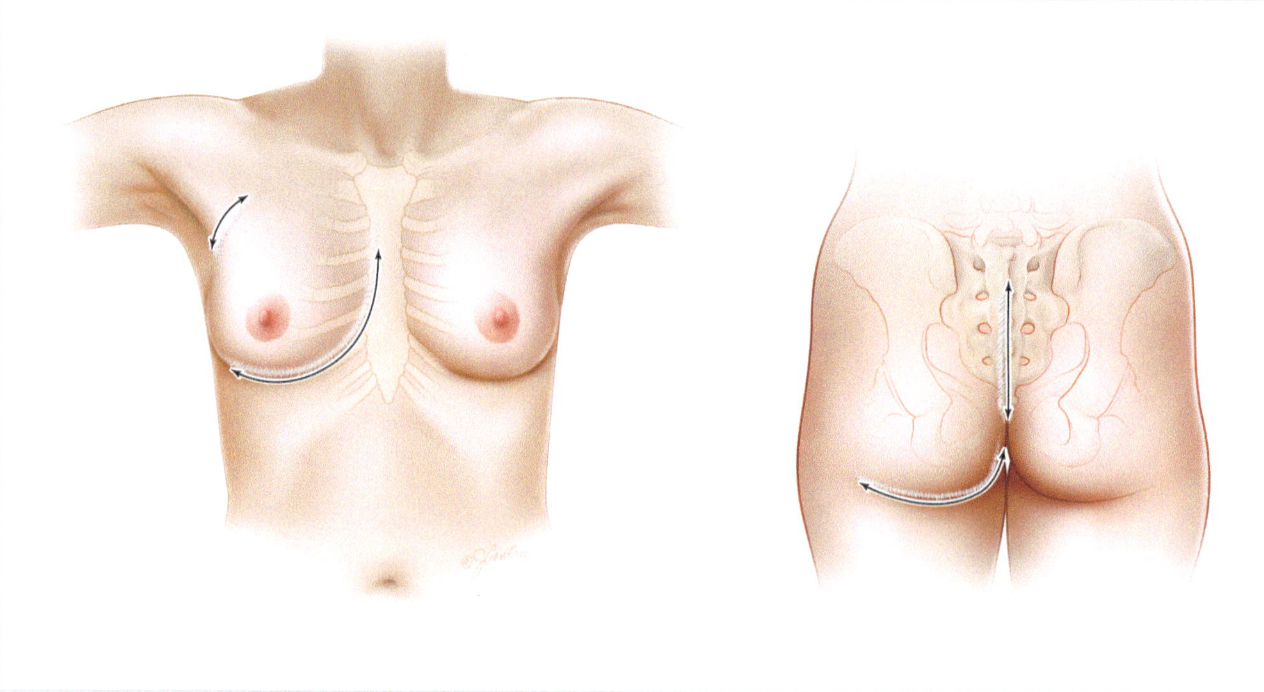

Fig. 8.7 Anatomy of breast. **(a)** The breast is a subcutaneous structure attached to the skin at the nipple; it is only loosely attached to the pectoralis fascia. The breast is held in place by skin–fascial attachments (zones of adherence) to the chest wall. **(b)** The inframammary fold and the attachments over the sternum are much like the attachments at the gluteal crease and the sacrum; they are not breast structures. (Reproduced from Hall-Findlay EJ. Aesthetic Breast Surgery: Concepts & Techniques. New York, NY: Thieme Medical Publishers; 2011.)

All tissue beyond the Wise pattern is removed in a breast reduction.[12] A vertical wedge of breast tissue and skin is removed inferiorly, and then any excess tissue beyond the limits of the Wise pattern is removed by direct excision, followed by tailoring out by peripheral liposuction. The pillars are brought together (without tension), giving good projection to the remaining breast. Note that lower pole tissue is recruited by this maneuver, while the inframammary fold rises. In a mastopexy, this inferior tissue is "moved" rather than "removed" (▶ Fig. 8.6c–f).

We have come to learn as plastic surgeons that we are much better at pulling excess tissue downward (abdominoplasty) than we are at pulling excess upward (facelifting). The key to successful breast surgery is to realize that we cannot "lift" the breast on the chest wall, and our most long-lasting results occur when we "remove" or "move" the heavy inferior pole and cone the remaining upper pole. Skin can act as a good brassiere when it is young and retains good elasticity, but we are often presented with patients with poor skin quality. We are well aware that our best clothing is made with good-quality fabric, but often in surgery we are forced to compromise with poor-quality material (skin). We must instead work against gravity, which means that we should address the lower pole tissue and not try to raise or lift or push tissue upward.

8.3 Anatomy

The breast is a subcutaneous fourth-intercostal-space structure that is attached to the skin at the level of the nipple. Posteriorly the breast has only loose attachments to the pectoralis fascia (which is why we used to sweep a subglandular pocket easily with our fingers for insertion of a breast implant).

The breast is only very loosely attached to the chest wall; it is instead held in place by skin–fascial attachments at the IMF and over the sternum (much like the gluteal fold and the sacrum for the buttocks; ▶ Fig. 8.7). When a woman lies on her side, the upper breast folds over the sternum and the lower breast slides out laterally. When a woman stands on her head, the breast slides toward her chin. There are no significant lateral or superior skin–fascial attachments. The zones of adherence are medial and inferior, and they are not attachments from the breast but separate skin–fascial attachments.[9,12]

Attempts to suture the breast tissue to the pectoralis fascia are unlikely to succeed. Any actual adherence to the fascia results in scar contracture and retraction of the breast tissue with muscle movement. McKissock stated that the concept of suturing up breast tissue to the chest wall is so seductive that it is doomed to be tried (and fail) repeatedly.[13] On the other hand, removal of weight inferiorly will allow the IMF to rise with aggressive resection above the fold with a breast reduction or re-reduction.[14]

The main blood supply consists of an artery and vein from the fourth intercostal space (from the internal mammary system) that enter the posterior surface of the breast just above the fifth rib just medial to the breast meridian. The rest of the blood supply is in the subcutaneous tissue superficial to the breast parenchyma, and it is pushed outward as the breast develops. The veins travel separately and drain mainly superomedially. The lateral aspect of the breast is supplied by the superficial branch of the lateral thoracic system, but the

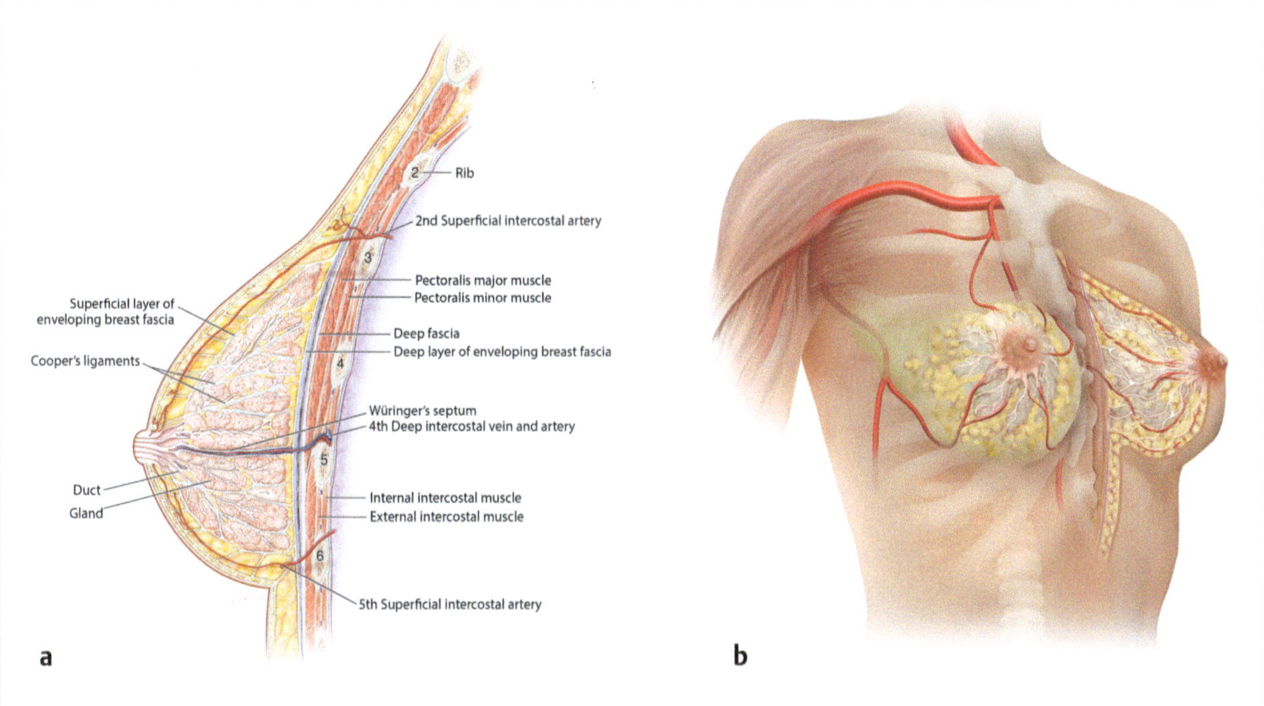

Fig. 8.8 Blood supply to the breast. **(a,b)** The blood supply to the breast is mainly in the subcutaneous tissue curving up around and superficial to the breast parenchyma. Most of the blood supply is from the internal mammary (thoracic) system with some input from the superficial branch of the lateral thoracic artery. The only deep artery that courses through the parenchyma (along with venae comitantes) to supply the nipple and areola comes from the internal mammary artery at the fourth (usually) intercostal space, and it passes along the internal aspect of the chest wall, pierces the intercostal and pectoralis muscles, and then travels through the parenchyma to the nipple. There are some lateral branches (in Würinger's septum), and of course there are vessels that supply the parenchyma itself. The rest of the blood supply starts deep around the edge of the sternum and then courses up in the subcutaneous tissue, not through the parenchyma. The veins travel separately from the arteries, and they course just under the dermis (as is seen during de-epithelialization of the pedicle). (Reproduced from Hall-Findlay EJ. Aesthetic Breast Surgery: Concepts & Techniques. New York, NY: Thieme Medical Publishers; 2010.)

major blood supply is from the internal mammary vessels (▸ Fig. 8.8).[15,16]

Innervation to the nipple is not just from the lateral fourth intercostal nerve (both deep and superficial) but also from the medial intercostal nerves as well.[17] In analyzing patient-reported sensation after vertical breast reduction, it was clear that the sensation from a medially based pedicle was about equal to that from an inferior pedicle (85% return of normal to near-normal sensation) but superior to both a lateral pedicle (76%) and a superior pedicle (67%).[8]

Breast reduction and mastopexy cut through the ducts, but many of them reconnect. Cruz-Korchin has carefully studied breastfeeding after a medial-pedicle vertical breast reduction and found that the results were the same as in patients with large breasts and no surgery: about 60% were able to breastfeed, and 25% of those patients needed to supplement with formula.[18]

8.4 Mastopexy Design

Knowledge of the anatomy will allow us to design methods to "move" that ptotic gland. Usually, the nipple needs to be moved, and knowledge of the various blood supplies to the pedicle is important. Most mastopexies, as described in this chapter, involve a superior or superomedial pedicle to move the nipple and an inferior flap to move or rearrange the ptotic gland.

There are various designs available to move the redundant gland, but the most effective is the inferior flap of Ribeiro described in Section 8.4.4.[4,5] A medial pedicle extension flap can be effective, but it does not allow much movement of the inferior parenchyma. A superior pedicle extension flap is turned up under the superior pedicle, but the breast can be difficult to close, and there is very little upward advancement of the parenchyma. None of these methods work as well as the inferior flap.[19,20]

8.4.1 Medial Pedicle Extension Flap

The design and execution of a medial pedicle extension flap are shown in ▸ Fig. 8.9. Note that it is somewhat difficult to inset, thereby achieving only minimal glandular ptosis correction. For this patient, the result shows that the extension flaps did not make much, if any, difference.

8.4.2 Superior Pedicle Extension Flap

The superior pedicle has an excellent blood supply, and the extension can be created from the inferior wedge that would be removed in a breast reduction. It can then be turned up under the areola to give the breast more fullness. Unfortunately it is difficult to inset without pulling the areola under with it, as shown in ▸ Fig. 8.10. There is also tension on the flap, and it can

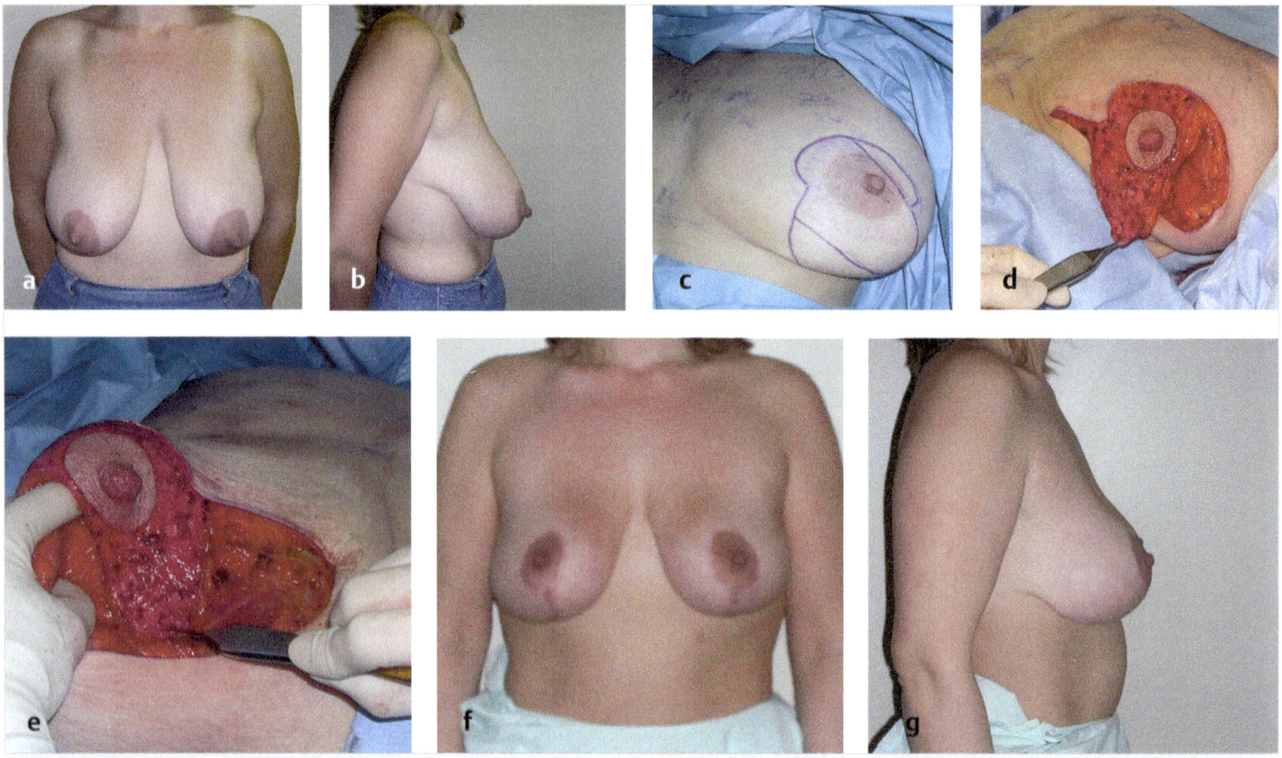

Fig. 8.9 Medial pedicle extension flap. **(a,b)** Patient aged 44 at presentation. She weighed 173 lb (78 kg), and was 5 ft 8 in. (173 cm) tall. She had a medial pedicle extension flap in addition to removal of 240 grams from the right and 255 grams from the left breast. **(c)** Breast markings. **(d)** The flap elevated and de-epithelialized. **(e)** The flap being rotated into position. **(f,g)** Postoperative at 9 months.

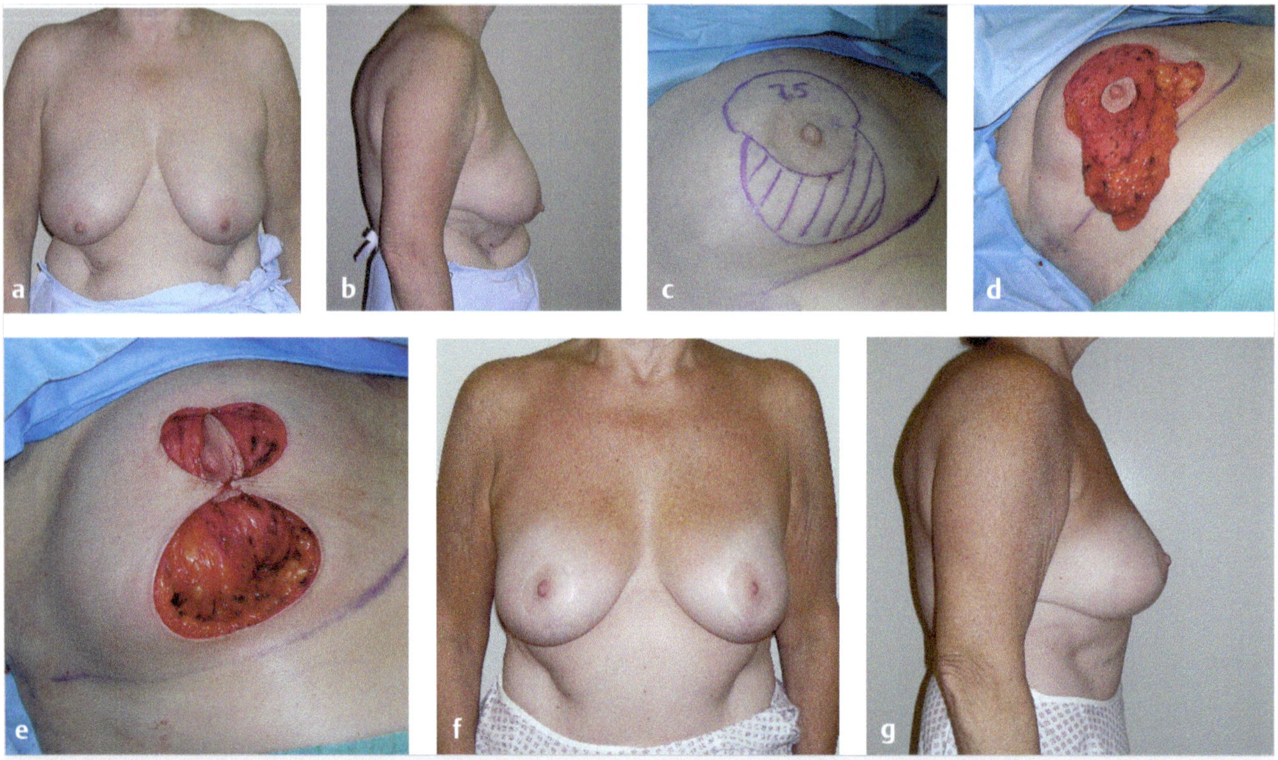

Fig. 8.10 Superior pedicle extension flap. **(a,b)** Patient aged 68 at presentation. She was 5 ft 3 in (160 cm) tall and weighed 135 lb (61 kg). **(c)** Breast markings. **(d)** The flap elevated and de-epithelialized. **(e)** The flap being rotated into position. **(f,g)** Patient at 4 years postoperative.

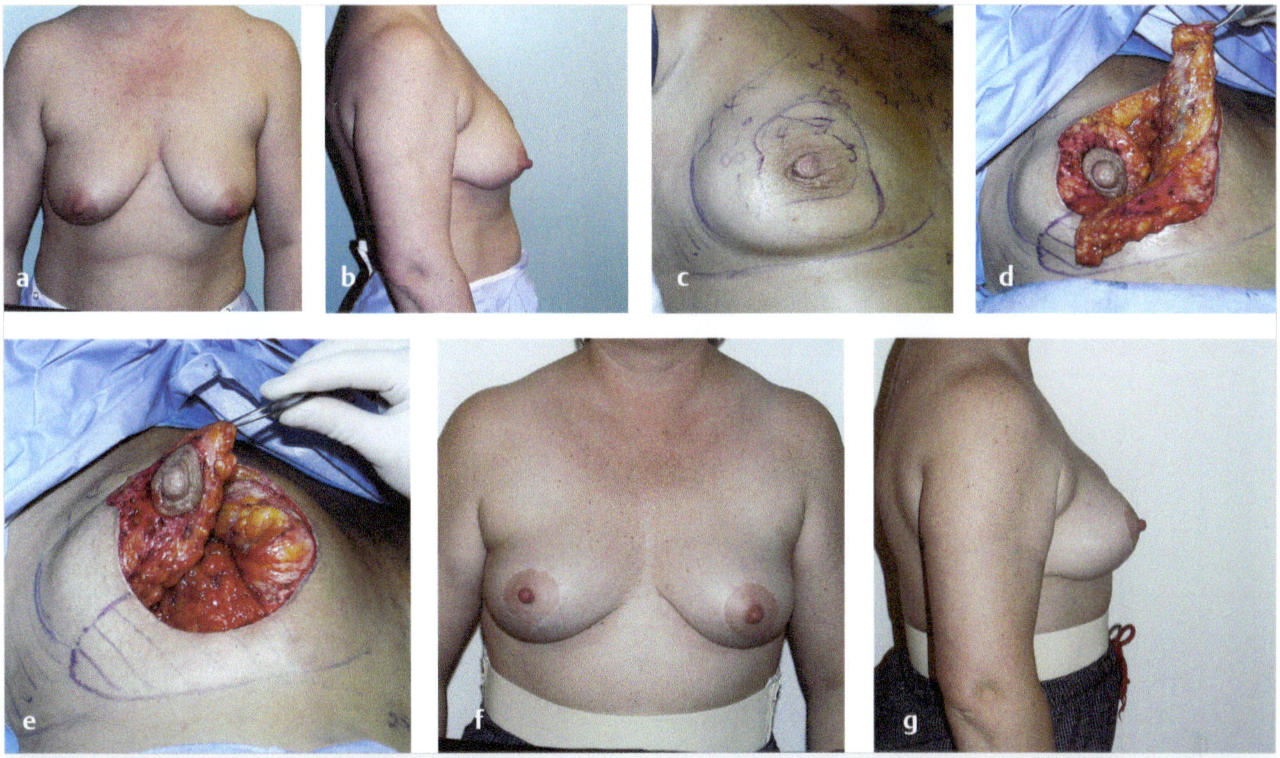

Fig. 8.11 Lateral pedicle with two medial flaps. **(a,b)** Patient aged 44 years at presentation. She was 5 feet 4 inches (163 cm) tall and weighed 170 lb (77 kg). **(c)** Breast markings. **(d)** The medially based flaps de-epithelialized and elevated. **(e)** The flaps mobilized. The medially based upper flap was used in an attempt to fill the upper pole, and the medially based lower flap was used to correct the glandular ptosis. **(f,g)** The patient shown 1 year postoperatively.

give way. The patient shown felt both breasts "drop" at 3 months postoperatively.

8.4.3 Other Rearrangement Flaps

After realizing that the skin brassiere (including dermal flaps) was not effective at correcting glandular ptosis, the author tried multiple different methods of rearranging the breast parenchyma before finding that the inferior flap, discussed in the next section, was the most reliable. The patient in ▶ Fig. 8.11 underwent a lateral pedicle along with two medial flaps (one above the pedicle into the upper pole and one below the pedicle to the midpoint of the breast) to rearrange the breast tissue.

8.4.4 Inferior Chest Wall–Based Flap (Ribeiro)

The inferior flap, as described by Liacyr Ribeiro,[5] has proven to be the most effective method of rearranging breast tissue for a mastopexy. The flap can be mobilized better than the other flaps described. This is the tissue that would be "removed" in a breast reduction and can be "moved" in a mastopexy. The flap can be better mobilized than any of the other flaps described in the preceding sections, and the breast and the flap move together. The flap does not heal to pectoralis fascia; rather, the anterior surface of the flap heals to the posterior surface of the pedicle. Later, if the patient decides to have an implant, there is still a good plane between the pectoralis fascia and the inferior flap. Unfortunately Ribeiro's article was entitled "inferior pedicle," so it was missed in the English literature, but in fact he used a *superior* pedicle with an inferior flap.

This is the type of flap used in the patients shown in ▶ Fig. 8.1 and ▶ Fig. 8.3; ▶ Fig. 8.12 shows the interoperative photos from the latter. Both patients did have an inferior flap held up with a pectoralis sling, as described by Daniel and Graf,[6,7] but the pectoralis strip is not necessary. The author no longer uses the sling because sometimes the breast tissue descends around the flap, especially in a massive-weight-loss patient, leaving an unsightly bump. The original description provided by Ribeiro is the method that gives the author the best result.[4,5] It is best if both the breast and the flap settle together.

8.5 Operative Technique

There have been numerous descriptions of inverted **T** and vertical mastopexy techniques, and all have their merits.[21,22,23,24,25,26,27,28,29,30,31,32,33,34,35,36,37,38] The best mastopexy for a surgeon to perform is the mastopexy that individual surgeon performs the best. All of the long-lasting results involve rearrangement of the breast parenchyma. The following approach describes the technique that has worked the best in the author's hands.[5] The author believes that it is important to move the excess breast tissue where it is in excess (inferior and lateral). It is important in a breast reduction to "remove" the glandular ptosis, and in a mastopexy it is important to "move" the glandular ptosis.[8]

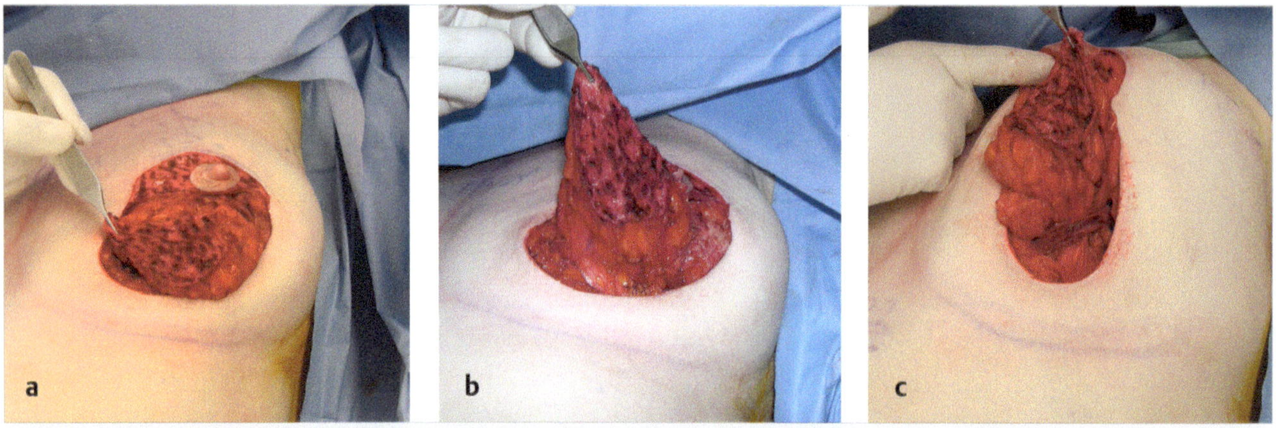

Fig. 8.12 Inferior flap of Ribeiro. I have used the pectoralis strip[6,7] to hold the flap up but it is not necessary. **(a)** The inferior flap (the wedge of skin and parenchyma that would be removed in a breast reduction) is de-epithelialized. **(b)** The flap is mobilized by separating it on all four sides but leaving it as a chest wall–based flap (blood supply is the same as that for an inferior pedicle coming up through the muscles at the fourth intercostal space just medial to the breast meridian). **(c)** The superior pedicle is elevated off the chest wall, and the flap is sutured to pectoralis fascia to hold it until the anterior surface of the flap can heal to the posterior surface of the pedicle. The flap does not end up healing to the pectoralis fascia.

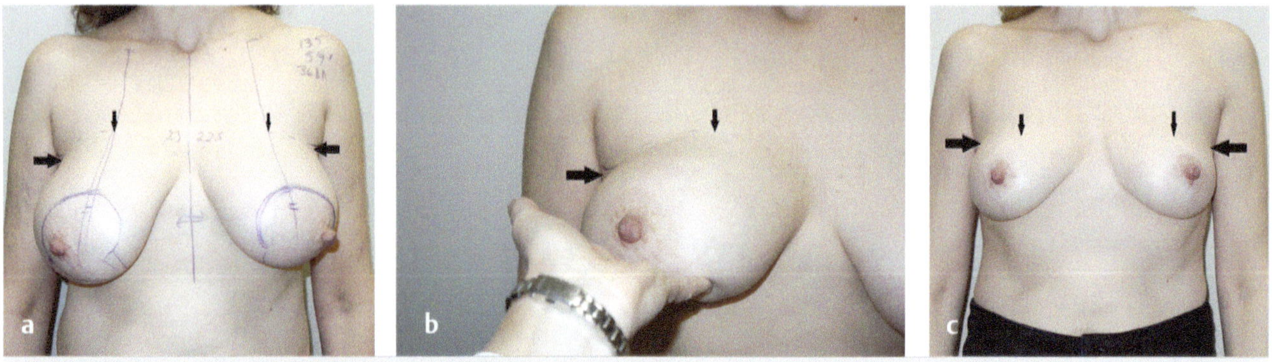

Fig. 8.13 Principles of marking. The principles of marking for a breast reduction (removal of inferior wedge) and for a mastopexy (moving of the inferior wedge) are much the same. This breast reduction/mastopexy patient shows how the upper breast border does not change after surgery and how the new breast meridian should be drawn though the ideal position, not through the existing nipple position. Aged 53 at presentation, the patient was 5 ft 9 in (175 cm) tall and weighed 140 lb (63 kg). **(a)** Marking showing the upper breast border and ideal breast meridian. **(b)** The upper breast border can be demonstrated by folding up the breast (not pushing it up). The upper breast border starts laterally at the junction of the preaxillary fold and the outward curve of the breast. **(c)** The final result at 18 months after removal of 230 grams from the right breast and 190 grams from the left breast.

8.5.1 Markings

Upper Breast Border

The upper breast border is a better landmark for determining new nipple position than the IMF, as Scott Spear also maintained (Spear S, personal communication). The upper breast border will not change after surgery from its preoperative position with either a breast reduction or a mastopexy. The IMF, on the other hand, is quite variable from patient to patient (▶ Fig. 8.1). Some patients have a long vertical breast footprint, and other patients have a very narrow vertical footprint. Although the upper breast border remains the same after a breast reduction or a mastopexy, the IMF can be adjusted.

The upper breast border (small vertical arrows in ▶ Fig. 8.13a) is the junction between the chest wall and the takeoff of the breast. It starts at the junction of the preaxillary fullness (large horizontal arrows) and the outward curvature of the breast. If it is not obvious, the breast can be folded up (not just pushed up), as shown in ▶ Fig. 8.13b, and the line of demarcation will become more clear (smaller vertical arrows).

The patient in ▶ Fig. 8.13 shows that the surgeon needs to evaluate not only glandular ptosis but also nipple position in all directions, not just elevation. Note that in the postoperative (18 months) photo (▶ Fig. 8.13c), the upper breast border has not changed from its original position.

Breast Meridian

The new breast meridian should not be drawn through the existing nipple position but in its ideal location, which is usually about 8–10 cm from the chest midline (as drawn through the air, not around the breast). The new breast meridian should be placed slightly more laterally in an inverted **T** breast reduction because the breast base ends up wider than in most vertical breast reductions.

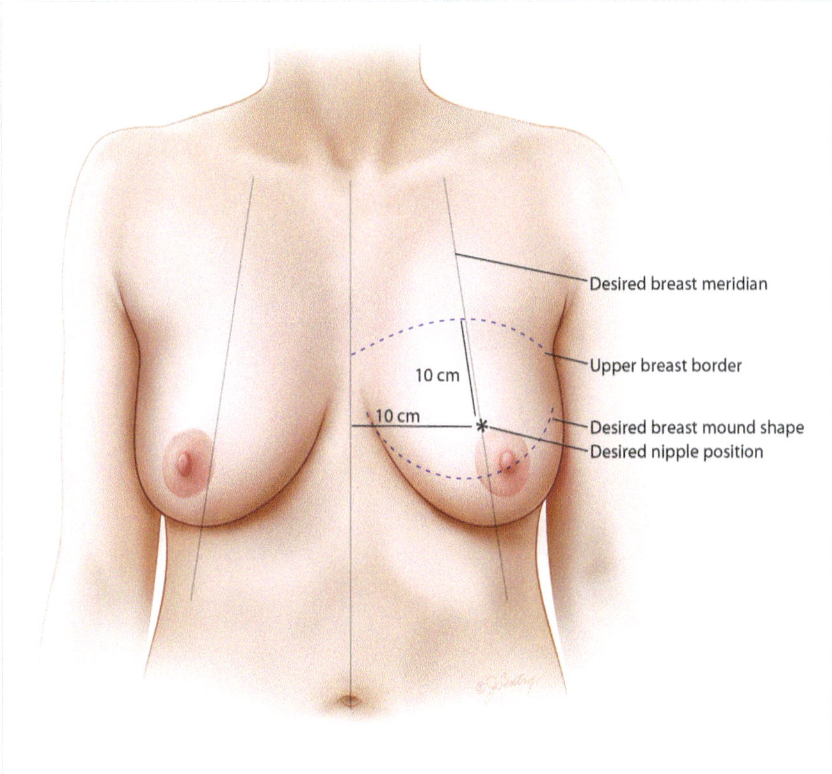

Fig. 8.14 Ideal nipple position. The ideal nipple position on an average 5 ft 6 in (168 cm)-tall patient is about 10 cm down from the upper breast border and about 10 cm from the chest midline (as measured with a straight ruler, not measured around the curve of the breast). (Reproduced from Hall-Findlay EJ. Aesthetic Breast Surgery: Concepts & Techniques. New York, NY: Thieme Medical Publishers; 2011.)

Note that in the patient shown in ▶ Fig. 8.13a, the nipples are very asymmetric and very lateral. The new breast meridian is not drawn through the existing nipple position; otherwise the nipples would have remained asymmetric and too lateral.

New Nipple Position

Because the upper breast border will not change postoperatively, it is easy for the surgeon to visualize the final result (see line drawn on the left breast in ▶ Fig. 8.14). The ideal nipple position on most average sized patients with a C-cup breast is about 8–10 cm down from the upper breast border and along the intended breast meridian, about 8–10 cm (as drawn through the air, not around the breast) from the chest midline. From this starting point, the surgeon can stand back and visualize the ideal landmarks. The final choice between 8 and 10 cm will depend on the height and size of the patient and the desired final outcome. Surgeons should start measuring their patients both before and after surgery to determine their own measurement system.

The new nipple position should be one-third to one-half the distance up the final breast mound; otherwise the areola will slip up and become exposed in bathing suits or undergarments. Although the IMF can be a good landmark for the new nipple position, it can be misleading. As previously discussed, the upper breast border is a more accurate landmark because it does not change postoperatively.

Areolar Opening

The new areolar opening is marked 2 cm above the new nipple position. It should be about 16 cm in length to match a 5-cm-diameter areola. A 14-cm circumference matches a 4.5-cm-diameter areola. It is not the marking of the areola itself that matters the most, because the areola skin will tend to stretch out to match the skin opening. It is also important to mark the new nipple and areola slightly lower on the larger breast.

The upper breast border is marked with a dotted line. The breast meridian is marked in its ideal position – which is close to the original position in the patient shown in ▶ Fig. 8.15. A line is drawn over the right breast to illustrate how the surgeon can visualize the final result.

Photos are taken of the patient at the time of consultation and drawings made (▶ Fig. 8.15e–h) to show the patient what to expect. The postoperative images (▶ Fig. 8.15b,d) show how close the results are to what was drawn.

Pedicle Design

The vertical limbs of the skin resection pattern are similar to the vertical limbs of an inverted **T**, but they do not need to be as precise, because this is not a skin brassiere operation. The design resembles a snowman, and the two vertical limbs are then joined together at least 2–4 cm above the IMF. Note that the new nipple position is marked well above the IMF level in the patient shown in ▶ Fig. 8.4c; in some patients it will need to be marked well below the IMF. The upper breast border is a far better landmark than the IMF for determining new nipple position.

A superior (▶ Fig. 8.16a) or superomedial (▶ Fig. 8.16b,c) pedicle can be used with either a vertical skin resection pattern or an inverted **T** pattern. In a very large breast, the skin resection pattern may well need to be an inverted **T** pattern, but there should be no tension on the skin because the more extensive skin resection pattern is dictated by the need to remove

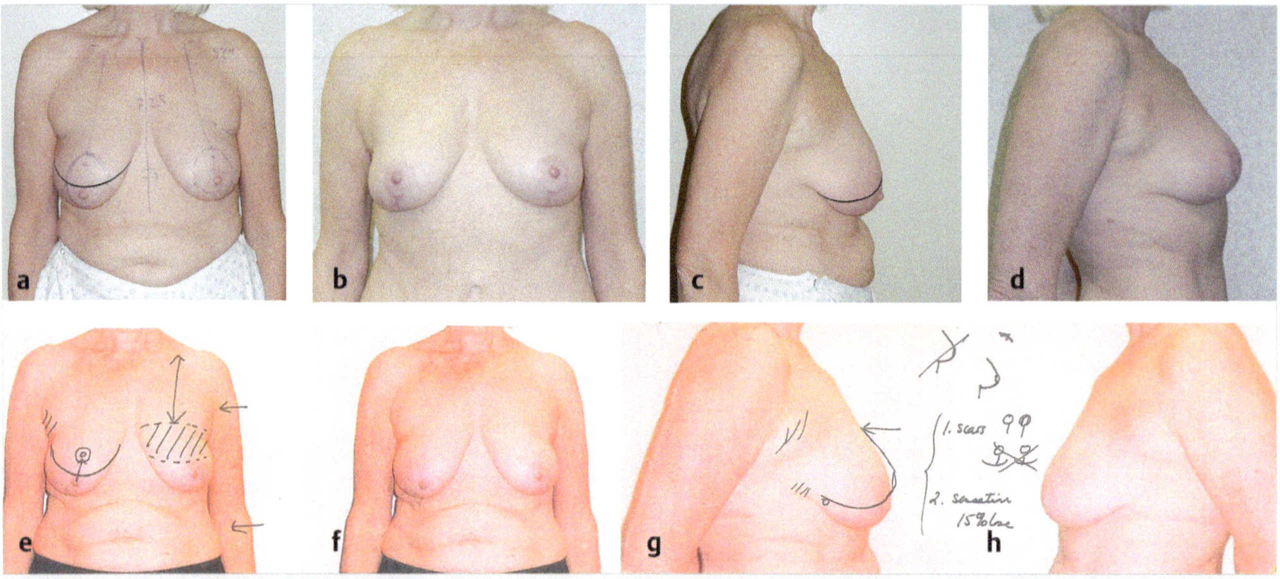

Fig. 8.15 Mastopexy consultation planning. This patient aged 59 at presentation had an inferior flap (Ribeiro) type mastopexy with removal of only skin from her left breast and 22 grams from her right breast. She was 5 ft 6 in (168 cm) tall and weighed 145 lb (66 kg). **(a,b)** Preoperative (showing markings) and 1-year postoperative frontal views. **(c,d)** Preoperative and 1-year postoperative lateral views. **(e–h)** Markings on consultation photos show how the results can be predicted for managing patient expectations.

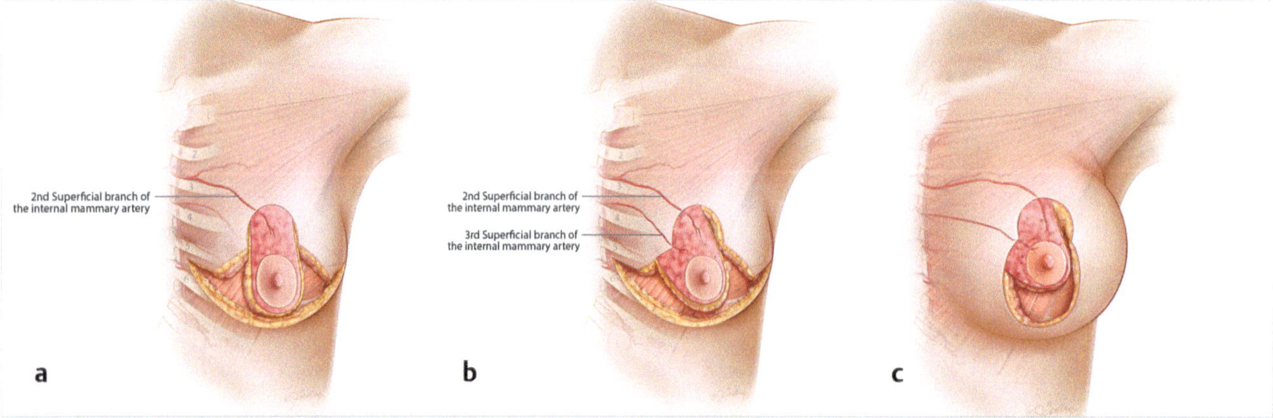

Fig. 8.16 Pedicle design considering blood supply. **(a)** A superior pedicle is often used with an inferior flap for a mastopexy. It has a strong reliable blood supply anterior to the parenchyma in the subcutaneous tissue. It usually arises from the second intercostal space from the internal mammary (thoracic) artery. **(b)** A true superomedial pedicle has a dual-axial blood supply. The base of the pedicle should be carried across just lateral to the breast meridian to be certain of including the artery from the second intercostal space. A pencil Doppler can be used if needed. The pedicle is shown with an inverted-T skin resection pattern. **(c)** True superomedial pedicle with a vertical skin resection pattern. (Reproduced from Hall-Findlay EJ. Aesthetic Breast Surgery: Concepts & Techniques. New York, NY: Thieme Medical Publishers; 2011.)

redundant skin, not by the need to use the skin as a brassiere to hold up heavy inferior breast tissue.

A superior pedicle has an excellent blood supply that courses in the subcutaneous tissue to the nipple and areola. A superior pedicle not only can be safely lifted away from the pectoralis fascia, but it can also be thinned as needed. When the nipple does not need to be moved very far in a mastopexy, a superior pedicle is the best choice.

A true superomedial pedicle can be used when the nipple needs to be significantly elevated in a mastopexy. A superomedial pedicle has a dual-axial blood supply, as it includes the descending artery from the second intercostal space as well as the artery from the third intercostal space. It can be more difficult to inset a true superomedial pedicle than a pure medial pedicle (which is easier to rotate), but deep tissue can be removed if needed to allow the pedicle to be inset without compression. The descending artery from the second intercostal space enters the areolar opening close to the breast meridian in the subcutaneous tissue (pencil Doppler tested in 85 patients[8]), and it is only about 1 cm deep to the skin surface, so deeper tissue can be safely debulked. The only blood supply that travels through the breast parenchyma to reach the nipple is at the fourth intercostal space (supplying an inferior pedicle and not necessary for a medial or superomedial pedicle); the rest of the blood supply travels up and around the parenchyma in the subcutaneous tissue.[12,16]

Inferior Flap Design

The inferior flap has the same blood supply as an inferior pedicle. The flap relies on the deep artery and venae comitantes that come directly from the chest wall at the fourth intercostal space. These are the only artery and vein that travel through the breast parenchyma to supply the nipple and areola. In this case, the nipple is supplied by a superior pedicle, and the inferior flap is supplied by chest wall–based vessels.

If an implant has been used previously, the blood supply to the flap is no longer available. It does not matter whether the implant was placed in the subglandular or the subpectoral pocket. Creation of an implant pocket damages that deep artery and vein.

The inferior flap needs to be detached on all sides while being left as a chest wall–based flap.[7] If the inferior flap is not completely mobilized, it will cause retraction and postoperative distortion. The surgeon needs to release the flap carefully until it can be advanced without pulling on inferior skin etc. The blood supply is usually just medial to the breast meridian just above the fifth rib (▸ Fig. 8.17a).

The patient in ▸ Fig. 8.17 underwent an inferior flap (Ribeiro) type of mastopexy. Only skin was removed from the right breast, and 48 g was removed from the left breast. She is shown at 3 years after her mastopexy in ▸ Fig. 8.17e,g. The key to avoiding recurrent glandular ptosis is to rearrange the breast tissue rather than relying on the skin brassiere. This inferior flap technique gives the best and most consistent long-lasting results.

8.5.2 Surgical Technique

Infiltration

Only the areas where liposuction is to be performed (if indicated) need to be infiltrated. Tumescent-type fluid is used in obese patients when liposuction needs to be more extensive. It is important not to infiltrate the skin where the incisions will be made, because the veins can be damaged.

Skin Incisions

The skin is incised along the preoperative markings. The mastopexy is not a skin brassiere operation, and it is important not to take too much skin, so that it does not need to be closed under tension. The inferior flap needs only to be wide enough to correct the glandular ptosis. More skin can be removed later if desired, but it is important to recognize that the skin is not needed to hold the breast up. If there is significant skin redundancy, an inverted **T** or **J** or **L** can be added to the skin resection pattern.

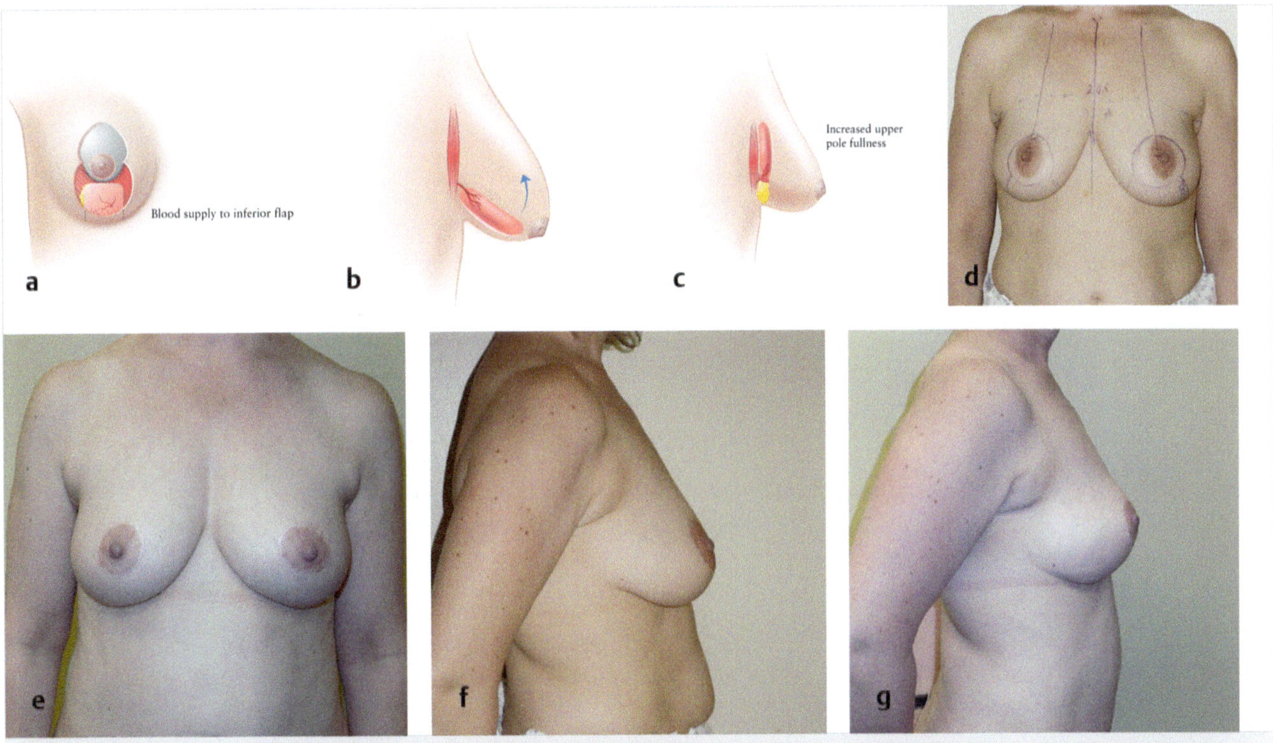

Fig. 8.17 Mastopexy design with inferior Ribeiro flap. **(a)** A superior pedicle is used with an inferior flap. **(b)** The lateral view shows how effective the inferior flap is in achieving rearrangement of the breast tissue to correct the glandular ptosis. **(c)** The inferior flap is sutured up the chest wall in order to hold it in place long enough that the anterior surface of the flap can heal to the posterior surface of the breast parenchyma. **(d,e)** Preoperative and 3-year postoperative frontal views of a patient, aged 49 at presentation, who had only skin removed from her right breast and 48 grams from her left breast. She was 5 ft 5 in (165 cm) tall and weighed 146 lb (66 kg). **(f,g)** Preoperative and 3-year postoperative lateral views showing good correction of the glandular ptosis. (Reproduced from Hall-Findlay EJ. Aesthetic Breast Surgery: Concepts & Techniques. New York, NY: Thieme Medical Publishers; 2011.)

Pedicle Creation

The superior pedicle is beveled upward slightly to help avoid damaging the blood supply to the inferior flap.

A true superomedial pedicle is carried just lateral to the new breast meridian in order to include the descending arterial branch from the second interspace. If the pedicle is short, then a pure superior pedicle can be used.

Inferior Flap Creation

The parenchyma that is excised as an inferior wedge in a breast reduction is preserved as an inferior chest wall–based flap (Video 9.1). It is important to keep the Wise pattern in mind as a template of how to shape the remaining parenchyma. The pillars will be about 7 cm in length, and liposuction can be used to tailor out any excess fat along the IMF. The lateral and medial skin flaps should be at least 1 cm thick, with enough fat attached to the dermis to prevent scar contracture.

Care needs to be taken to prevent the inferior flap from being detached from its chest wall–based blood supply. It is best to bevel out initially under the superior pedicle, then dissect the flap from the lateral pillar. The blood supply is more medial, so the inferior and medial dissection needs to be beveled out to preserve the artery and veins that come usually just above the fifth rib and just medial to the breast meridian. At the same time, it is important to release all tethering fascial attachments so that the flap moves easily and does not pull up on the inferior skin.

Flap Advancement under the Superior Pedicle

The mobilized flap is then sutured to pectoralis fascia up under the superior pedicle (Video 9.1). Attempting to use the flap for more upper pole fullness is likely to lead to a small bump that is not attractive. This is especially true in massive-weight-loss patients, in whom the breast tends to settle back down around the elevated flap. This problem is most likely to occur when the flap is held up too high with a pectoralis strip. It is best to assume that the flap will be used for correction of the glandular ptosis instead and to help give more breast projection, not to give more upper pole fullness.

The flap is sutured to pectoralis fascia, not in the expectation that it will heal to the fascia (it will not) but to hold it there long enough that it heals to the overlying breast tissue. The lack of healing to the pectoralis fascia can be seen when later an implant is added in patients who later decide that they want more upper pole fullness; the flap is healed to the overlying breast tissue, and it is easy to create a subglandular plane between the flap and the fascia.

Pillar Closure

The pillars are then sutured together caudal to the flap. Only a few sutures are needed to bring the pillars together so that they can heal together without tension.

The pillars do not extend down as far caudally as either the skin resection or the IMF. The lower end of the pillars actually is at the same level as the Wise pattern skin resection pattern.

Dermal Closure

The dermis is then closed without tension using deep interrupted sutures. Only enough are needed to just allow dermis-to-dermis apposition. The skin closure does not need to be tight because the skin is not being used as a brassiere.

Peripheral Liposuction

Once the dermis is closed, it is easier to assess any residual tissue that needs to be removed. Any excess glandular breast tissue needs to be directly excised, but any redundant fatty tissue can be removed with liposuction. It is important to suction laterally between the original IMF and the desired (curved) new IMF. Any pucker that results postoperatively is a problem of excess subcutaneous tissue and rarely a problem of excess skin.

Skin Closure

The skin is then closed with a loose subcuticular suture. The skin is not "gathered" or "cinched. That maneuver does not shorten the vertical scar, but instead leads to wound healing problems.[39] The excess vertical length is needed to accommodate projection, and it tucks up behind the pillars.

It is important, however, to leave enough fat deep to the dermis to prevent scar contracture. The skin needs to be free to slide over the deep tissues and the inferior flap. It may be tempting to suture the pucker down to the chest wall, but this can develop adherence that needs to be released several months later as a revision procedure.

Surgeons need to realize that a long vertical distance is needed to accommodate the increased projection that results from the vertical approach. We have been taught to leave the vertical limbs at 5–7 cm because of bottoming out when using an inferior pedicle, inverted **T** procedure, but that is because the skin in that case is being used to compress the breast in order to hold up the parenchyma. With the vertical approach, any bottoming out occurs because of inadequate parenchymal rearrangement. A good B-cup breast has a vertical distance from the inferior aspect of the areola to the IMF of 7 cm. A C-cup breast has a vertical distance of 9 cm, and a D-cup breast has a vertical distance of 11 cm.

If a **T** skin resection pattern is added, it is important to curve up the excision and to make sure that the scar lies well above the IMF. Postoperatively, the fold will rise, and it is important that the scar does not lie on the chest wall instead of on the inferior aspect of the breast.

Drains

Drains are usually unnecessary. They do not prevent a hematoma. It is important to look for the known arteries and make sure hemostasis is secure. Seromas do occur, but they resolve easily without aspiration. Drains would need to remain in place for over a week to take care of any potential seromas.

Tape, Bandages, and Brassieres

The incisions are covered with Micropore paper tape (3 M, St. Paul, MN). Patients are encouraged to shower the next day and pat the tape dry. It will stay in place for 3–4 weeks without needing to be replaced. Bandages are used initially, and a surgical brassiere applied to hold the bandages in place. Neither the tape nor the brassiere is used for compression or shaping. It is the nature of the surgical resection that gives the breast the final shape—not the skin, not the tape, and not the garment.

8.5.3 Complications

Complications with a vertical mastopexy using an inferior flap are very similar to those with other types of breast surgery, except that there are fewer wound healing problems when there is no tension on the skin closure.

Hematomas/Seromas

Significant hematomas need to be evacuated, but seromas tend to absorb on their own. A large hematoma might compress the pedicle. A specific bleeder is not always found. Hematoma rate should be less than 1–2%.

Fat Necrosis

There is a risk of the inferior flap becoming necrotic if the dissection interrupts the chest wall–based blood supply.

Infection

The breast ducts contain bacteria because they communicate with the outside world. One dose of preoperative cephalosporins is indicated, and the author has found that using Monocryl Plus sutures (embedded with the antibacterial triclosan; Ethicon Inc., Bridgewater, NJ) helps prevent suture spitting. Infection rate should be less than 1–2%.

Wound Healing Problems

Tension causes wound healing problems, especially at the **T** junction in an inverted **T** mastopexy when the skin is being used to hold the breast up. Allowing healing by secondary intention is often the best choice.

Bottoming Out

Recurrent glandular ptosis can still be a problem even with creation of the inferior flap. In large breasts, it is best to make them smaller when there is a significant amount of glandular ptosis that will respond to gravity.

Nipple Necrosis

The most feared complication in breast reduction surgery is nipple necrosis. A true superomedial pedicle has excellent blood supply because it has a dual-axial artery supply and much of the venous drainage is superomedial. Intervention should be undertaken only if there is any possible compression or the areola is distended with venous compression. Once nipple necrosis is inevitable, it is best to let it declare itself and avoid débridement unless absolutely necessary. The nipple and areola appear to be somewhat privileged, and watchful waiting can give a better outcome than expected.

Puckers

Excess skin and subcutaneous tissue is the most frequent complication with vertical breast procedures. Most puckers are caused by excess subcutaneous tissue, but enough fat needs to be left on the dermis to prevent scar contraction. It is not a good idea to suture the skin down to the chest wall, because it will remain adherent and require later revision. The breast should be able to slide freely over the chest wall while it is held in place by skin-fascial attachments to the chest wall. It is not a good idea to gather or cinch the vertical skin closure because that can actually cause a pucker that needs to be revised. Puckers that are above the IMF can be excised vertically, and puckers that are below the IMF should be excised horizontally.

8.6 Summary

The author has been able to achieve better, more lasting breast results using Liacyr Ribeiro's inferior flap approach to mastopexy. The key is to move the excess parenchyma where it is in excess—inferior and lateral. Skin stretches and causes bottoming-out if there is weight on the skin, and it is important to recognize that the skin should not be used as a brassiere. This procedure relies on parenchymal reshaping instead. By moving an inferior vertical flap of parenchyma, the glandular ptosis is corrected and the pillars can be brought together, which narrows the breast base diameter and gives increased projection. A long vertical skin distance is actually needed to accommodate this increased projection. Wound healing complications are far less when there is no tension on the skin closure, and long-lasting results are good when there is no tension on the parenchymal repair.

Key Points

- The upper breast border is a better landmark than the inframammary fold for planning a mastopexy.
- The actual attachment of the breast to the chest wall (footprint or base) varies significantly from patient to patient, and the breast borders can be changed only minimally with surgery.
- The surgeon needs to understand not only the footprint but what can and cannot be achieved with manipulating the breast mound in order to determine the ideal nipple position.
- The surgeon needs to determine how much of the gland is sagging or ptotic and correct it. Adjusting the skin brassiere will not correct glandular ptosis. Skin stretches and causes bottoming-out if there is weight on the skin, and it is important to recognize that the skin should not be used as a brassiere.
- The key to successful breast surgery is to realize that it is not possible to "lift" the breast on the chest wall, and the longest-lasting results occur when the surgeon "removes" or "moves" the heavy inferior pole and cones the remaining breast parenchyma.
- There have been numerous descriptions of inverted **T** and vertical mastopexy techniques, and all have their merits. The best mastopexy is the mastopexy that the individual surgeon performs the best.

- It is important to move the excess breast tissue where it is in excess (inferior and lateral). It is important in a breast reduction to "remove" the glandular ptosis, and in a mastopexy it is important to "move" the glandular ptosis.
- The author has been able to achieve better, more lasting breast results using Liacyr Ribeiro's inferior flap approach to mastopexy. The key is to move the excess parenchyma where it is in excess—inferior and lateral. This procedure relies on parenchymal reshaping.
- By moving an inferior vertical flap of parenchyma, the glandular ptosis is corrected and the pillars can be brought together, which narrows the breast base diameter and gives increased projection.
- The ideal nipple position on most average sized patients with a C-cup breast is about 8–10 cm down from the upper breast border and about 8–10 cm (as drawn through the air, not around the breast) from the chest midline.
- Attempting to use the inferior flap for more upper pole fullness is likely to lead to a small bump that is not attractive. It is best to assume that the inferior flap will be used for correction of the glandular ptosis instead and to help give more breast projection, not to try to give more upper pole fullness.
- With the vertical mastopexy approach, any bottoming-out occurs because of inadequate parenchymal rearrangement.
- A longer vertical skin distance is actually needed to accommodate this increased projection with the vertical mastopexy technique. A good B-cup breast has a vertical distance from the inferior aspect of the areola to the inframammary fold of 7 cm. A C-cup breast has a vertical distance of 9 cm, and a D-cup breast has a vertical distance of 11 cm.
- Complication management pearl: If nipple necrosis is inevitable, it is best to let it declare itself and avoid débridement unless absolutely necessary. The nipple and areola appear to be somewhat privileged, and watchful waiting can give a better outcome than expected.
- Wound healing complications are far less when there is no tension on the skin closure and, long-lasting results are good when there is no tension on the parenchymal repair.

References

[1] Regnault P. Breast ptosis. Definition and treatment. Clin Plast Surg. 1976; 3 (2):193–203

[2] Blondeel P, Hijjawi J, Depypere H, Roche N, Van Landuyt K. Shaping the breast in aesthetic and reconstructive breast surgery: an easy three-step principle. Plast Reconstr Surg. 2009; 123:455–462

[3] Hall-Findlay EJ. The three breast dimensions: analysis and effecting change. Plast Reconstr Surg. 2010; 125(6):1632–1642

[4] Ribeiro L. A new technique for reduction mammaplasty. Plast Reconstr Surg. 1975; 55(3):330–334

[5] Ribeiro L, Accorsi A, Jr, Buss A, Marcal-Pessoa M. Creation and evolution of 30 years of the inferior pedicle in reduction mammaplasties. Plast Reconstr Surg. 2002; 110(3):960–970

[6] Daniel MJB. Mammoplasty with pectoral muscle flap. Presented at the 64th Scientific Meeting of the American Society of Plastic and Reconstructive Surgeons; 1995; Montreal, Canada

[7] Graf R, Auersvald A, Bernardes A, Biggs TM. Reduction mammaplasty and mastopexy with shorter scar and better shape. Aesthet Surg J. 2000; 20:99–106

[8] Hall-Findlay EJ. A simplified vertical reduction mammaplasty: shortening the learning curve. Plast Reconstr Surg. 1999; 104(3):748–759, discussion 760--763

[9] Hall-Findlay E. Aesthetic Breast Surgery: Concepts & Techniques. New York, NY: Thieme; 2011

[10] Mallucci P, Branford OA. Population analysis of the perfect breast: a morphometric analysis. Plast Reconstr Surg. 2014; 134(3):436–447

[11] Wise RJ. A preliminary report on a method of planning the mammaplasty. Plast Reconstr Surg (1946). 1956; 17(5):367–375

[12] Hall-Findlay EJ, Shestak KC. Breast reduction. Plast Reconstr Surg. 2015; 136 (4):531e–544e

[13] McKissock PK. In discussion of: Mathes SJ, Nahai F, Hester TR. Avoiding the flat breast in reduction mammaplasty. Plast Reconstr Surg. 1980; 66:63–70

[14] Mistry RM, MacLennan SE, Hall-Findlay EJ. Principles of breast re-reduction: a reappraisal. Plast Reconstr Surg. 2017; 139(6):1313–1322

[15] Würinger E, Mader N, Posch E, Holle J. Nerve and vessel supplying ligamentous suspension of the mammary gland. Plast Reconstr Surg. 1998; 101(6): 1486–1493

[16] Hall-Findlay EJ. Discussion: the blood supply of the breast revisited. Plast Reconstr Surg. 2016; 137(5):1398–1400

[17] Schlenz I, Kuzbari R, Gruber H, Holle J. The sensitivity of the nipple-areola complex: an anatomic study. Plast Reconstr Surg. 2000; 105(3):905–909

[18] Cruz-Korchin N, Korchin L. Breast-feeding after vertical mammaplasty with medial pedicle. Plast Reconstr Surg. 2004; 114(4):890–894

[19] Losken A, Holtz DJ. Versatility of the superomedial pedicle in managing the massive weight loss breast: the rotation-advancement technique. Plast Reconstr Surg. 2007; 120(4):1060–1068

[20] Kim P, Kim KK, Casas LA. Superior pedicle autoaugmentation mastopexy: a review of 34 consecutive patients. Aesthet Surg J. 2010; 30(2):201–210

[21] Goulian D. Dermal mastopexy. Clin Plast Surg. 1976; 3(2):171–175

[22] Bartels RJ, Strickland DM, Douglas WM. A new mastopexy operation for mild or moderate breast ptosis. Plast Reconstr Surg. 1976; 57(6):687–691

[23] Whidden PG. The tailor-tack mastopexy. Plast Reconstr Surg. 1978; 62(3): 347–354

[24] Erol OO, Spira M. A mastopexy technique for mild to moderate ptosis. Plast Reconstr Surg. 1980; 65(5):603–609

[25] Benelli L. A new periareolar mammaplasty: the "round block" technique. Aesthetic Plast Surg. 1990; 14(2):93–100

[26] Chiari Júnior A. The L short-scar mammaplasty: a new approach. Plast Reconstr Surg. 1992; 90(2):233–246

[27] Botti G. Vertical scar mammaplasty: stable padding of the superior pole by means of a posteriorly based pedicle autoprosthesis. Aesthet Surg J. 1999; 19: 116–123

[28] Spear SL, Giese SY, Ducic I. Concentric mastopexy revisited. Plast Reconstr Surg. 2001; 107(5):1294–1299, discussion 1300

[29] Exner K, Scheufler O. Dermal suspension flap in vertical-scar reduction mammaplasty. Plast Reconstr Surg. 2002; 109(7):2289–2298, discussion 2299–30

[30] Sampaio Góes JC. Periareolar mammaplasty: double-skin technique with application of mesh support. Clin Plast Surg. 2002; 29(3):349–364, v

[31] Qiao Q, Sun J, Liu C, Liu Z, Zhao R. Reduction mammaplasty and correction of ptosis: dermal bra technique. Plast Reconstr Surg. 2003; 111(3):1122–1130

[32] Becker H. Subareolar mastopexy: update. Aesthet Surg J. 2003; 23(5):357–363

[33] Rubin JP. Mastopexy after massive weight loss: dermal suspension and total parenchymal reshaping. Aesthet Surg J. 2006; 26(2):214–222

[34] Foustanos A, Zavrides H. A double-flap technique: an alternative mastopexy approach. Plast Reconstr Surg. 2007; 120(1):55–60

[35] Stevens WG, Stoker DA, Freeman ME, Quardt SM, Hirsch EM. Mastopexy revisited: a review of 150 consecutive cases for complication and revision rates. Aesthet Surg J. 2007; 27(2):150–154

[36] Hammond DC, Alfonso D, Khuthaila DK. Mastopexy using the short scar periareolar inferior pedicle reduction technique. Plast Reconstr Surg. 2008; 121 (5):1533–1539

[37] Colwell AS, Breuing KH. Improving shape and symmetry in mastopexy with autologous or cadaveric dermal slings. Ann Plast Surg. 2008; 61(2):138–142

[38] Corduff N, Taylor GI. Rotation mastopexy: an anatomical approach. Aesthetic Plast Surg. 2009; 33(3):377–385, discussion-386-387

[39] Matthews JLK, Oddone-Paolucci E, Lawson DM, Hall-Findlay EJ. Vertical scar breast reduction: does gathering the incision matter? Ann Plast Surg. 2016; 77(1):25–31

9 Augmentation and Mastopexy—Basic Principles to Develop a Treatment Plan and Technical Pearls

Alan Serure, Renee Gasgarth, and Alan Matarasso

Summary

This chapter describes the operative technique for single-stage breast augmentation with mastopexy. The preoperative evaluation of the patient, including musculoskeletal, nipple areolar, inframammary fold, skin type, ptosis, and volume, assessment, is detailed. Three techniques for the mastopexy are then described in depth: circumareolar, vertical or "lollipop," and Wise pattern. The chapter concludes with a brief description of useful adjunctive procedures (liposuction and nipple reduction) and postoperative care.

Keywords: augmentation mastopexy, breast augmentation with mastopexy, single-stage augmentation-mastopexy, circumareolar mastopexy, vertical mastopexy, Wise pattern mastopexy

9.1 Introduction

Single-stage augmentation mastopexy remains a key operation in plastic surgery because there are no effective nonsurgical modalities to lift the breast. The authors present an overview that represents the senior author's personal techniques, which have evolved over three decades of experience with the benefit of long-term follow-up and revisiting existing literature.[1,2,3,4,5,6] This chapter is in no way intended to discard alternative procedures that may prove to be useful in the future. For example, acellular dermal matrix and other scaffolds are being developed that may be proven to provide long-term additional support and better outcomes. The authors recognize that techniques will continue to evolve.

The tendency toward using shortened scars has often pushed surgeons to the brink and beyond, sacrificing breast shape and long-term results to avoid a few additional centimeters of scar. A wise man once said, "If there are many ways to perform a procedure, there is usually no perfect answer" (Melvin Spira, M.D. F.A.C.S., personal communication). This chapter describes three different techniques for augmentation mastopexy: circumareolar, vertical "lollipop," and a Wise-pattern mastopexy. In the opinion of the authors, the surgeon should be well versed in all techniques to avoid stretching indications and producing poor results. When indications are stretched, techniques that are good become techniques that do not work. For example, a circumareolar lift that attempts to overcome excess ptosis and poor skin quality will result in a stretched, deformed areola with minimal or no improvement in glandular ptosis (▶ Fig. 9.1). A vertical "lollipop" mastopexy, which extends the circumareolar mastopexy to incorporate a vertical skin excision, represents a middle ground between the circumareolar and the Wise-pattern mastopexy. If overused, the vertical mastopexy can result in scars that are too long, a too-high-nipple deformity, redundant glandular ptosis, and the need for lower-pole horizontal skin excision. The Wise pattern is the "go-to" for breast excellence in the majority of cases because it is predictable, consistent, and versatile. In the authors' experience, a small minority of patients present with good skin elasticity and minimal ptosis, and these are the patients that benefit from circumareolar or vertical mastopexies. All techniques can be overused or exaggerated, therefore creating suboptimal results with any of them. Consequently, the preoperative plan and realistic expectations are the keys to quality outcomes.

9.2 Preoperative Evaluation

9.2.1 Patient Evaluation

Images of the ideal youthful breasts found in popular fashion advertising, most notably Victoria's Secret, have simultaneously created the best- and worst-case scenario for plastic surgeons. The best-case scenario is an increased desire for breast enhancement. The worst-case scenario is that all women expect their breasts to be round, full, without any element of ptosis.

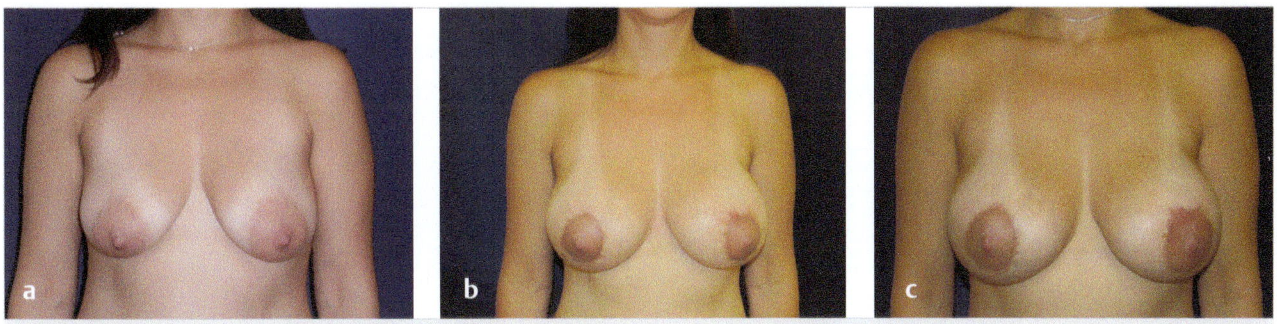

Fig. 9.1 Limits of circumareolar mastopexy. **(a)** 48-year-old woman who elected to undergo circumareolar lift with augmentation despite extensive counseling regarding the need for additional scars to improve the glandular ptosis and reduce the areola. **(b)** Two months post augmentation with 370-mL silicone implants and circumareolar mastopexy. **(c)** One year post circumareolar mastopexy: note the widening and elongation of the nipple areolar complex and recurrent glandular ptosis.

The patients often fail to recognize that these are painstakingly selected models who are naturally anatomically blessed and/or often have had breast enhancement. When a surgeon fails to match reality and patient expectations, unhappiness ensues for both patient and surgeon. Skin type, breast tissue type, body habitus, age, skeletal issues, postpartum status, and menopause will all influence outcomes. Moreover, all results are subject to forces of time, gravity, and the aging process. Skin may not "hold up" because of inherent loss of elasticity in spite of a perfectly executed procedure. A critical part of the preoperative evaluation, therefore, involves listening to the patient's concerns and setting realistic expectations. This includes reviewing photos of what they can expect, discussing how realistic their expectations are, and explaining how results can change over time (▶ Fig. 9.2).

The authors' preference is to meet with patients while they are fully clothed. This allows a neutral setting to discuss concerns regarding size, ptosis, and any existing asymmetry. A detailed past medical history is taken, with particular attention paid to weight fluctuations, pregnancies, breastfeeding, menopause, hormonal replacement therapy, oral contraceptives, age of onset of breast growth/rapid breast growth in younger women, personal or family history of breast cancer, and appropriate radiographic breast evaluation. The authors recommend an early baseline mammogram for patients 35 years of age or older. The risks of needing further imaging or even biopsies, as well as the current recommendations for screening guidelines, are discussed. If patients younger than 40 years old refuse mammograms, this is documented in the chart. Patients who are 40 years of age or older must have imaging within 1 year of the surgery to proceed. All patients are evaluated within 30 days of surgery because weight changes and skin changes can occur rapidly, significantly altering the preoperative appearance and potentially requiring a different operative technique.

9.2.2 Examination

Musculoskeletal Assessment

Examine the patient's skeletal framework and look for scoliosis and other skeletal abnormalities: pectus deformities, prominent ribs, or a downward and laterally sloping chest wall. All skeletal abnormalities and asymmetries can and will be exaggerated postoperatively following implant placement. Excess lateralization of implants is frequently a consequence of a common chest wall variant, which we refer to as a sloping chest wall. In this variant, the sternum is the peak of the "roof," and the laterally sloping ribcage does not provide a level platform to support the implant (▶ Fig. 9.3). These skeletal asymmetries cannot be emphasized enough. Patients are often unaware of them and do not comprehend the challenges that their unique anatomy presents and cannot be overcome.[7]

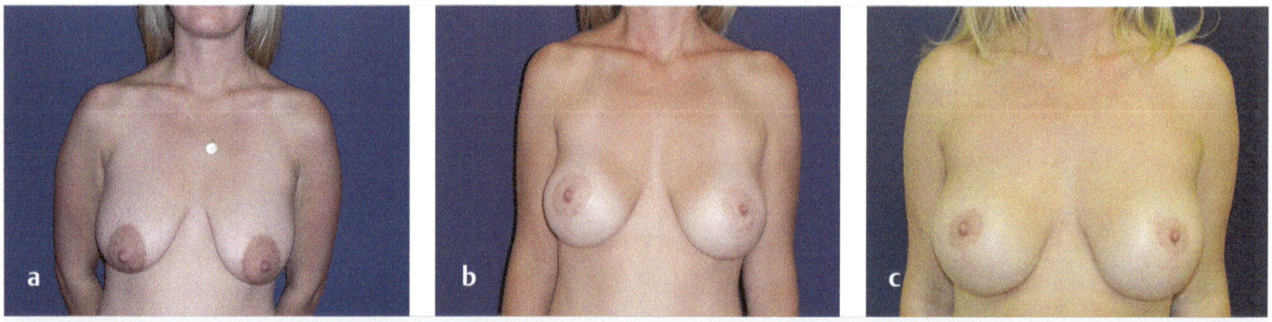

Fig. 9.2 Expected postoperative changes over a decade. **(a)** 42-year-old woman who elected to undergo mastopexy augmentation with Wise-type pattern. **(b)** Three years post mastopexy augmentation with 250 mL saline implant on the left and 325 mL on the right. **(c)** Eight years postoperative.

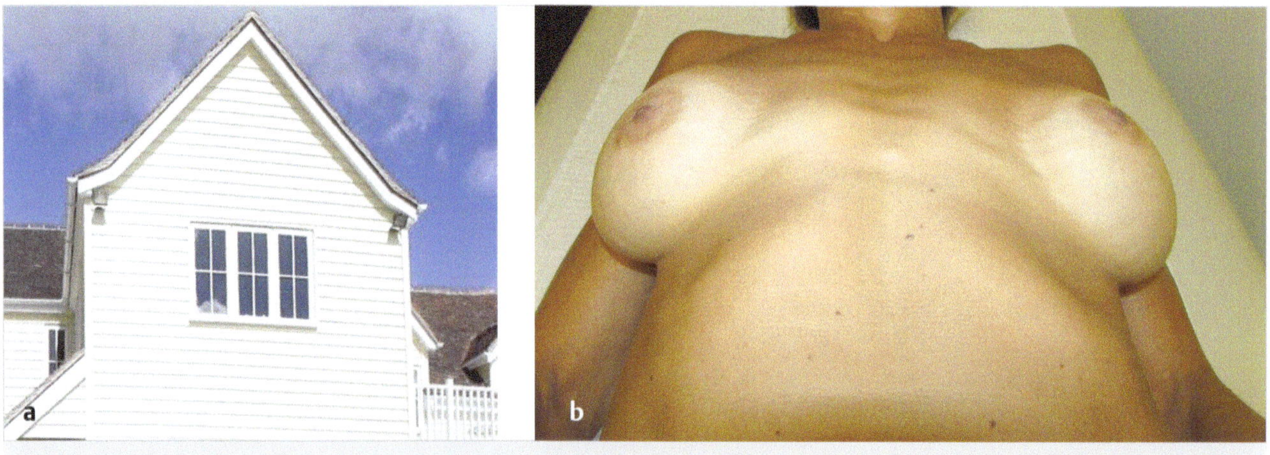

Fig. 9.3 Sloping chest wall deformity. **(a)** The sternum is the peak, and the ribcage slopes away from it like the roof's eaves. **(b)** 59-year-old woman with sloping chest wall deformity and excessive lateralization of the silicone implants.

Nipple Areolar Assessment

Measure the distance from the sternal notch to the nipple bilaterally and also from mid-sternum to nipple. Point out any asymmetries. The youthful ideal nipple position is an equilateral triangle of 21 cm on each side, but this is rarely seen in patients requiring a mastopexy.[8] Markings of nipple position should be made by simultaneously palpating the inframammary fold (IMF) and the breast tissue to approximate the new nipple position. Lowering the nipple position based on the location of the IMF and the patient's individual anatomy will lessen the likelihood of a "too-high-nipple deformity." Nipples can be long and ptotic, or overly projecting.

Nipple reduction should be discussed with the patient as a possible adjunct, much as a chin implant or genioplasty may be mentioned to a rhinoplasty patient to correct facial imbalance.

Inframammary Fold

Note the medial take-off (D1) and lateral extent of the IMFs (D2). The diameter of each and the position of the IMF on the chest wall are frequently asymmetric, and these asymmetries should be pointed out to the patient. Patients are asked to lift their breasts to reveal the true height of the IMFs that are concealed by existing glandular ptosis. The presence and adjunctive treatment of axillary fat deposits may be discussed at this time.

Patients may present with a long torso, and thus have a long breast footprint.[9] The patient often perceives this as ptosis, when it really reflects a lowered position of the breast itself and the IMF. It exacerbates ptosis and the perception of ptosis. The position of the IMF cannot be raised in a routine mastopexy, and attempting to correct the long breast footprint with raising the nipple areolar complex (NAC) will result in a too-high-nipple deformity.

Skin Type

Skin type is evaluated by visual examination and palpation. Shiny thin skin, telangiectasias, and striae indicate atrophy. Sun damage and wrinkles in the décolletage should be noted, as well. The pinch test can also be used to evaluate for elasticity, as well as the traditional 1 inch (2.5 cm) of breast glandular tissue to cover an implant. If patients with minimal glandular ptosis but poor elasticity receive a circumareolar lift, they will be doomed to bottom out once the implant weight asserts itself.

Degree of Ptosis

The surgeon must evaluate pseudoptosis (glandular ptosis) and ptosis of the NAC. There are more nuances than the classic grading system of mild/moderate/severe ptosis defines.[10] Recognizing these subtleties and patient specific factors (skin type, chest wall length, etc.) helps determine the best type of mastopexy to perform.

Volume Assessment

Bra size is subjective. Sizes vary between bra manufacturers: for example, European bras are sized much smaller than bras manufactured in the United States. Many women also do not understand the relationship between base diameter and cup size. For example, a broad-chested woman may want an A or B cup, but this is an anatomic impossibility because her wide base size precludes a small cup size. Showing bras to the patient helps illustrate this. Furthermore, women often wear the incorrect bra size to accommodate redundant skin with a larger cup or band size. They may also wear a smaller cup size to push the breasts up, or they may refuse to increase the band or cup size because of a reluctance to wear a bigger number.

As an aid in evaluating breast volume without the impact of ptosis, paper tape is used to simulate the mastopexy by taping the breasts "up" (▶ Fig. 9.4). At this time, the surgeon can re-emphasize skin elasticity, skin type, skeletal issues, NAC position, and any other asymmetries. Implant sizers with a soft bra are tried on by the patient to demonstrate implant volume. This is critical, because patients often have a false idea of volume and will refer to a "friend's" implant volume and subsequent bra size without understanding their own preoperative

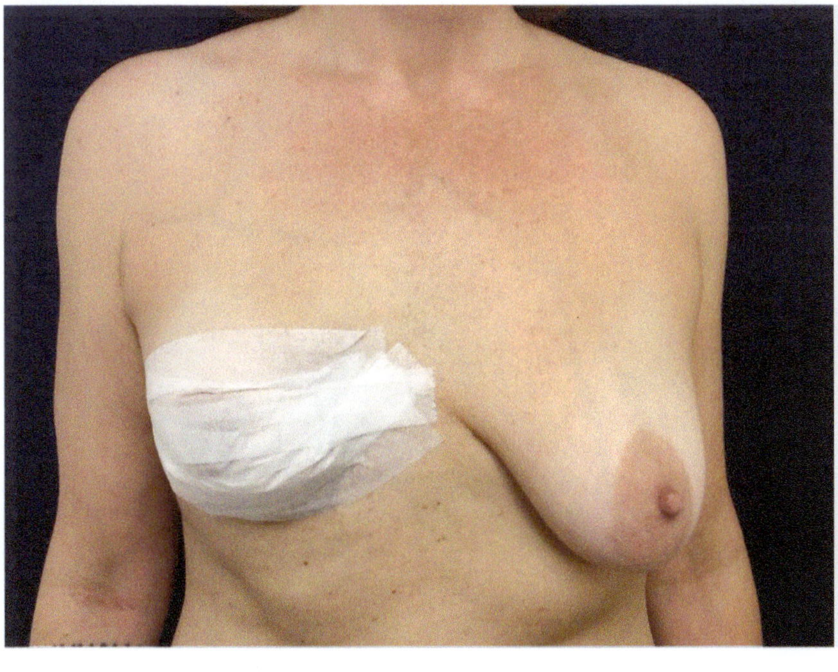

Fig. 9.4 45-year-old woman with mastopexy taping of third-degree ptosis to illustrate the predicted size after mastopexy without augmentation.

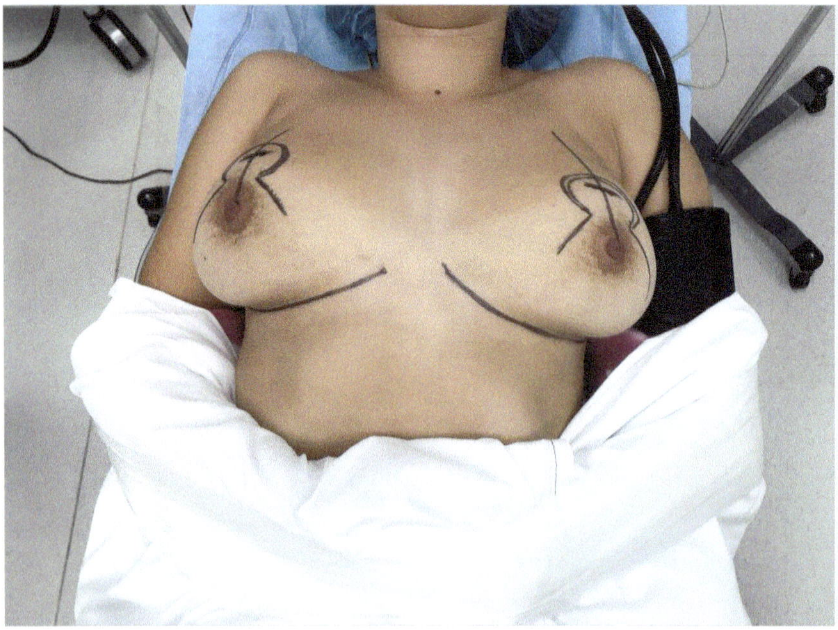

Fig. 9.5 Intraoperative patient positioning. Patient positioning for breast augmentation and Wise-pattern mastopexy with the arms crossed across the abdomen and elbows padded.

anatomy. The surgeon also explains that the exact implant size is less important than the range, and there is an "artistic license" that the surgeon must have. Patients should not fixate on a specific number. It is perfectly reasonable for patients to have an idea of what volume they will be receiving, but a single size option will "handcuff" the surgeon and compromise the aesthetic result. Ideally the surgeon has an assortment of priles and sizes available. If this is not possible, the surgeon should work with the implant manufacturer to have an adequate range of sizes available for each case.

Summarizing the Procedure for the Patient

At the end of each consultation, review the patient's unique anatomy and review the proposed surgical plan and implant size range. Take your finger or a marker and draw on the patient the extent and length of scars. Give her the benefit of your experience regarding the unpredictability of hypertrophic scarring and keloidal scarring. Recommend any adjunctive procedures at this time.

9.3 Techniques

9.3.1 Circumareolar Mastopexy

Circumareolar mastopexy is best employed in patients who have good skin quality and minimal glandular ptosis/pseudoptosis and require minimal nipple areolar elevation. The planned elevation should be 1.5–2 centimeters or less.[11] The patient is marked in a standing position, placing the nipple 1–2 cm above the IMF.

The operating table should be tested to verify 90° flexion before the patient enters the room. The patient must be placed symmetrically on the table with shoulders and hips aligned. Poor alignment can result in an iatrogenic asymmetry when the patient is placed in a sitting position. Procedures can be effectively done with monitored anesthesia care (MAC) or general anesthesia with laryngeal mask airway (LMA) versus endotracheal tube (ETT) depending on the preference of the anesthesiologist. Our preference is general anesthesia with an ETT to allow muscle relaxation when the pectoralis is elevated. A long circuit is required to enable the patient to be placed in a sitting position during the procedure. Intravenous antibiotics are administered, and sequential compression devices (SCDs) are applied. After induction of anesthesia, the arms are adducted, flexed gently at the elbow, and placed across the abdomen. Elbow pads are used, and a sheet with tape is then used to secure the arms (▶ Fig. 9.5). This prevents unnecessary stretching of the pectoralis and better simulates the expected postoperative position of the implants. Note that if liposuction of the axilla is planned, the arms are placed abducted on padded arm boards and secured in place with 6-inch Ace wraps (3 M, St. Paul, MN). The chest is prepped with povidone-iodine and then draped in the standard sterile fashion.

In all mastopexies, the surgeon must have a fixed point on which to base the skin resection. The superior aspect of the planned new areolar position is this fixed A point, and it is predetermined at the time of marking with the patient standing (▶ Fig. 9.6). The extent of the circumareolar skin excision is determined intraoperatively with tailor tacking and temporary skin staples. The final skin excision, however, occurs after the implant has been placed. A cookie cutter template is used to mark the areola size, which is between 4 and 5 cm, based on the patient's breast diameter to maintain appropriate proportions. A solution of 0.5% lidocaine with 1:200,000 epinephrine is injected at the site of the incision and as a local field block. At the end of the procedure, this block is repeated with 0.25% marcaine with 1:200,000 epinephrine. The intraareolar incision is made into, but not through, the deep dermis with the breast under tension. The tension applied by the surgical assistant to the breast must be the same on each side to prevent asymmetries between areolar sizes. The breast parenchyma is entered between 3 and 9 o'clock, preserving adequate blood supply to the NAC. Dissection proceeds meticulously with electrocautery. The vast majority of

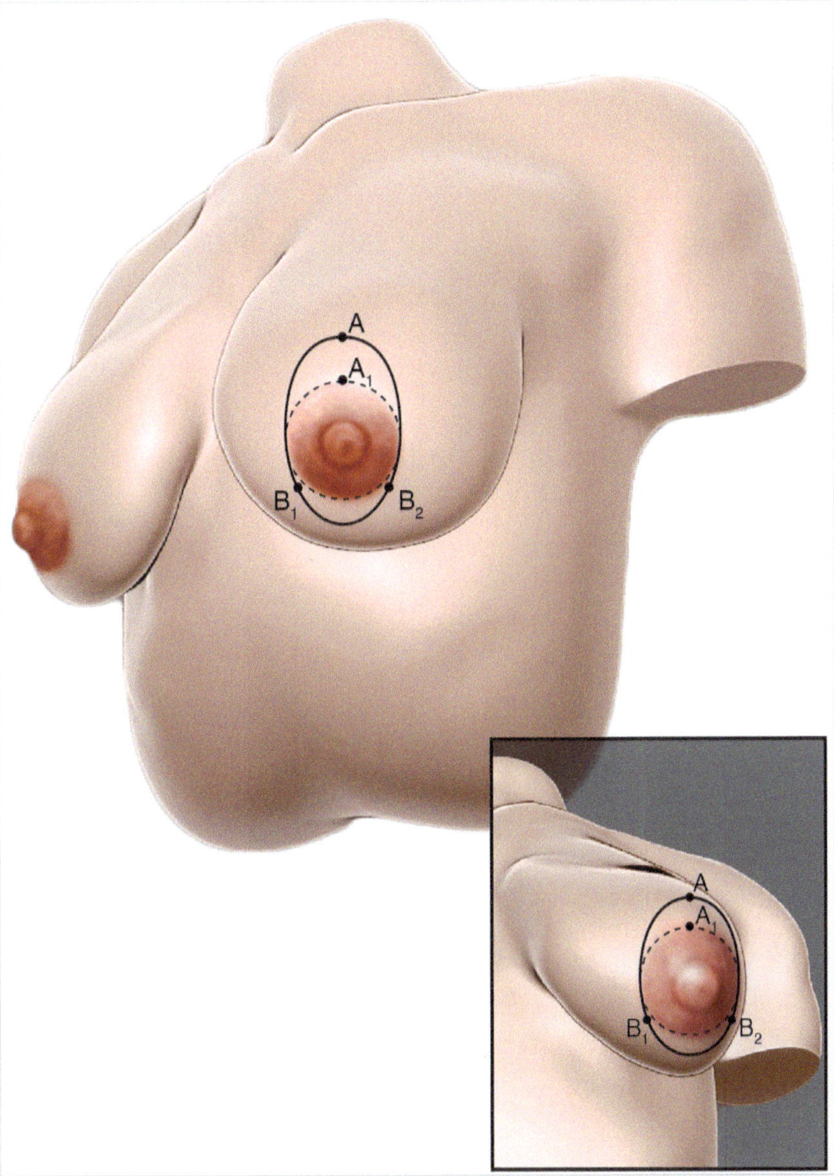

Fig. 9.6 Circumareolar mastopexy markings. A is the superior aspect of the planned areolar position. This is the fixed point that is determined preoperatively. Note that the circle is drawn eccentrically with more tissue removed from the superior aspect of the resection. A_1 is the upper aspect of the areolar. B_1 and B_2 correspond to the inferior lateral borders of the skin excision that may be modified as needed.

implants are placed in the subpectoral plane, superiorly covered by the pectoralis major muscle and inferiorly subglandular. Exceptions are patients who present for secondary surgery to address size change and ptosis with previously placed subglandular implants without capsular contracture or rippling. Body builders are another example of patients who may be candidates for subglandular placement. Avoid blunt dissection or the avulsion of muscle from the rib cage, as this leads to an increase in bleeding and postoperative pain.[6] Avoid extensive lateral dissection and overdissection of the pocket. When necessary, correct for constricted IMFs by dissecting more inferiorly to lower the fold. After completion of dissection and inspection for hemostasis, sizers are utilized to determine the appropriate final implant size. The mastopexy is then tailor-tacked, and the implant selection is finalized. The authors use smooth gel implants given the association of textured implants with breast implant–associated anaplastic large cell lymphoma.[12]

After the implants are placed, a small crescent of breast tissue may be resected inferiorly to plicate redundant breast tissue internally to assist with glandular ptosis. The pocket is irrigated copiously with triple antibiotic solution (cefazolin, bacitracin, gentamicin), and the patient's chest is again prepped with povidone-iodine. Povidone-iodine is placed directly in the pocket, as well. The surgical assistant partially opens the implant package and bathes the implant in the triple antibiotic solution combined with povidone-iodine. Gloves are changed. Then the permanent implants are placed, minimizing any contact between the prepped skin and the implant. The breast issue is then reapproximated with 4–0 absorbable braided sutures (Vicryl, Ethicon, Bridgewater, NJ). The mastopexy skin resection is then tailor-tacked with staples and finalized by placing the patient in the sitting position. After any needed adjustments are made, the patient is placed in the supine position to complete the final skin excision. The areola is then closed with a 3–0 polytetrafluoroethylene (PTFE) suture (Cytpolast, Osteogenics Biomedical, Lubbock, TX) on a Keith needle in a "purse-string" fashion, paying careful attention to start the suture deep in the dermis and end deep. The knot is prepped with povidone-iodine prior to burying it. The final layer is a 5-0 monofilament absorbable suture (Monocryl, Ethicon, Bridgewater, NJ) run subcuticularly. Approximate the incision as needed with 6-0 simple interrupted sutures using permanent suture (nylon or polypropylene). If the patient has not had previous surgery, Mastisol liquid adhesive (Ferndale Laboratories, Ferndale, MI) and Steri-Strips (3 M, St. Paul, MN) are applied. In secondary cases, skin adhesive is avoided because of numerous allergic reactions. Pleating of the areolar edge usually resolves within 6 months. The patient is placed in a soft surgical bra on the day of surgery with gauze padding placed lightly over the incisions.

Two cases are illustrated in ▶ Fig. 9.7 and ▶ Fig. 9.8.

9.3.2 Vertical "Lollipop" Mastopexy

The patient is marked in a standing position. The IMF is marked in its natural position while the breast is held in the appropriate position, as it tends to rise a bit higher in a vertical mastopexy. By palpating the IMF, the new nipple position is translocated at the level of the IMF. A 4- to 5-cm cookie cutter is placed with its center at the new nipple position, and the superior border of the skin resection is determined. This is the fixed A point in all mastopexies. Next, the inferior aspect of the areola, which is the also the superior aspect of the vertical limb, is marked (B_1 and B_2 in ▶ Fig. 9.9). These marks are adjusted to excise the areola completely and adjust the length of the vertical limb. The most inferior point of the vertical limb (C) is marked either at or 1 cm below the IMF, which tends to be lowered at least a centimeter with the placement of implants. The width of the vertical skin excision is gently tapered in a **V** excision to the C point. This width also is adjusted intraoperatively, and all pigmented areolar tissue should be excised. Unlike breast reductions, where the envelope is significantly reduced, mastopexy augmentation expands the envelope, requiring a more conservative skin resection (▶ Fig. 9.10).

After the patient has been marked, the previously described operative protocol for circumareolar mastopexy is followed. The skin incision, however, is made vertically within the center of the **V** skin excision (B_1/B_2 to C), and the muscle is accessed

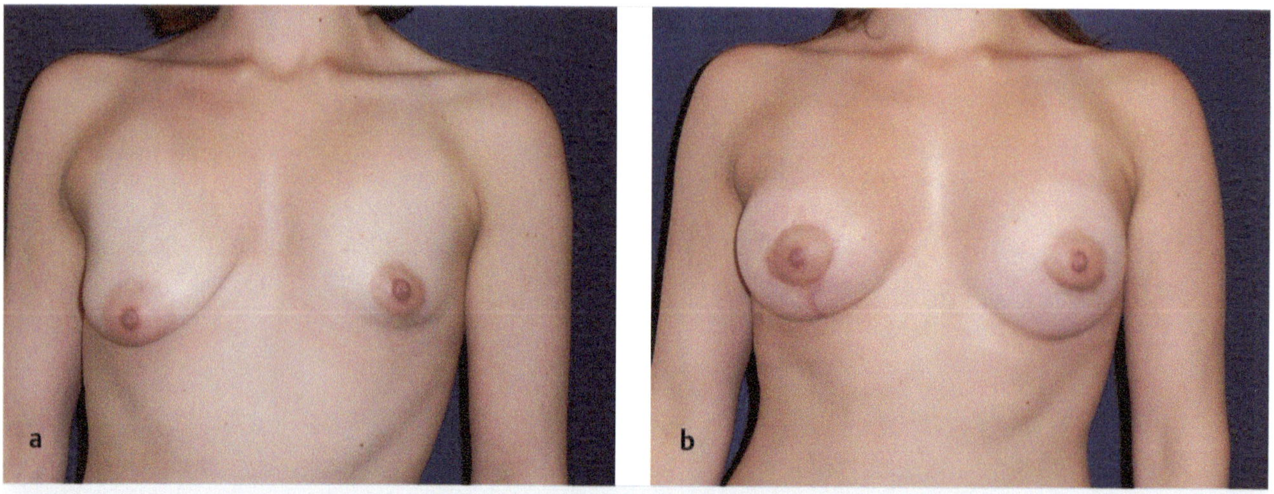

Fig. 9.7 Right vertical "lollipop" mastopexy augmentation. **(a)** 30-year-old woman with asymmetry who underwent right vertical mastopexy and bilateral circumareolar mastopexy. **(b)** One-year follow-up after right vertical mastopexy with 265 mL silicone implant and left augmentation 295 mL silicone implant.

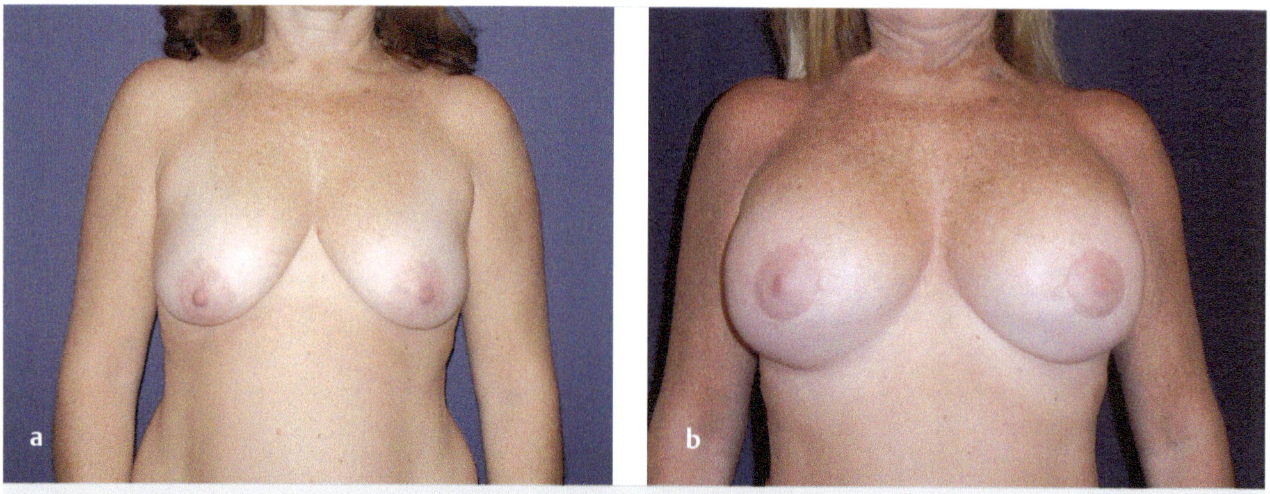

Fig. 9.8 Circumareolar mastopexy with 5-year follow-up. **(a)** 55-year-old woman with ptosis more of nipple areolar complex than of glandular tissue. **(b)** Five years post circumareolar mastopexy with silicone implants (400 mL on the right, 425 mL on the left).

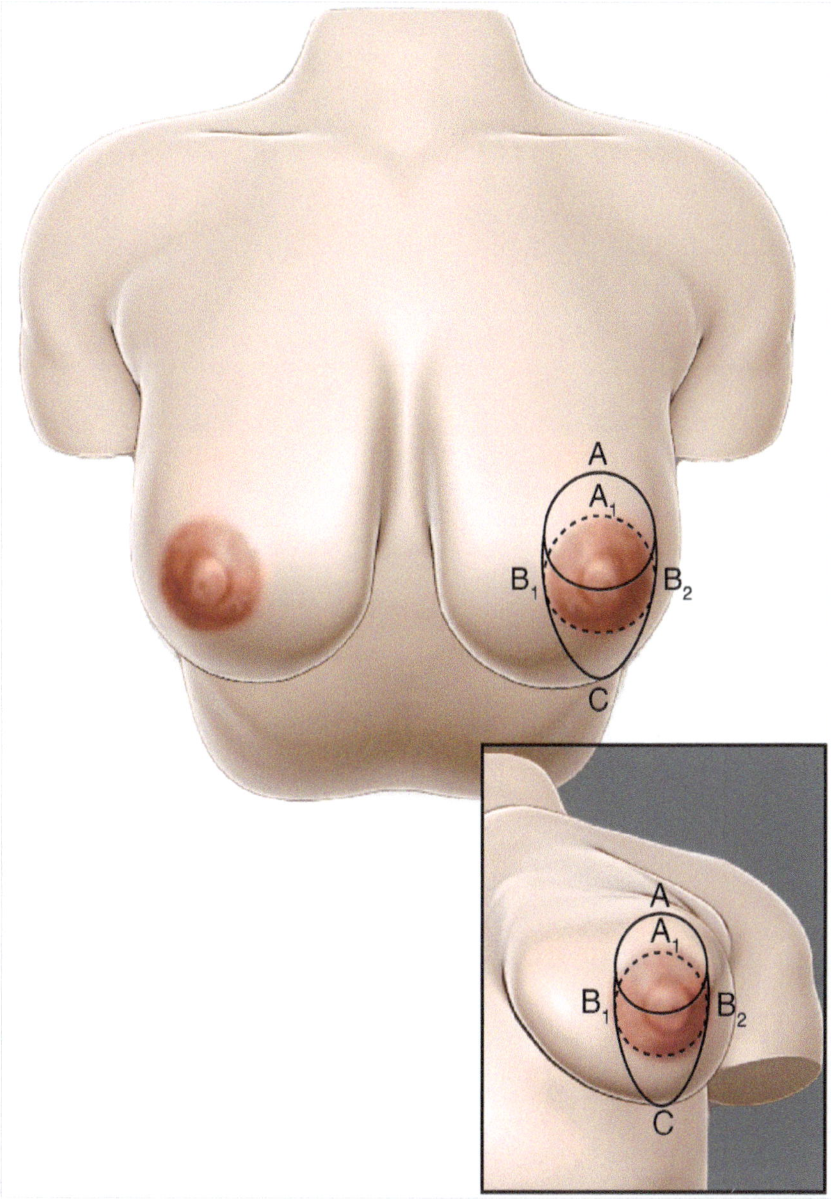

Fig. 9.9 Vertical "lollipop" mastopexy markings. Point A: Fixed position determined preoperatively based on new areolar height. Points B_1 and B_2: Superior aspect of the vertical limbs marked to ensure complete excision of areola. Point C: Most inferior point of vertical limb marked at or 1 cm below the inframammary fold.

transversely through the inferior aspect of this incision. The muscle is elevated with electrocautery in an identical fashion to the circumareolar mastopexy. Sizers are utilized to determine the appropriate volume replacement. Tailor-tacking is used at this point. Often there is redundant, ptotic breast tissue at the central inferior aspect of the lower pole, which may be seen as a bulge once the mastopexy is tailor-tacked. It is the authors' practice to resect this redundant breast tissue (▶ Fig. 9.11). Removing the tissue and suturing the pillars of the breast tissue together internally gives another layer of support for the implants and creates a more youthful shape. After the redundant breast tissue is removed and the mastopexy is tailor-tacked with skin staples, the patient is again placed in seated position to confirm the implant sizes and final skin resection. Marcaine is again injected as a field block, the pockets are irrigated, and sterile implants are placed. The breast tissue is then approximated with 3–0 absorbable braided suture (Vicryl) to carefully close the pocket and the pillars that were created from resection of redundant tissue. The areola and skin incisions are closed as previously described for the circumareolar mastopexy.

Two cases are shown in ▶ Fig. 9.12 and ▶ Fig. 9.13.

9.3.3 Wise-Pattern Mastopexy

The incisions are marked with a modified Wise pattern, using a template, with the patient in standing position (▶ Fig. 9.14).[1] The template's keyhole is 5 cm in diameter, which is the same size as the cookie cutter used to mark the vertical mastopexy. The IMFs are also marked preoperatively, and the medial and lateral extent of the marks should not be violated, because these scars are more conspicuous and heal poorly. Patients with extensive axillary skin redundancy (i.e., massive weight loss patients) are possible exceptions. The new nipple position

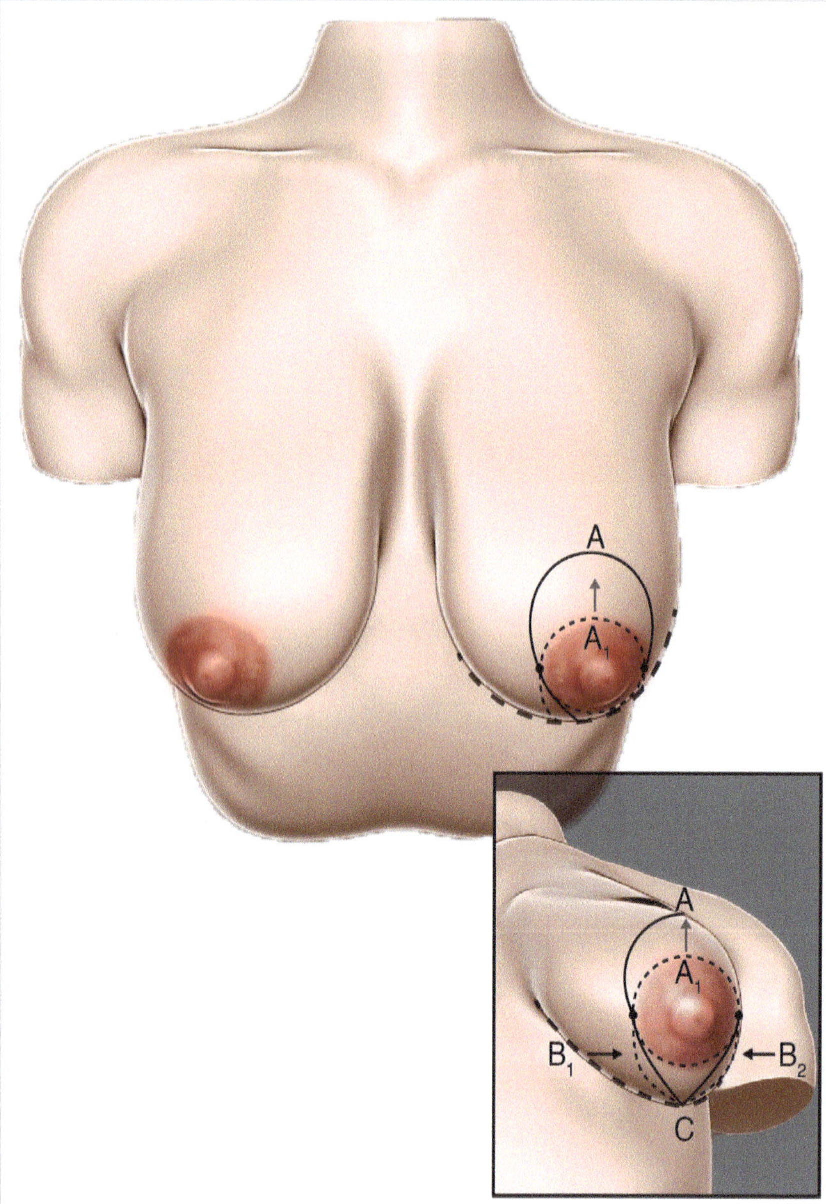

Fig. 9.10 Adjustment of the vertical mastopexy markings. The width of the vertical skin excision is less when a mastopexy is combined with augmentation. The vertical skin excision is tapered gently to a narrower **V** excision instead of a wider more elliptical pattern.

should be at the level of the IMF, or a centimeter above, and the template is adjusted on the breast so that the most superior aspect of the keyhole is the fixed point A. Careful attention should be made to marking the breast meridian as well. The vertical limbs are marked 5–6 cm in length, but given that the augmentation will expand the tissue envelope, have a low threshold for adjusting more obliquely the angles of B_1 to C_1 and B_2 to C_2 in ▶ Fig. 9.15, which results in a smaller skin resection. This adjustment is a key factor. The lateral horizontal limbs (C_1 to D_1 and C_2 to D_2) are next marked; ensure that the most medial and lateral extent of the incision stays within the natural IMF and the breast shadow. The lateral resection can be adjusted to be more elliptical in shape (C_1 to D_1) rather than like a **V** to resect excess redundant tissue toward the axilla.

After the patient has been marked, she is taken to the operating room and placed in supine position with arms abducted if she has extensive lateralization of her breast tissue. The patient is prepped and draped in the standard fashion, and the mastopexy marks are verified with tailor tacking. The B to C limbs are often adjusted intraoperatively because a tension-free closure between C_1 and C_2 to the IMF is essential. The skin incision is made along the IMF, and electrocautery is again used to elevate the pectoralis. Sizers are placed prior to tailor-tacking the mastopexy to ensure appropriate resection of skin. The implants are placed prior to cutting the mastopexy in order to provide tension on the breast. The pocket is closed with 3–0 braided absorbable suture prior to the resection. As with the vertical mastopexy, there is often redundant tissue inferiorly and centrally. It is resected as a central vertical ellipse and an inferior horizontal crescent. In the authors' experience, it is often the redundant breast tissue along the IMF that is the first to fall in recurrent ptosis cases. The skin is then closed in a similar fashion to the vertical mastopexy. However, there is usually less tension on the circumareolar closure; therefore, the areola is closed with 4–0 interrupted absorbable deep dermal

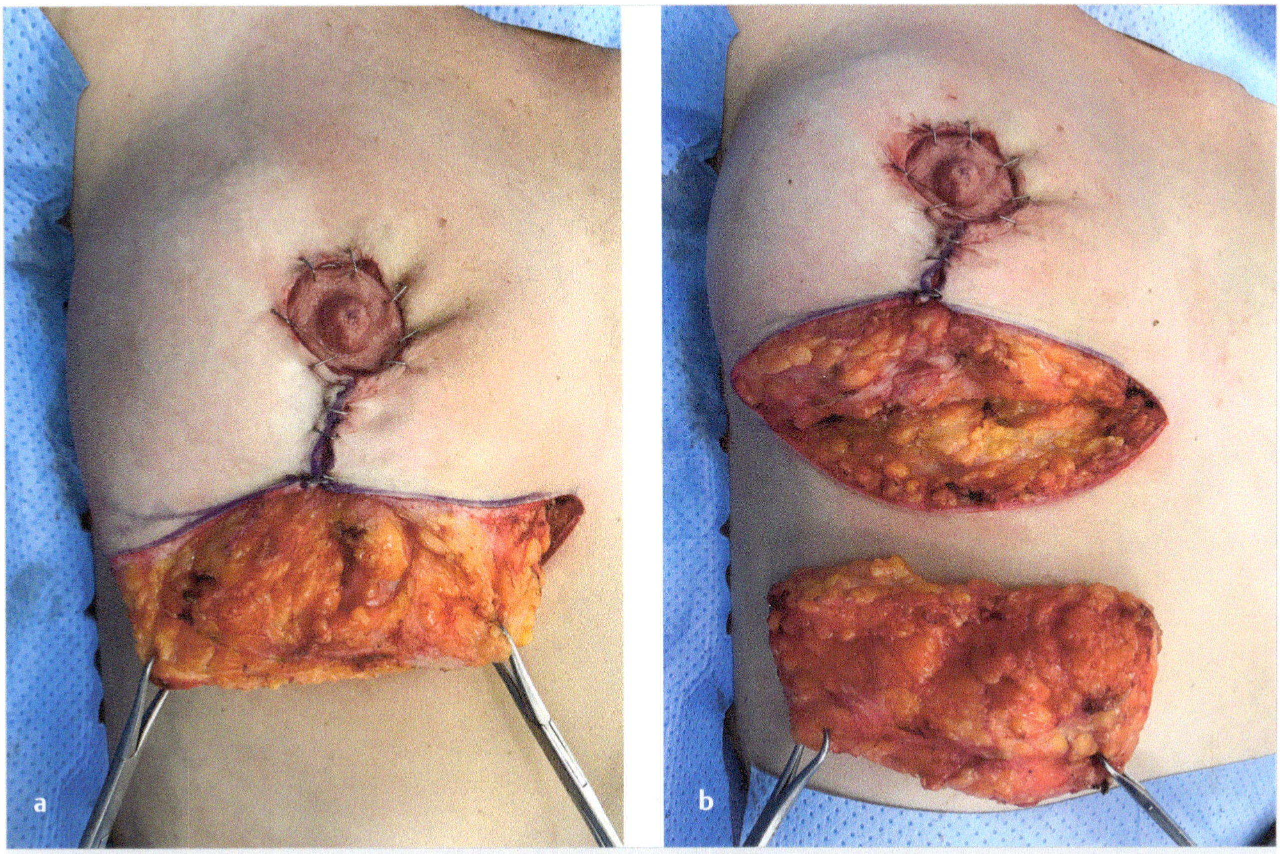

Fig. 9.11 Resection of redundant breast tissue. **(a)** The inferior and central portion of the glandular breast tissue is often redundant and requires resection during a vertical or Wise-pattern mastopexy. **(b)** Intraoperative photograph after resection of a crescent of redundant breast tissue along the inferior pole.

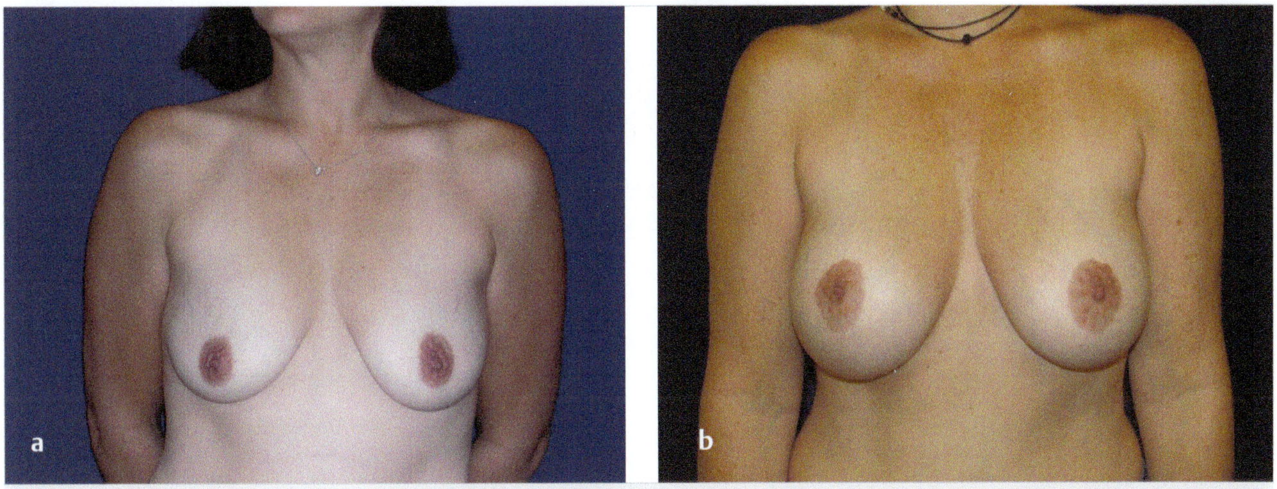

Fig. 9.12 Vertical "lollipop" mastopexy augmentation. **(a)** 41-year-old woman preoperative of a vertical mastopexy augmentation. **(b)** Twelve years post vertical mastopexy with 125 mL silicone implants.

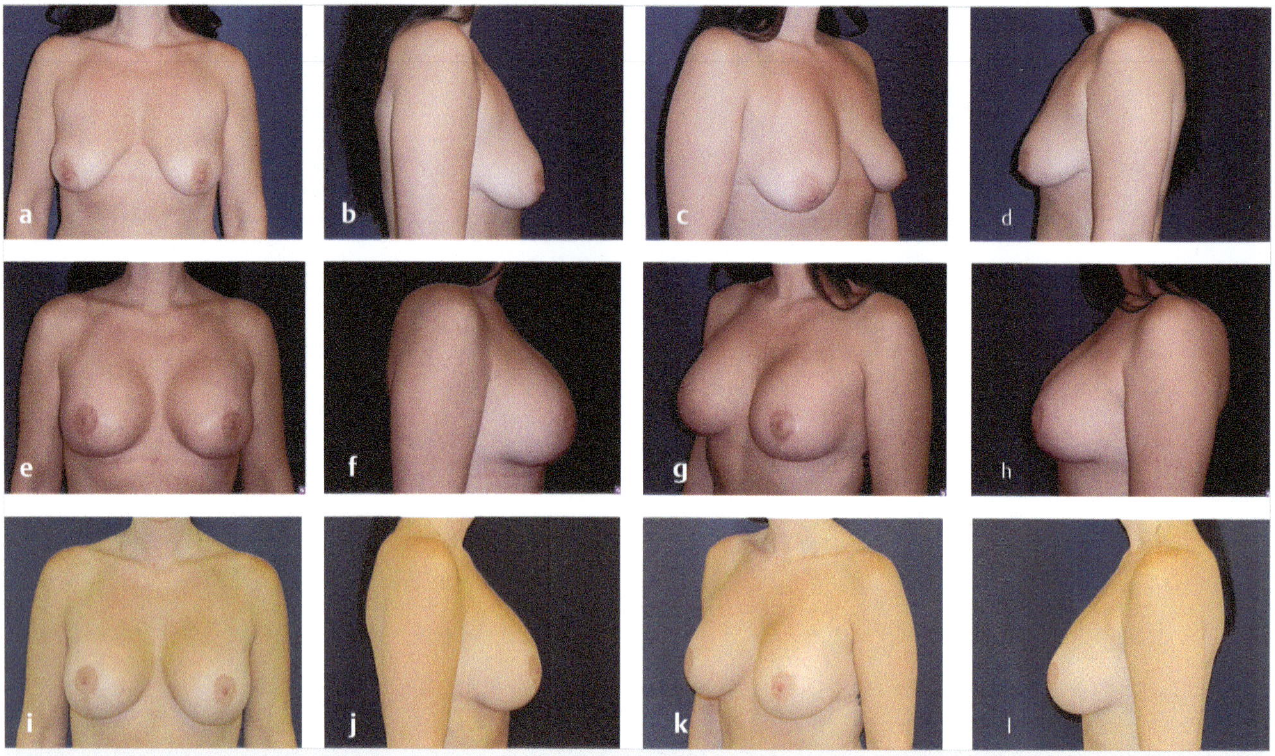

Fig. 9.13 (a–d) Preop of a 34-year-old patient for vertical mastopexy augmentation. **(e–h)** Early 2-month follow-up of vertical mastopexy augmentation with smooth round silicone; right 325 mL, left 350 mL. **(i–l)** Three-year follow-up of the same patient.

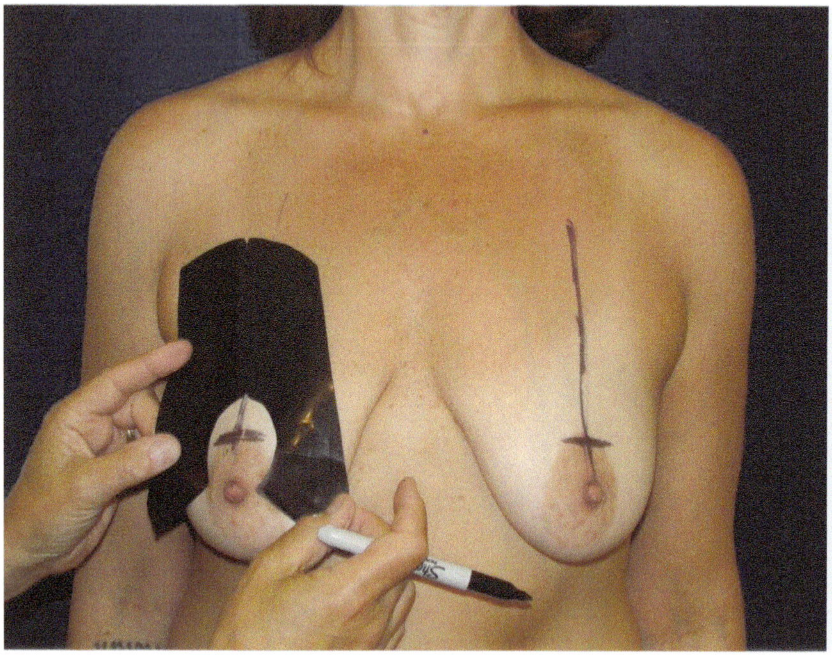

Fig. 9.14 Preoperative patient marking of a modified Wise pattern using a template. The width of the vertical limbs are adjusted as needed.

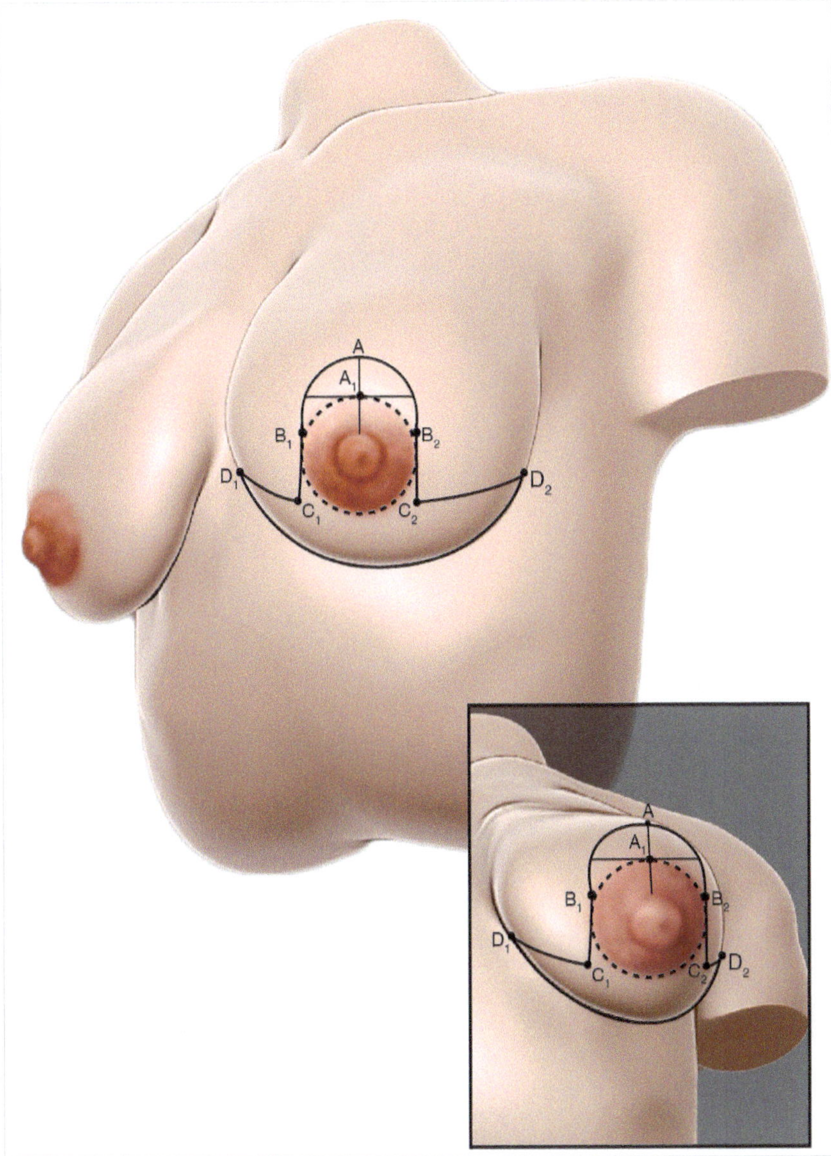

Fig. 9.15 Wise-pattern mastopexy markings. Point A: Most superior aspect of planned areolar position and fixed point. Points B_1 and B_2: Medial and lateral superior aspect of the vertical resection; they are adjusted to excise all remaining areolar tissue completely. The width of the vertical limbs B_1 to B_2 and C_1 to C_2 are adjusted according to skin excess and elasticity. Points C_1 and C_2: Medial and lateral aspects of the most inferior aspect of the vertical resection. Points D_1 and D_2: Medial and lateral aspects of the horizontal skin resection; these points should remain within the shadow of the breast.

sutures and then a running 5–0 Monocryl. In rare cases of tension, a PTFE deep dermal suture may be used.

Two cases are illustrated in ▸ Fig. 9.16, ▸ Fig. 9.17.

9.4 Adjunctive Procedures

9.4.1 Liposuction

Liposuction is an excellent adjunct to mastopexy augmentation. It can be used along the upper abdomen to define a sharper IMF. It narrows the chest when performed on the lateral axillary area, colloquially called the "bra fat" area. The posterior axillary fatty deposits (the "back-xilla") cannot be addressed appropriately in the supine position; therefore, a position change to prone is necessary. Liposuction is accomplished through the lateral IMF incision or areolar incision. The area is infiltrated with a modified Hunstad tumescent formula in a 1/2:1 or 1:1 ratio of infiltration fluid to aspiration.[13] Power-assisted liposuction is then performed with a 3- or 4-mm triple-hole cannula; the holes always face away from the skin. Occasionally an additional incision is needed in the axillary fold for cross-tunneling. Any additional incisions are closed with simple interrupted 5–0 polypropylene suture. The mastopexy incisions are otherwise closed as previously described. After Steri-Strips are applied, Topifoam (Byron Medical, Tucson, AZ) is placed within the bra to allow for uniform compression at the sites of liposuction and left in place for one week.

9.4.2 Nipple Reduction

Patients with ptotic or elongated nipples are candidates for simultaneous nipple reduction. A portion of the inferior aspect of the nipple is amputated in full thickness. The incision should be flush with the areola, and it may remove as much as 50% of the nipple. The superior portion of the nipple is then inset into the edge of the nipple-areolar junction with simple interrupted sutures using absorbable 5–0 twisted gut (chromic). Antibiotic ointment is applied, and

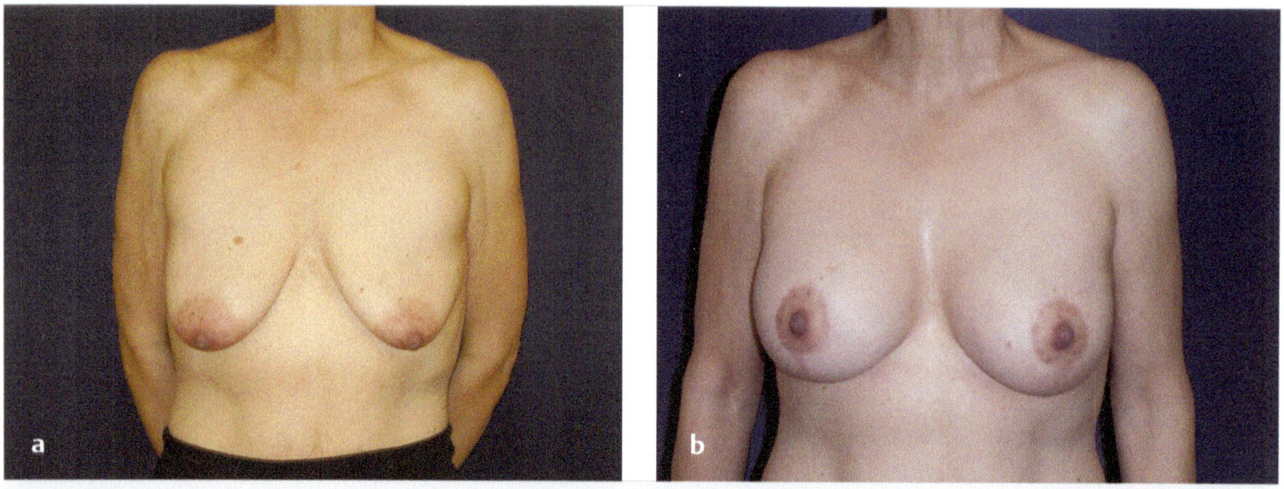

Fig. 9.16 Wise-pattern mastopexy with 3-year follow-up. **(a)** 51-year-old woman preoperative for Wise-pattern mastopexy with augmentation. **(b)** Three years post Wise-pattern mastopexy with 421 mL silicone implants bilaterally.

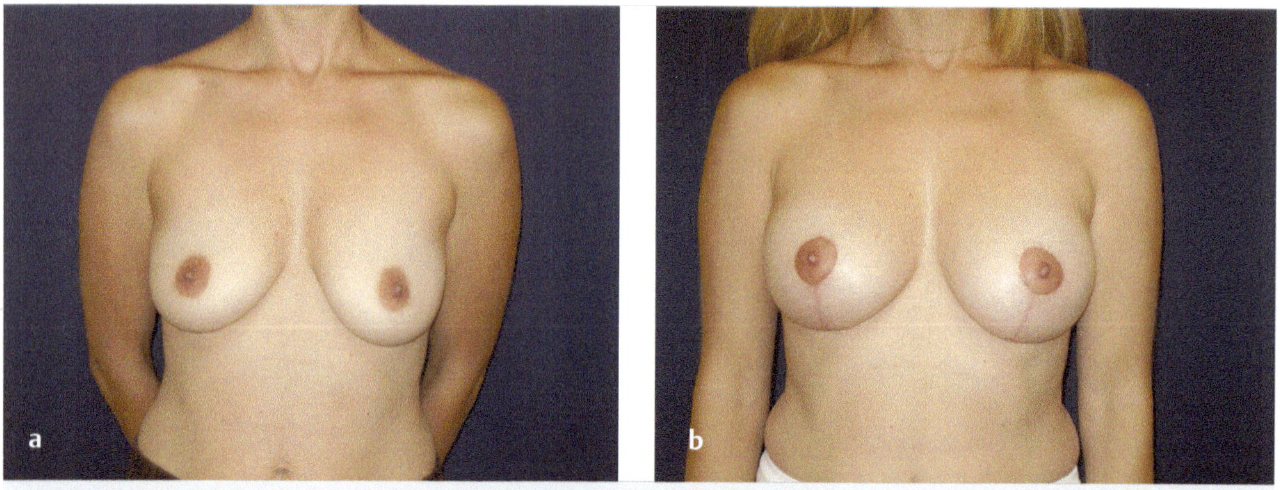

Fig. 9.17 Wise-pattern mastopexy augmentation with 5-year follow-up. **(a)** 41-year-old woman preoperative for Wise-pattern mastopexy with augmentation. **(b)** Five years post Wise-pattern mastopexy with 213 mL bilateral silicone implants.

then the nipple is covered by a nonadherent bandage (Telfa, Covidien, Minneapolis, MN) and gauze.

9.5 Postoperative Instructions

Patients are given prescriptions for oxycodone/acetaminophen 7.5/325 mg (8 tabs), lorazepam (8 tabs, one per night), odansetron, and cefadroxil (1-week supply). It is very rare that patients require additional narcotics. The patients are seen often, including postoperative day 1 and again postoperative day 3 or 5. They are placed in a soft surgical bra at the time of surgery and given an additional soft bra to alternate for the first month. After 1 month, they may resume using underwire bras. Steri-Strips are removed at the 2-week postoperative visit to allow for suture removal; they are then replaced and kept in place until 3 weeks postoperative. At this point, patients are instructed on scar care. They are reminded to avoid sun exposure and to use topical silicone gel twice a day. If there is evidence of poor scarring, triamcinolone acetonide (Kenalog, Bristol-Myers Squibb, Buffalo, NY) injections to target scar thickness and laser treatment to target hyperpigmentation can begin as early as 2 weeks postoperatively. A Nd:YAG laser set with spot 8, 12 J, and 0.25 msec is administered monthly for four treatments.

Key Points

- Single stage augmentation mastopexy is challenging procedure because of the multiple variables that affect patient outcomes.
- Preoperative planning and realistic expectations are the key to quality outcomes.
- The Wise pattern remains the most versatile, predictable, and consistent pattern for skin resection.
- The circumareolar mastopexy is best employed for patients with good skin quality and minimal glandular ptosis/pseudoptosis who require less than 2 cm of nipple areolar elevation.

- The most critical portion of the preoperative marking is marking the height of the new nipple areolar position. Commit to the A point and the new nipple position, even as the skin resection and implant size are adjusted intraoperatively.
- Augmentation expands the tissue envelope, therefore, the vertical limbs of the vertical and Wise-pattern mastopexy are often adjusted to resect a smaller amount of skin than marked preoperatively.
- There is often some redundant inferior breast tissue that requires resection to achieve the optimal contour of the lower pole.
- Liposuction of the axilla and nipple reduction can be useful adjunctive procedures.

References

[1] Wise RJ. A preliminary report on a method of planning the mammaplasty. Plast Reconstr Surg (1946). 1956; 17(5):367–375

[2] Erol OO, Spira M. A mastopexy technique for mild to moderate ptosis. Plast Reconstr Surg. 1980; 65(5):603–609

[3] Benelli L. A new periareolar mammaplasty: the "round block" technique. Aesthetic Plast Surg. 1990; 14(2):93–100

[4] Hall-Findlay EJ. A simplified vertical reduction mammaplasty: shortening the learning curve. Plast Reconstr Surg. 1999; 104(3):748–759, discussion 760–763

[5] Hammond DC. Short scar periareolar inferior pedicle reduction (SPAIR) mammaplasty. Plast Reconstr Surg. 1999; 103(3):890–901, discussion 902

[6] Tebbetts JB. Achieving a predictable 24-hour return to normal activities after breast augmentation: part I. Refining practices by using motion and time study principles. Plast Reconstr Surg. 2002; 109(1):273–290, discussion 291–292

[7] Martinovic ME, Blanchet NP. BFACE: A framework for evaluating breast aesthetics. Plast Reconstr Surg. 2017; 140(2):287e–295e

[8] Penn J. Breast reduction. Br J Plast Surg. 1955; 7(4):357–371

[9] Hall-Findlay EJ. The three breast dimensions: analysis and effecting change. Plast Reconstr Surg. 2010; 125(6):1632–1642

[10] Kirwan L. Augmentation of the ptotic breast: Simultaneous periareolar mastopexy/breast augmentation. Aesthet Surg J. 1999; 19:34–39

[11] Puckett CL, Meyer VH, Reinisch JF. Crescent mastopexy and augmentation. Plast Reconstr Surg. 1985; 75(4):533–543

[12] Knight R, et al. Epidemiology and risk factors for breast implant-associated anaplastic large cell lymphoma (BIA-ALCL) in Australia and New Zealand. Plast Reconstr Surg Glob Open. 2016; 9:82–83

[13] Hunstad JP. Tumescent and syringe liposculpture: a logical partnership. Aesthetic Plast Surg. 1995; 19(4):321–333

10 Management of the Massive-Weight-Loss Breast

Sharona Czerniak, Jeffrey A. Gusenoff, and J. Peter Rubin

Summary
The massive-weight-loss patient can present with severe deformities of the breast, including major deflation of skin, loss of upper pole fullness, medialization of the nipple areolar complex, loss of the lateral curvature of the breast with prominent lateral chest roll, and loose and inferiorly displaced inframammary fold. Deformities of the breast can be complicated by surrounding soft tissue laxity of adjacent aesthetic units such as the upper abdomen, arm, lateral chest, or back. The dermal suspension, parenchymal reshaping mastopexy is the authors' method of choice for restoring the breast to a youthful shape and normalized breast position on the chest wall. This chapter includes a review of careful patient selection for the procedure, discussion of staging of breast reshaping procedures relative to other aesthetic units, advantages and disadvantages, relative contraindications, and results from outcomes studies utilizing the dermal suspension technique. A step-by-step approach to marking the dermal suspension, parenchymal reshaping mastopexy will be described along with surgical tips and pearls to optimize results and reduce complications. Other surgical options for the massive-weight-loss breast will be discussed.

Keywords: massive weight loss, postbariatric, breast, mastopexy, dermal suspension, parenchymal reshaping, body contouring

10.1 Introduction

The most effective and durable method to treat morbid obesity is bariatric surgery.[1] The landscape of bariatric procedures has changed over the past several years. According to the American Society for Metabolic and Bariatric Surgery (ASMBS), the number of bariatric procedures continues to increase, from 158,000 in 2011 to 228,000 in 2017. Popularity of procedures has shifted from the Roux-en-Y gastric bypass to the sleeve gastrectomy, which accounted for 59.4% of procedures in 2018.[2] After massive weight loss (MWL) resulting from such measures, thousands of patients present for breast-contouring procedures every year: 15,360 procedures in 2018, according to the American Society of Plastic Surgeons (ASPS).[3]

The MWL breast presents a distinct surgical challenge. The deformities observed in the MWL breast are severe, far beyond what plastic surgeons usually see in the regular cosmetic patient, and present a great technical challenge. The MWL breast is not just ptotic and deflated but has specific unique features[4,5]:

- Poor tissue quality, with redundancy and loss of skin elasticity.
- Severe volume loss, especially in the upper pole, which may be asymmetric, with an enormous skin excess relative to parenchymal volume.
- Ptosis (usually third-degree) and medialization of the nipple-areola complex (NAC).
- Loss of lateral curvature of the breast and, occasionally, prominent lateral chest wall excess that merges with the breast.
- Low and loose inframammary fold (IMF), especially laterally.

The breast deformities are often seen in concert with other upper body deformities after MWL, with surrounding aesthetic units of the lateral chest wall, arm, back, and upper abdomen also in need of concurrent evaluation (▶ Fig. 10.1).

There are several goals of breast reshaping after MWL: to obtain a youthful, well-contoured breast; to restore volume, especially in the upper pole, with central projection; to position the nipple properly on the chest wall; to improve the lateral curvature of the breast; and, most importantly, to maintain the longevity of the result, which is especially relevant in patients after MWL because of their poor skin quality and tendency for recurrent skin laxity.

Most of the breast reduction and mastopexy techniques (with or without breast implants or added autologous tissue) fall short in addressing the deformities associated with the MWL breast because of progressive skin laxity with loss of projection, loss of upper pole fullness, bottoming-out and implant malposition. To choose the correct surgical procedure to achieve these goals, the surgeon must assess the volume, shape, degree of ptosis, laxity/excess tissues surrounding the breast, the patient's desires, and what extent of scars she is willing to accept.

This chapter focuses mainly on the dermal suspension and parenchymal reshaping mastopexy pioneered by the senior author.[6] Several surgical procedures have been developed to aid in contouring the MWL breast, and these will be mentioned briefly.

10.2 Preoperative Assessment

10.2.1 Weight Stability

Patients after bariatric surgery lose most of their weight during the first and second year after the procedure.[7] Patients typically reach a nadir and then plateau at a slightly higher weight. Body contouring after weight loss typically is deferred until the patient is at least 12–18 months out from her weight loss surgery or start of self weight loss and has been stable for 3 months with only approximately 5 lb (2.25 kg) of weight fluctuation over that time.[8,9] Patients who are not yet weight stable or who have residual obesity are typically referred to weight loss specialists or their bariatric team, with a scheduled follow-up in 3 months for re-evaluation.

10.2.2 Nutrition

Certain bariatric procedures, such as the Roux-en-Y gastric bypass, have a malabsorptive component in addition to the restrictive nature of the surgery. Care must be taken to assess

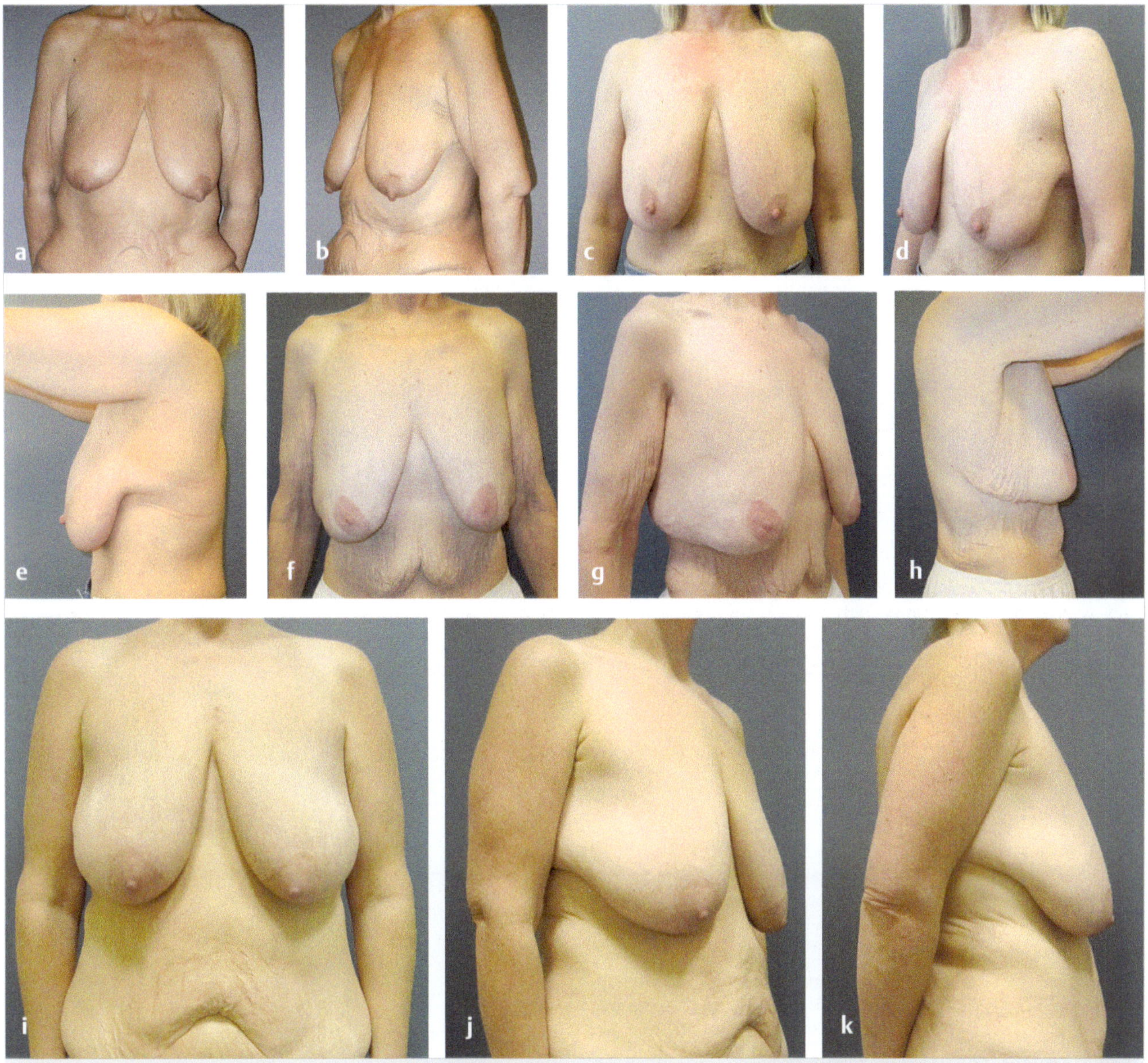

Fig. 10.1 (a–k) Variations of the massive weight loss breast include third-degree ptosis, loss of upper pole fullness, loss of the lateral curvature of the breast, medialized nipple areolar complex, and descent of the inframammary fold. Surrounding deformities include laxity of the lateral chest, arms, back, and upper abdomen.

and correct nutritional deficiencies, as this is crucial for wound healing and minimizing the need for blood transfusion. All patients should have a thorough evaluation including albumin, prealbumin, iron, and vitamins A, D, E, K, and B_{12}. Protein malnutrition may be present, especially for patients with malabsorptive procedures or fad diets. Patients are guided to increase their protein intake perioperatively with a goal of 75–100 grams per day.

10.2.3 Body Mass Index

Obesity is defined as body mass index (BMI) greater than 30 kg/m^2. Several investigators have reported an increased risk for complications in patients undergoing body contouring procedures with a body mass index greater than 30 kg/m^2.[10,11,12,13,14] A large cohort study of MWL patients undergoing multiple procedures demonstrated complications associated with maximal BMI prior to weight loss and change in BMI, or delta BMI. However, the exact etiology of this is not well understood, as many factors can contribute to complications. In addition, no strict BMI cutoff was determined to influence complications.[15] For this reason, the authors advocate for examining patients for breast contouring procedures on an individual basis, as a patient with a high BMI may have very deflated breasts but carry most of her excess weight in a pannus or thighs, which are not the patient's priority or goal. Patients with lower BMI around the time of surgery typically obtain better cosmetic results, and patients with a BMI greater than 35 kg/m^2 are not uncommonly referred for further weight loss prior to proceeding with surgery.

10.2.4 Preoperative Assessment and Comorbidities

At consultation, a complete medical and surgical history is obtained, including any personal or familial history of coagulopathies or thrombotic events; former problems with anesthesia; and history of breast cancer, breast disease, or prior breast surgery. Detailed medication history includes all prescription, over-the-counter, and herbal medications and specifically the use of aspirin, other nonsteroidal anti-inflammatory drugs (NSAIDs) or any other medication that might increase the risk of bleeding postoperatively. A history of substance abuse or need for chronic pain medication is obtained. Many of the comorbidities associated with obesity will resolve or improve with bariatric surgery, such as diabetes, sleep apnea, hypertension, heart disease, and gastroesophageal reflux disease (GERD) [16,17,18]; however, depression and anxiety may not improve. Patients are often referred for consultation for various residual comorbidities, such as hematology evaluation for iron deficiency anemia, or to medical specialists for clearance for surgery (such as internal medicine, cardiology, or psychology).

Smoking increases the risk for surgical complications, and all patients should stop smoking for at least 4 weeks prior to and after surgery.[10,19,20,21] This is especially important for flap survival and prevention of distal flap necrosis. Urine cotinine prior to surgery is routinely measured in patients who state they have recently quit smoking.

Complete physical examination with a comprehensive breast exam and assessment of the position of the IMF, quality of skin, degree of ptosis and nipple position, amount of breast tissue, asymmetry, and adjacent tissue excess is mandatory.

Preoperative laboratory workup includes complete blood count with platelets, complete metabolic panel (including albumin), prothrombin, and activated partial prothrombin time within 30 days of surgery. Urine pregnancy testing is done in all reproductive-age women on the morning of surgery.

Chest radiograph and electrocardiograms are ordered as indicated by age and medical profile. All patients above 40 must obtain a mammogram prior to surgery.

Preoperative photography is obtained in standing position with anterior, lateral, and oblique views from the lower neck to the waist. Photographic documentation is important to analyze and plan the procedure properly as well as to document preoperative asymmetry and surrounding soft tissue deformities that may become more noticeable after the breasts are contoured.

During the consent process, it is important to make sure the patient has realistic goals and understands the limitations of plastic surgery, including possible asymmetry postoperatively and recurrent skin laxity despite how tight the tissues are in surgery. Managing expectations ahead of surgery can avoid significant patient and surgeon disappointment postoperatively.

10.2.5 Staging and Combination of Body-Contouring Procedures

Breast contouring after MWL is often done as a solo procedure; however, adjacent body areas may need contouring as well. Patients and the surgeon may opt to perform multiple procedures, depending on the patient's desires, financial abilities, comorbidities, nutritional status, and ability to withstand a lengthy operation and recovery and on the surgeons' experience and the available team.

When combining procedures, keep in mind the following:[22,23]

- Pulling in opposite vectors at the same time can limit results.
- Patient safety comes first: if medical comorbidities preclude a lengthy operation, the surgical plan may need to be changed.
- Consider the magnitude and stress of recovery when combining procedures.
- Optimal staging and combination of procedures may not correspond with patient's preferences.

Favorable procedure combinations including the breast are[10]

- Abdominoplasty + mastopexy: a common combination that gives the patient a powerful transformation.
- Circumferential lower body lift + mastopexy.
- Upper body lift + mastopexy: eliminating the upper body lift "dog-ears" while merging the incisions together.
- Brachioplasty + mastopexy: curving the lateral chest incision into the axilla.
- Vertical thigh lift + mastopexy.

Caveats for combining breast and other body contouring procedures:

- Mastopexy may be safely combined with an abdominoplasty with excellent results. Since the IMF on the MWL breast is very loose and mobile, especially laterally, it may be displaced inferiorly upon completion of the abdominoplasty, requiring the surgeon to adjust the mastopexy markings.[10,22] Similarly, addition of a fleur-de-lis vertical extension to an abdominoplasty can mobilize the inframammary fold inferomedially. Hence, it is wise to complete the abdominoplasty before proceeding with the mastopexy. In cases where the IMF is completely nonadherent to the chest wall, it would better serve the patient to separate these two procedures completely.
- Be careful of fresh triple point incisions, such as when combining an upper body lift + dermal suspension parenchymal-reshaping mastopexy + brachioplasty; these areas tend to break down and cause wound healing problems.[10,22] The mastopexy can be performed merging in the brachioplasty scar at the lateral chest, or merged into the upper body lift, delaying either the upper body lift or brachioplasty until a later time.

10.3 Dermal Suspension Parenchymal Reshaping Mastopexy

The dermal suspension and parenchymal reshaping mastopexy is based on an extended deepithelialized Wise pattern. The lateral and medial extensions, which would ordinarily be discarded in a breast reduction, are mobilized and incorporated into the breast mound as dermoglandular flaps for auto-augmentation. These help enhance the breast volume and improve shape while redefining the contour of the lateral chest wall. The dermoglandular flaps are suspended to the chest wall in multiple fixation points to ensure longevity of the result and secure the new nipple position, while plication of the broad dermal surface enables the surgeon to reshape the breast parenchyma and reposition the breast on the chest wall. This technique is very versatile in addressing and correcting the patient's specific anatomy, as the surgeon can titrate the amount of breast tissue needed for the auto-augmentation by elongating the lateral extension or shortening it. The Wise pattern can be laterally extended beyond the borders of the **T** (lateral dermoglandular) flap to improve the contour of the lateral chest wall effectively, as needed.

This technique was developed based on previous publications discussing breast reconstruction, reduction, and mastopexy. In 1986, Holmström described breast reconstruction using a lateral thoracodorsal fasciocutaneous flap for auto-augmentation with or without an implant, based on redundant tissue of the lateral chest wall.[24] In 1999, Frey published his technique of a bralike dermal suspension method for breast reduction, which was secured to the deep fascia of the chest wall, with a **B**-formed incision, eliminating the medial inframammary scar.[25] Lockwood described superficial fascial system (SFS) suspension with nonabsorbable sutures to improve scarring and achieving long-lasting results.[26] Gulyás developed a periareolar dermal cloak, relying on dermis for glandular support.[27] In 2002, Graf and Biggs described creating an inferiorly based de-epithelialized flap, which was mobilized superiorly and held in place by a loop of pectoralis muscle, to maintain upper pole fullness with added support by suturing the dermal edges of the flap to pectoralis muscle fascia.[28] In 2003, Qiao et al published their technique for breast reduction with a crescent glandular resection excluding the inferior quadrant of the breast, with creation of a dermal bra, secured to the pectoralis muscle fascia.[29] Several other investigators have published reports on their experience with auto-augmentation of the MWL with local flaps.[30,31,32,33,34,35]

Patients who would benefit most from this technique are MWL patients, with ptotic, deflated, and flattened breasts, an excess of inelastic skin, and prominent axillary folds, providing sufficient tissue for auto-augmentation.

Those patients with inadequate amounts of tissue for auto-augmentation may be candidates for an implant-based augmentation-mastopexy or other auto-augmentation methods. Patients with ptosis and significant excess parenchymal breast tissue would be better served with a formal breast reduction, as described in the algorithmic approach to the MWL breast by Colwell et al.[36]

10.3.1 Advantages of This Technique

- The method is safe with reliable, long-lasting, reproducible results and a low complication rate.
- It uses all the available breast tissue and surrounding autologous tissue (as needed), avoiding the need to use breast implants with their associated morbidity and tendency to descend over time or develop ptosis of natural tissues over the implant.
- It repositions the NAC on the chest wall, securing its position intraoperatively with ease, with less chance of bottoming out thanks to the secure suspension to the chest wall.
- It enables the surgeon to shape the breast parenchyma, restoring upper pole fullness and mammary projection.
- It enables the surgeon to reshape the skin envelope of the breast without relying on it for support of the breast tissue and NAC position.
- It improves the lateral chest contour by eliminating the lateral skin roll and re-creating a discrete lateral curvature.
- It may be combined with other body-contouring procedures safely.

10.3.2 Disadvantages of This Technique

- It requires longer operation times because of extensive de-epithelialization and intraoperative tailoring (a two-team approach increases efficiency and decreases operative time).
- It cannot be easily combined with an implant for further augmentation. The patient must have enough autologous tissue available for auto-augmentation. Should the patient desire additional volume, a subpectoral augmentation may be added in a separate future procedure.

10.3.3 Relative Contraindications

- Active tobacco users are at risk of flap necrosis.
- Patients with previous breast surgery are at risk of inadequate perfusion to undermined tissues.
- In non-MWL breasts, tight parenchymal reshaping or skin closure can increase risk of parenchymal or skin necrosis.

10.3.4 Markings

The patient is marked in a standing position, based on an extended Wise pattern marking with a central pedicle.

1. Mark the sternal notch and midline.
2. Mark the breast meridian: at the midclavicle (approximately 6 cm from the sternal notch), a line is dropped toward the IMF. In many MWL patients, the breast meridian will not be in line with the nipple, as the nipple is often medialized.
3. Mark the new nipple position on the breast meridian: Pitanguy's point is projected forward by placing a hand at the level of the IMF and projecting the point forward. In patients with very descended IMFs, this point may need to be elevated slightly, but care should be taken not to overelevate the IMF and thus the new nipple position. Check for symmetry.
4. Mark the extended Wise pattern:
    a) The superior part of the keyhole (representing the new upper border of the areola) is placed 2 cm above the new nipple position.
    b) 7-cm vertical limbs are drawn from the new nipple position. The keyhole is then designed extending from the point 2 cm above the new nipple position to 2 cm down each vertical limb. This maintains a 5-cm vertical limb that represents the new inferior nipple-to-IMF distance. An 8-cm base (angle of divergence) is planned. If the patient has more dense breast parenchyma, the angle of divergence may be narrowed, reducing the amount of parenchyma internally for reshaping and increasing the amount of skin externally. In addition, the vertical limbs can be extended to increase the estimated length from the bottom of the nipple to the IMF (▶ Fig. 10.2).

c) Mark the medial point of the extended Wise pattern: typically, at the takeoff of the breast.
d) Mark the IMF: a "cheat" may be marked at the middle part of the central pedicle (along the breast meridian) to further reduce tension at the T point junction further. If not needed, it can be de-epithelialized prior to incision closure.

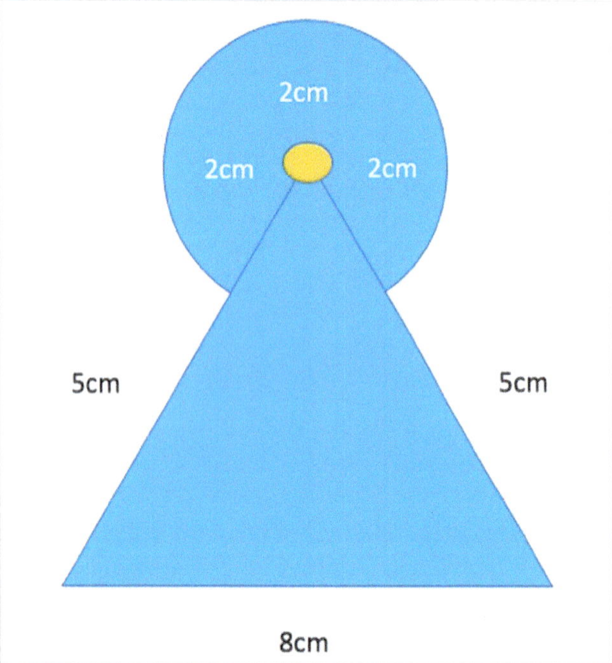

Fig. 10.2 Keyhole for the extended Wise pattern.

e) Mark the lateral point of the Wise pattern: this will determine how much of the axillary roll will be de-epithelialized and incorporated into the breast for auto-augmentation. Tissue is routinely taken and consistently reliable to the mid-axillary line. Excision may be extended to the posterior axillary line and farther to improve contour of the lateral chest wall.
f) Connect the lateral point to the vertical limb of the Wise pattern in a curvilinear line: this conserves more tissue medially and creates a larger takeout laterally.

5. Mark the second and third ribs bilaterally.
6. Mark the superior footprint of the breast by pushing up on the breast to simulate the upper boundary of the breast.
7. Check for symmetry in the markings between the breasts (▶ Fig. 10.3).

Preoperative asymmetry in nipple position is taken into consideration during the markings to avoid asymmetric nipple placement during the dermal suspension. To correct for the asymmetry, the keyhole markings are the same bilaterally, but less tissue is de-epithelialized on the side of the lower nipple to account for the discrepancy. The excess skin above this new point is excised (▶ Fig. 10.4).

10.3.5 Surgical Technique

The patient is placed in the supine position, arms abducted to 90°. Care is taken to secure the arms to padded arm boards, as the patient will be in a near-sitting position for a large part of the surgery.

1. Mark the areola with a 42-mm nipple washer or cookie cutter.

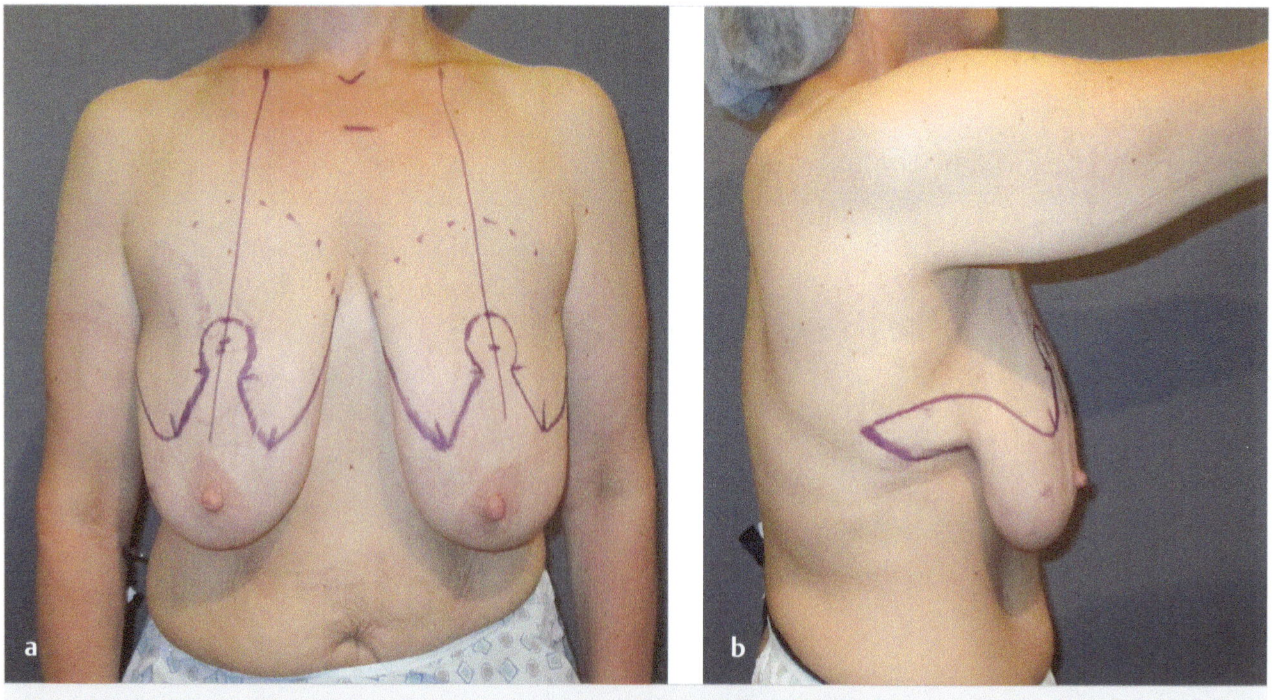

Fig. 10.3 Markings for dermal suspension parenchymal rearrangement mastopexy. **(a)** Anterior. **(b)** Lateral.

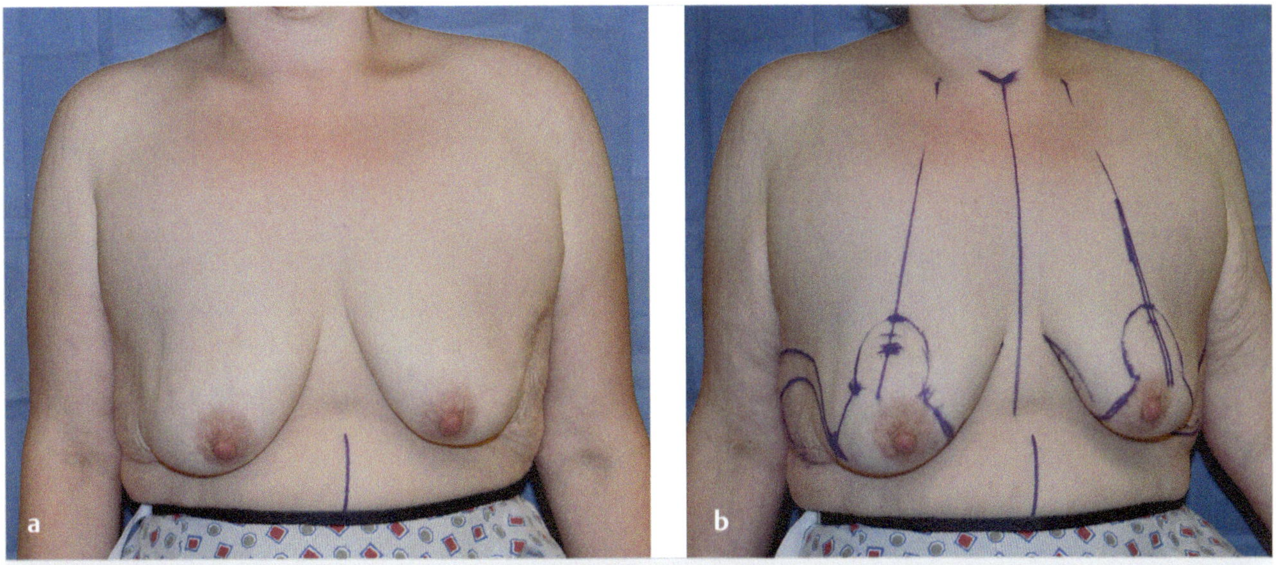

Fig. 10.4 Markings for dermal suspension parenchymal rearrangement mastopexy in cases of asymmetry. **(a)** Note the difference in nipple height. Here the right nipple is lower than the left. **(b)** Mark the projected inframammary fold to set nipple height (similar on both sides), draw keyhole for the extended Wise pattern (similar on both sides), measure the nipple areola complex discrepancy. To correct the discrepancy, less tissue will be de-epithelialized on the right (lower nipple) at the superior part of the keyhole and will be discarded, shortening the sternal notch–to-nipple distance and elevating the right nipple more.

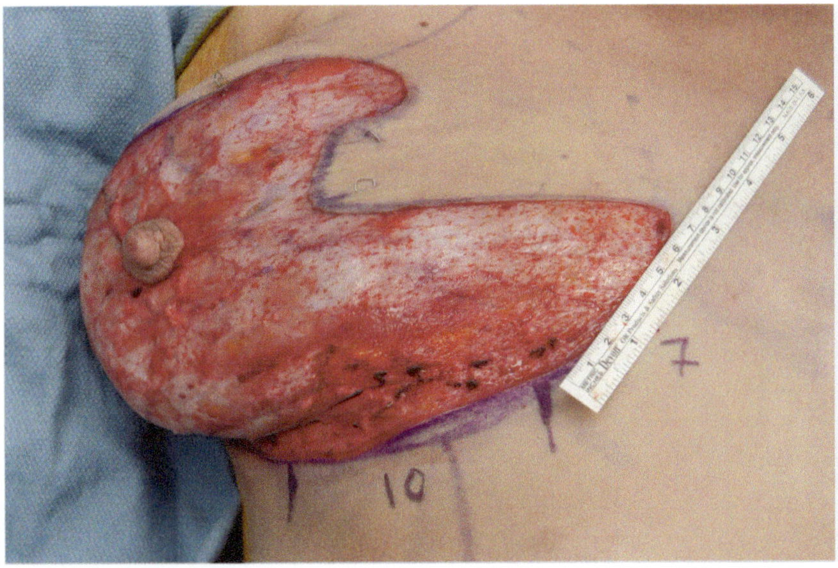

Fig. 10.5 Marking a 10 cm wide central pedicle: Determine the location of the central pedicle, approximately 7 cm from the most medial point of the extended Wise pattern. These measurements can be altered based on breast size or chest width.

2. Superficially inject a local anesthetic solution (epinephrine 1:100,000) to areas of de-epithelialization (the entire region within the Wise pattern, excluding the NAC).
3. De-epithelialize the entire extended Wise pattern with its extensions medially and laterally.
4. Mark a 10-cm-wide central pedicle at the base of the breast starting 7 cm from the most medial point of the extended Wise pattern (▶ Fig. 10.5).
5. Use electrocautery to score all around the Wise pattern markings to reach breast parenchyma, excluding the 10-cm base of the central pedicle inferiorly (▶ Fig. 10.6).
6. The upper breast flap is then raised with a 1- to 1.5-cm thickness until the chest wall is reached. Undermining along the breast meridian continues until the second rib is clearly palpable. A subcutaneous pocket is created, into which the breast tissue—which is now isolated on a central mound as a dermoglandular flap (with robust blood supply)—will be transposed as it is being shaped. Care should be taken not to overdissect medially, as this can result in a symmastia appearance of the breasts. Similarly, the lateral attachments of the upper flap should be released only as needed to accommodate the newly constructed breast mound (▶ Fig. 10.7).
7. The lateral and medial dermoglandular flaps are then elevated off the chest wall at the level of the fascia over the chest muscles, preserving as many significant perforating vessels as possible near the flap base. Care is taken to check routinely that the 10-cm central pedicle thickness is

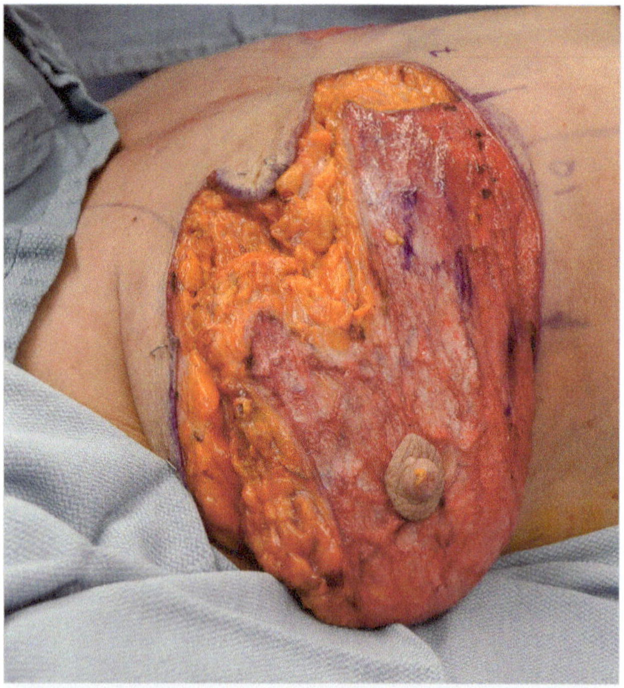

Fig. 10.6 Scoring all around the extended Wise pattern, excluding the central pedicle 10-cm base.

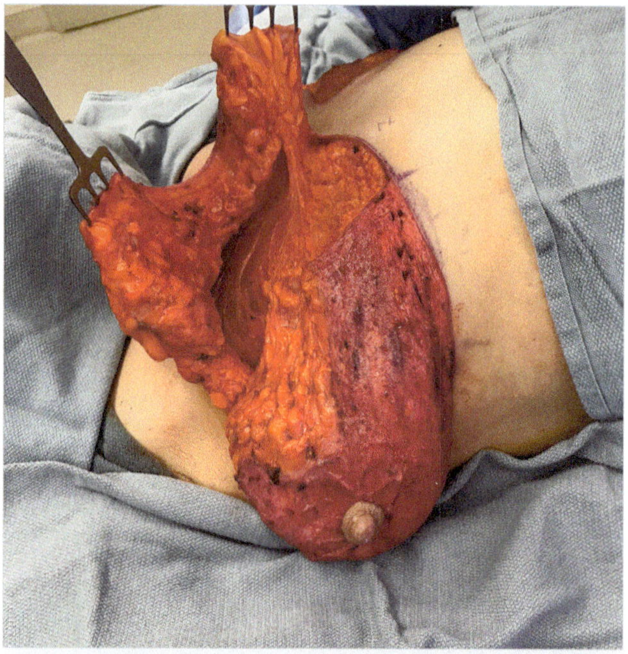

Fig. 10.7 Elevation of the upper breast flap, keeping it 1–1.5 cm thick, and additional pocket creation along the breast meridian, taking care not to overdissect medially and laterally, up to the level of the clavicle.

preserved, as it can easily be undermined unconsciously in a much-deflated breast. The authors typically limit the lateral extent of the dermoglandular flap to the mid- or posterior axillary line, since incorporating tissue distal to that point carries the potential risk of fat necrosis. Trim the lateral flap as needed for auto-augmentation, discarding distal tissue removed for contour purposes (▶ Fig. 10.8).

Dermal Suspension

Reposition the patient in a near-sitting position. The upper flaps are elevated with Deaver retractors. The desired height of suspension is determined intraoperatively, usually the second rib. In a very ptotic breast, reaching the second rib is usually simple. However, if the NAC was relatively well positioned on the breast mound preoperatively, it is suggested to move the central mound down to the third rib to avoid a difficult nipple inset at the end of the case.

1. Suspend the superior dermal edge of the keyhole on the central pedicle to rib periosteum (usually the second rib) using a permanent 0 braided nylon suture in a mattress fashion along the breast meridian. Reinforce with a second similar suture, next to the first one. This sets the axis of the breast on the chest wall. To perform safely, place your fingers in the intercostal spaces and feel the rib between your fingers, passing the needle between them, making sure to take a good bite including rib periosteum.
2. Redrape and check nipple height. If it is too high because of a short distance on the keyhole pattern, drop the suspension suture down to the third rib. If the NAC is very ptotic at the second-rib position, you may plicate the dermis superior to the NAC to help elevate nipple position more (▶ Fig. 10.9).
3. Suspend the distal edge of the lateral flap one rib below the central flap (usually the third rib), and directly underneath it (essentially positioning it behind the central flap) along the breast meridian. This avoids a breast shape that is too wide (▶ Fig. 10.10).
4. The medial flap is often not very robust in size. It is typically suspended to the fourth rib periosteum to provide medial fullness once the breast flaps are redraped (▶ Fig. 10.11, ▶ Fig. 10.12).

Plication, Shaping, and Adding Multiple Suspension Points to the Chest Wall

1. Approximate the lateral and central flaps dermis to dermis with single 2–0 absorbable, braided sutures, reinforcing with a running 2–0 absorbable, braided suture. Connect the medial flap to the central flap in a similar fashion. The medial flap is often small, so sometimes only a few stitches are needed to approximate it to the central pedicle (▶ Fig. 10.13).
2. Shorten the nipple-to-IMF distance with plication sutures so that the distance from the inferior edge of the areola to the IMF is 5 cm (the same as the length of the vertical limb of the Wise pattern): measure 2 cm down from the inferior areolar edge and 3 cm up from the IMF. This is a starting point for planning the crescent-shaped plication that is performed to round out the breast mound construct. The planned markings can then be tailor-tacked with staples to see whether the overall contour is round and smooth. The plication is then performed using single 2–0 absorbable, braided sutures, reinforcing with 2–0 absorbable, braided running suture. Care is taken to remove any staples used for

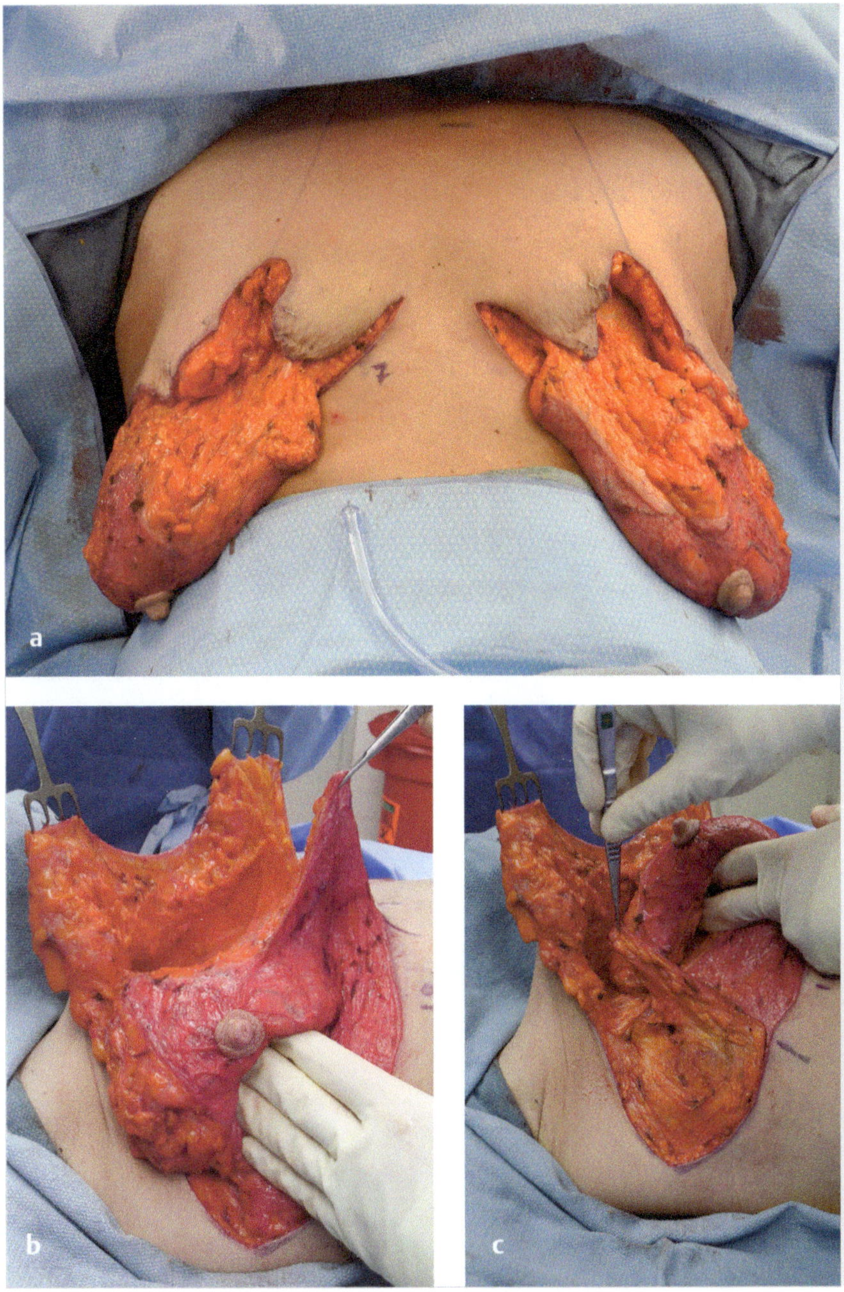

Fig. 10.8 **(a)** After elevation of the central, medial, and lateral dermoglandular flaps. **(b)** The medial flap. **(c)** The lateral flap.

the tailor tack during the suturing process. The skin is redraped frequently to check for contour and symmetry. While work is being done in the upright position, the skin flaps can be stapled up to the drapes so that they are out of the way during plication (▶ Fig. 10.14).

3. The lateral curvature of the breast is restored by placing several (5 to 8) horizontal mattress sutures with 0 braided nylon from the lateral dermal edge of the lateral dermoglandular flap to the fascia of the lateral chest wall overlying the musculature. Care is taken not to take deep bites that may injure deeper blood vessels or nerves. It is important to try and tuck the breast parenchyma in as the sutures are placed, creating the lateral curvature desired and increasing projection. This portion of the operation can be done before or after the parenchymal reshaping (▶ Fig. 10.15).
4. More sutures may be added to plicate and contour the breast shape further as needed. At the end of this part of the surgery, the breast resembles the appearance of a breast implant or baseball firmly affixed to the chest wall (▶ Fig. 10.16).

Skin Closure and Positioning the NAC

1. After meticulous hemostasis, the new T-point is determined. This may not correlate with the original breast meridian line marked at the beginning of the case but may be a bit more medial. The limiting factor in the location of the T-point is

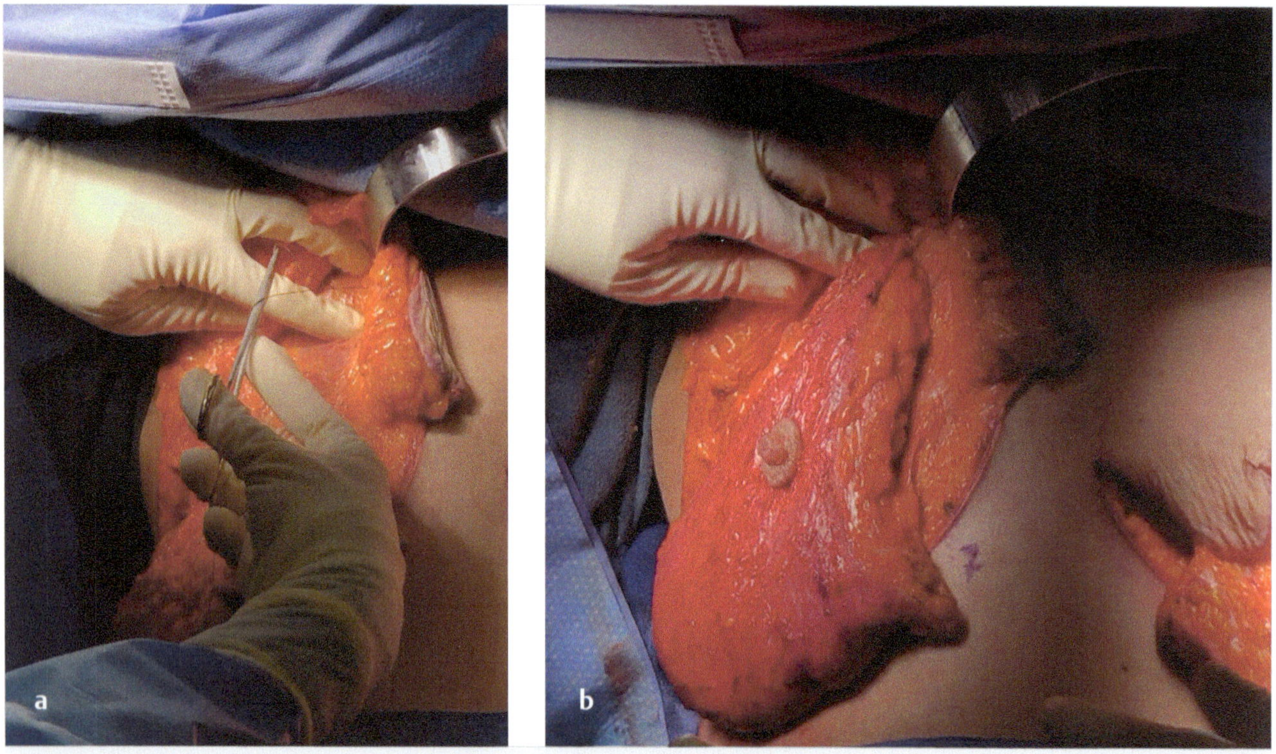

Fig. 10.9 **(a)** Suspension of the central flap (and the nipple areola complex) to the second-rib periosteum along the breast meridian using a permanent 0 braided nylon horizontal mattress suture. It is important to support the breast while tying the suture. Patient is in a near sitting position. **(b)** After suspension of the central flap.

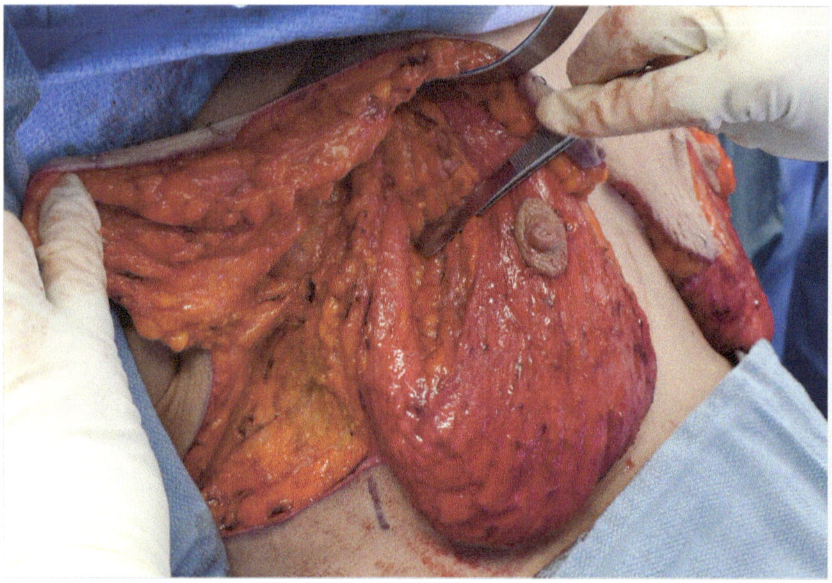

Fig. 10.10 Suspension of the lateral flap one rib below the central flap, exactly underneath the central pedicle suspension suture, using a permanent 0 braided nylon suture.

the medial breast skin flap. This is brought down toward the IMF, and at the point of maximal positioning without distorting the medial corner of the breast incision, a new location of the T-point is marked. Then the lateral breast flap can often reach this point, since it is larger and can be undermined further to assist in reaching. Another tip to reduce tension on the T-point closure is to have an assistant elevate the abdominal wall tissues, as there is often excess laxity here, to aid in recruiting the IMF up to aid in closure. The T-point is closed with a buried 2–0 absorbable, braided suture or half-buried nylon 2–0 mattress suture over a Xeroform gauze pledget (Medtronic, Minneapolis, MN). The vertical, medial, and lateral incisions are approximated with staples. The vertical limb is closed using buried 3–0 monofilament absorbable sutures (▶ Fig. 10.17).

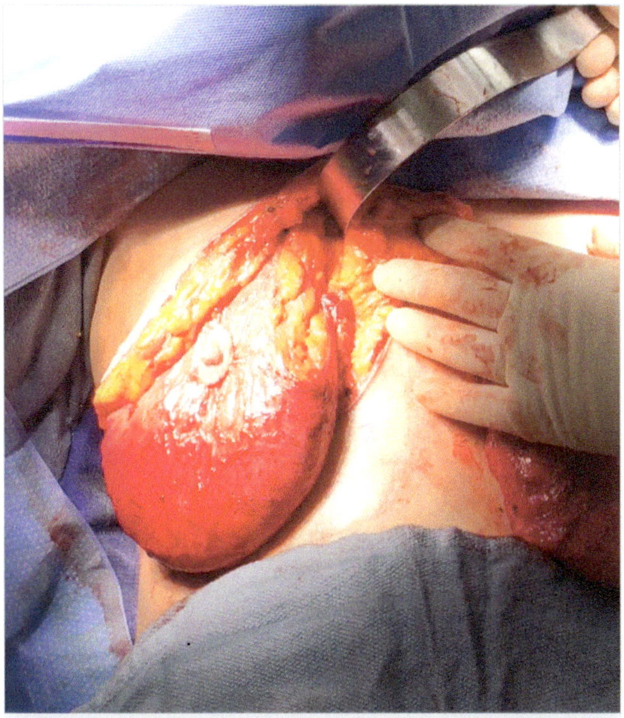

Fig. 10.11 Suspension of the medial flap, usually to the fourth rib, using a permanent 0 braided nylon suture.

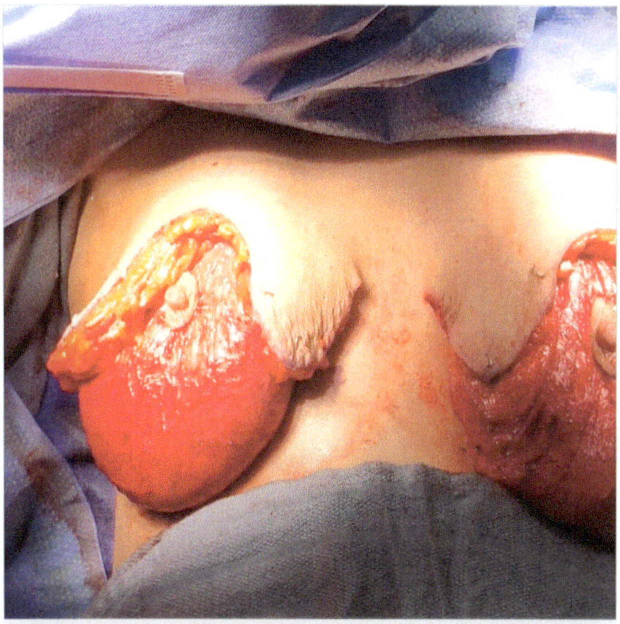

Fig. 10.12 After completing suspension of the central, lateral and medial flaps, redrape the skin to check for obvious asymmetries and discrepancy in volume so that the excess parenchyma can be resected before reshaping if needed.

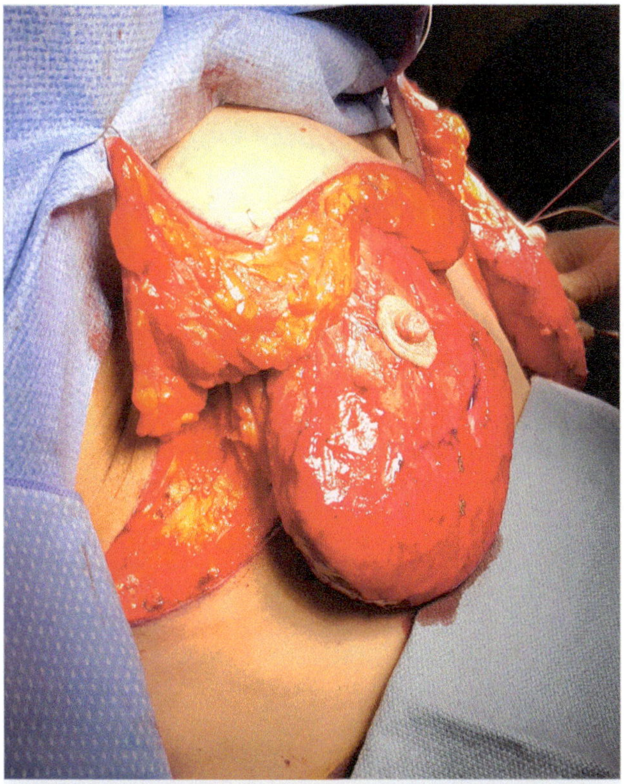

Fig. 10.13 Approximating the lateral and central flaps, using interrupted and running absorbable 2–0 braided sutures.

2. If the nipple is tethered or pulled inappropriately, electrocautery is selectively used to release dermal tethering points around the NAC, allowing it to slide nicely into the keyhole. This is a safe maneuver to perform, since the NAC has a robust central pedicle blood supply. A double hook is placed on the tethered NAC position, and the keyhole skin is retracted with an Army Navy retractor to gain exposure to the dermis around the NAC. Try to avoid releasing the NAC circumferentially. Suture the NAC to its new position using 3–0 buried monofilament absorbable sutures (▶ Fig. 10.18).
3. Layered skin closure over a suction drain is performed with an absorbable monofilament 3–0 suture and absorbable barbed intradermal suture. Skin glue is applied to all incisions (▶ Fig. 10.19).
4. This operation can have a slight reverse abdominoplasty effect from the pull of the lateral wing as it is mounted to the chest wall. This may cause some tethering of the dermis at the IMF that causes difficulty with incisional closure. This can also be released using a double hook and the electrocautery to free the dermal edge of the upper abdomen IMF incision (▶ Fig. 10.20).

During the operation, it is important to redrape the skin and check for symmetry regarding volume, shape and nipple position frequently, as well as to perform the suspension and plication simultaneously on both breasts with the use of a second surgical team, to promote achieving a symmetrical result.

Keep in mind that no two breasts are alike and the plication pattern may differ between breasts and between patients. The versatility of this technique is what makes it powerful.

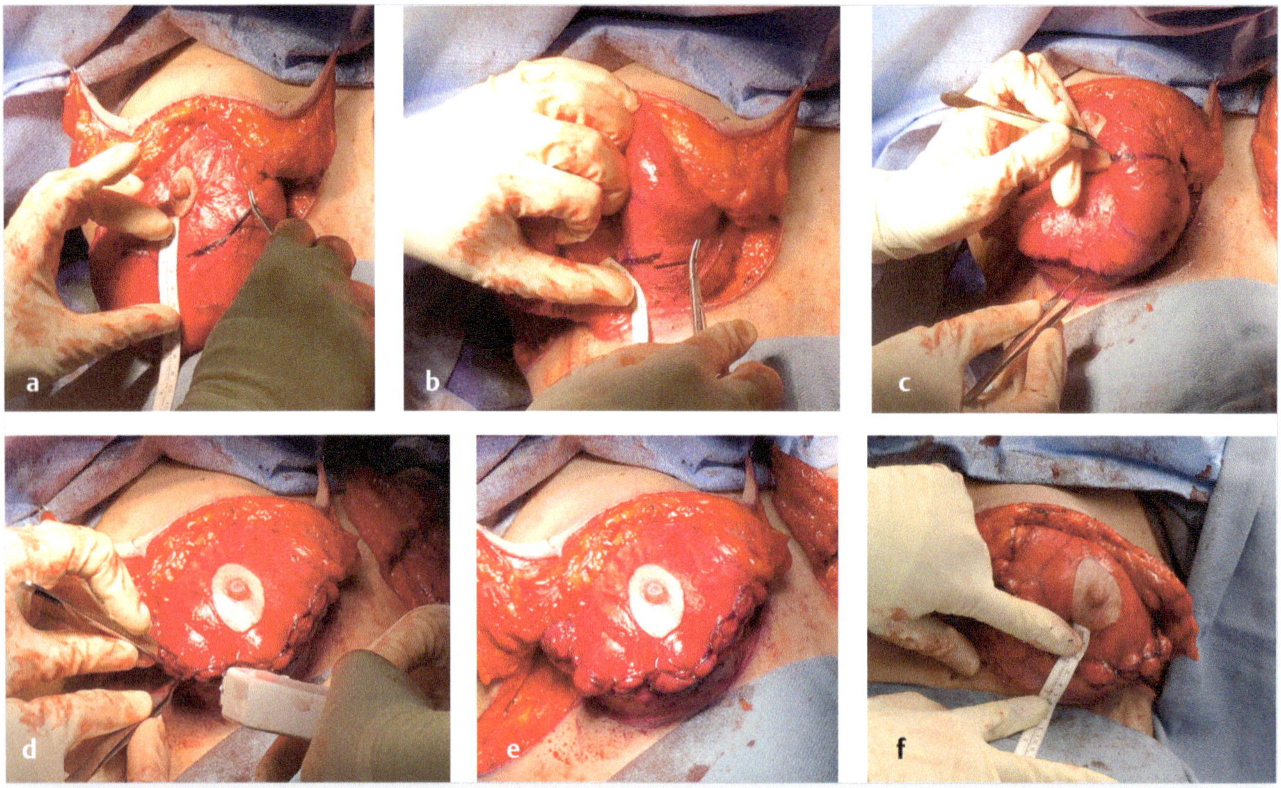

Fig. 10.14 Plication and shaping of the breast. Mark the plication to shorten the nipple areola complex–to–inframammary fold distance to 5 cm: **(a)** Measuring 2 cm from the inferior border of the areola. **(b)** Measuring 3 cm from the inframammary fold. **(c)** Marking the borders of the plication in a crescent-shaped design to capture medial and lateral excess. **(d,e)** Use staples to tailor-tack the markings to evaluate contour before plication. **(f)** Distance from nipple areola complex to inframammary fold is 5 cm.

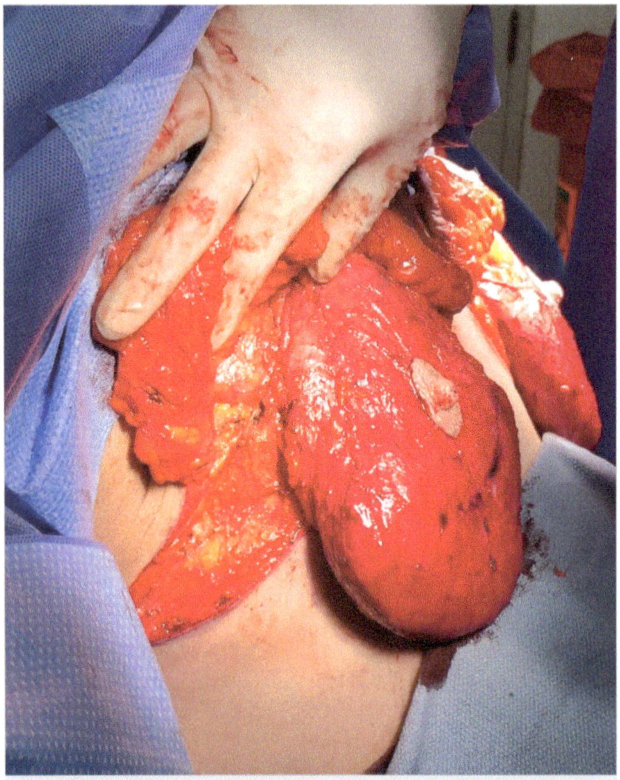

Fig. 10.15 Defining the lateral curvature of the breast using several permanent 0 braided nylon horizontal mattress sutures to the chest wall fascia.

Patients should be advised that the breasts will be very high and firm after surgery, like baseballs on the chest. By 6 weeks, they soften and become much more natural-appearing. Any small asymmetries in the breasts at closure are often not noticeable by 6 weeks as they soften and mature.

10.3.6 Postoperative Care

This procedure can often be done as outpatient surgery. If it is combined with other procedures, patients are often kept overnight.

1. Immediate postop, a surgical bra is applied with fluffs and abdominal pads, or Ace wrap. Patient is instructed not to remove dressings or shower until the first postop visit at postoperative day (POD) 7.
2. Drains are usually removed on the first post-operative visit (POD 7), when output is < 30 mL per day.
3. A surgical/sports bra with no underwire is worn for 6 weeks.
4. Antibiotics are given for 1 week postoperatively.
5. Follow-up visits occur at 1, 2, and 4 weeks after the procedure and at 3, 6, and 12 months.

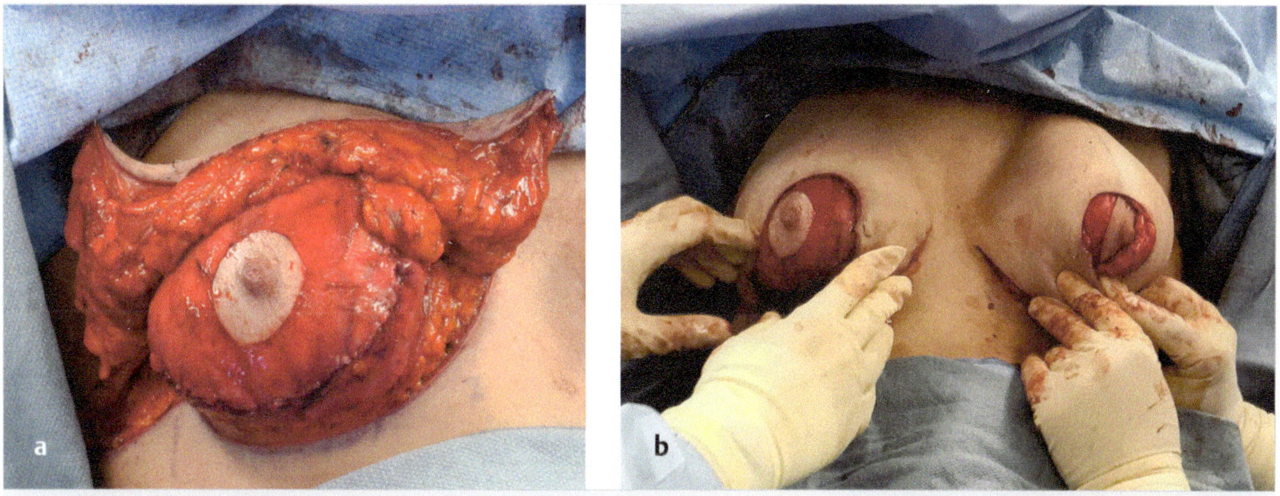

Fig. 10.16 (a) After plication and contouring, the breast is firmly affixed to the chest wall. (b) Redrape the skin and check for symmetry.

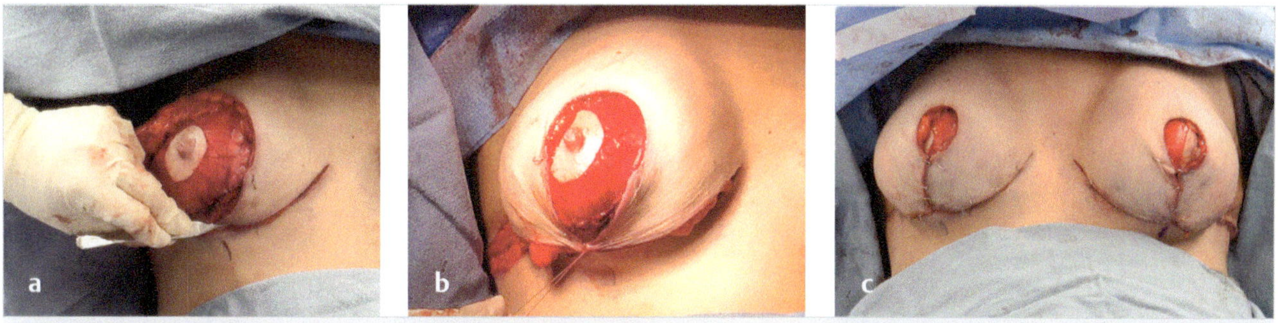

Fig. 10.17 (a,b) Determine the position and secure the T-point. (c) Approximate the vertical, medial, and lateral incisions with staples, and re-assess symmetry.

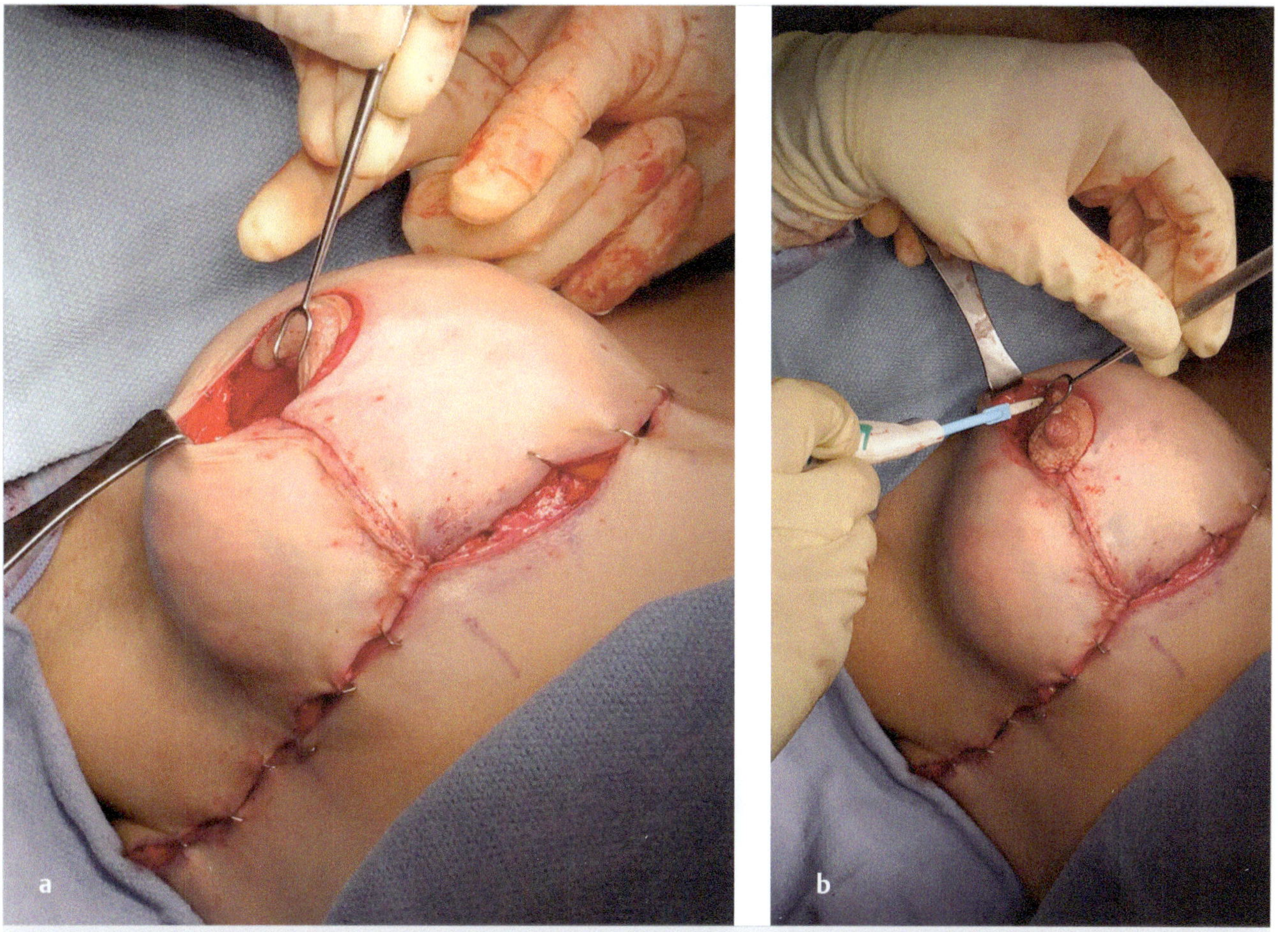

Fig. 10.18 (a,b) Release the nipple from tethering points as needed. Use an Army Navy retractor and a double hook to expose the dermis surrounding the areola, use electrocautery to release the dermis selectively 2–3 mm from the areola. Avoid releasing around the entire areola.

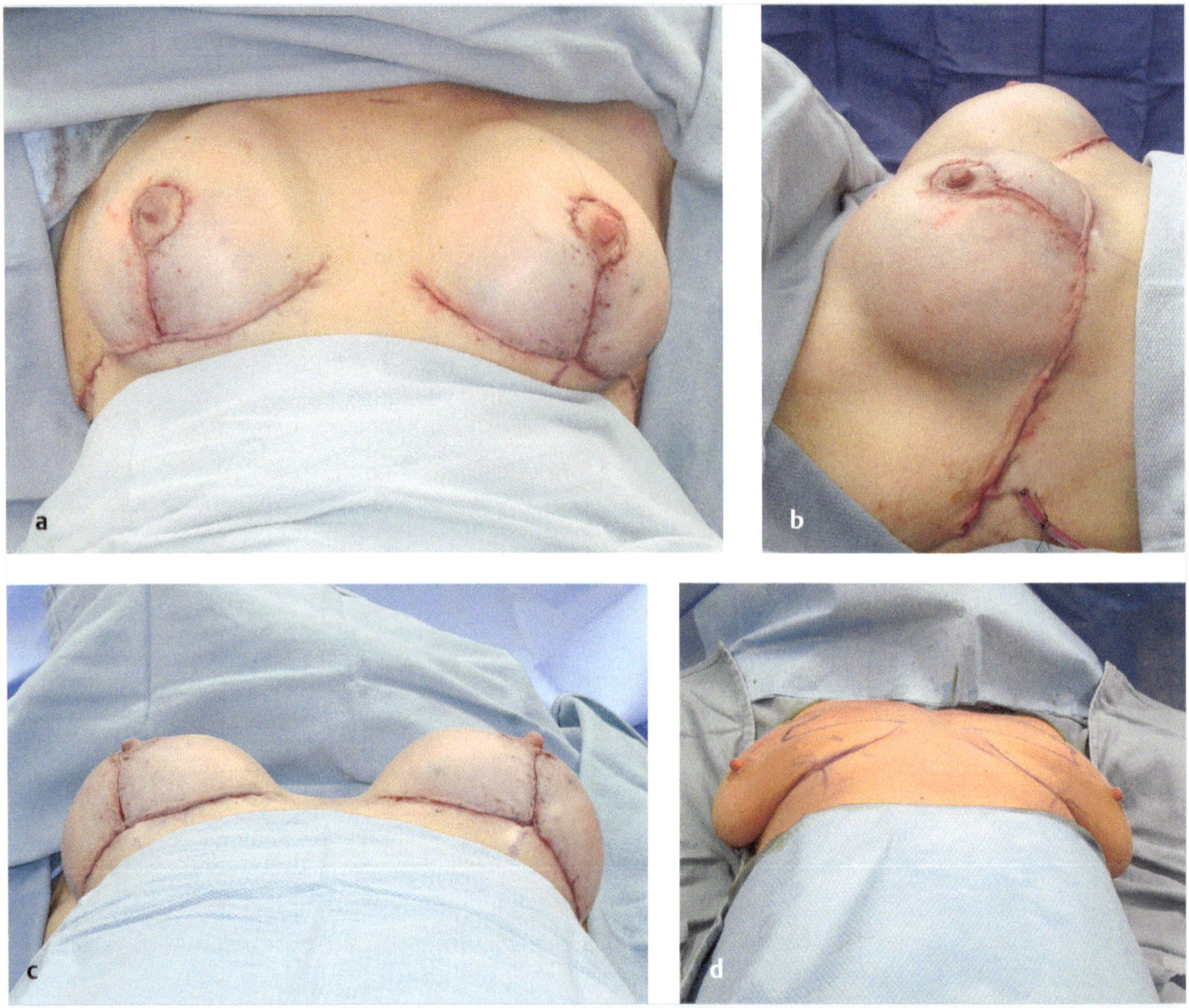

Fig. 10.19 (a–c) Layered skin closure over drains. Skin glue applied to all incisions. (d) Preoperative inferior view is provided for comparison.

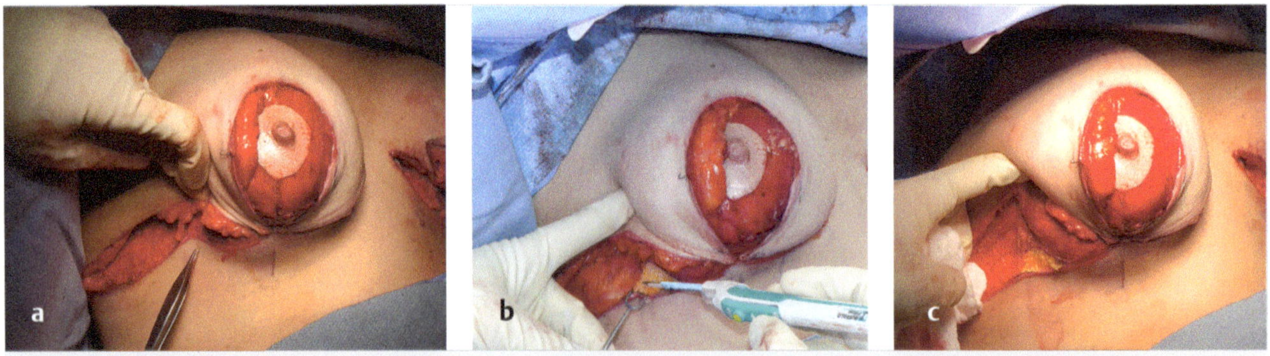

Fig. 10.20 (a–c) Releasing tethering of the dermis at the inframammary fold. Use a double hook and electrocautery to release.

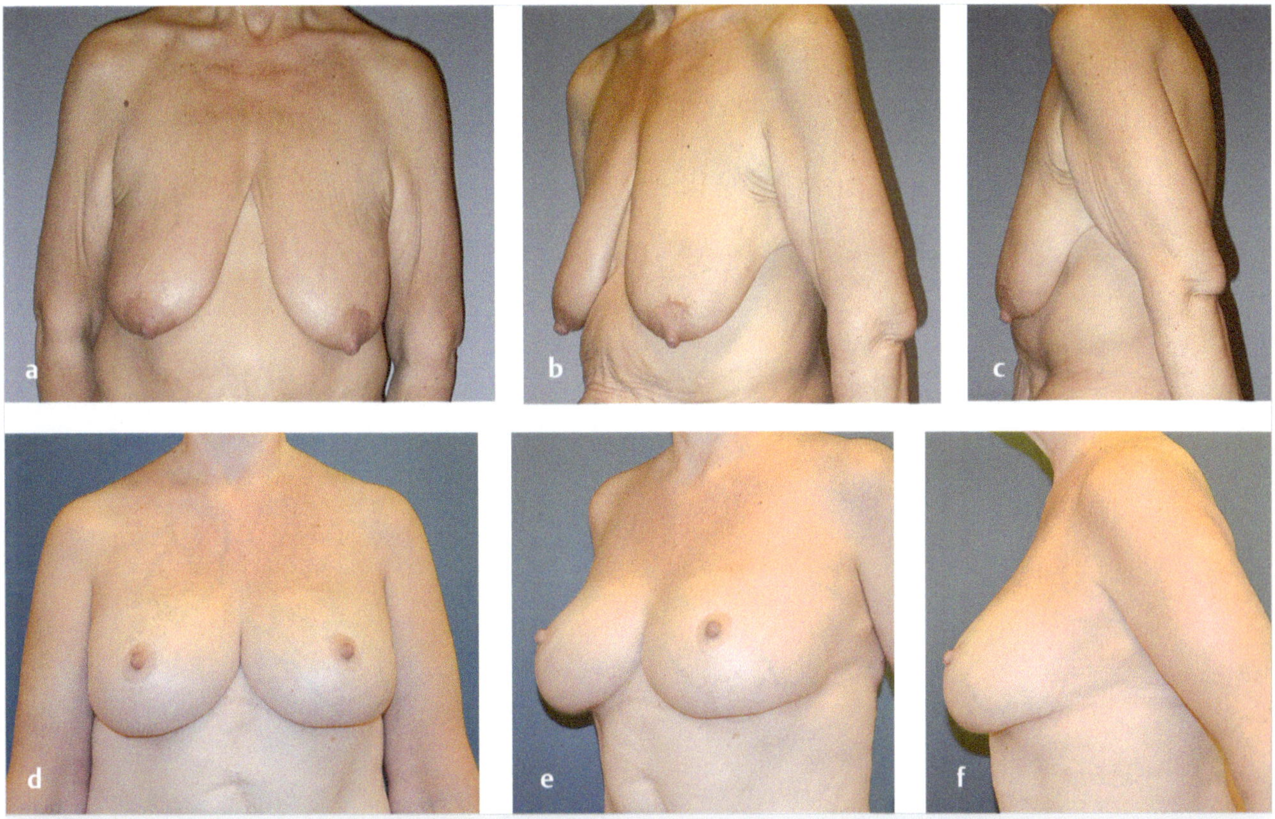

Fig. 10.21 Patient is a 52-year-old woman s/p 100 lb weight loss from bariatric surgery. She underwent a dermal suspension, parenchymal reshaping mastopexy. Preoperative: (a) anterior, (b) anterolateral, and (c) lateral; 6 years postoperative: (d) anterior, (e) anterolateral, and (f) lateral.

10.3.7 Preoperative and Intraoperative Safety Measures

Deep Vein Thrombosis/Pulmonary Embolism Prophylaxis

Sequential compression devices are used before, during, and after surgery. Chemoprophylaxis is considered for higher-risk patients according to their Caprini risk score. Early ambulation is encouraged.

Hypothermia

Every effort is made to prevent hypothermia with body warmers and blankets, before, during, and after the operation, as it has been found to be an independent factor for seroma formation.[37]

Surgical Site Infection

Prophylaxis is afforded by perioperative and postoperative antibiotics for all patients, appropriate skin preparation with povidone-iodine or chlorhexidine, and close glycemic control when necessary.

10.3.8 Potential Complications

The following potential complications have been reported.[22,38,39,40]

- Minor wound dehiscence, with delayed healing at the T point in less than 5% of patients.
- Seroma.
- Fat necrosis.
- Unaesthetic scars.
- NAC necrosis.

10.4 Example Photos

The dermal suspension, parenchymal reshaping mastopexy in massive weight loss patients provides long-lasting results with restoration of a youthful-appearing breast (▶ Fig. 10.21, ▶ Fig. 10.22, ▶ Fig. 10.23).

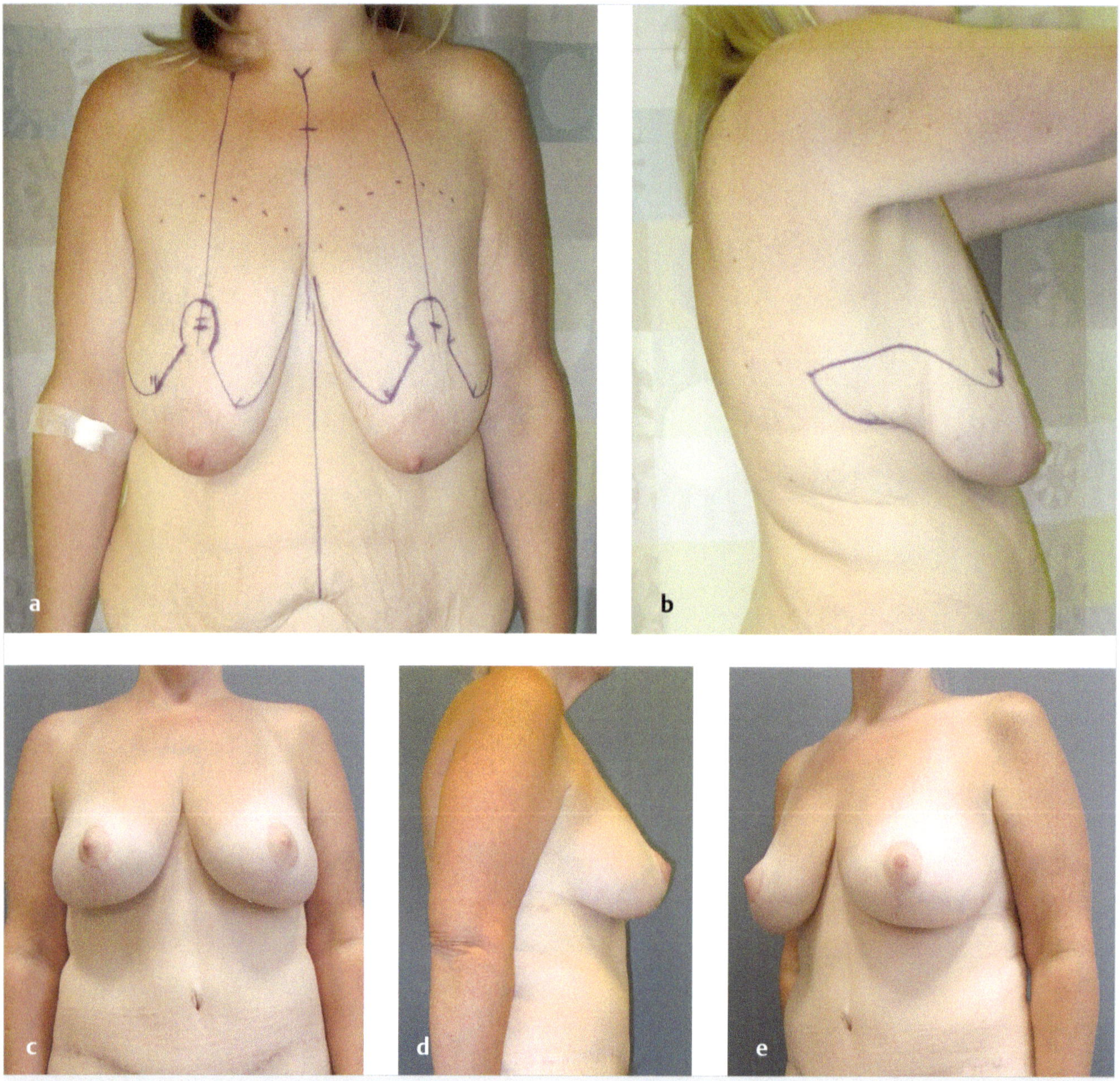

Fig. 10.22 Patient aged 42 after laparoscopic Roux-en-Y gastric bypass, maximal weight 246 lb (112 kg), minimal and current weight 146 lb (66 kg), BMI 25. Preoperative markings **(a)** anterior and **(b)** lateral; 1 year postoperative **(c)** anterior, **(d)** lateral, and **(e)** anterolateral. Patient also had an abdominoplasty.

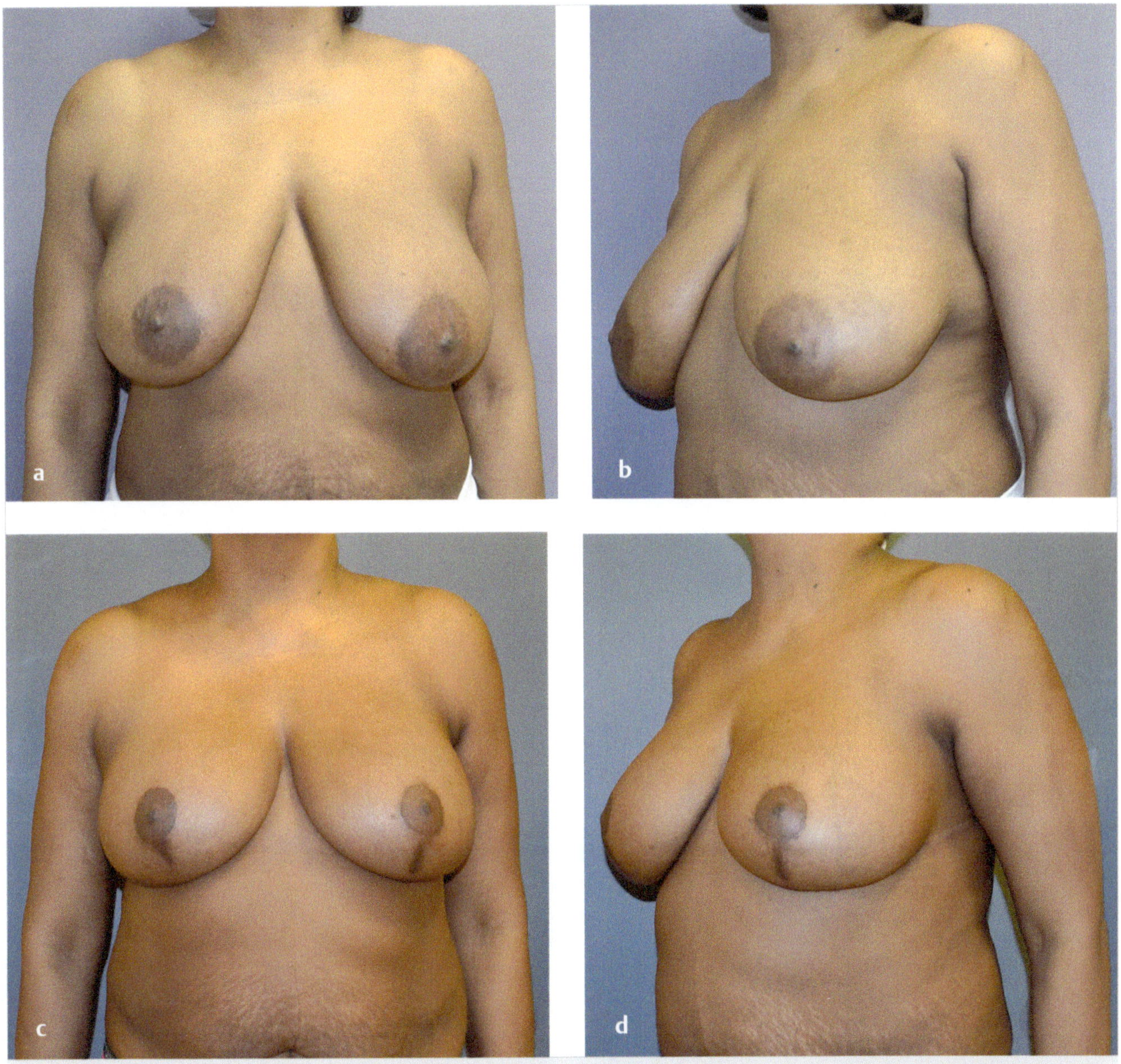

Fig. 10.23 Patient is a 55-year-old woman s/p 60 lb weight loss from diet and exercise. She underwent a dermal suspension, parenchymal reshaping mastopexy. Preoperative **(a)** anterior and **(b)** anterolateral views; 15 months postoperative **(c)** anterior **(d)** and anterolateral views.

Key Points

- The breast after massive weight loss (MWL) presents with challenging deformities.
- The dermal suspension and parenchymal reshaping mastopexy is a safe and reliable means of restoring the youthful shaped breast in patients after MWL.
- For patients who have enough autologous tissue, this procedure avoids potential malposition problems with implants and provides a durable result without the need for reoperation.[22]

References

[1] Weiner RA. Indications and principles of metabolic surgery [in German]. Chirurg. 2010; 81(4):379–394, quiz–395

[2] American Society For Metabolic and Bariatric Surgery (ASMBS). Estimate of Bariatric Surgery Numbers, 2011–2017. ASMBS; 2018. URL: https://asmbs.org/resources/estimate-of-bariatric-surgery-numbers. Accessed July 15, 2019

[3] American Society of Plastic Surgeons (ASPS). 2018 Plastic Surgery Statistics Report. ASPS; 2019. https://www.plasticsurgery.org/documents/News/Statistics/2018/plastic-surgery-statistics-full-report-2018.pdf. Accessed July 15, 2019

[4] Song AY, Jean RD, Hurwitz DJ, Fernstrom MH, Scott JA, Rubin JP. A classification of contour deformities after bariatric weight loss: the Pittsburgh Rating Scale. Plast Reconstr Surg. 2005; 116(5):1535–1544, discussion 1545--1546

[5] Rubin JP, Hurwitz DJ. Breast reshaping after massive weight loss: Autologous tissue techniques. In: Rubin JP, Jewell ML, Richter DF, Uebel CO, eds. Body Contouring and Liposuction. Philadelphia, PA: Saunders; 2013;122–138

[6] Rubin JP, Khachi G. Mastopexy after massive weight loss: dermal suspension and selective auto-augmentation. Clin Plast Surg. 2008; 35(1):123–129

[7] Buchwald H, Estok R, Fahrbach K, et al. Weight and type 2 diabetes after bariatric surgery: systematic review and meta-analysis. Am J Med. 2009; 122(3): 248–256.e5

[8] Rubin JP, Nguyen V, Schwentker A. Perioperative management of the post-gastric-bypass patient presenting for body contour surgery. Clin Plast Surg. 2004; 31(4):601–610, vi

[9] Gusenoff JA, Rubin JP. Plastic surgery after weight loss: current concepts in massive weight loss surgery. Aesthet Surg J. 2008; 28(4):452–455

[10] Almutairi K, Gusenoff JA, Rubin JP. Body contouring. Plast Reconstr Surg. 2016; 137(3):586e–602e

[11] Matory WE, Jr, O'Sullivan J, Fudem G, Dunn R. Abdominal surgery in patients with severe morbid obesity. Plast Reconstr Surg. 1994; 94(7):976–987

[12] Vastine VL, Morgan RF, Williams GS, et al. Wound complications of abdominoplasty in obese patients. Ann Plast Surg. 1999; 42(1):34–39

[13] Arthurs ZM, Cuadrado D, Sohn V, et al. Post-bariatric panniculectomy: pre-panniculectomy body mass index impacts the complication profile. Am J Surg. 2007; 193(5):567–570, discussion–570

[14] Nemerofsky RB, Oliak DA, Capella JF. Body lift: an account of 200 consecutive cases in the massive weight loss patient. Plast Reconstr Surg. 2006; 117(2): 414–430

[15] Coon D, Gusenoff JA, Kannan N, El Khoudary SR, Naghshineh N, Rubin JP. Body mass and surgical complications in the postbariatric reconstructive patient: analysis of 511 cases. Ann Surg. 2009; 249(3):397–401

[16] Kokkinos A, Alexiadou K, Liaskos C, et al. Improvement in cardiovascular indices after Roux-en-Y gastric bypass or sleeve gastrectomy for morbid obesity. Obes Surg. 2013; 23(1):31–38

[17] Chikunguwo SM, Wolfe LG, Dodson P, et al. Analysis of factors associated with durable remission of diabetes after Roux-en-Y gastric bypass. Surg Obes Relat Dis. 2010; 6(3):254–259

[18] Kaplan LM. Body weight regulation and obesity. J Gastrointest Surg. 2003; 7 (4):443–451

[19] Rohrich RJ, Coberly DM, Krueger JK, Brown SA. Planning elective operations on patients who smoke: survey of North American plastic surgeons. Plast Reconstr Surg. 2002; 109(1):350–355, discussion 356–357

[20] Coon D, Tuffaha S, Christensen J, Bonawitz SC. Plastic surgery and smoking: a prospective analysis of incidence, compliance, and complications. Plast Reconstr Surg. 2013; 131(2):385–391

[21] Krueger JK, Rohrich RJ. Clearing the smoke: the scientific rationale for tobacco abstention with plastic surgery. Plast Reconstr Surg. 2001; 108(4):1063–1073, discussion 1074–1077

[22] Rubin JP, Gusenoff JA, Coon D. Dermal suspension and parenchymal reshaping mastopexy after massive weight loss: statistical analysis with concomitant procedures from a prospective registry. Plast Reconstr Surg. 2009; 123 (3):782–789

[23] Gusenoff JA, Coon D, Rubin JP. Brachioplasty and concomitant procedures after massive weight loss: a statistical analysis from a prospective registry. Plast Reconstr Surg. 2008; 122(2):595–603

[24] Holmström H, Lossing C. The lateral thoracodorsal flap in breast reconstruction. Plast Reconstr Surg. 1986; 77(6):933–943

[25] Frey M. A new technique of reduction mammaplasty: dermis suspension and elimination of medial scars. Br J Plast Surg. 1999; 52(1):45–51

[26] Lockwood T. Reduction mammaplasty and mastopexy with superficial fascial system suspension. Plast Reconstr Surg. 1999; 103(5):1411–1420

[27] Gulyás G. Mammaplasty with a periareolar dermal cloak for glandular support. Aesthetic Plast Surg. 1999; 23(3):164–169

[28] Graf R, Biggs TM. In search of better shape in mastopexy and reduction mammoplasty. Plast Reconstr Surg. 2002; 110(1):309–317, discussion 318–322

[29] Qiao Q, Sun J, Liu C, Liu Z, Zhao R. Reduction mammaplasty and correction of ptosis: dermal bra technique. Plast Reconstr Surg. 2003; 111(3):1122–1130

[30] Graf RM, Mansur AE, Tenius FP, Ono MC, Romano GG, Cruz GA. Mastopexy after massive weight loss: extended chest wall-based flap associated with a loop of pectoralis muscle. Aesthetic Plast Surg. 2008; 32(2):371–374

[31] Hurwitz DJ, Agha-Mohammadi S. Postbariatric surgery breast reshaping: the spiral flap. Ann Plast Surg. 2006; 56(5):481–486, discussion 486

[32] Akyurek M. Vertical mastopexy and lateral intercostal artery perforator (LICAP) flap with pectoralis muscle sling for autologous tissue breast augmentation in the bariatric patient. Ann Plast Surg. 2011; 66(1):29–35

[33] Hamdi M, Van Landuyt K, Blondeel P, Hijjawi JB, Roche N, Monstrey S. Autologous breast augmentation with the lateral intercostal artery perforator flap in massive weight loss patients. J Plast Reconstr Aesthet Surg. 2009; 62(1): 65–70

[34] Kwei S, Borud LJ, Lee BT. Mastopexy with autologous augmentation after massive weight loss: the intercostal artery perforator (ICAP) flap. Ann Plast Surg. 2006; 57(4):361–365

[35] Persichetti P, Tenna S, Brunetti B, Aveta A, Segreto F, Marangi GF. Anterior intercostal artery perforator flap autologous augmentation in bariatric mastopexy. Plast Reconstr Surg. 2012; 130(4):917–925

[36] Colwell AS, Driscoll D, Breuing KH. Mastopexy techniques after massive weight loss: an algorithmic approach and review of the literature. Ann Plast Surg. 2009; 63(1):28–33

[37] Coon D, Michaels J, V, Gusenoff JA, Chong T, Purnell C, Rubin JP. Hypothermia and complications in postbariatric body contouring. Plast Reconstr Surg. 2012; 130(2):443–448

[38] Eisenhardt SU, Nienhueser H, Braig D, Penna V, Bannasch H, Torio-Padron N. Comparison of the Rubin dermal suspension sutures and total parenchymal reshaping technique with a traditional inverted T-scar reduction mammaplasty technique using a superior pedicle. Aesthetic Plast Surg. 2013; 37(6): 1153–1160

[39] Losken A. Breast reshaping following massive weight loss: principles and techniques. Plast Reconstr Surg. 2010; 126(3):1075–1085

[40] Rubin JP. Mastopexy after massive weight loss: dermal suspension and total parenchymal reshaping. Aesthet Surg J. 2006; 26(2):214–222

11 Internal Bra Technique in the Breast with Poor Soft Tissue Support

C. Bob Basu and Nirav Bipin Patel

Summary
The chapter discusses use of a mesh scaffold "internal bra," which has been previously described for mastopexy alone. These constructs also have utility in addressing breast implant malposition or for patients desiring substantial upper pole fullness, especially when there is a low inframammary fold crease or poor soft tissue support. Examples include AlloDerm (Bio-Horizons, Birmingham, AL), or other acellular dermal matrices, and GalaFLEX (poly-4-hydroxybutyrate, or P4HB; Galatea Surgical, Lexington, MA) bioresorbable mesh. Combining mesh with breast shaping and implants can help obtain a durable aesthetic result attributable to a resistant support system. One should be cognizant of the complexity of these internal bra techniques, especially in cases of severe tissue weakening, including the risk for delayed healing, implant extrusion, skin necrosis, residual asymmetry, and need for a secondary procedure to fine-tune results. However, when executed correctly in the right indications, the use of surgical mesh in revisional aesthetic surgery can yield safe, reliable, and excellent outcomes, particularly for the patient seeking upper pole volume and improved cleavage when the soft tissues are too weak to provide requisite support.

Keywords: mastopexy augmentation, periareolar mastopexy, mesh scaffold, internal bra

11.1 Introduction

One of the limitations of any cosmetic breast procedure is the patient's baseline anatomy, including the quality of the patient's skin and breast tissue (soft tissue support) and the overall position of the inframammary fold (IMF) crease. In patients with poor soft tissue support, achieving and maintaining upper pole volume can be challenging. What ultimately holds up the breast in any cosmetic procedure is the *quality* of the patient's tissue, despite techniques to tighten loose skin or manipulate an existing capsule. The position of the IMF crease also helps determine how high the augmented breast sits on the chest wall. What can a plastic surgeon do to achieve desired upper pole fullness in cases where there is evidence of poor soft tissue support,[1] there is a low IMF crease (i.e., tall chest wall height),[2] or both? Although internal capsulorraphy is a well-established option, the authors find this approach limited in cases of suboptimal soft tissue support (poor tissue quality), especially when the patient is opting for larger or heavier implants.

Single-stage mastopexy–augmentation presents unique challenges in aesthetic breast surgery, in attempting simultaneously to counterbalance the gravitational forces of the breast implant with skin and parenchymal reshaping to correct ptosis.[1,2,3] The additional variable of poor underlying soft tissue support—whether secondary to age, repeated surgery, postpartum changes, or weight loss history—only increases the potential for recurrent ptosis and rates of complications.[4,5]

Use of de-epithelialized dermoglandular flaps for breast reshaping formed the basis for Sampaio Góes' periareolar approach, described in 1989.[6] However, in following patients longitudinally, surgeons noted that this tissue construct was inadequate in preserving an optimal shape of the remodeled breast. Thus, an internal support construct was deemed necessary for stability and prevention of soft tissue relaxation, which enables increases in breast base and areolar diameter. Sampaio Góes began to utilize mesh placed in between the external, intact skin envelope and the de-epithelialized internal layer.[7] The innovation helps provide a longer-lasting aesthetic result that is reliant on a more resistant support system. The mesh maintains the ideal gland position postoperatively and facilitates tissue fixation, opposing gravitational forces on the breast.

Internal bra meshes have been fabricated from different kinds of materials. For instance, some surgeons have used acellular dermal matrices (ADMs) for internal bras. Polyglactin 910 was among those absorbable meshes first described and was found to preserve aesthetic results for up to 2 years, after which partial loss was reported. Thereafter, mixed mesh composed of polyglactin 910 and polyester was utilized, showing durable results for several years' follow-up.[8] Other described mesh polymers include Vypro, made of polypropylene and polyglactin (Ethicon, Bridgewater, NJ); UltraPro, made of polypropylene and Monocryl (poliglecaprone 25; Ethicon, Bridgewater, NJ); SERI scaffold, made of raw silk protein filaments (Sofregen Medical, Medford, MA); and more recently GalaFLEX, made of poly-4-hydroxybutyrate (P4HB; Galatea Surgical, Lexington, MA).[9] Importantly, nonabsorbable meshes have not directly shown complications attributable to their inherent material, which heuristically is sensible, as routine suture threads similarly are well-tolerated in general.

11.2 Patient Selection

Indications for use of the internal bra technique for augmentation mastopexy include but are not limited to

- Severely loose skin with poor soft tissue support; tissue quality unable to support an implant in the desired position (upper pole fullness).
- Low-riding breasts with very low IMFs or tall chest wall height.
- Bottomed-out breasts with low IMFs.
- Fold restoration following a total capsulectomy of a severely calcified breast implant capsule.
- Implant malposition (lateral or inferior malposition).
- Symmastia reconstruction.
- Breast asymmetries (fold asymmetry).

Combined with mastopexy, use of a mesh scaffold with an internal bra technique facilitates breast elevation, raises the patient's IMF, and addresses lateral malposition. In milder cases of ptosis, a mastopexy may not be warranted. A mastopexy also may not be warranted in the case of a younger patient seeking upper pole volume with good tissue quality but very low IMF crease position (i.e., tall chest wall height)

In cases with significant asymmetries of the breasts as well as IMFs, coupled with extensive prior breast surgeries, patients must be counseled extensively regarding their challenging anatomy as well as on surgical risks, limitations of the procedure, and possible need for secondary revisions. Even with the senior author's extensive experience with internal bra technique procedures in revisional augmentation mastopexy, the authors advise all patients of an up to 20% chance of needing a secondary procedure to refine the result. It is important to educate the patient that the internal bra technique is not merely an augmentation mastopexy; it is an advanced technique to essentially reengineer breast anatomy. Often, surgeons are addressing multiple variables in one case: implant size, lateral malposition, inferior malposition, fold asymmetries, excess skin, ptosis and nipple position, and symmetry. Hence, the patient must be made aware of the need to fine-tune results, which should be part of a detailed informed consent process. Furthermore, we strongly advise including a separate consent for the surgeon's choice of surgical mesh/ADM for proper informed consent.

11.3 Patient Assessment and Markings

The authors routinely mark the patient midline and current IMF crease. All markings are done in the upright position, with the patient observing all markings in the mirror. During the initial consultation, we document any fold asymmetries that may exist at baseline. It is important to re-highlight baseline fold asymmetries to the patient during preoperative marking. We advise the patient to use her hands to mimic the effect of a push-up bra to demonstrate how she wants her breasts to sit on her chest wall. While the patient is pushing her current/old implants up demonstrating her desired "cleavage takeoff point," or the point at which the upper pole of breast volume begins, it is important to mark out this new upper pole border (▶ Fig. 11.1). Now the surgeon must estimate the base width of the new implant and estimate where the neo-IMF should sit. A key question is to what extent the surgeon needs to raise the IMF? It is important to mark out the medial and lateral borders of the desired neo-IMF. These markings will be utilized intraoperatively and will help to ensure symmetry when reconstructing or raising the patient's IMF (▶ Fig. 11.2).

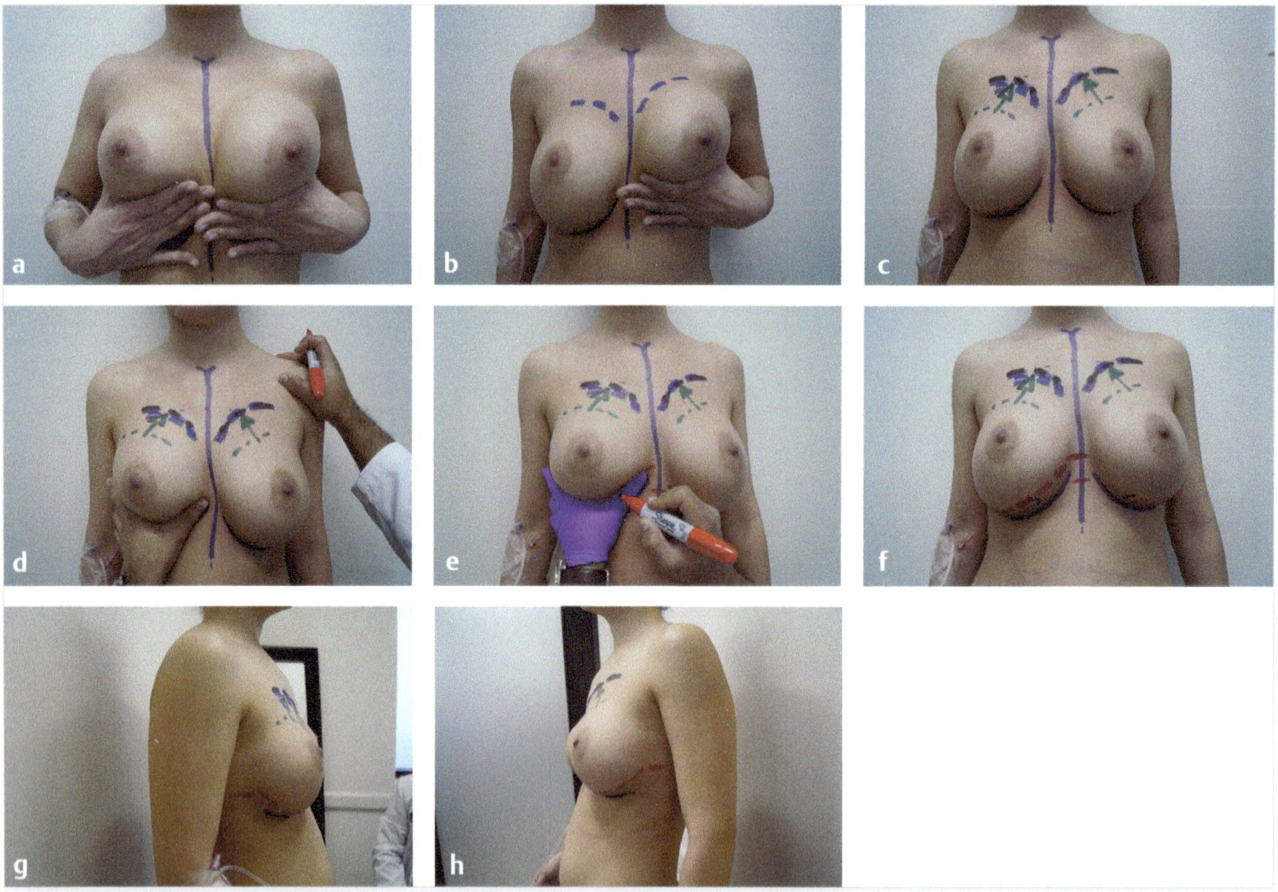

Fig. 11.1 **(a,b)** Patient demonstrates her desired upper pole volume. **(c,d)** This desired upper pole border (*blue thick dashes*) sets the goal to be achieved intraoperatively. The red markings illustrate the position **(e-h)** of the neo-inframammary fold crease (desired fold position).

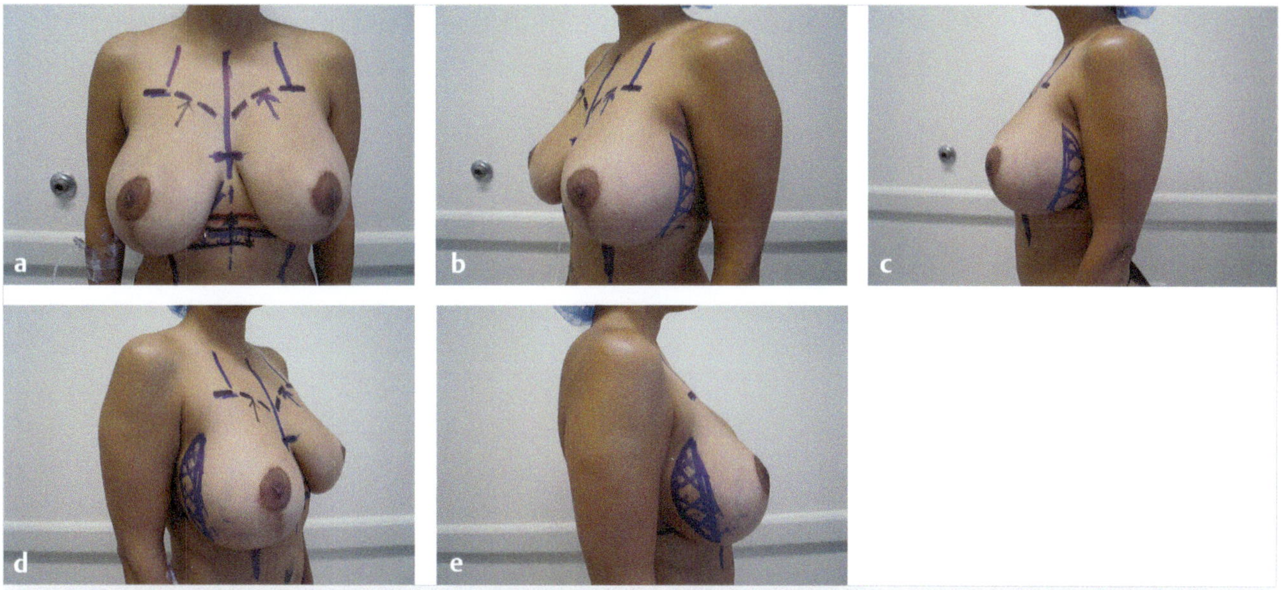

Fig. 11.2 (a-e) Preoperative markings illustrate baseline fold position, the neo-inframammary fold crease (desired fold position where the fold crease needs to be raised), and the desired upper pole of the breast. Lateral cross marks illustrate where internal bra can treat lateral malposition.

11.4 Surgical Technique

11.4.1 Considerations

Local anesthetic is infiltrated along the patient's IMF and around any anticipated mastopexy incisions to aid in hemostasis and facilitate pain control. In secondary cases, an IMF crease approach is typically utilized. If the patient presents with severe loose skin that will require a circum-vertical or full mastopexy, a generous 4- to 5-cm vertical incision along the breast meridian, below the nipple areola complex (NAC), can be utilized for access to the patient's original implants; this incision will later be buried into the subsequent mastopexy. In cases that will require only a periareolar mastopexy, the authors have utilized an IMF crease approach, occasionally utilizing a limited inferior periareolar access incision if needed.

11.4.2 Planning the Neo-IMF Crease Position

The degree to which the IMF will need to be elevated is estimated based on preoperative markings, and the IMF incision marked appropriately to minimize visible scarring. Preoperatively, the authors recommend having the patient demonstrate her desired result: have the patient show you where she wants the upper border of her breast to be. Then, based on this position, mark where you think the neo-IMF crease needs to be to achieve the desired result (▶ Fig. 11.1).

11.4.3 Management of the Breast Capsule in Revisional Cases

If the capsule is benign and nonpathologic, a total capsulectomy is not warranted. If there is lateral malposition present, a lateral capsulorraphy can be performed. The surgical mesh or ADM product can also be utilized to prevent lateral malposition as well. A total capsulectomy is indicated, by contrast, when capsules demonstrate thickening or calcification. In some revisional cases, the IMF crease and structure are notably low on the chest wall and occasionally extend into the upper abdominal space. In severe cases of capsular contracture and/or in cases of poor soft tissue support or quality, the patient can be left with a weakened IMF when the capsule is removed from the inferior gutter of the implant pocket. In these cases, the patient may be at increased risk for bottoming out or inferior malposition, especially if a larger implant is placed. Use of the internal bra technique is an option in these cases to restore the integrity of the fold and/or raise its position on the chest wall.

11.4.4 Mesh Application

On each side, the chest wall is marked above the current IMF, delineating where the mesh scaffold is to be anchored. If lateral malposition is present, the chest wall can be additionally marked where the mesh is to be anchored laterally to correct lateral malposition. If a lateral capsulorraphy has been performed, simply placing the surgical mesh as an overlay can suffice. Mesh scaffold is selected and soaked in antibiotic solution per manufacturer and product specifications. Intraoperative paper templates may be used to estimate mesh size needed to accommodate the contour of the patient's anticipated new implants. It is important to remember the natural curvature of the new implant to be placed. If the mesh is too small to accommodate the curvature of the implant, this can blunt and distort the lower pole of the breast. The choice of mesh is otherwise prepped per industry recommendations, including any irrigation fluid soaks and washes to clear retained preservative, if needed.

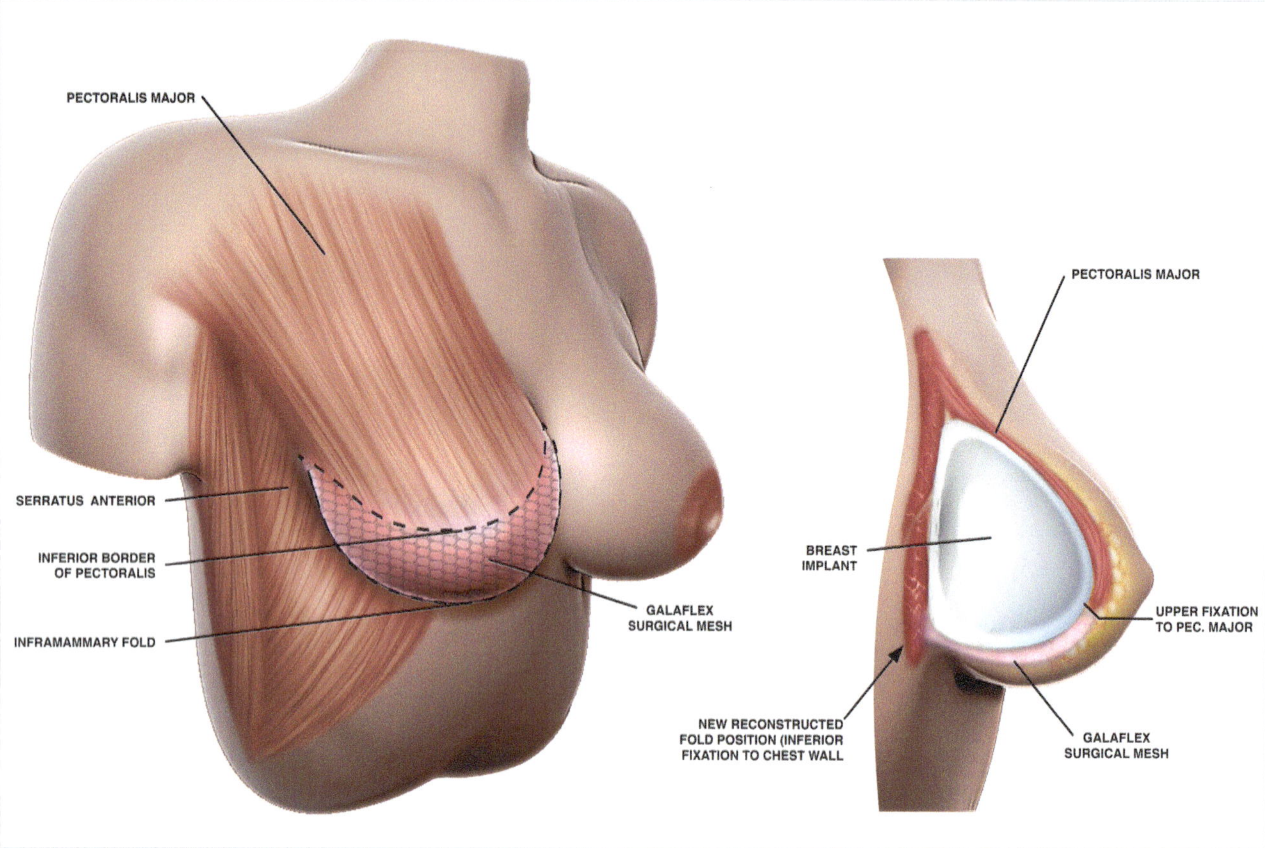

Fig. 11.3 Lateral view illustrates placement of internal bra surgical mesh/acellular dermal matrix with lower insetting to the chest wall at the level of the new inframammary fold and the upper insetting to the inferior edge of the pectoralis major muscle. If the muscle is not available due to previous surgery or severe retraction, then the upper insetting can be completed to a segment of the old capsule.

At this time, the authors' preferred surgical mesh is GalaFLEX, made of poly-4-hydroxybutyrate (P4HB). The advantages of GalaFLEX include but are not limited to (1) use of a long-standing safe suture material that dissolves over 18–24 months, (2) relatively low cost compared to other ADM or surgical mesh products, (3) reliable safety profile with low risk of extrusion, and (4) rapid integration and adherence to surrounding tissue.

11.4.5 The Internal Bra

Mesh is trimmed for each pocket to suit the patient's chest wall anatomy and accommodate the anterior surface of the new implant. The basic framework involves the inferior edge of the mesh, which is inset along the neo-IMF markings along the chest wall with buried interrupted absorbable monofilament sutures (2–0 PDS [polydioxanone suture; Ethicon, Bridgewater, MA] or equivalent). The upper border of the mesh should be inset to the inferior border of the pectoralis major muscle to achieve essentially a dual-plane placement of the new implant. Centrally, an opening is maintained to facilitate passage of the patient's final implants. Once the implant has been placed in the new pocket, the remainder of the insetting is completed. We recommend upper fixation to the pectoralis muscle to ensure longevity of support. In the extremely rare instance where the pectoralis muscle is unavailable due to prior surgery or severe retraction, it is advised to preserve a small segment of anterior pocket capsule for upper mesh insetting (▶ Fig. 11.3).

There are two technical options to inset the internal bra mesh: (1) a top-down technique and (2) a bottom-up technique.

Top-Down Technique

In the top-down technique, the upper border of the mesh is inset to the inferior edge of the pectoralis major muscle using interrupted buried 2–0 PDS sutures. If the vertical length of the mesh needs to be determined, an intraoperative implant sizer can be utilized. Once the inferior edge of the mesh is marked and trimmed, the implant sizer is removed and the inferior edge of the mesh is then inset to the neo-IMF medially and laterally using two figure-of-eight 2–0 PDS sutures. These medial and lateral sutures are not tied down yet. They are placed as "parachute" sutures to be tied down later. The free ends of these sutures are secured with a hemostat. Now the center portion of the inferior mesh remains not secured to the neo-IMF crease. This will be the passage to introduce the final implant (▶ Fig. 11.4).

The breast pocket is irrigated with antibiotic mixed saline solution as per the surgeon's preferred protocols, and the final implant is introduced into the subpectoral and "sub-mesh" pocket. Once the implant position has been confirmed, the authors tie down the medial and lateral figure-of-eight sutures.

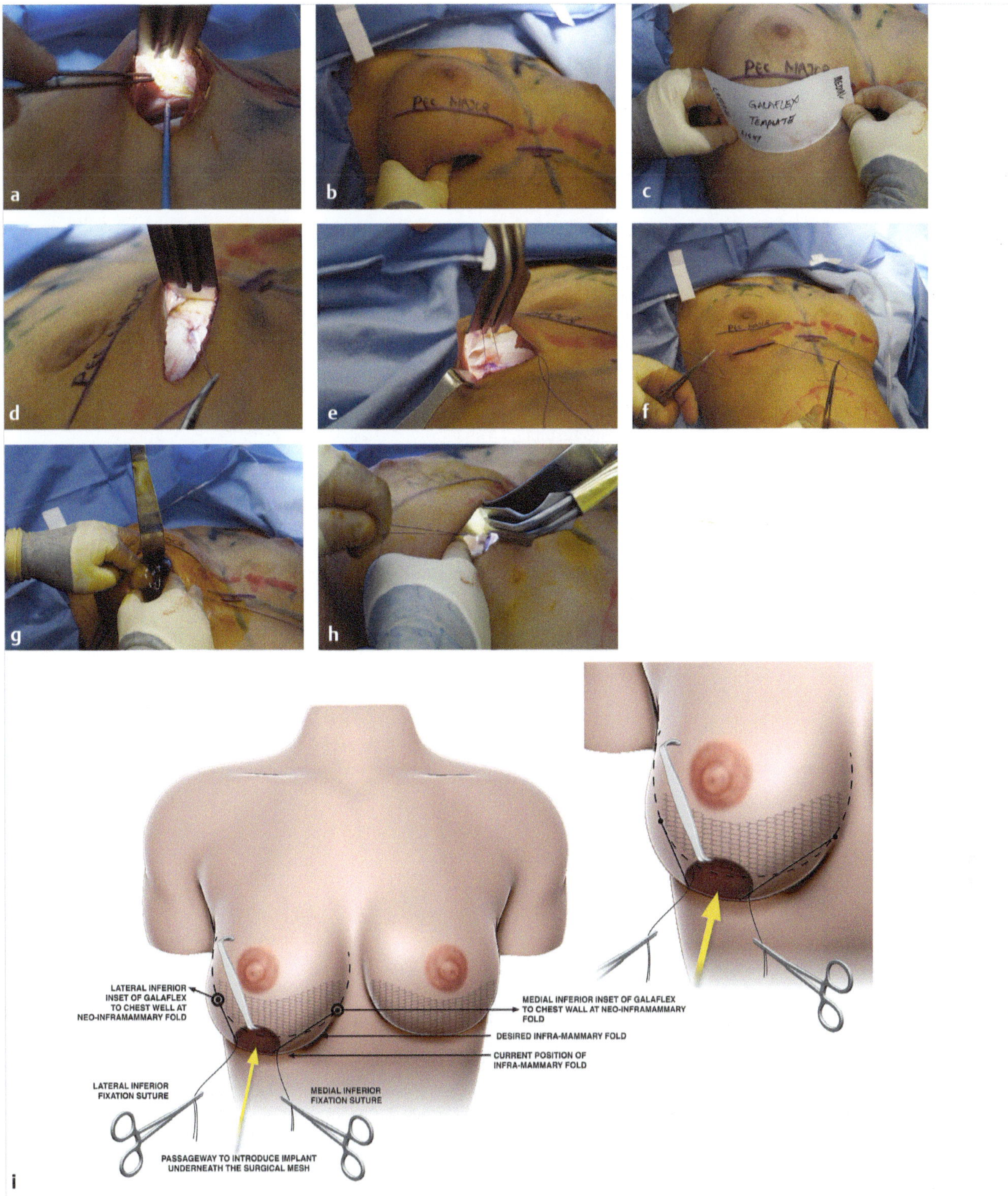

Fig. 11.4 **(a)** Illustrates and dissection of the inferior edge of the pectoralis major muscle as it is separated from the anterior capsule. The bovie tip is pointing to the free edge of the muscle. **(b)** Has a temporary implant sizer in place to help determine the size of the surgical mesh. **(c)** Illustrates a sterile paper template that is used to determine the exact size of the mesh to lay over the anterior surface/dome of the new implant. **(d,e)** After the sizer is removed and after fixation of the upper edge of the surgical mesh to the inferior edge of the pectoralis major muscle, we then inset the inferior edge of the mesh to the neo-IMF medially and laterally using "parachute" sutures. **(f)** Illustrates the medial and lateral inferior sutures retracted by a hemostat. **(g)** Final implant is introduced into the subpectoral and "sub-mesh" dual plane pocket. **(h)** Tie down the inferior medial and lateral mesh fixation sutures anchoring the mesh down to the neo-IMF. **(i)** This diagram illustrates the passageway to introduce the implant into the subpectoral-submesh pocket before final insetting using medial and lateral "parachute" sutures which are tied down after the final implant has been placed.

Now, under direct visualization and with mechanical protection of the implant, the central 2–0 PDS sutures are placed to complete insetting of the mesh to the central portion of the neo-IMF crease. The senior author places a 10- or 15-French Jackson-Pratt drain in the fold crease gutter. Drain placement can vary depending on the surgeon's selection of mesh product or ADM. The authors prefer a short course of a drain, as they feel the continuous suction accelerates adherence of the GalaFLEX surgical mesh to the adjacent tissue.

Bottom-Up Technique

In the bottom-up technique, the mesh is first inset along the neo-IMF crease using interrupted 2–0 PDS sutures. Then a figure-of-eight suture is placed medially and laterally to inset the mesh temporarily to the inferior border of the pectoralis muscle. Here, the medial and lateral sutures are not tied down but kept as "parachute" sutures that will be tied down later. Free suture ends are secured with hemostat clamps. This results in a central passageway through which the implant can be passed. Once the implant has been placed, the central sutures are then placed to complete upper fixation of the mesh to the muscle. When larger implants are to be placed, visualization of the central segment of the pectoralis major muscle can be quite difficult. If one opts for the bottom-up technique, then a counterincision (periareolar) may be necessary. For instance, if all the work is being done just through an IMF crease incision, a limited periareolar incision may be needed to achieve proper exposure to complete insetting of the mesh to the central segment of the pectoralis major muscle. Based on their experience, the authors recommend the "top-down" technique to facilitate exposure and expedite surgical times. Trimming of the mesh is done laterally to eliminate redundancy in the horizontal axis. Importantly, completing a lateral inset also prevents recurrent lateral migration or malposition.

11.4.6 Evaluation of the Internal Bra Position for Symmetry

Once the internal bra mesh has been inset on each side, it is very important to sit the patient upright on the operating room table to assess symmetry. Often with raising the fold position, there will be loose skin that will need to be addressed with either a periareolar, circum-vertical. or full mastopexy. With the patient in the upright position, we recommend a tailor-tack mastopexy to address the loose skin and nipple position. At this point, the implant position should achieve the upper pole volume as designated by the surgeon's desired preop markings. If one breast is sitting higher than the other, determine which side achieves the desired result. Make adjustments on the contralateral breast to achieve intraoperative symmetry. Once the best possible symmetry has been achieved, it is important to take intraoperative photos to document the result in the upright position. We also advise a final photo once the mastopexy has been completed to document an on-table final result. During the postoperative phase, if swelling manifests, these intraoperative photos provide the patient with a "light at the end of the tunnel": she can see what her end result will be once postoperative swelling subsides. Photos can provide the patient with great emotional support and reassurance during the healing process.

With final implants in position and mesh properly inset, the internal bra technique is complete, and shape and symmetry are reassessed with the patient upright. ▶ Fig. 11.5 illustrates a patient who had unsuccessfully undergone two breast

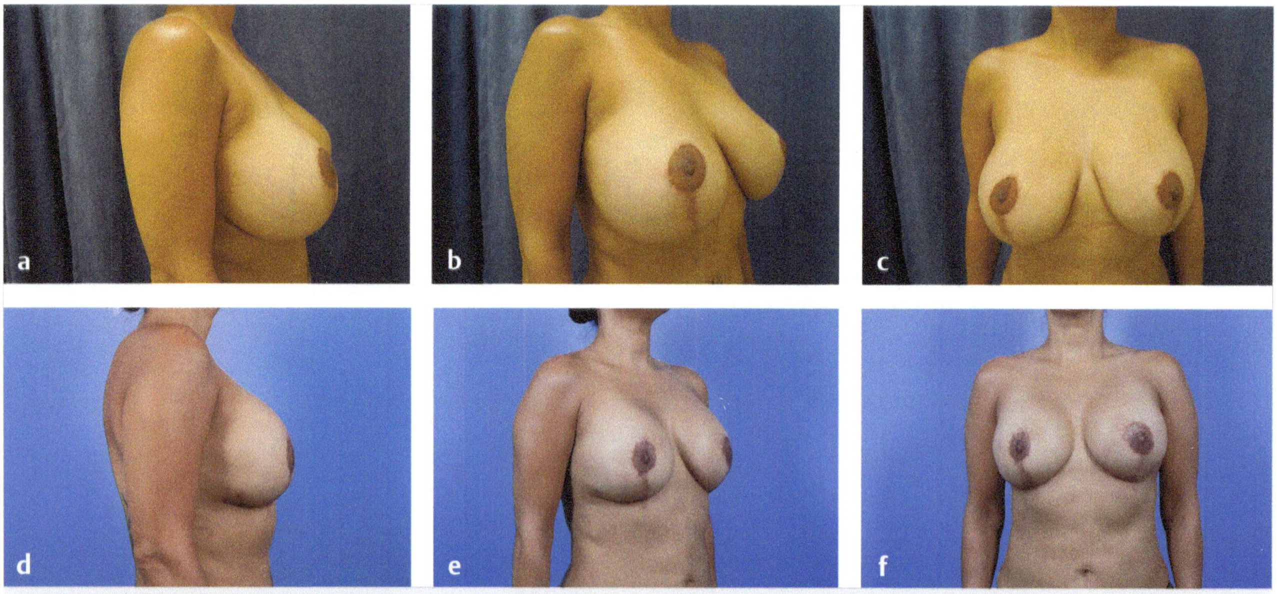

Fig. 11.5 Patient who had unsuccessfully undergone two breast augmentation mastopexy procedures at an outside institution. She presented seeking a downsizing of her large silicone gel implants and sagging. She had bilateral bottoming out (inferior malposition) and lateral malposition. She was also seeking more upper pole volume. She had very poor tissue quality. **(a)** Preoperative lateral view. **(b)** Preoperative anterolateral view. **(c)** Preoperative anterior view. She underwent a revision breast augmentation with a downsizing to smaller Inspira SoftTouch silicone gel implants and an internal bra technique with GalaFLEX surgical mesh and a full revisional mastopexy. **(d)** Three months postoperative lateral view. **(e)** Postoperative anterolateral view. **(f)** Postoperative anterior view.

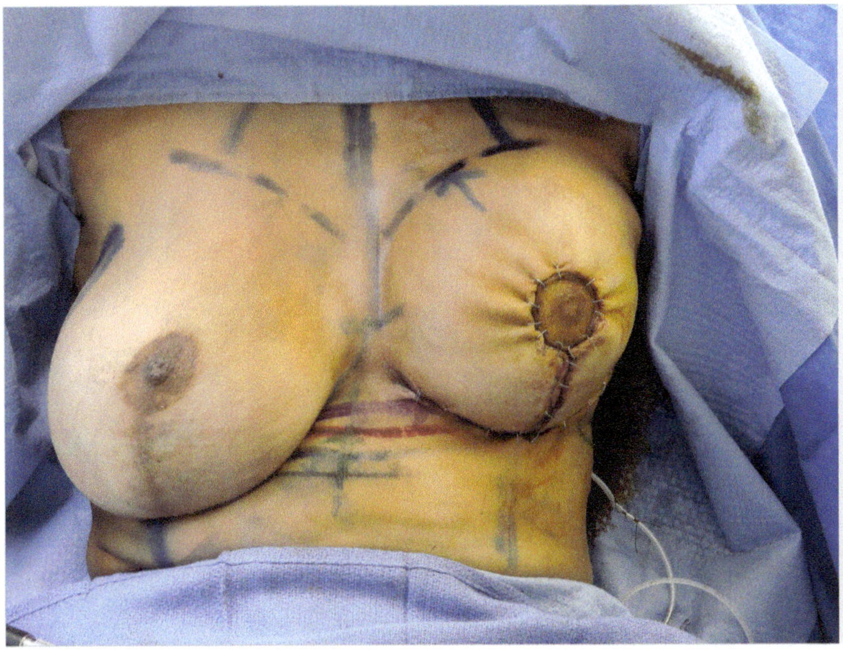

Fig. 11.6 Patient shown in Fig. 11.5 in the upright position after her left side was tentatively done with the internal bra technique and the contralateral breast not yet touched. This clearly demonstrates and documents the intraoperative change achieved for the patient.

augmentation mastopexy procedures at an outside institution. She presented seeking a downsizing of her large silicone gel implants and correction of her sagging. She has bilateral bottoming out (inferior malposition) and lateral malposition. She was also seeking more upper pole volume. She has very poor tissue quality. She underwent a revision breast augmentation with a downsizing to smaller Inspira SoftTouch (Allergan, Dublin, Ireland) silicone gel implants and an internal bra technique with GalaFLEX surgical mesh and a full revisional mastopexy. The internal bra technique raised her IMF crease (▶ Fig. 11.6) by over 2 inches (5 cm) and helped treat her inferior and lateral malposition. Given the downsizing, a full revisional mastopexy was required to address nipple position and excess skin. As the 3-month postop lateral view in ▶ Fig. 11.5d illustrates, the result has established upper pole volume with a more youthful breast shape.

11.4.7 Mastopexy

The tailor-tack periareolar mastopexy described is revised as needed to confirm ideal shape and symmetry. Additional adjustments are made to ensure symmetric nipple position. For instance, to improve breast shape, the nipple-to-IMF distance may require reduction through a horizontal component to the mastopexy with an IMF crease incision. Nipple-to-IMF distance is set symmetrically and based on dimensional planning.

Triangular measurements on the breast (i.e., bilateral sternal notch to new nipple position and nipple to midline) are confirmed. The tailor-tacking staples' positions are reinforced with a surgical marker prior to removal. Mastopexy incisions are then made, and the intended buried dermoglandular tissue is de-epithelialized, taking care to preserve the vascularity of the subdermal plexus. The authors advise against violation of the subdermal blood supply and advise against any undermining, in order to preserve the blood supply to the NAC. Wound edges are reapproximated with deep dermal and skin monofilament sutures (3–0 and 4–0 Monocryl or PDS, respectively). Meticulous tissue reapproximation is crucial for cases utilizing the inverted-**T** incision pattern. Definitive skin closure is achieved with subcuticular suturing coupled with skin adhesive or Steri-Strips (3 M, St. Paul, MN) application. Both NACs are assessed for perfusion prior to placement of the patient in a compressive chest wrap garment, extubation, and recovery room transfer.

11.5 Some Example Results

▶ Fig. 11.7 illustrates a revision breast augmentation using the internal bra technique with GalaFLEX surgical mesh in a patient who was seeking to improve the hollowing in her upper chest (more upper pole volume and cleavage).

▶ Fig. 11.8a shows a lateral view of a patient who presented with the complaint that her augmented breasts were too low and she had no upper pole volume. She knew she had a tall chest wall, but she wanted "not to have to wear a push-up bra all the time to look normal." Her IMF crease was low on her chest wall, and she had bottoming out with pseudoptosis. She underwent a revision breast augmentation with the internal bra technique with GalaFLEX surgical mesh. No mastopexy was required. The "fresh" postop result, 8 days after surgery, in ▶ Fig. 11.8b illustrates her breast sitting much higher on her chest wall with her nipple position almost centered vertically on her breast mound. ▶ Fig. 11.8c illustrates the long-term result of this patient at 18 months postop with sustained support and resolution of bottoming-out and her pseudoptosis.

11.6 Complications

From the senior author's operative series, over 75 cases have been performed utilizing the internal bra technique for revisionary mastopexy-augmentation. Implants selected have generally been large-volume, ranging 400 to 800 mL. The longest

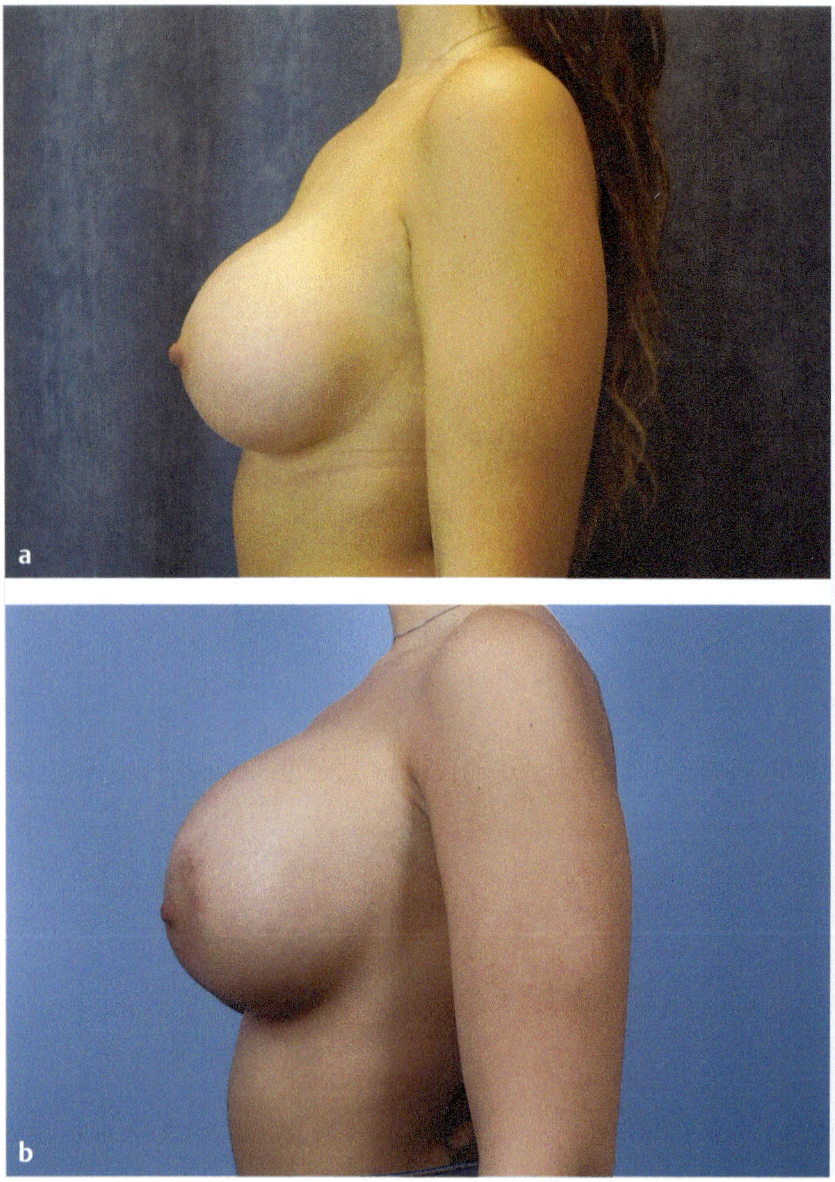

Fig. 11.7 Revision breast augmentation using the internal bra technique with GalaFLEX surgical mesh in a patient who was seeking to improve the hollowing in her upper chest (more upper pole volume and cleavage). **(a)** Preoperative. **(b)** Six months postoperative.

follow-up has been for over 3.5 years with only one known recurrence. The single case of recurrence was the patient's fourth revisional surgery. The patient had a history of massive weight loss and presented with severe weakness in tissue with poor soft tissue support, and she was seeking large implants. In this case, the pectoralis major muscle had been either resected or damaged in previous operations by another surgeon. The mesh was inset to the patient's soft, benign capsule. Although the patient was pleased with her overall long-term result and improvement, the authors feel there was some mild recurrence of implant inferior malposition. No cases of recurrence were noted when the internal bra mesh was inset to the pectoralis major muscle.

In cases of severe poor tissue quality (e.g., paper-thin breast tissue, history of massive weight loss, or history of multiple previous breast implant surgeries), it is important to advise the patient that the internal bra technique is a powerful way to support the implant position. However, in the most challenging cases where the tissue has severe weakness (poor soft tissue support), the patient's thin breast tissue or skin may still require a secondary skin tightening. The majority of these revisional procedures have been mastopexy scar revisions done under local anesthesia. It is important to make patients aware that the internal bra technique is far more complex than a revisional breast augmentation–mastopexy. This technique enables the surgeon to "re-engineer" the patient's natural breast anatomy, raising her IMF crease and natural footprint of her breast on her chest wall. In these cases, the surgeon is juggling multiple variables at once: implant size/symmetry, fold position, lateral position, nipple position, breast skin, breast projection, and so on. It is important for patients to understand and accept that in up to 20% of cases, a secondary procedure may be needed to

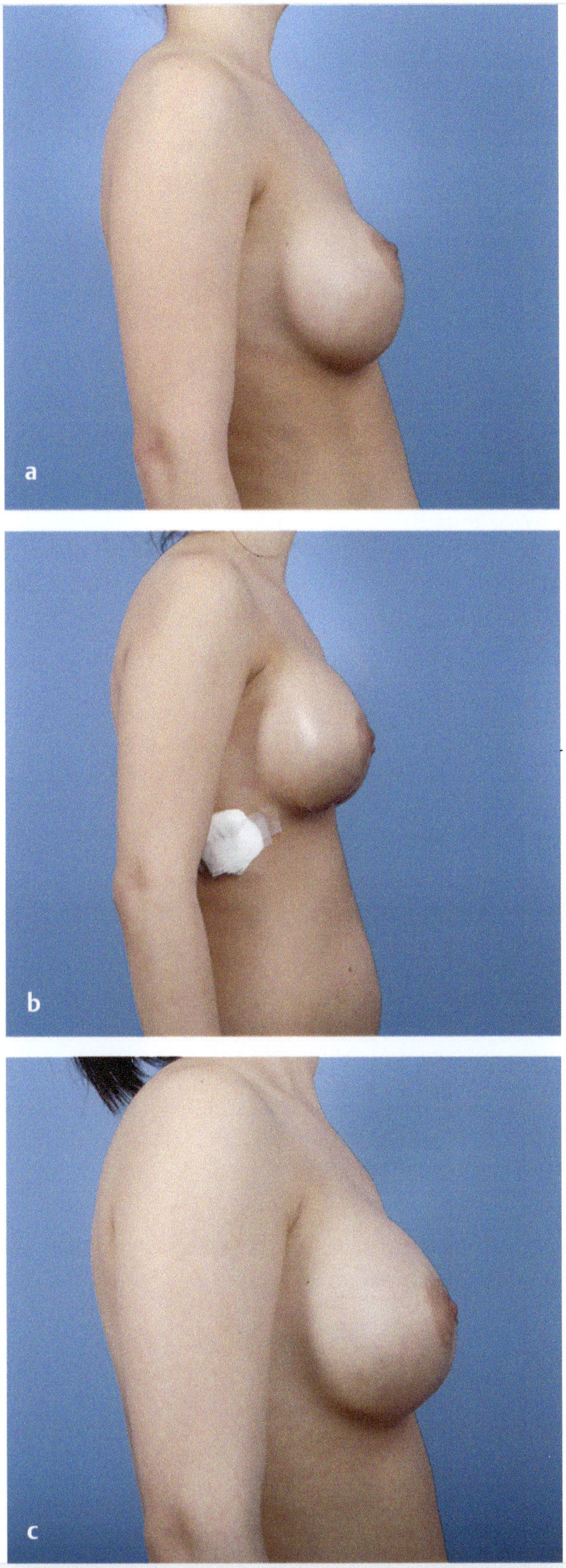

Fig. 11.8 Lateral view **(a)** before, **(b)** "fresh" postop result 8 days, and **(c)** 18 months after surgery.

fine-tune results; disclosing this potential scenario is important to set patient expectations correctly. Done correctly, the internal bra technique with revisional breast augmentation–mastopexy affords our patients transformative results that simply cannot be achieved using their tissue alone.

Key Points

- Internal bra techniques using an acellular dermal matrix product or resorbable surgical mesh (GalaFLEX) in augmentation–mastopexy can help maintain upper pole volume in cases of poor soft tissue support (weak breast tissue) or low breast inframammary fold position.
- The internal bra technique is a reliable option for fold repositioning or restoration in revisional breast implant surgery.
- The internal bra technique can provided additional support in primary or secondary cases involving large-volume implants.
- Internal bra techniques can be complex, particularly in cases of weakened soft tissues. Patient expectations should be managed accordingly regarding the need for possible secondary procedures to fine-tune aesthetic results.

References

[1] Doshier LJ, Eagan SL, Shock LA, Henry SL, Colbert SH, Puckett CL. The subtleties of success in simultaneous augmentation-mastopexy. Plast Reconstr Surg. 2016; 138(3):585–592

[2] Lee MR, Unger JG, Adams WP, Jr. The tissue-based triad: a process approach to augmentation mastopexy. Plast Reconstr Surg. 2014; 134(2):215–225

[3] Nahabedian MY. Breast deformities and mastopexy. Plast Reconstr Surg. 2011; 127(4):91e–102e

[4] Coombs DM, Srivastava U, Amar D, Rubin JP, Gusenoff JA. The challenges of augmentation mastopexy in the massive weight loss patient: technical considerations. Plast Reconstr Surg. 2017; 139(5):1090–1099

[5] Rubin JP, Khachi G. Mastopexy after massive weight loss: dermal suspension and selective auto-augmentation. Clin Plast Surg. 2008; 35(1):123–129

[6] Sampaio, Góes JC. Periareolar mammaplasty: double skin technique with application of polyglactin 910 mesh [in Portuguese]. Rev Bras Cir Plast. 1992; 7: 1–3

[7] Sampaio Góes JC. Periareolar mammaplasty: double-skin technique with application of mesh support. Clin Plast Surg. 2002; 29(3):349–364, v

[8] de Bruijn HP, ten Thije RH, Johannes S. Mastopexy with mesh reinforcement: the mechanical characteristics of polyester mesh in the female breast. Plast Reconstr Surg. 2009; 124(2):364–371

[9] Adams WP, Jr, Moses AC. Use of poly-4-hydroxybutyrate mesh to optimize soft-tissue support in mastopexy: a single-site study. Plast Reconstr Surg. 2017; 139(1):67–75

12 Reduction Mammaplasty

Clark Schierle and Megan Fracol

Summary

Reduction mammaplasty is one of the most rewarding procedures performed in plastic surgery, for both the patient and the surgeon. Patients express high satisfaction rates after reduction mammoplasty, and surgeons who perform this procedure can provide both aesthetic and functional improvements to the patient's life. This chapter will focus on historical perspective, pertinent breast anatomy, breast physiology relevant to performing breast reduction at various ages, the history and physical exam, common techniques, and complications.

Keywords: mammoplasty, reduction mammoplasty, breast reduction, breast hypertrophy, gigantomastia

12.1 Introduction

Reduction mammaplasty is one of the most rewarding surgical procedures performed by plastic surgeons. Patients report high levels of satisfaction after reduction mammaplasty, with significant improvement in pain and lifestyle.[1] Most complications are minor and easily manageable. In this chapter, we will review the anatomy of the breast relevant to parenchymal resection patterns, considerations in the initial workup of a patient presenting for reduction mammaplasty, preoperative markings, skin resection patterns, pedicle options, variations in surgical technique, and common postoperative complications with associated management.

In these cases, there is an excess of skin, fat, and parenchyma, usually coupled with an overall breast shape that is less than ideal aesthetically. Patients with mammary hypertrophy can also present with a variety of symptoms. Typical complaints include neck and back pain, shoulder grooving from bra straps, inframammary intertrigo, and limited ability to exercise. Psychosocial issues surrounding excessively large breasts also exist, creating embarrassment for women, especially teenagers and elderly women.[2] Netscher et al encourage a focus on the constellation of symptoms of a patient rather than absolute volume as an arbitrary criteria for reduction mammaplasty. Further, their work shows that disease-specific group of physical and psychosocial complaints are more directly related to large breast size than to being generally overweight.[3] Kerrigan et al demonstrated the superiority of surgical intervention over conservative measures such as weight loss and special bras.[4] The main purpose of breast reduction is to improve the quality of life of the women who suffer from mammary hypertrophy. Blomqvist et al used a standardized quality of life questionnaire to demonstrate the long lasting positive impact on women's quality of life.[5] In addition to improvement in quality of life, creation of an aesthetically pleasing breast is clearly an important consideration as well. Spear may have put it best when he said that breast reduction represents "the clearest example of the interface between reconstructive plastic surgery and aesthetic plastic surgery."[2]

12.2 History of the Practice

One of the first cases of reduction mammaplasty was reported by Dieffenbach in 1848, who reduced the lower two-thirds of the breast via an inframammary fold (IMF) incision.[6] Over the next century there were many approaches to reducing breast tissue and correcting ptosis. Schwarzmann suggested that the perfusion and viability of the nipple areolar complex (NAC) could be improved by maintaining a ring of dermis around it, allowing more reliable transposition.[7] Penn in 1955 noted that sternal notch–to-nipple distances should be 21 cm and the nipple-to-nipple distance should be the same, to form an equilateral triangle.[8] Wise reported his keyhole pattern of skin resection in 1956.[9] Ultimately resulting in an inverted-**T** scar, the Wise pattern of breast reduction remains one of the most reliable and popular breast reduction techniques to this day.

Subsequent decades have seen continued evolution of techniques involving choice of blood supply and skin resection and scar patterns. Pitanguy and Weiner described the superiorly based dermoglandular pedicle in 1973.[10] Orlando and Guthrie devised the technique of the superomedial dermoglandular pedicle shortly thereafter in 1975.[11] McKissock described a vertical bipedicle technique.[12] Claude Lassus developed his technique in 1970 using a vertical scar.[13] Many other plastic surgeons around the world further developed short-scar, superior pedicle techniques for reduction mammoplasty in the 1980s and 1990s, including Lejour, Marchac, Peixoto, Sampaio Góes, and Benelli.[14,15,16,17,18,19] Techniques to avert the vertical scar, such as the technique of Passot, have been refined by various authors in the 1990s and 2000s, including Lalonde, Matloub, and Pribaz.[20,21,22] Hammond's short-scar periareolar inferior pedicle reduction (SPAIR) technique for breast reduction combines a short-scar skin resection with an inferior pedicle, in contrast to most other short-scar techniques, which implement a superior or superomedial pedicle.[23] Hall-Findlay describes a medial pedicle technique with minimal skin undermining.[24] The overall goal of these techniques is to fight the tendency to bottom out while reducing overall scar burden.

12.3 Anatomy

In reviewing the anatomy of the breast relevant to reduction mammaplasty, this section will focus particularly on blood supply. The parenchymal resection pattern is less important in planning the operation than focusing on the parenchymal pattern that is left behind and what pedicle remains to provide robust blood supply to this residual breast tissue. In particular, the NAC not only is a key aesthetic landmark of the breast but unfortunately is also the tissue the farthest away from any given pedicle and thus most prone to necrosis in case of vascular insufficiency.

The landmarks of the breast commonly referred to in oncologic surgery include the latissimus dorsi muscle laterally, the clavicle superiorly, the sternum medially, and the inframammary fold (IMF) inferiorly. Given the rich, overlapping vascular network to the breast, it is possible to design a pedicle from virtually any direction. There are four major arterial networks supplying the breast: the internal mammary medially, the lateral thoracic laterally, the thoracoacromial superiorly, and the intercostal perforators arising both medially and laterally (▶ Fig. 12.1). The NAC is supplied by both glandular perforators and the subdermal plexus; hence the importance of leaving dermis behind when de-epithelializing around the NAC. The skin is supplied only by the subdermal plexus, likewise pointing to the importance of leaving thick skin flaps. Venous drainage occurs primarily via the axillary vein but also via internal mammary and intercostal veins. There can be considerable anatomic variability between breasts, and our understanding of these variations is still evolving.[25]

12.4 Physiology

Mammary hypertrophy is primarily the result of an abnormal sensitivity of the breast to circulating estrogens, causing breast proliferation that is predominantly adipose and connective tissue rather than glandular parenchyma. Most women with

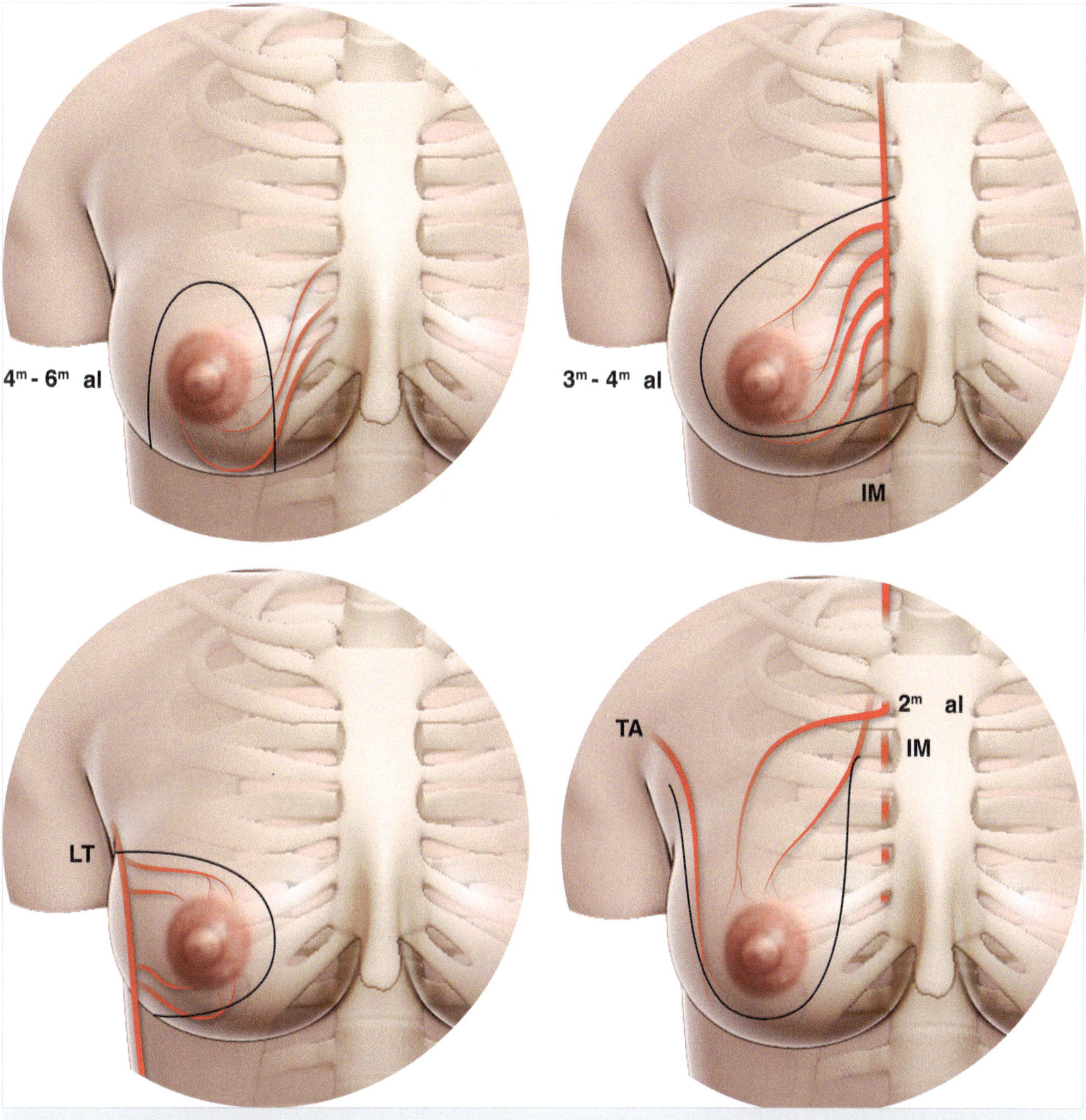

Fig. 12.1 Examples of pedicle options in breast reduction based on blood supply to the breast. Major pedicles to the breast include the internal mammary perforators medially, intercostal perforators both medially and inferiorly, lateral thoracic perforators laterally, and the thoracoacromial perforators and internal mammary/anterior intercostals superolaterally.

mammary hypertrophy have normal levels of serum estrogen as well as normal amounts of estrogen receptors in the breast tissue.[26,27]

Cases of true juvenile virginal hypertrophy of the breast can present in the age range of 11–14 years.[27] Durston reported the first case of juvenile virginal breast hypertrophy in 1670. The woman in his case report died at age 24 and was found to have a 64-pound (29-kg) right breast with no evidence of disease.[28] Recurrence in these patients is common, and they should be counseled for the likely need for secondary reduction mammaplasty.[29]

12.5 Patient History and Physical Exam

Preoperative evaluation of the patient presenting for reduction mammaplasty should focus on symptoms caused by the macromastia and any medical comorbidities that may impair wound healing or otherwise increase surgical risk. For insurance to cover reduction mammaplasty, certain symptoms not amenable to medical management should be documented.[30] These include chronic back pain requiring the use of pain medications, bra strap grooves in the shoulders, nerve pain, breast pain, intertrigo or rash within the IMFs, and restriction of physical activities. While not always necessary, a history of attempted weight loss with diet control and exercise shows patient motivation and failure of nonsurgical management. It is important to inquire whether the patient has a history of gastric bypass surgery or is considering weight loss surgery, as this may affect breast volume. If a patient is planning to undergo weight loss surgery then reduction mammaplasty may be better delayed until 6 months to 1 year after the patient's weight is stable and there is less risk of nutritional deficiencies that may impair wound healing.

Other comorbidities that are important to ask about include anything that would impair wound healing, such as diabetes or history of immunosuppression; anything that may increase risks associated with general anesthesia, such as significant cardiac or pulmonary history; and anything that may increase risk of postoperative complications, such as hypertension and coagulopathies.

While a physical exam is helpful to get a sense of the volume of breast tissue the patient would like removed, it is important to counsel the patient that it is impossible to give her an exact bra size she will be postoperatively. That will depend on how much breast tissue is removed in the operation, but it may also change somewhat as postoperative swelling goes down. Additionally, bra size is not standardized across retailers. The patient's height, weight, and body habitus are often mandatory for insurers to calculate the amount of breast tissue they require for the reduction procedure to be covered. This amount can vary from insurer to insurer. Some insurers use an absolute mass based on the patient's height. Others use calculations involving the patient's height and weight, such as the Schnur sliding scale, to approve or reject patients' insurance claims for breast reduction. Schnur et al developed this scale in 1991 after analyzing surveys of plastic surgeons.[31] In their study, women whose removed breast weight was under the fifth percentile sought the procedure for cosmetic reasons, while women whose resected breast weight was above the 22nd percentile reported medical reasons. Many U.S. health insurers approve only patients whose predicted resected weights fall above the 22nd percentile based on the Schnur scale.[32] Most plastic surgeons agree that such a formulaic approach is flawed and that greater emphasis should be placed on individual patient characteristics and symptomatic considerations.

As part of the physical exam, it is also helpful to show the markings of where the final scars will be on the breast, as most patients are not aware of the scarring to be expected afterward. The degree of ptosis can be noted, and the patient should be shown where to expect the new nipple position. Body mass index (BMI) should also be documented as part of the physical exam. The risk of postoperative complications increases with increasing weight of breast resection and increasing BMI.[33,34]

Finally, it is important to document any family history of breast cancer. While American College of Surgeons and the American Cancer Society recommend screening mammograms starting at age 40, the United States Preventative Task Force recommends screening mammograms starting at age 50.[35] Most plastic surgeons will order a preoperative screening mammogram in any patients aged 40 or greater. In patients with a significant family history of breast cancer or *BRCA*-positivity, it may be reasonable to order a screening mammogram even in patients less than 40 years old.

12.6 Operative Technique

12.6.1 Preoperative Markings

The preoperative breast markings are perhaps the most important step of the operation. These markings help ensure symmetry between the breasts and guide the surgeon once anatomic landmarks get displaced as the patient lies supine on the operating table. Additionally, these markings help remind the patient of the scars to expect postoperatively so that there are no surprises afterward.

The breast markings should be made with the patient in the upright position. Ensure that the patient's shoulders are relaxed, she is not leaning to one side or the other, and her legs are not crossed. First, mark the sternal notch (1 in ▶ Fig. 12.2). From there, mark the midline of the chest down the sternum (2 in ▶ Fig. 12.2). Next, mark the meridian of each breast extending from approximately the junction of the medial and middle thirds of the clavicle down through the nipple, typically 6–8 cm from the midline (3 in ▶ Fig. 12.2). This breast meridian will help to determine placement of the new nipple position. Next, mark the IMF (4 in ▶ Fig. 12.2). This can be done by gently raising the breast with the back of your nondominant hand and allowing the marking pen to fall gently into the crease between breast and upper abdominal wall. Once the IMF is marked, the new position of the nipple is ready to be placed. This can be done by placing your four fingers of your nondominant hand into the IMF and using your thumb to mark where this position translates onto the top of the breast. This is called Pitanguy's point, and the new nipple position will lie approximately at the intersection of the IMF translation onto the breast and the line created previously by the breast meridian (5 in ▶ Fig. 12.2). The final markings are to be placed around the new nipple position

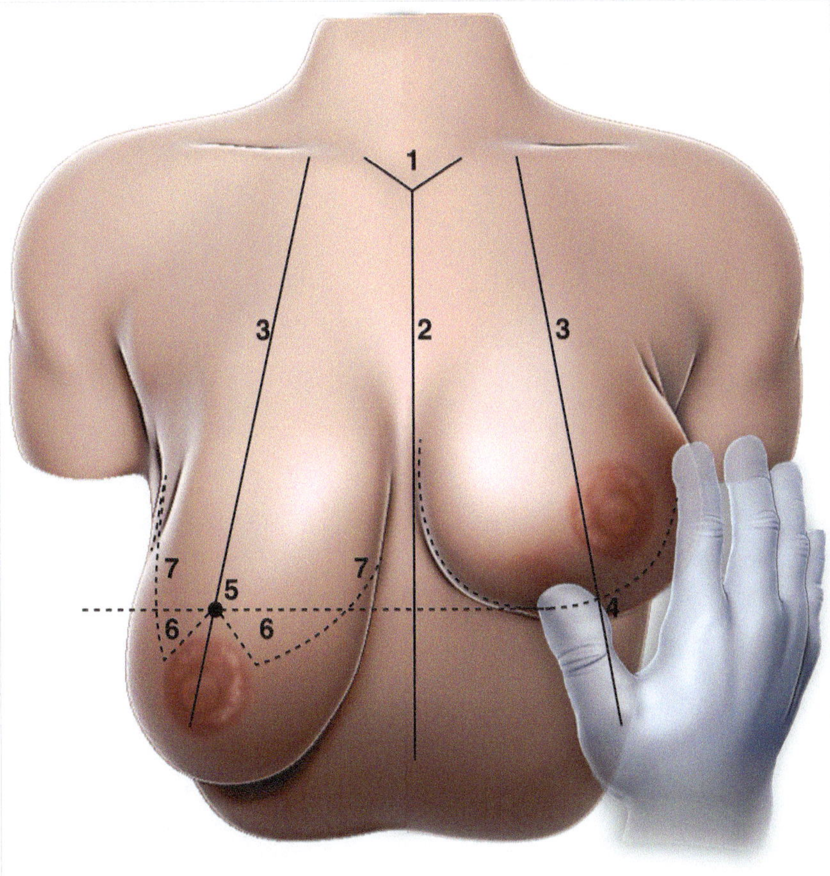

Fig. 12.2 Preoperative markings in a patient undergoing breast reduction. 1: sternal notch; 2: midline of chest; 3: breast meridian; 4: inframammary fold; 5: new nipple position; 6: vertical skin resection lines; 7: horizontal skin resection lines.

and depend on the skin resection pattern that has been decided upon. The most traditional and common, the Wise pattern, consists of both vertical and horizontal limbs of skin resection. These can be extended from a preset keyhole pattern that is marked using a template. The round part of the keyhole template marks the new position of the areola and is centered around the new nipple position. Oblique limbs extending from the round part of the keyhole mark the vertical skin resection pattern. From these limbs, horizontal extensions should be marked that meet at either end of the previously marked IMF to create the horizontal skin resection pattern. Alternatively, instead of using the preset keyhole pattern, the surgeon can mark an equilateral triangle with its superior point at the position of the new nipple. The limbs of the triangle should range between 7 and 10 cm, and these limbs extending obliquely will be the vertical skin resection pattern (6 in ▶ Fig. 12.2). Again, from these limbs, markings can be extended horizontally to connect to each end of the IMF marking to create the horizontal skin resection pattern (7 in ▶ Fig. 12.2). The new areolar position is then decided upon in the operating room after the reduction is complete and is marked with a cookie cutter at that time.

Finally, the pedicle itself can be outlined as markings on the breast. The base of the pedicle should be approximately 8–10 cm. This base can be measured on the breast and the pedicle subsequently outlined.

If an alternative pattern of skin resection is chosen, such as a vertical skin reduction mammaplasty or a periareolar skin reduction mammaplasty, then these markings will need to be modified accordingly to reflect the skin resection pattern.

12.6.2 Skin Resection Patterns

Various skin resection patterns exist for tightening the skin envelope over the reduced breast. Commonly used patterns include the Wise pattern (inverted **T**), vertical only, short-scar periareolar, and no-vertical-scar (▶ Fig. 12.3).

The Wise pattern is probably the most common (▶ Fig. 12.3a). This is frequently performed in conjunction with an inferior pedicle. The Wise pattern can be marked out either using a Mosque template, which resembles a keyhole pattern, to mark out the new NAC, or with a simple equilateral triangle whose side lengths will become the new nipple-to-IMF distance. With the former, it is important not to place the new nipple position too high, as this is very difficult to correct. With the latter, the nipple position is chosen intraoperatively after the skin flaps have been closed.

The vertical-scar-only incision is best used in smaller breast reductions (▶ Fig. 12.3b). The incision resembles a snowman, with a periareolar incision and a larger ellipse inferior to this. It is important with this incision pattern to keep the lower border of the elliptical incision at least 2 cm above the IMF. Once the ellipse is closed, the incision will lengthen and can potentially fall below the IMF if placed too close.

The no-vertical-scar technique utilizes both a periareolar skin excision and a separate IMF excision (▶ Fig. 12.3c). The breast

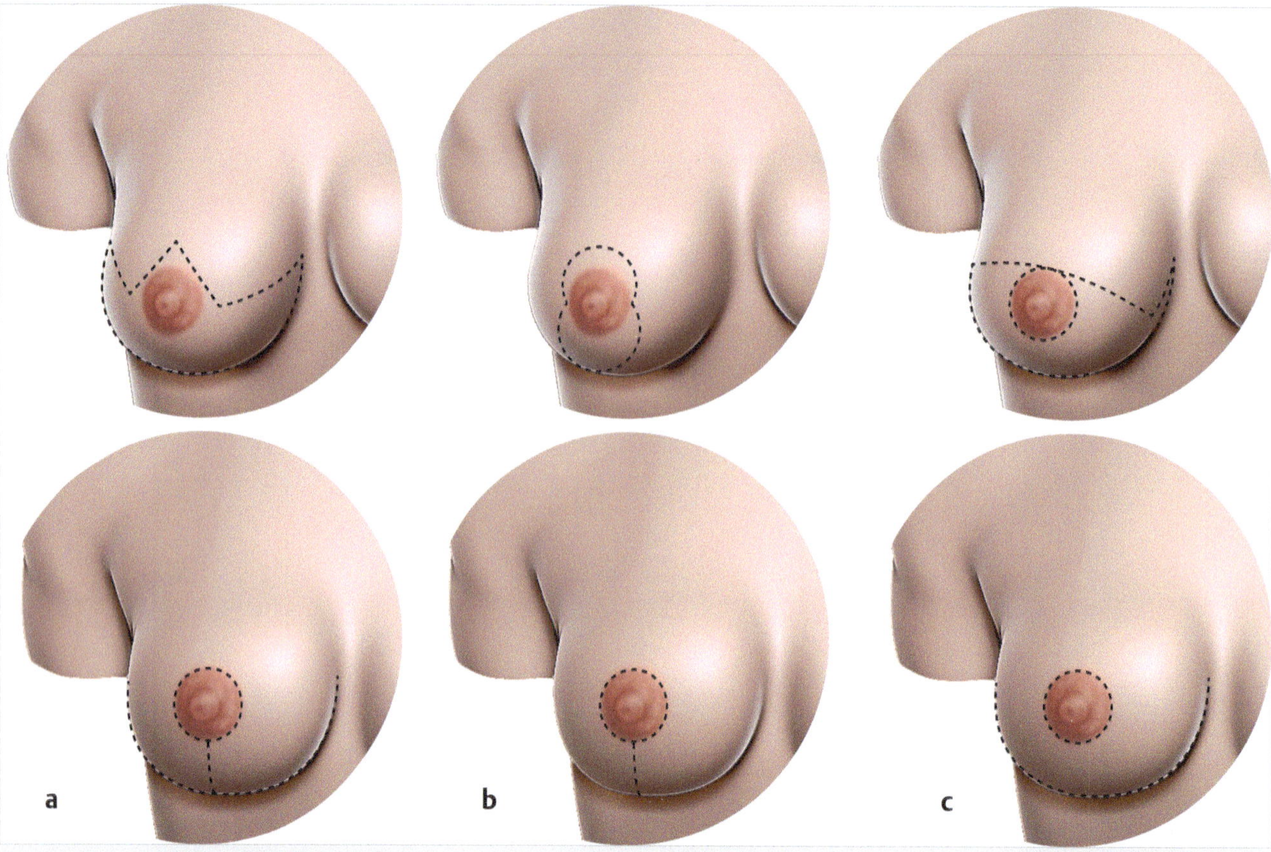

Fig. 12.3 Skin resection patterns in breast reduction. **(a)** Wise-pattern breast reduction. **(b)** Vertical-scar breast reduction, better for small resections. **(c)** No-vertical-scar breast reduction, best utilized for very ptotic or pendulous breasts.

skin flaps act as an apron that is then pulled down and over the breast parenchyma after resection. With this technique, it is imperative not to overresect skin from the IMF excision. Ideally, the excision width should not exceed 7 cm; otherwise, one risks not being able to close the skin over the breast parenchyma. See ▶ Fig. 12.4 for an example of a no-vertical-scar breast reduction.

12.6.3 Pedicle Options

Pedicle selection should be based on the surgeon's understanding of the most reliable blood supply to the NAC as well as considerations involving long-term maintenance of superior pole projection. Most proponents of the superior or superomedial pedicle techniques will argue that retaining the more cephalic breast tissue encourages long-term maintenance of superior pole fullness while ameliorating the phenomemon of pseudoptosis or "bottoming out." Proponents of the inferior pedicle will point out that, particularly in a more ptotic breast, this is likely to be the most reliable blood supply to the NAC. Superior or superomedial pedicles tend to be associated with short-scar or vertical-scar techniques as an additional consideration of pedicle selection. If a short or vertical scar is being utilized, the decision between a superior or medial pedicle will typically be determined by the position of the NAC relative to the planned location of the new areola. As this is marked preoperatively in the mosque or keyhole pattern, assessment can be made as to whether the NAC will translate easily into its final position with a simple vertical advancement or whether more significant ptosis would benefit from the 90° rotation associated with a medial pedicle to allow the areola to rotate into its final, more cephalic position.

12.6.4 Free Nipple Grafts

Free nipple grafts may be indicated in larger breasts. The utility of a free nipple graft is that it allows a greater amount of parenchymal resection when needed. While there are no hard cutoffs for when a free nipple graft is necessary, commonly accepted indications include gigantomastia, very large parenchymal resection (i.e., greater than 2 kg), long sternal notch–to-nipple distance (i.e., greater than 30 cm), and inverted nipples.[36] When using an inferior pedicle, which is often necessary in larger breasts, a free nipple graft allows the surgeon to shorten the pedicle and resect more tissue for a less bulky result, which would otherwise be hampered by the nipple at the apex of the pedicle.

Free nipple grafts are taken as a full-thickness graft. To enhance nipple projection and prevent inversion, it is useful to take the areolar portion as a dermal graft and then to tunnel down to take a wedge of tissue directly underneath the nipple to enhance projection in its final position. The position of the graft is determined after the final skin closure. Many surgeons will use a larger cookie cutter pattern to take the nipple graft, followed by a smaller cookie cutter pattern at the site chosen

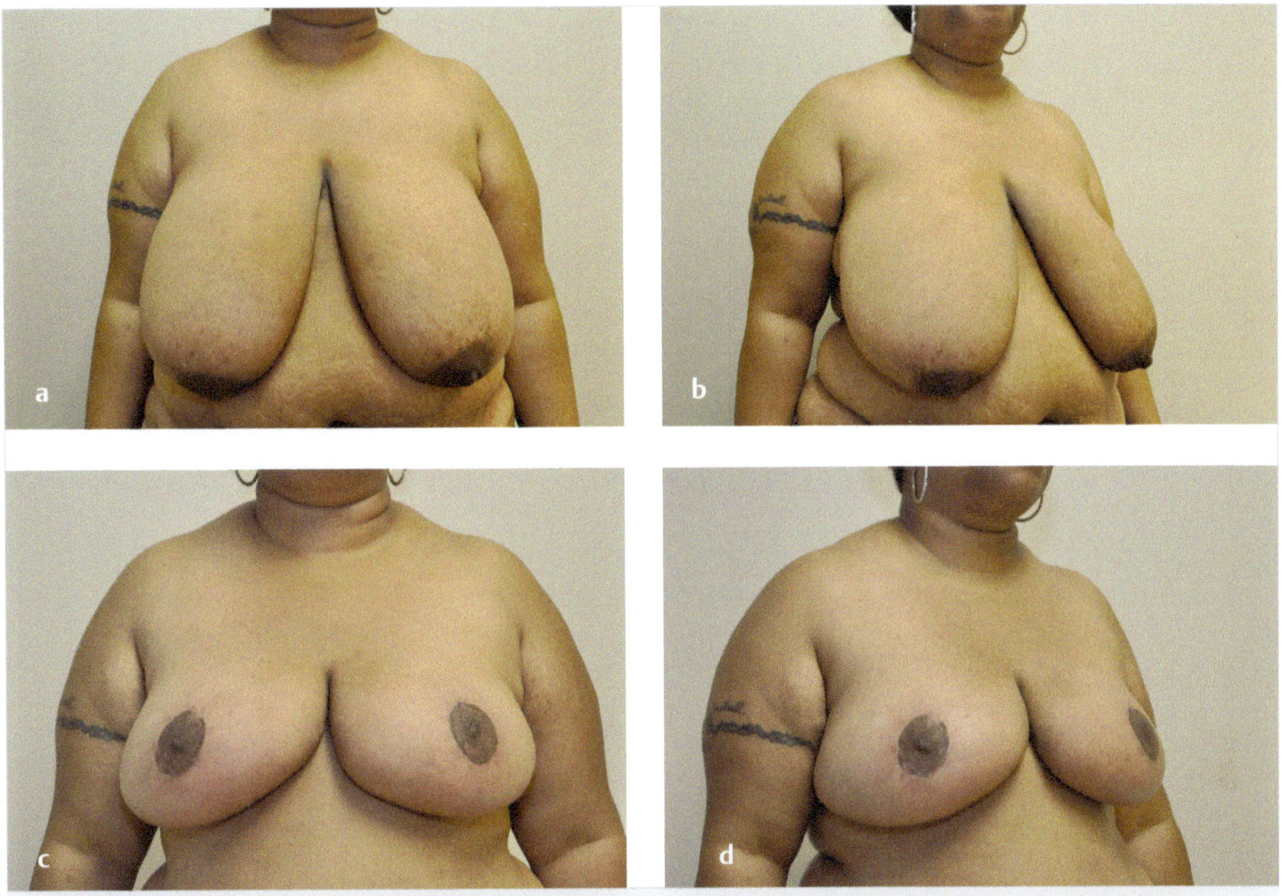

Fig. 12.4 (a,b) Preoperative and **(c,d)** postoperative photos demonstrating a patient before and after a no-vertical-scar breast reduction. In this case, the scar extends only around the areola and secondarily along the inframammary fold, where it is hidden.

for inset of the graft. This will take tension off the inset of the nipple graft and prevent widening of the NAC over time. A bolster dressing is then applied to prevent hematoma formation underneath the graft and improve graft take.

It is important to advise patients of the drawbacks of free nipple grafts. These include loss of nipple sensation, inability to breastfeed, possible NAC necrosis, and hypopigmentation of the NAC.[36] Loss of nipple sensation is unavoidable. Inability to breastfeed limits this technique to women who have no future plans for childbearing and lactation. Complete NAC necrosis is rare, but partial NAC necrosis occurs more commonly and may be managed with local wound care. Hypopigmentation is more common in darker-skinned patients and can be addressed with tattooing if desired.

12.6.5 Surgical Technique

Prepping and Draping

There are many variations in the surgical approach to breast reduction, but the overall sequence of steps is similar in all. To start, the patient should be positioned supine with the arms abducted as symmetrically as possible to avoid any differential effect on the bilateral breast mounds. It is important to ensure that the arms are well secured to arm boards, as the patient will be sat up several times during the case. A trial of sitting up before prepping the patient is useful to avoid intraoperative problems with positioning or breaks in sterility. When prepping and draping, it is useful to drape above the clavicles as an anatomic landmark and to include the umbilicus in the field as a midline marker.

Local Anesthetic

Once the patient is prepped and draped, local anesthetic can be infiltrated subcutaneously over the incision lines. Alternatively, some surgeons prefer to use a wetting solution and tumescent technique in the breast. This provides vasoconstriction in addition to pain control throughout the breast parenchyma and allows the resection to be performed with a knife instead of electrocautery, which can decrease operating times. The downside to using tumescent technique is that it can be more difficult for the novice surgeon to assess accurately how much breast volume needs resection given the addition of the solution. As such, it is important to ensure that equal volumes of solution are placed in each breast to avoid subsequent asymmetry once the solution has been reabsorbed postoperatively. Tumescent technique may be utilized laterally with suction-assisted lipectomy (liposuction) for lateral breast shaping and to debulk any unwanted fullness on the lateral chest wall that does not require skin resection. If tumescent technique is not used, then the parenchymal resection is better performed with electrocautery or a breast tourniquet to minimize blood loss.

Inferior Pedicle Wise Pattern

Once the local anesthetic of choice has been utilized, the peri-areolar incision is marked with a cookie cutter and then scored with a no. 15 blade while circumareolar retraction is applied. The rest of the skin incisions are then scored with a knife. Some surgeons prefer to score the IMF incision and tailor-tack the final skin excision with the patient in an upright position intra-operatively. The skin over the pedicle that will end up beneath the skin flaps is then de-epithelialized. In the inferior pedicle Wise pattern, the area requiring de-epithelialization tends to be larger than with other pedicle/skin resection patterns. Once this area has been freed of epidermis, skin flaps are raised. It is helpful to raise skin flaps prior to dissecting out the pedicle, as the weight of the breast tissue helps provide tension against the skin flaps to speed this dissection. Some surgeons prefer to outline the pedicle first, however, which is also reasonable. It is important to remember that skin flaps in a breast reduction should be much thicker than those performed in a mastectomy, aiming for 1- to 2-cm-thick flaps. The skin flap dissection needs to proceed high enough for the skin flaps that will remain after skin resection to be able to tack over and cover the residual parenchymal pedicle. It is important to keep in mind that the parenchymal pedicle containing the nipple will also be raised and tacked higher on the chest wall to combat long-term bottoming out, so the skin flaps should be high enough to allow tacking of the pedicle as well. Sometimes this requires raising skin flaps as high as the clavicle, but not always. Thus, one advantage of the inferior pedicle Wise pattern is that it allows greater lifting of the breast. This may seem counterintuitive, but by eliminating the superior breast parenchyma, a pocket is created for the remaining breast parenchyma to be lifted and inset into, thereby improving ptosis and bottoming out. Another pearl that assists with the aesthetic outcome includes keeping the inferomedial skin flap much thicker, such that the surgeon is almost dissecting perpendicular to the skin nearly straight down to chest wall. Keeping this inferomedial skin flap thicker than the other portions of the skin flap prevents hollowing of this medial breast region.

Once skin flaps are raised, the parenchymal resection then proceeds around the inferior pedicle, cutting straight down through the breast down to chest wall (▶ Fig. 12.5). As a general rule of thumb, the base width of any pedicles in the breast should be around 8 cm to ensure adequate perfusion to the NAC and distal breast parenchyma. When dissecting down to chest wall, it is important to leave pectoralis fascia down on the chest wall to reduce postoperative pain and to remain in an avascular plane as the parenchymal resection is lifted off the chest. This also optimizes the probability of preserving the deep branch of the fourth intercostal nerve, as it provides sensory innervation to the NAC. In the lateral breast, it is easy to get lost in the parenchymal resection. When this happens, go back to the mid-clavicular line of the breast parenchyma and find the pectoralis fascia. Follow pectoralis fascia laterally until the lateral border. This lateral border can serve as a marker for how far down the lateral breast parenchymal resection should proceed.

Once the parenchymal resection is complete, the remaining breast tissue is tacked into position. As mentioned, an advantage of the inferior pedicle is that removal of superior breast tissue creates a pocket giving significantly increased room to lift the NAC and eliminate breast ptosis. Some surgeons tack the breast with permanent suture such as nylon or polypropylene, while others will use absorbable suture such as polydioxanone (PDS). To tack the breast, take bites through fibrotic glandular tissue to gain a strong bite and then through pectoralis fascia. Some surgeons will perform a running suture laterally, sometimes with a barbed suture, to help round out the lateral breast tissue and improve cosmesis. Much of the tacking process is dependent on surgeon preference and variation.

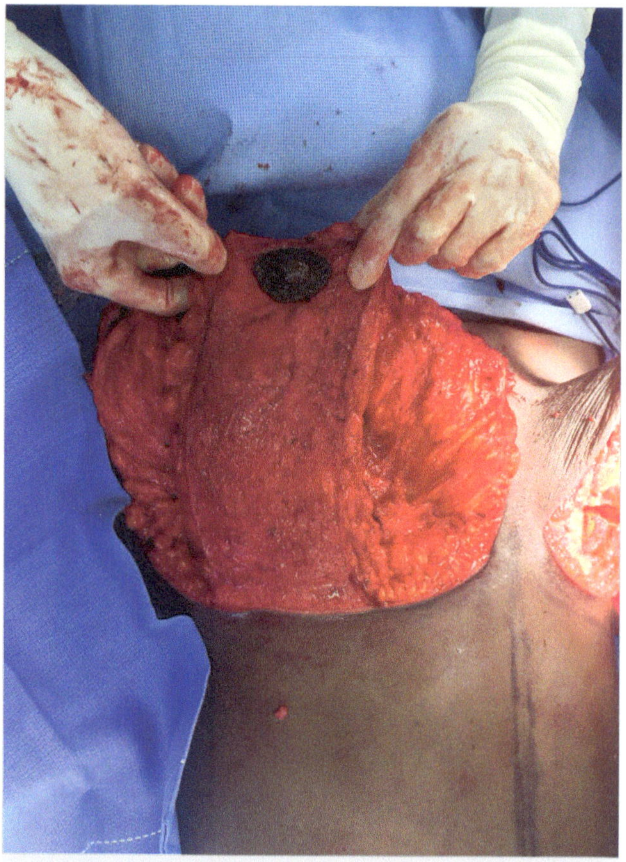

Fig. 12.5 Intraoperative photo demonstrating an inferior pedicle technique.

See ▶ Fig. 12.6 for long term post-operative outcome after an inferior pedicle Wise-pattern breast reduction.

Superomedial Pedicle Vertical-Scar

After the patient has been prepped, draped and local anesthetic applied, the superomedial pedicle vertical-scar technique proceeds similar to any other breast reduction, starting with marking the NAC with a cookie cutter. The NAC is then scored with a knife, and the pedicle and skin incisions are also scored with a knife. De-epithelialization of the superomedial pedicle, which will end up beneath skin flaps, is then performed. This area tends to be smaller in the superomedial pedicle vertical-scar technique.

In contrast to the inferior pedicle Wise-pattern technique, large skin flaps do not have to be raised with a superomedial

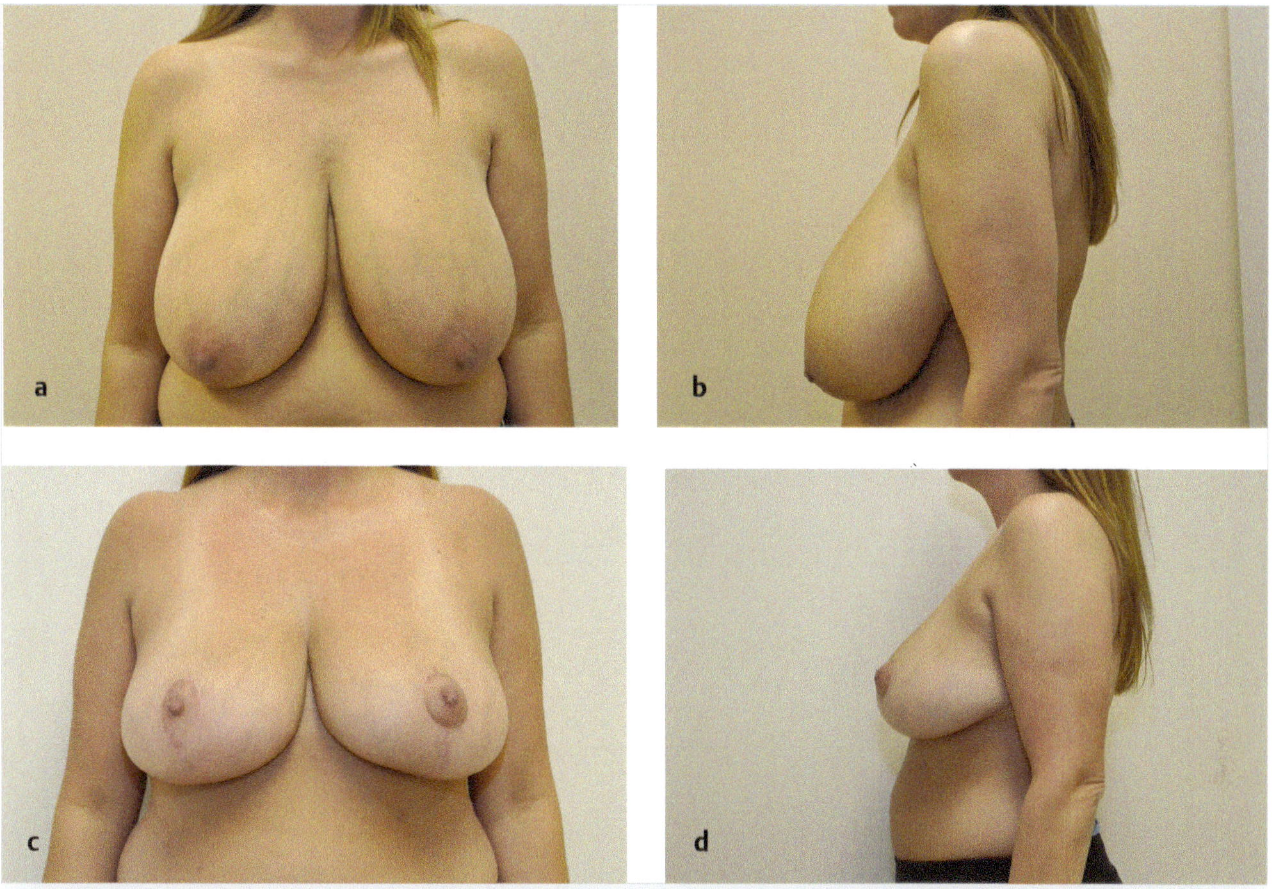

Fig. 12.6 (a,b) Preoperative and **(c,d)** postoperative photos demonstrating a patient before and after an inferior pedicle Wise-pattern breast reduction. Notice that the scar extends around the areola, then vertically down to the inframammary fold, and is hidden along the fold (not seen).

pedicle. Rather, the operation proceeds straight to outlining the pedicle and dissecting through parenchyma straight down to chest wall. In a particularly ptotic breast or where there is concern about blood supply to the nipple, preserving the breast parenchyma at the 12 o'clock position (superior) to the NAC preserves the blood supply from the second intercostal space, which travels about 1 cm deep in the skin at this point.[37] If the 12 o'clock position is undercut, this blood supply may be disrupted, making the breast reduction based on a medial pedicle only. Once the pedicle is outlined, dissection proceeds inferomedial to the inferior border of the pedicle. In this most inferomedial portion of the breast, parenchyma will be resected, since it is inferior to the outlined pedicle. In this region, a small skin flap will need to be raised to remove this breast tissue. Often, this requires dissecting through the IMF down to chest wall. The dissection can then proceed laterally through the IMF (keeping 1- to 2-centimeter-thick skin flaps inferiorly) until the lateral skin incision is reached. Using the lateral skin incision as a border, the breast parenchyma is again dissected straight down to chest wall and all parenchyma from the inferomedial breast to the lateral skin incision, proceeding superiorly to where the new NAC will be rotated, is removed en bloc off the chest wall. Frequently the area into which the new NAC will be rotated (the head of the snowman) requires additional parenchymal resection to create enough room into which to rotate the pedicle. With a superomedial pedicle, the parenchyma needs to be rotated approximately 90–120° so that the apex of the pedicle points superiorly and brings the nipple into good position. After rotation of the pedicle, the inferior border of the pedicle becomes the new medial breast pillar. With rotation of the pedicle, the new location of the IMF becomes visible where it falls medially. This location can be transposed to the lateral breast parenchyma, and, if necessary, additional inferolateral breast parenchyma can be removed such that the new location of the medial IMF is a continuous line with where it should fall laterally on the breast. It is important to keep in mind that the IMF is raised when performing a superomedial pedicle vertical-scar technique. As such, it is important to design the inferior skin resection (body of the snowman) carefully, keeping it several centimeters above the pre-existing IMF, since both the IMF will be raised *and* the vertical scar will lengthen when closed in a straight line. If the inferiormost portion of the skin resection is too close to the pre-existing IMF, then the scar will likely fall onto the upper abdomen when skin is closed. Once the breast parenchyma is resected, the new medial pillar of the breast (the inferior edge of the parenchymal pedicle) is sutured to the lateral pillar of the breast (the lateral border of the skin incision).

See ▶ Fig. 12.7 for long-term outcome after a superomedial pedicle with vertical scar technique.

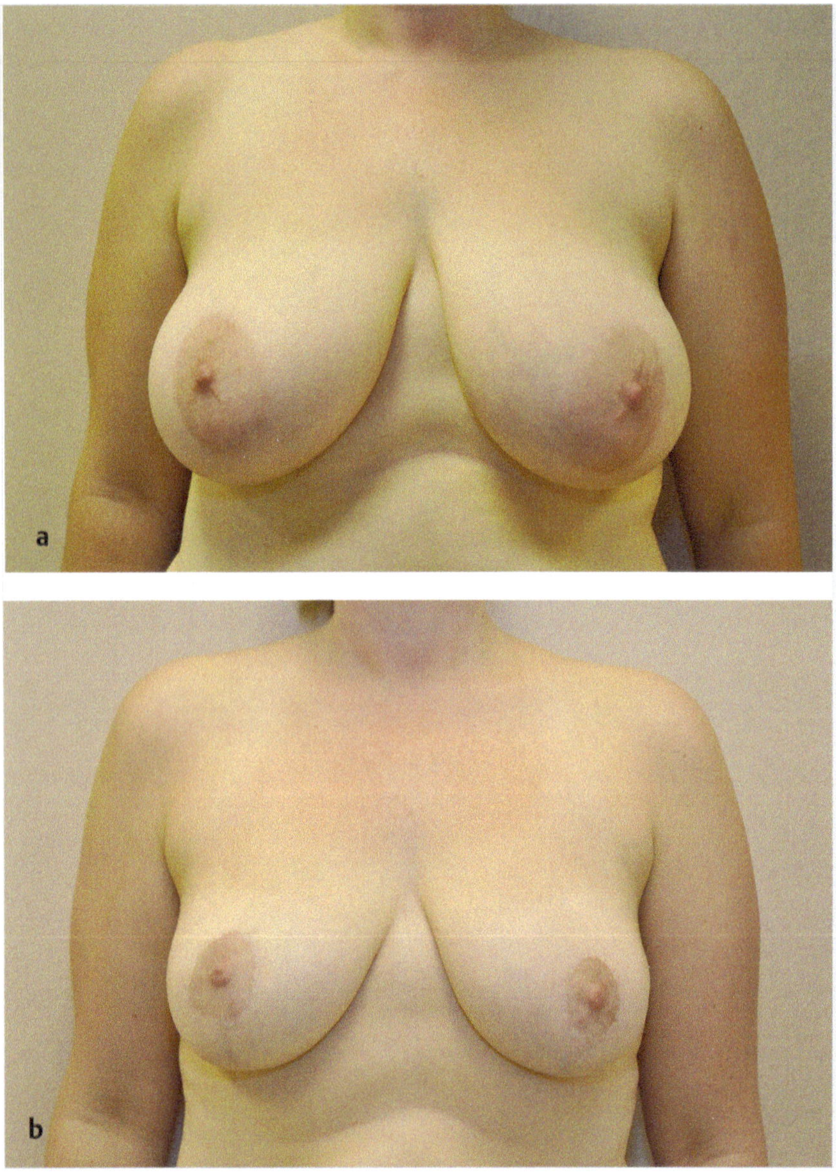

Fig. 12.7 **(a)** Preoperative and **(b)** postoperative photos of a small-volume breast reduction that is ideal for a superomedial pedicle vertical-scar technique.

Closing

Once the parenchyma is appropriately positioned, the skin incisions are brought together temporarily and the patient is sat up to evaluate for symmetry and overall result. Any asymmetries in breast volume are addressed by additional resection from the more voluminous breast as needed. Once the team is satisfied with the result with the patient in the upright position, the incisions can be closed. Drains are unnecessary and increase patient discomfort.

All resected tissue should be sent for pathologic examination. Reported rates of occult breast cancer (both invasive breast cancer and ductal carcinoma in situ) in resected specimens are around 1%.

12.7 Postoperative Complications

Up to one third of patients will experience a postoperative complication; however, the majority of complications are minor and easily managed in the clinic setting. Common postoperative complications include hematoma, seroma, wound dehiscence (particularly at the **T** junction in the Wise-pattern skin resections), fat necrosis, skin flap or NAC necrosis, surgical site infection, decreased nipple sensation, and inability to breast feed.[1,38,39,40]

Hematoma usually requires a return to the operating room for washout. This improves wound healing and prevents infection. Rarely is an actively bleeding vessel found at the time of return. Seroma can be managed with aspiration in clinic as needed. Aggressive aspiration may help to prevent infection, particularly in areas of the breast that are associated with significant fat necrosis or dead space.

Perhaps the most common complication that patients should be advised to expect is breakdown at the **T** junction in Wise-pattern skin resections. This is generally managed with conservative wound care in the outpatient setting, such as topical silver sulfadiazine or simple wet-to-dry dressing changes daily. This area tends to heal with time. Skin flap and NAC necrosis can be prevented by creating thick skin flaps in the operating room. If there is any concern for impending necrosis, topical nitropaste can be applied and may help to limit the amount of necrosis; however, this needs to be recognized and started expeditiously.

Surgical site infections are more common in obese patients and those with significant comorbidities, such as diabetes. Most infections can be managed with antibiotics without the need to return to the operating room.

Although some women report decreased nipple sensation postoperatively, others have even reported increased nipple sensation, possibly due to the release of tension and stretching that was present in the hypertrophic breast.

Key Points

- Breast reduction overall has one of the highest patient satisfaction rates in all of plastic surgery. The outcome is often satisfying not only for the patient but also for the surgeon, who can see immediate relief at the first postoperative visit.
- Various techniques, combining various pedicles and skin resection patterns, are available and widely described. Surgeon preference, with some component of patient anatomy, often dictates the chosen technique.
- While complications may be frequent, these tend to be minor and easily managed in the outpatient setting.

References

[1] Daane SP, Rockwell WB. Breast reduction techniques and outcomes: a meta-analysis. Aesthet Surg J. 1999; 19(4):293–303

[2] Spear SL. Breast reduction: inverted-T technique. In: Thorne CH, Beasley RW, Aston SJ, Bartlett SP, Gurtner GC, Spear SL, eds. Grabb and Smith's Plastic Surgery. 6th ed. Philadelphia, PA: Lippincott Williams & Wilkins; 2007:593–603

[3] Netscher DT, Meade RA, Goodman CM, Brehm BJ, Friedman JD, Thornby J. Physical and psychosocial symptoms among 88 volunteer subjects compared with patients seeking plastic surgery procedures to the breast. Plast Reconstr Surg. 2000; 105(7):2366–2373

[4] Kerrigan CL, Collins ED, Striplin D, et al. The health burden of breast hypertrophy. Plast Reconstr Surg. 2001; 108(6):1591–1599

[5] Blomqvist L, Eriksson A, Brandberg Y. Reduction mammaplasty provides long-term improvement in health status and quality of life. Plast Reconstr Surg. 2000; 106(5):991–997

[6] Dieffenbach JF. Die operative Chirurgerie. Leipzig, Germany: Brockhaus; 1848

[7] Schwarzmann E. Die technik der mammaplastik. Chirurg. 1930; 2:932

[8] Penn J. Breast reduction. Br J Plast Surg. 1955; 7(4):357–371

[9] Wise RJ. A preliminary report on a method of planning the mammaplasty. Plast Reconstr Surg (1946). 1956; 17(5):367–375

[10] Pitanguy I. Surgical treatment of breast hypertrophy. Br J Plast Surg. 1967; 20 (1):78–85

[11] Orlando JC, Guthrie RH, Jr. The superomedial dermal pedicle for nipple transposition. Br J Plast Surg. 1975; 28(1):42–45

[12] McKissock PK. Reduction mammaplasty with a vertical dermal flap. Plast Reconstr Surg. 1972; 49(3):245–252

[13] Lassus C. A technique for breast reduction. Int Surg. 1970; 53(1):69–72

[14] Lejour M, Abboud M. Vertical mammaplasty without inframammary scar and with breast liposuction. Perspect Plast Surg. 1990; 4(2):67–90

[15] Lejour M. Vertical mammaplasty and liposuction of the breast. Plast Reconstr Surg. 1994; 94(1):100–114

[16] Marchac D, de Olarte G. Reduction mammaplasty and correction of ptosis with a short inframammary scar. Plast Reconstr Surg. 1982; 69(1):45–55

[17] Peixoto G. Reduction mammaplasty: a personal technique. Plast Reconstr Surg. 1980; 65(2):217–226

[18] Sampaio, Góes JC. Periareolar mammaplasty: double skin technique with application of polyglactine or mixed mesh. Plast Reconstr Surg. 1996; 97(5): 959–968

[19] Benelli L. A new periareolar mammaplasty: the "round block" technique. Aesthetic Plast Surg. 1990; 14(2):93–100

[20] Lalonde DH, Lalonde J, French R. The no vertical scar breast reduction: a minor variation that allows to remove vertical scar portion of the inferior pedicle Wise pattern T scar. Aesthetic Plast Surg. 2003; 27(5):335–344

[21] Yousif NJ, Larson DL, Sanger JR, Matloub HS. Elimination of the vertical scar in reduction mammaplasty. Plast Reconstr Surg. 1992; 89(3):459–467, discussion 468

[22] Movassaghi K, Liao EC, Ting V, et al. Eliminating the vertical scar in breast reduction—Boston modification of the Robertson technique. Aesthet Surg J. 2006; 26(6):687–696

[23] Hammond DC. Short scar periareolar inferior pedicle reduction (SPAIR) mammaplasty. Plast Reconstr Surg. 1999; 103(3):890–902

[24] Hall-Findlay EJ. A simplified vertical reduction mammaplasty: shortening the learning curve. Plast Reconstr Surg. 1999; 104(3):748–759, discussion 760–-763

[25] van Deventer PV, Graewe FR. The blood supply of the breast revisited. Plast Reconstr Surg. 2016; 137(5):1388–1397

[26] Jabs AD, Frantz AG, Smith-Vaniz A, Hugo NE. Mammary hypertrophy is not associated with increased estrogen receptors. Plast Reconstr Surg. 1990; 86 (1):64–66

[27] Govrin-Yehudain J, Kogan L, Cohen HI, Falik-Zaccai TC. Familial juvenile hypertrophy of the breast. J Adolesc Health. 2004; 35(2):151–155

[28] Sperling RL, Gold JJ. Use of an anti-estrogen after a reduction mammaplasty to prevent recurrence of virginal hypertrophy of breasts. Case report. Plast Reconstr Surg. 1973; 52(4):439–442

[29] Hoppe IC, Patel PP, Singer-Granick CJ, Granick MS. Virginal mammary hypertrophy: a meta-analysis and treatment algorithm. Plast Reconstr Surg. 2011; 127(6):2224–2231

[30] Becker H. Breast reduction insurance denials. Plast Reconstr Surg. 2004; 114 (6):1687

[31] Schnur PL, Hoehn JG, Ilstrup DM, Cahoy MJ, Chu CP. Reduction mammaplasty: cosmetic or reconstructive procedure? Ann Plast Surg. 1991; 27(3):232–237

[32] Schnur PL. Reduction mammaplasty—the Schnur sliding scale revisited. Ann Plast Surg. 1999; 42(1):107–108

[33] Zubowski R, Zins JE, Foray-Kaplon A, et al. Relationship of obesity and specimen weight to complications in reduction mammaplasty. Plast Reconstr Surg. 2000; 106(5):998–1003

[34] Shah R, Al-Ajam Y, Stott D, Kang N. Obesity in mammaplasty: a study of complications following breast reduction. J Plast Reconstr Aesthet Surg. 2011; 64 (4):508–514

[35] Warner E. Clinical practice. Breast-cancer screening. N Engl J Med. 2011; 365 (11):1025–1032

[36] Colen SR. Breast reduction with use of the free nipple graft technique. Aesthet Surg J. 2001; 21(3):261–271

[37] Hall-Findlay EJ. Vertical breast reduction using the superomedial pedicle. In: Spear SP, ed. Surgery of the Breast: Principles and Art. Philadelphia, PA: Lippincott Williams & Wilkins; 2011: 1045–1062

[38] Makki AS, Ghanem AA. Long-term results and patient satisfaction with reduction mammaplasty. Ann Plast Surg. 1998; 41(4):370–377

[39] Meshulam-Derazon S, Barnea Y, Zaretski A, et al. Large-volume breast reduction: Long-term results. Scand J Plast Reconstr Surg Hand Surg. 2009; 43(2): 65–70

[40] Dabbah A, Lehman JA, Jr, Parker MG, Tantri D, Wagner DS. Reduction mammaplasty: an outcome analysis. Ann Plast Surg. 1995; 35(4):337–341

Part IV

Management of the Undesirable Result and Revisional Breast Surgery

IV

13 Management of Acute Complications of Aesthetic Breast Surgery Part I—Local and Systemic Complications

Christodoulos Kaoutzanis, Julian Winocour, James C. Grotting, and Kent K. "Kye" Higdon

Summary
This book chapter provides a thorough discussion on the incidence, diagnosis, and management of the most commonly encountered acute complications following aesthetic breast surgery. Local complications discussed include hematoma, seroma, surgical site infection, delayed wound healing, fat necrosis, nipple areolar complex necrosis, and Mondor's disease (superficial thrombophlebitis of the thoracoepigastric veins). Systemic complications reviewed include venous thromboembolism and pneumothorax.

Keywords: aesthetic breast surgery, aesthetic plastic surgery, augmentation mastopexy, breast augmentation, breast reduction, cosmetic surgery, mastopexy, postoperative complications, reduction mammoplasty, surgical complications

13.1 Introduction

Aesthetic breast surgery has seen a tremendous growth over the last few decades and currently represents one of the most commonly performed cosmetic surgical interventions in North America. According to the American Society for Aesthetic Plastic Surgery (ASAPS) statistical reports, the annual number of breast cosmetic surgical procedures has increased significantly over the years with procedures performed in 2018 exceeding 670,000.[1] In 5 years, the annual number of breast augmentations increased by 15.2%, mastopexy by 55.9%, reduction mammaplasty in women by 27.6%, and male breast reduction for correction of gynecomastia by 47.9%.[1]

Unfortunately, not all breast surgical procedures result in a favorable outcome. When complications occur, they can be dealt with in the office setting, but more severe cases may require emergency room visits, hospital admissions, or even reoperations. More importantly, whether minor or major complications, they can result in a potentially devastating cosmetic outcome and pose significant financial burden on the patient and the surgeon. The cosmetic surgeon can be faced with numerous unfavorable situations following aesthetic breast surgery, and likewise there are many ways to treat these problems. As such, the focus of this chapter is to review the acute complications encountered following aesthetic surgical procedures and discuss their management.

13.2 Local Surgical Complications

13.2.1 Hematoma

Postoperative bleeding and hematoma represent one of the most common complications in aesthetic breast surgery. Several risk factors predisposing toward hematoma formation following these procedures have been previously identified, including age, medical comorbidities such as high blood pressure and malignancy, anticoagulant and antidepressant medications, operative and anesthetic techniques, as well as postoperative management.[2,3,4,5] As a result, postoperative hematoma rates vary. Although the incidence is less than 2% in the majority of the studies on aesthetic breast surgery, some series have reported rates as high as 8%.[5,6,7,8,9,10,11,12,13,14]

Postoperative hematomas typically develop within the first 24 hours after surgery. Less commonly, hematomas can present days, weeks, or even months after surgery and may be associated with minor injury or trauma to the breast, overactivity, or clotting disorders. Hematomas may present with a variety of symptoms and signs, some of which may be nonspecific. Suspicion should arise if there is increasing unilateral pain or tenderness, edema, extensive ecchymosis of the skin, or new volume discrepancy. Other signs include erythema or warmth, especially if complicated by an infectious process, and in some instances hemodynamic changes.

Small hematomas can be observed and usually resolve without intervention. However, larger hematomas should be taken back to the operating room for evacuation under sterile conditions. Reoperation should involve removal of the implant if present, evacuation of the clot, and irrigation of the breast pocket, followed by meticulous hemostasis and identification of any causative vessels if possible, reirrigation of the pocket, implant replacement, and incision closure. Any underlying coagulation abnormality must also be addressed and corrected. Prompt identification and management of these hematomas is crucial, because if left untreated they can result in a variety of negative long-term sequelae. In cases of delayed presentation with a liquefied hematoma, the hematoma may be aspirated by the physician or with imaging guidance. The compressive effect of a sizable fluid collection or clot can cause wound dehiscence, flap compromise, or even necrosis of the nipple areolar complex (NAC). These complications can further lead to exposure of an underlying implant and subsequent implant loss. Poor cosmesis and asymmetries may also become an issue. In addition, periprosthetic hematomas have been associated with increased risk of both subclinical infection and capsular contracture (▶ Fig. 13.1).[15,16,17] As our knowledge of capsular contracture risk factors grows, as well as its link to implant-associated anaplastic large cell lymphoma, the plastic surgeon must be aware how hematoma formation plays a role. It has also been shown that submuscular implant placement in breast augmentation has a higher hematoma incidence compared with the subglandular position.[10] If surgeons attempt to mitigate the risk of capsular contracture by choosing to place the implant in the submuscular plane, they must be more vigilant with hemostasis to prevent hematoma formation.

Hematoma risk can be generally minimized with careful pocket dissection using direct vision and, if needed, special lighted retractors, with special attention to hemostasis. Patients should be advised to abstain from certain medications and supplements that may predispose to bleeding for at least a week preoperatively, such as platelet inhibitors, anticoagulants,

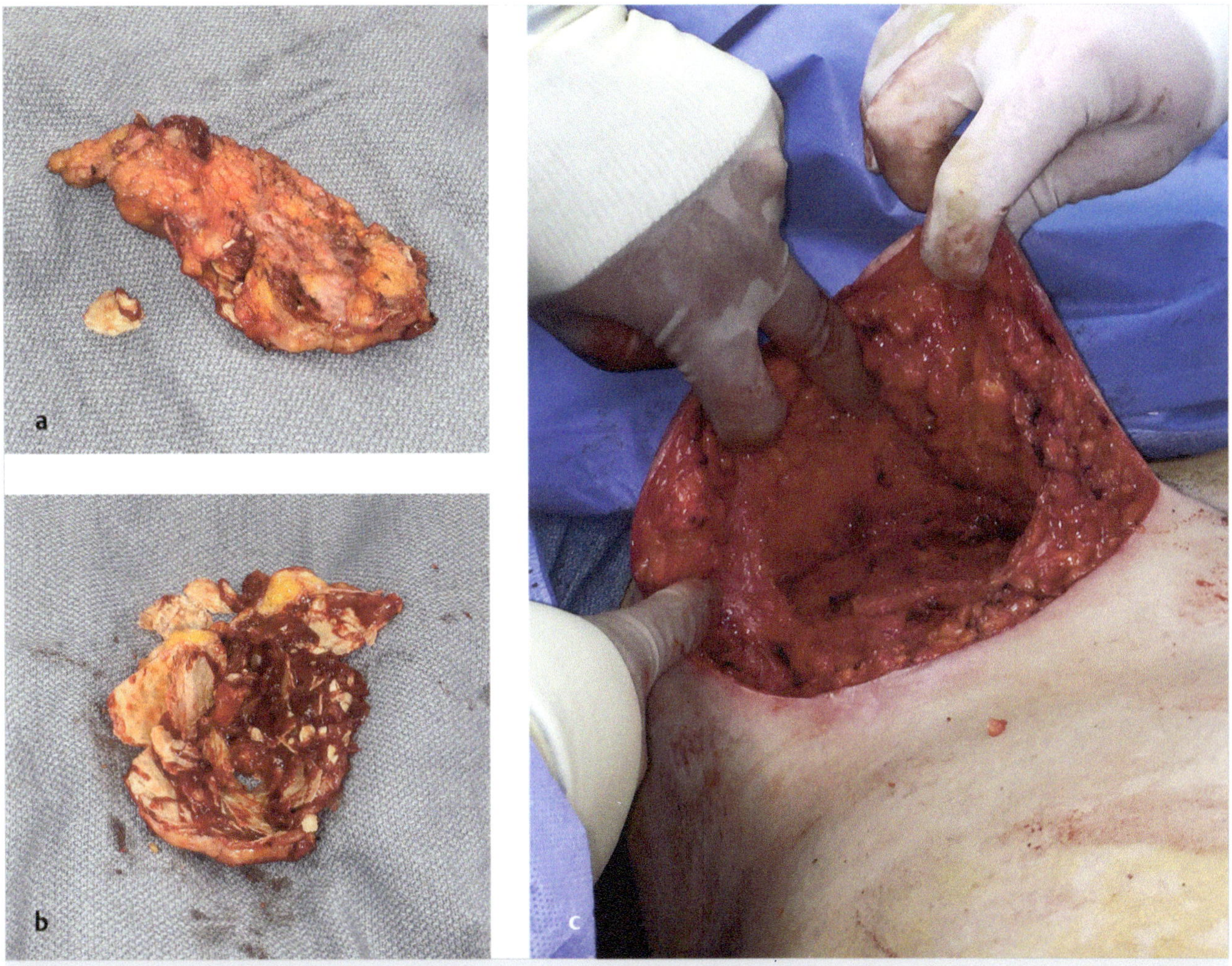

Fig. 13.1 (a) External aspect of calcified breast capsule. (b) Internal aspect of calcified breast capsule with residual hematoma. (c) Breast pocket following total capsulectomy in a patient with calcified capsular contracture as a result of a chronic hematoma.

androgenic hormones, nonsteroidal anti-inflammatory drugs (NSAIDs), and vitamin E. The use of drains in the breast pocket is controversial, with no convincing evidence in the literature to support decreased hematoma recurrence rates.[18] Postoperative breast compression after breast augmentation is still practiced by some surgeons; however, in a randomized study of 130 patients it was not shown to reduce the frequency of postoperative bruising or hematoma formation.[19] In fact, 37.5% of the patients complained about the use of compression. Also, although supportive mild compression with a surgical bra or wrap is used for breast reductions and mastopexies, excessive compression should be avoided, as it can compromise the circulation of the breast flaps and the NAC.

13.2.2 Seroma

Seroma is not frequently observed following primary aesthetic breast procedures, but its reported incidence ranges from 0.2 to 5.5%.[8,12,13] It is more common for troublesome seromas to occur after revisionary implant surgery, especially after capsulectomy or extensive capsulotomy.[20] Likewise, the use of acellular dermal matrix, mostly in revisionary surgery, has been advocated to increase the incidence of seroma formation, which if not treated may in its turn lead to non-adherence of the acellular dermal matrix. Significant fluid accumulation within the breast implant pocket or breast cavity after mastopexy and reduction mammoplasty may cause breast enlargement and asymmetries, discomfort, pain or tenderness, or wound dehiscence with drainage of clear/yellowish fluid. Occasionally, an undrained seroma may cause ongoing cellulitis in the absence of infection, and has to be excluded.

When an early seroma is detected, percutaneous aspiration should be considered if it is palpable or ballotable. This can be done with ultrasound guidance. If an implant is present, extreme care must be taken not to puncture it during aspiration. A safe approach involves positioning the patient in the lateral decubitus position and performing the aspiration through the skin of the lateral aspect of the breast at the most dependent aspect of the fluid collection, while manually protecting the implant by displacing it medially.[20] A sample of the drained fluid should be sent to the microbiology laboratory for culture if an infection is suspected, as well as for histology in the case of a late seroma if anaplastic large cell lymphoma is suspected. At times, a short-term catheter may be left in place for continuous drainage. If repeated aspirations do not effectively resolve the seroma, open drainage in the operating room under sterile conditions may be required. If surgical exploration reveals a seroma capsule, then the surgeon should perform complete capsulectomy, implant removal (with possible placement of a new implant), and possible drain placement.

One should be aware that different surgical approaches might lead to different outcomes. For example, Hall-Findlay and Shestak suggested that seromas after breast reduction are less likely to resolve spontaneously with the inverted-T skin resection pattern than with the vertical pattern because the inframammary scar can block drainage.[21] Significant drainage may also result from increased movement of the implant, due either to an excessively large pocket or, more likely, to too much activity by the patient. The patient should be cautioned to reduce activity if seroma develops while a drain is still in place. It is important to remember that undrained seromas can have other untoward consequences such as implant rotation, malposition, and infection. To our knowledge, the current literature does not identify prognostic factors associated with conversion of simple seroma to infected seroma and possible implant loss. Furthermore, if a recurrent seroma is not regularly drained, it can sometimes form a hardened mass of scar tissue.

There is no strong evidence in the literature to support the placement of drains to reduce the occurrence of seromas after primary aesthetic breast procedures. In the United States, common practice is not to leave a drain in the breast pocket after breast augmentations or augmentation mastopexies. Drain placement after mastopexies and breast reductions is less standardized and comes down to surgeon's preference. Other authors prefer to leave a drain after significant liposuction to the breast or lateral axillary roll has been performed, as this appears to contribute to seroma formation.[20] In the authors' practice, they are more likely to leave a drain after revisionary implant surgery that involves substantial modification of the capsule, such as capsulectomy or extensive capsulotomy. Typically, the authors allow removal of the drain catheter when drainage is less than 20 mL over a 24-hour period for 2 consecutive days. The timing of drain removal is critical, but can become tricky if there is persistent drainage. If the drain is removed too early, there is a risk of fluid reaccumulation, but if it is left in place for a prolonged period of time, there is a risk of introducing infection into the breast pocket.

13.2.3 Surgical Site Infection

Surgical site infection (SSI) is also one of the most frequently encountered complications following aesthetic breast surgery. Published rates of SSI have been shown to be lowest in breast augmentation, ranging from 0.001% to 7%, and highest in breast reduction, ranging from 0.11% to 24.5%.[5,10,12,16,22,23,24,25,26,27,28,29,30] Although minor SSIs might be common, the incidence of major SSIs that require emergency room visit, admission to the hospital, or reoperation is very low and less than 1% in two of the largest studies analyzing the CosmetAssure database over different time intervals.[5,22] Hanemann et al reviewed 51,235 cosmetic breast surgery procedures between 2003 and 2009, and revealed a major SSI rate of 0.22%.[22] Similarly, Gupta et al found an overall major infection rate of 0.25% in over 73,608 aesthetic breast procedures.[5] This was broken down to an infection risk for breast augmentation of 0.19%, augmentation–mastopexy of 0.43%, mastopexy of 0.32%, and breast reduction of 0.55%. Another significant study by Fisher et al analyzed the American College of Surgeons National Surgical Quality Improvement Program (ACS-NSQIP) database for complications following reduction mammoplasty.[31] This study included 3,538 patients and found an overall postoperative complication rate of 5.1%, and specifically an SSI rate of 3.0% (superficial infection: 2.7%, deep infection: 0.2%, organ space infection: 0.1%). As advocated by prior studies, the impact of surgical technique may play an important role on infection rates including meticulous hemostasis and dissection, avoiding the use of drains, use of antibiotic/antimicrobial irrigations, careful handling of the implants, and avoidance of external exposure of the implant to the air and patient skin.[10,32] Several other factors play a role in influencing postoperative SSIs after cosmetic breast procedures, and it is not surprising that many of these have a synergistic effect. These include age, increased body mass index, smoking, diabetes, steroids and other immunosuppressive medications, pregnancy, vigorous exercise, prolonged operative times, and combining procedures such as augmentation with mastopexy.[5,29,30,33,34,35,36,37,38]

The majority of SSIs manifest within the first month after surgery, but there is usually a lag of at least 5 days and up to 2 weeks postoperatively before the SSI appears.[39] Some infections, especially related to implants, can occur months or even years after the initial operation.[16,36,40] In rare occasions, SSIs manifest within the first 48 hours after surgery and are almost always due to *Clostridium* species or *Streptococcus pyogenes*. These infections can progress very rapidly if not addressed in a timely fashion and can have devastating consequences. For such necrotizing infections, serial aggressive surgical débridements may be required. Postoperative toxic shock syndrome caused by *Staphylococcus aureus* wound infection can also be observed within the first 48 hours after surgery.[41] In these cases, the incision appearance can be deceptively benign on examination, and diagnosis is based upon fulfillment of the following six criteria: fever, rash, desquamation, hypotension, multisystem organ involvement, and negative culture results and serologies.[39,42]

Local signs of swelling, pain, erythema, and purulent drainage are usually reliable in diagnosing an SSI. However, in morbidly obese patients or those with deep, multilayer wounds, external signs of SSI may be delayed.[43] Other adjunct tests, such as laboratory or imaging studies (such as ultrasound), can assist with the diagnosis. Certainly, any fluid collections around a breast implant should be drained and cultured, whenever possible. The causative organisms may be different, depending on the type of surgical procedure, but are mostly bacteria. For example, the most frequently isolated bacteria following breast augmentations include *S. aureus*, *S. epidermidis*, streptococci A and B, *Klebsiella pneumoniae*, *Bacillus*, and *Propionibacterium*, whereas *Corynebacterium* species, *Propionibacterium acnes*, *Pseudomonas aeruginosa*, *Escherichia coli*, and Enterobacteriaceae are less common.[36,44,45,46,47] Sporadic cases of mycobacteria have been described and should be suspected for late infections with an indolent course when common techniques fail to isolate a cause.[14,46,48,49,50] Acid-fast stains and cultures should be obtained in all cases of subacute infection, even when routine culture reveals skin flora.[51] It is not unusual to observe some erythematous skin changes around or near the surgical incision during the first week after surgery without the other symptoms and signs of infection. Most of these changes resolve without any treatment and may be related to tape sensitivity or other local tissue insult not involving bacteria. In fact, previous data suggest that antibiotics begun immediately postoperatively or continued for long periods after the procedure do not prevent or cure this inflammation or infection.[52,53,54,55] Special attention should be paid among individuals who underwent implantation of acellular dermal matrix (ADM) during revisionary breast surgery, as erythema of the breast within the first weeks postoperatively could also reflect "red breast syndrome."[56,57] This is self-limited and believed to be related to an immune response. Unlike an infection, it is not associated with significant leukocytosis or systemic signs of infection, and the erythema only overlies the ADM.[57]

Management of breast infections in the setting of implants is slightly different compared to infections without implants, and it will thus be discussed separately. In patients without implants, simple cellulitis from a suspected infectious etiology can be managed with an oral course of antibiotics. If a deeper infection is suspected, typically the first and most important step in the management is incision and drainage. The incision should be opened, the infected material should be evacuated, the cavity should be thoroughly washed out, and appropriate dressing changes should be initiated to promote wound healing by secondary intention. Incision and drainage of superficial abscesses rarely cause bacteremia; hence prophylactic antibiotics are not necessary.[58] Making the incision too small may fail to control the infection. It is critical to open the incision adequately, not only to control the infection but also to diagnose and treat associated problems such as necrosis of the subcutaneous tissue and fascia that require debridement. However, there is a fine balance between effective debridement and unnecessary overexcision; this balance is particularly important in the aesthetic surgery population, where cosmetic outcomes are crucial to the success of the operation. The latest practice guidelines for the management of skin and soft tissue infections published by the Infectious Diseases Society of America (IDSA) states that adjunctive systemic antimicrobial therapy is not routinely indicated but, in conjunction with incision and drainage, may be beneficial for SSIs associated with a systemic response such as erythema and induration extending > 5 cm from the wound edge, temperature > 38.5 °C, heart rate > 110 beats/min, or white blood cell count > 12 000/µL.[43] The antibiotic choice is usually empiric but can be supported by Gram stain, culture of the wound contents, and the site of surgery.

When implants are present, infections tend to occur late (months and occasionally years after surgery) and are often associated with limited clinical manifestation.[59] A high level of suspicion is thus required. Management remains challenging, and it is still not clearly defined given the absence of high-level evidence in the literature. In the past, immediate removal of infected prostheses was standard practice. However, nowadays it is not uncommon for the patient and the surgeon to be unwilling to accept the loss of the implant, with its associated physical and financial consequences, until they are convinced that an attempt at medical therapy has failed. As a result, plastic surgeons have explored other options in an attempt to salvage these devices, such as systemic antibiotics combined with either conservative wound drainage, antibiotic lavage, capsulotomy with implant exchange, and capsule curettage with implant exchange.[60,61,62,63,64,65] In 2004, Spear et al proposed treatment guidelines for breast implant salvage in the setting of infection with and without implant exposure (▶ Fig. 13.2).[62] Patients with mild infections can be started immediately on oral antibiotics, whereas patients with severe infections should be started on parenteral antibiotics. Those patients who respond completely require no further treatment. However, surgical intervention is recommended for persistent infections or threatened or actual exposure. In these cases, drainage of the fluid collection is indicated. This is followed by partial or total capsulectomy, debridement, pocket lavage, site change, implant exchange, and possible local tissue and/or flap coverage, which is chosen based on the surgeon's experience and clinical judgment. Salvage attempts for implant infection and exposure depend on the degree of infection, response of the infection to initial antibiotic therapy, and availability of adequate soft tissue coverage. In addition, if aggressive salvage measures must be taken, both the patient and the surgeon should be prepared to go through this process together. In some occasions, implant salvage is contraindicated. Examples include identification of atypical pathogens on wound culture (such as nontuberculous mycobacteria), fungal infections, and persistence of systemic signs of sepsis despite appropriate antibiotic therapy.[51,63] In these cases, timing of implant replacement depends on the degree of infection and the causative organisms.[16] Some experts recommend waiting 3 to 6 months before reimplantation, but there is no good evidence to support this approach.

Over the years, a variety of perioperative prevention measures have been proposed to assist in reducing the incidence of SSIs. Although aesthetic breast procedures are not required to follow the Surgical Care Improvement Project (SCIP) guidelines, the prophylactic use of antibiotics by board-certified plastic surgeons, as shown by prior surveys, has steadily increased over the last few decades.[66,67,68] In 2015, the American Association of Plastic Surgeons selected experts to evaluate the evidence for efficacy and safety of antibiotic prophylaxis in plastic surgery procedures, and consensus recommendations were published.[69] Meta-analysis of randomized controlled trials has shown that routine antibiotic prophylaxis for patients undergoing clean cosmetic breast surgery results in a significant reduction in the risk of SSIs (2.5% versus 11.4%; odds ratio 0.16; 95% confidence interval 0.04–0.61; $p = 0.01$). Further subgroup analyses of patients undergoing breast reduction and breast augmentation with implants suggested that both groups benefit from antibiotic prophylaxis, but it was not possible to determine the best antibiotic and optimal dose from the available data. Irrigation of a surgical pocket at the time of implant placement is commonly performed by most plastic surgeons despite the lack of high-level evidence that this technique is actually effective in preventing SSIs. There are, however, a few retrospective and limited prospective cohort studies that demonstrated lower rates of SSIs following irrigation of the implant pocket with a combination of antibiotics (e.g., cefazolin, gentamicin, and bacitracin) and antiseptics (povidone-iodine).[70,71,72] Finally, several regimens have been tested for their decolonization efficacy to prevent methicillin-resistant *Staphylococcus aureus* (MRSA)

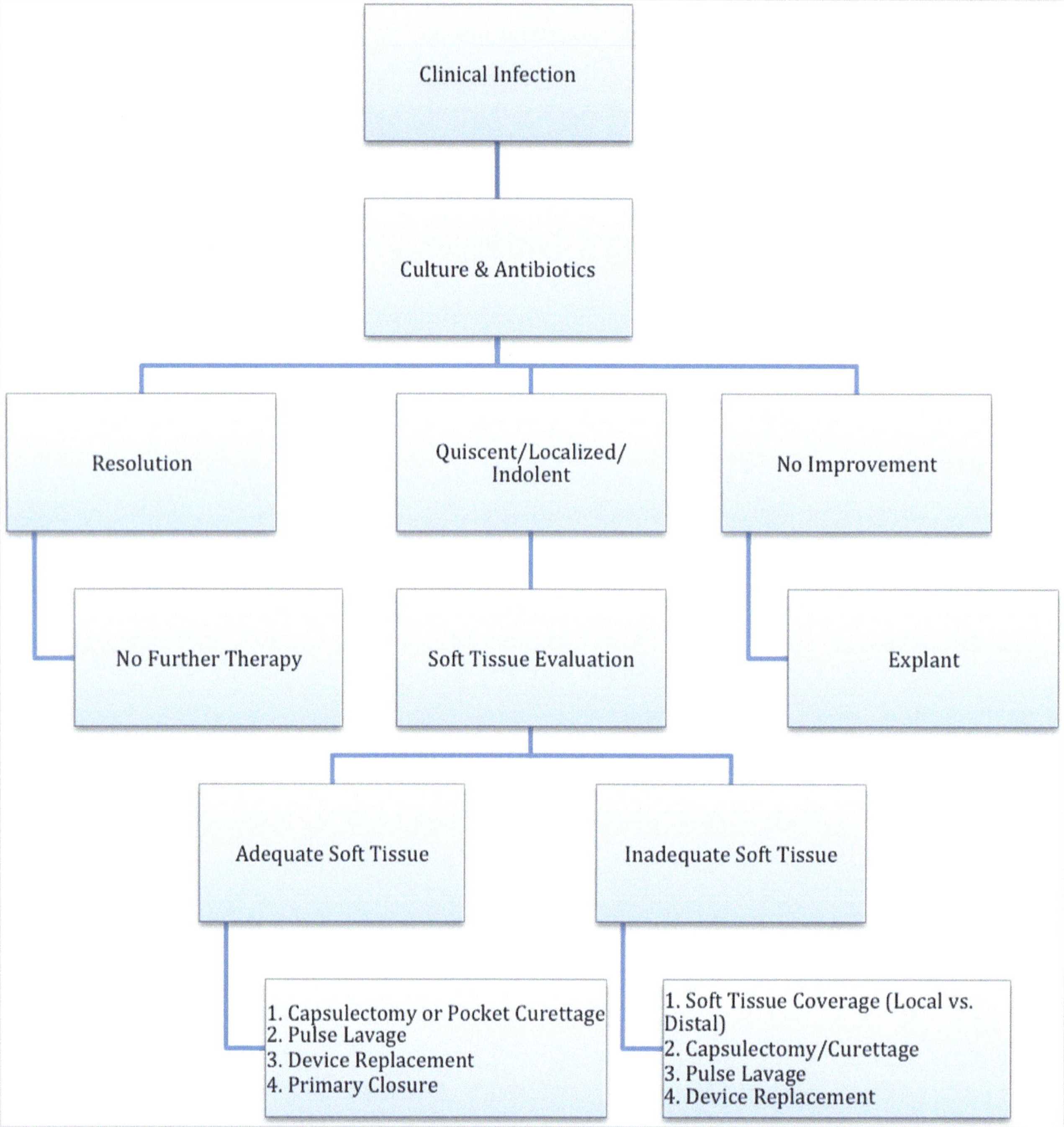

Fig. 13.2 Possible pathways for the treatment of periprosthetic infections.

infections, including chlorhexidine body washes, povidone-iodine body washes, mupirocin nasal ointment, and oral antibiotics.[73,74] Of those, prophylactic use of intranasal mupirocin was shown to reduce the rate of postoperative *S. aureus* infections significantly among carriers,[75] but it did not provide long-term MRSA control, and it did not prevent recolonization or subsequent infections.[76,77] Therefore, since the optimal decolonization regimen is unclear at this point in time, it should be reserved for patients who are colonized with MRSA or are known to have had a MRSA infection in the past.

13.2.4 Delayed Wound Healing

Delayed wound healing, although not frequently seen after mastopexy, it is the most common complication after breast reduction with reported incidences ranging from less than 1% to approximately 65%.[12,13,78,79,80] Perhaps one of the main reasons for this wide variation in the range of reported incidence is the different inclusion criteria for this complication among different studies. The majority of delayed wound healing complications are minor and can be managed in the outpatient setting with local wound care. However, a small proportion of these cases has extensive tissue involvement and may require reoperation to debride the devitalized tissue and create a more favorable environment for healing by secondary intention. If an unsightly scar develops, it can be revised at a later date. Another reason for the wide variation in the range of reported incidence of delayed wound healing and skin necrosis following reduction mammaplasty and mastopexy is the broad variety of techniques used. The Wise pattern of skin resection compromises the skin flaps to a greater degree than a vertical or periareolar reduction does.[81] Tension on the skin flaps at the time of the closure can lead to ischemia at the areas that are most remote from the blood supply; this includes the distal skin flaps at the central lower breast and at the point of convergence of the vertical and horizontal suture lines, commonly referred to as the inverted **T** point.[81] Even for the vertical reduction pattern, wound healing problems commonly occur where the NAC meets the vertical limb. This becomes more of a concern with augmentation mastopexy patients because of the risk of implant exposure. In these patients, a thorough assessment of the wound will determine imminent exposure of the implant, which may change the approach to the management and may prompt earlier implant removal and plan for delayed replacement, if at all. The incidence of these complications, as shown by several studies, is also affected by other factors such as age, obesity, cigarette smoking, and increased resection weights.[13,21,78,81,82,83]

Wound healing problems and skin flap necrosis following breast reduction and mastectomy are vexing complications to both the patient and the surgeon; thus, minimizing their occurrence is in the best interest of both. Ways to achieve this include preservation of the subdermal plexus, gentle retraction of the skin flaps, and minimization of thermal damage.[84] This is especially important in all revisional or reoperative breast surgery. Inherently, when a mastopexy is done in conjunction with a revision breast augmentation, the increased pressure on the flaps by the implant can lead to higher rates of skin necrosis and delayed wound healing. Techniques that involve wide skin undermining should be avoided in these cases, especially if the original augmentation was in the subglandular plane.[20]

Following breast augmentation, wound healing problems are rare. When wound dehiscence occurs in the early postoperative period, it is usually due to a technical error related to closure or an inappropriately selected heavy implant (▶ Fig. 13.3). In these cases, reoperation should be considered to salvage the implant by irrigating the pocket and reclosing the wound. During closure of the incision, particularly with the inframammary approach, the superficial fascial system of the breast should be identified and carefully approximated, not only to provide soft tissue coverage of the inferior aspect of the implant but also to prevent transmission of the weight of the implant directly to the incision.[20] If dehiscence occurs after the first postoperative week, an infectious process should be suspected. As previously discussed, management of these cases remains challenging. Implant removal is frequently required; however, in recent years several options to salvage these devices have been proposed by several groups.[60,61,62,63,64,65,85]

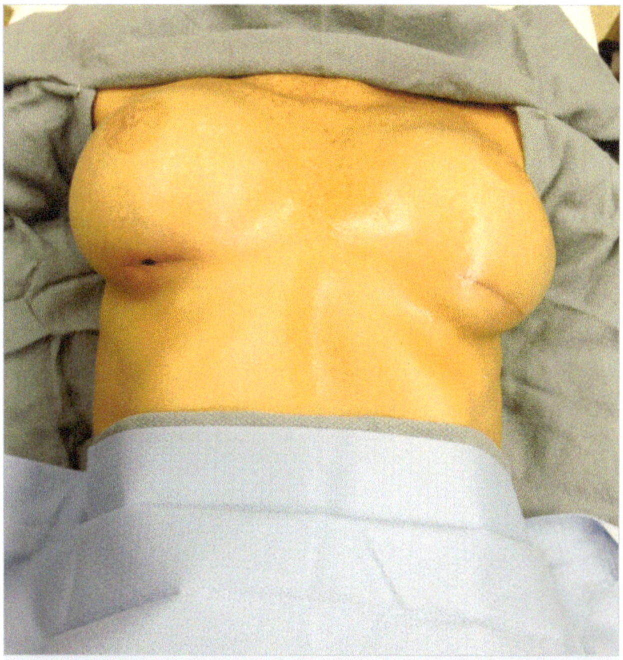

Fig. 13.3 Right breast wound dehiscence with associated implant exposure following primary breast augmentation.

13.2.5 Fat Necrosis

Fat necrosis is predominantly seen after reduction mammaplasty but can occasionally be seen after mastopexy. Although not very common, it can lead to anxiety for the patient and the surgeon. It results from vascular compromise of the adipose tissue of the breast parenchyma or from ischemic necrosis. For example, when large suture bites are used to approximate the breast parenchyma under tension, the perfusion of the adipose tissue can be disrupted, leading to fat necrosis. Likewise, the blood flow to the fatty component of the breast parenchyma may not be as robust at the distal end of the chosen pedicle, leading to necrosis.

In the vast majority of patients, fat necrosis presents as a breast lump. A firm, discrete, mobile breast mass can be found on physical examination. Occasionally, yellow drainage may be expressed from the incision in the early postoperative period without other signs of infection. Associated skin changes are not usually present. Examination can resemble other benign or even malignant breast pathology; therefore, the physician should take such findings seriously. Imaging studies, such as mammography and ultrasound, may be obtained to evaluate the lesion and establish a baseline for future follow-up. If any concerning features are noted on imaging, the lesion must be excised. Excision can also be done if it is bothersome to the patient. Resection can be accomplished through a pre-existing scar. Otherwise, such a mass can be observed for at least a year, since a fair number of these lesions will become softer or even resolve with time and massaging.

13.2.6 NAC Necrosis

Partial or total necrosis of the NAC represents one of the most feared complications following breast reduction and mastopexy, especially after revisionary cases. It is not only disappointing for patients but can also be discouraging for the surgeons. Its incidence ranges from 0 to 10%.[12,78,86,87,88] The spectrum of NAC ischemia spans from spontaneous, completely reversible nipple congestion to total loss of the nipple with extensive necrosis of subadjacent breast tissue.[89] Vascular compromise of the NAC can be caused by arterial insufficiency but is more commonly due to venous congestion.[88] Understanding the vascular anatomy of the breast is thus critical not only to preserving the arterial inflow but also to maintaining an adequate venous drainage system for the NAC. As demonstrated from previous studies, the most reliable blood supply to the NAC comes from the inferomedial aspect of the breast via the internal thoracic–anterior intercostal system, and less so from the superolateral aspect of the breast via the lateral thoracic artery and other minor branches.[88] The most reliable pattern of venous drainage, as shown with breast venograms, is located in the superomedial, medial, and inferior pedicles.[90]

Arterial compromise of the NAC manifests with delayed capillary refill, dark discoloration, and pale nipple that is cool to touch (▸ Fig. 13.4). On the other hand, signs of venous congestion include excessively brisk capillary refill and dark, rapid bleeding on pinprick, as well as cyanotic and edematous nipple. Causes of venous congestion include inadequate preservation of venous drainage, long pedicles, kinking or compression of the pedicle, excessively tight skin closure, and hematoma.[89] In addition, other factors have been shown to increase the risk of NAC ischemia, such as obesity, cigarette smoking, diabetes, large-volume tissue removal, and long distance of transposition of the NAC (more than 15 cm).[91] Patients who have had breast augmentation previously and wish to undergo secondary mastopexy are also at increased risk of ischemic complications.[92] Breast implants can cause tissue stretching and thinning that primarily affect the inferior pole of the breast, which has to be taken into consideration when selecting a pedicle for the secondary mastopexy. For instance, choice of an inferior pedicle will be more prone to vascular compromise because of thinning of the soft tissue of the inferior pole. For this patient population, it is wise to select the least aggressive mastopexy that will achieve the desired result. It is also important to avoid insertion of excessively large implants, which can lead to undue pressure on the tissues and possible ischemic changes.

Meticulous preoperative planning is also critical for patients undergoing revision breast reduction or mastopexy. Previous patient records, including the previous surgeon's operative report, should be obtained to determine which technique and pedicle were utilized. Special attention should be paid to the effect of the prior skin incisions on the blood supply of the nipple and the skin flaps. The safest approach during revision surgery is to reuse the pedicle that was used in the previous surgery. However, often surgeons do not have access to the previous operative report and do not have information regarding the previous pedicle used. In these cases, safe options include the use of bipedicled techniques and breast reduction by liposuction alone with skin-only mastopexy.[20] Techniques that involve wide undermining of skin flaps, especially in situations where the integrity of the vascular supply is unclear, should be avoided.

The viability of the nipple and areola should be evaluated frequently intraoperatively. Generally, the decision is made clinically, but if there is uncertainty, other techniques can be used, such as intravenous fluorescein and indocyanine green videofluorography.[93,94] The advantages of the latter method include repeated use during the same operation and simultaneous evaluation of both the arterial microcirculation and venous drainage. If it becomes obvious that the NAC is nonviable, it is advisable to convert it from a pedicle flap to a full-thickness graft. Fundamentally, the free nipple graft should be affixed to a healthy dermal bed with good blood supply, but not directly onto breast tissue or fat. Even though free nipple grafts have a higher incidence of projection loss and depigmentation, these consequences are preferable to frank necrosis.[20] If viability is questionable, either intraoperatively or immediately postoperatively, a few simple maneuvers can be attempted to improve the perfusion. Releasing the dermal and subdermal sutures around the periphery of the areola can improve the venous outflow significantly within minutes.[89] Application of vasodilating ointments to the area may also help. In our experience, Venelex ointment (balsam Peru and castor oil; Stratus Pharmaceuticals, Miami, FL), applied 5–6 times per day, offers promising results.

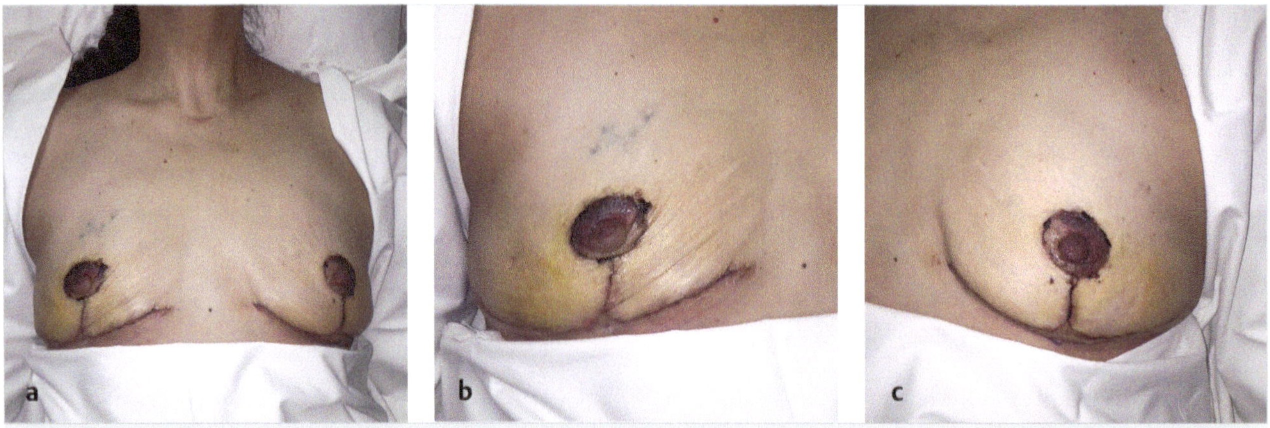

Fig. 13.4 **(a)** Bilateral partial necrosis of the nipple areolar complex following mastopexy on a patient with insulin-dependent diabetes. **(b)** Right nipple-areolar complex close up. **(c)** Left nipple-areolar complex close up.

Steroids such as methylprednisolone (Medrol Dosepak, Pfizer, New York, NY) have also been advocated to reduce local tissue edema and promote venous outflow.[89] Other methods that are not commonly used include leeches and hyperbaric oxygen therapy.[95,96] Although ischemia of the nipple and areola are a source of great angst for both the patient and the surgeon, it is not easy initially to gauge how much tissue will ultimately survive; thus, patience from both parties is required, and aggressive treatment should be avoided until the tissues demarcate.

Depending on the size of the necrotic area, one could either allow the nonviable tissue to slough or debride it. The remaining defect will then be managed with local wound care to promote healing by secondary intention.

NAC reconstruction should be considered, but it is advisable to delay the process for 3 to 6 months in order to allow for resolution of inflammation and improvement in local circulation as well as maturation and softening of the scar tissue.[89] Several reconstructive options are available. The choice is usually made based on the nature of the defect and the preference of the surgeon. For partial loss of the nipple or the areola, the contralateral NAC is the ideal donor site for a natural-appearing result. A full-thickness skin graft can be used for areola reconstruction and a composite nipple graft for nipple reconstruction, assuming there is enough tissue for sharing. If the damage is more extensive, a type of local flap is elevated and rotated or folded to create a nipple of desirable size and shape. Full-thickness skin graft for areolar reconstruction can also be obtained from other body regions, such as the upper inner thighs and labia minora. It is very common for the grafted areola to lose pigmentation over time, leaving behind a circular scar around the nipple. Intradermal tattooing is a simple method to restore that pigmentation.[97,98] More recently, three-dimensional tattooing has gained popularity. Prior authors have also advocated tattooing the intact contralateral NAC to provide the best possible color match between the two sides.[89]

13.2.7 Mondor's Disease

Mondor's disease, or thrombophlebitis of the thoracoepigastric system of veins, is an unusual condition that can be seen after breast augmentation. It has also been reported following breast reduction.[99] The literature for aesthetic surgery is scarce, but it is probably more prevalent than is commonly thought. In the largest series reported to date, there were 13 cases of Mondor's disease, involving 11 patients, in 2,052 breasts (0.63%), for an incidence of 1.07% in 1,026 cases of breast augmentation.[100] It is believed to occur more commonly after a transverse inframammary incision, which results in division of the vertically oriented superficial veins. As a result, retrograde blood flow is prevented because of the presence of valves in these superficial veins, causing venous stasis followed by thrombosis. Physicians should be familiar with several other etiologies linked with this diagnosis, including breast cancer, hypercoagulability disorders, connective tissue diseases, and extensive physical activity as well as external compression by tight-fitting dresses and tight bras.[101,102]

The disease presents as a firm or painful cord on the thoracoabdominal wall and can be visible when the arms are abducted.[100] Typically, it appears within the first 6 weeks after surgery, but it can occur even months later.[100,102] It generally resolves after a short period of time since the thrombus becomes organized, and the veins eventually recanalize after a few weeks. Treatment includes reassurance and supportive care with warm compresses and NSAIDs. While anticoagulation has been proposed by some authors in the context of concomitant prothrombotic risk factors, there is no robust evidence to support its use at this point in time.[100,101]

13.3 Systemic Complications

13.3.1 Venous Thromboembolism

Venous thromboembolism, defined as either deep venous thrombosis (DVT) or pulmonary embolus (PE), is an important patient safety issue among aesthetic surgery patients and undeniably represents one of the most feared complications in cosmetic surgery. In a small percentage of patients, PE can be rapidly fatal or lead to debilitating chronic cardiac dysfunction.[103,104] DVT can also damage the vein wall and the venous valves, predisposing patients to chronic venous reflux and the postthrombotic syndrome.[105] Although the incidence of venous thromboembolism in aesthetic breast surgery is reported to be less than 1%, this rate is believed to be underestimated.[5,13,80,87,104,106,107,108]

As previously advocated by many, including the Joint Commission and the American College of Chest Physicians, venous thromboembolism prevention is the most effective strategy to minimize its associate morbidity and mortality.[109,110,111,112,113] Individualized risk stratification by using the patient's personal characteristics (e.g., age, body mass index, hypercoagulable state) to conceptualize and quantify her venous thromboembolism risk has been proposed. As a result, several individualized risk stratification tools have been developed, but the 2005 Caprini score is currently the most widely used and well-validated among various surgical populations.[114,115,116,117,118,119,120,121,122] It contains 40 risk factors, some of which can be potentially modified before elective surgery, such as obesity, use of estrogen-based contraceptives, and history of prior major surgery within 1 month. Of note, the 2005 Caprini score has also been compared with the modified 2010 Caprini score and was found to provide superior risk stratification for adult plastic surgery patients.[123] Although the 2005 Caprini score has not previously been validated among the outpatient surgery population, theoretically there should be no reason why it would predict risk differently between these two populations. This is important for the aesthetic breast procedures, since they are typically performed in ambulatory surgery centers or outpatient surgical suites. Certainly, there are high-risk patients within this patient population who would benefit from individualized risk stratification to better conceptualize their venous thromboembolism risk and enable surgeons to propose risk modification and risk reduction strategies. Numerous other factors may affect the risk of venous thromboembolism. For instance, Kim et al examined more than 1.4 million cases from the ACS-NSQIP database and showed a clear relation between increased operative time and venous thromboembolism risk.[110] Likewise, other studies have suggested that general anesthesia, and particularly paralysis, may predispose patients to lower-extremity venous stasis by eliminating the positive action of the calf muscle pump.[124,125,126,127]

The existing plastic surgery literature recommends the use of mechanical devices and chemoprophylaxis for high-risk patients, as stratified by the 2005 Caprini score.[128,129] A meta-analysis comparing sequential compression devices (SCDs) and elastic compression stockings has demonstrated superiority of the sequential compression stockings for venous thromboembolism risk reduction.[130] To further support this finding, SCDs are believed to affect two limbs of Virchow's triad (stasis and hypercoagulability) by re-creating the calf muscle pump and stimulating the body's endogenous fibrinolytic system, as opposed to elastic compression stockings, which affect only one limb of the triad (stasis) by shunting blood from the superficial to the deep system.[105] It is for these reasons that the latest American Association of Plastic Surgeons guidelines favor the use of SCDs for all patients.[128] The same guidelines did not support the use of chemoprophylaxis in the overall plastic surgery population. Instead, chemoprophylaxis was recommended based on risk stratification for perioperative venous thromboembolism using the 2005 Caprini score. Specifically, chemoprophylaxis should be considered for patients with Caprini score greater than 8. In addition, the American Society of Plastic Surgeons recommendations state that chemoprophylaxis should be strongly considered for patients with 2005 Caprini scores of 7 or greater.[131] Based on these data, it is felt that chemoprophylaxis should be provided for patients with a 2005 Caprini score 7 or greater. Unfortunately, there is no strong data with regard to the optimal duration of chemoprophylaxis, especially for outpatient surgeries. In certain occasions, such as in patients with a recognized hypercoagulable state not clearly characterized by the 2005 Caprini score, a preoperative hematology consultation may be extremely valuable to assist with hypercoagulability workups, as well as perioperative venous thromboembolism risk modification and chemoprophylaxis.[132] Although the apparent risk of bleeding is a concern for plastic surgeons, several studies have shown increased rates of reoperative hematomas to be less than 1% after use of chemoprophylaxis, with only a minority of studies demonstrating statistically significant differences.[128,133,134]

Diagnosis of DVT is an ongoing clinical challenge. Accurate and timely diagnosis in patients with suspected DVT is critical because, if left untreated, thrombi can break off and travel into the pulmonary circulation, resulting in detrimental PE, whereas anticoagulation in the absence of thrombosis is medically inappropriate. In fact, previous studies have shown that more than 40% of patients with DVT have asymptomatic PE on imaging, and the majority of patients with a fatal PE have a detectable DVT on autopsy, mostly asymptomatic before death.[135,136,137] DVT classically presents with leg pain and edema. The pain can be worse with dorsiflexion of the foot (Homans's sign). Occasionally, warmth and erythema of the skin over the area of thrombosis are noted. PE presentation varies from nonspecific fatigue to gradually progressive dyspnea to sudden onset of pleuritic chest pain, cough, hemoptysis, hypoxia, or even cardiopulmonary collapse. Unfortunately, the majority of patients with a pulmonary embolus do not have a typical presentation, but rather nagging symptoms, which makes diagnosis more challenging. This is why a high index of suspicion is required, particularly when a patient has predisposing risk factors for the condition. Routine laboratory tests are not very useful diagnostically but may provide clues as to the underlying cause and may also influence treatment decisions if a thrombus is detected. D-dimer has been consistently demonstrated to have high sensitivity but poor specificity in postoperative patients with acute DVT.[137,138,139,140,141] Although it is an adjunct test for ruling out DVT, especially in those with a low to moderate suspicion of thrombosis, it can be elevated in many other conditions, which makes it a nonspecific test. Compression ultrasonography with Doppler is currently the imaging modality of choice for diagnosis of DVT given its high sensitivity and specificity.[142,143] Contrast-enhanced computed tomographic (CT) venography and magnetic resonance (MR) venography are rarely used unless there is uncertainty about iliac vein or inferior vena cava thrombosis after ultrasonography. These diagnostic tests are considered less well validated, have associated complications of radiation and contrast exposure, and are costlier.[144] For PE, the diagnostic study of choice is CT pulmonary angiography. Ventilation-perfusion (*V*/*Q*) lung scan is reserved for patients in whom CT is unavailable or contraindicated (e.g., history of moderate or severe contrast allergy, high risk of contrast nephropathy, difficulty lying flat). Other imaging modalities that are less commonly used include MR pulmonary angiogram and catheter-based pulmonary angiography.

Treatment of venous thromboembolism should be individualized, and numerous factors have to be taken into consideration. The primary objectives are to prevent propagation of the thrombus and recurrence, to reduce morbidity, and to minimize the risk of complications. For many decades, the mainstay of treatment has been anticoagulation. However, especially in surgical patients, the risk of bleeding from anticoagulation should be carefully balanced against the risk of recurrent thrombosis. Placement of an inferior vena cava filter, pharmacologic thrombolysis, and catheter-assisted or surgical thromboembolectomy may also be considered in some circumstances.

13.3.2 Pneumothorax

Pneumothorax is a rare complication after aesthetic breast surgery with an incidence of less than 1%, but it appears to be more common than it is generally thought following augmentation mammaplasty.[78,145] In most cases, it is difficult to determine the exact etiology, but various mechanisms have been proposed. They can be related to iatrogenic injury by the surgeon or the anesthesiologist, or even pre-existing pulmonary pathology. Examples include accidental needle penetration of the pleura during local anesthetic infiltration, direct damage or thermal damage to the pleura during dissection with electrocautery, rupture of a pre-existing bleb, raised air pressure within the surgical pocket during implant insertion, high-pressure ventilation or intubation maneuvers, a rush of air created while changing oxygen tanks during surgery, and a plugged exit valve.[145,146]

A pneumothorax can present immediately, hours, or even days after surgery. Presentation may range from completely asymptomatic to cardiopulmonary collapse. Typically, symptoms include pleuritic chest pain (with possible radiation to the ipsilateral shoulder and back), shortness of breath, diaphoresis, and anxiety. There have been reports of bilateral tension pneumothoraxes after breast augmentation, which represent a medical emergency.[147] Patients will present with severe dyspnea, cyanosis, tachypnea, tachycardia, and hypoxia. Pneumothorax can lead to decreased cardiac output as a result of compromised venous return due to compression of the vena cava and right atrium, which may potentially be life-threatening. Physical examination may reveal asymmetric lung expansion and distant or absent breath sounds on the affected side.

If the intercostal fascia and pleura are traumatized during the pocket dissection and the small defect is noted intraoperatively, this should be communicated with the anesthesiologist and managed immediately. The defect should be closed using a purse-string or interrupted suture over a catheter, if possible. The catheter is withdrawn during deep inspiration delivered by positive pressure ventilation or with a Valsalva maneuver if performed under intravenous sedation and local anesthesia.[145] If the parietal pleura and intercostal fascia cannot be reapproximated, other methods can be utilized to close the defect. These techniques would also be used in conjunction with the placement and removal of a catheter as just described. These other techniques include using a patch of breast implant capsule from another part of the posterior capsule, a de-epithelialized skin graft, or a biologic matrix patch, and covering with fibrin glue or similar material to create a seal. A postoperative chest radiograph is always obtained to ensure that there is no residual pneumothorax. If the patient is discharged home, the family or caregiver are instructed to observe for symptoms and signs of pneumothorax and have a low threshold to call or return to the emergency department.

Postoperatively, when pneumothorax is suspected, chest radiography will not only allow for confirmation of the diagnosis, but it will also act as a baseline study, determine the extent of the pneumothorax and potential causes, and assist with the treatment plan. Occasionally, a CT scan is needed to diagnose an occult pneumothorax. Tension pneumothorax is primarily a clinical diagnosis based on patient's presentation, and obtaining imaging may delay treatment, resulting in a detrimental outcome. In these cases, needle decompression should be performed, followed by tube thoracostomy. In general, the decision to observe or to treat with an immediate intervention (such as aspiration, small-bore catheter, or chest tube placement) should be guided by a risk stratification that takes into account the patient's presentation and the likelihood of spontaneous resolution and recurrence.[148]

13.4 Conclusion

Aesthetic breast surgery can achieve excellent outcomes with high patient satisfaction rates. However, as with any other surgery, acute complications may be encountered even in the most suitable candidates. Such complications can have lasting emotional and physical consequences for patients, their families, and the surgeon. As physicians we should never forget the tremendous sense of responsibility for the care of our patients that comes with taking the Hippocratic Oath, and correcting a possible medical error is part of our duty. Although fear of litigation, shame, blame, and concern about reputation are just a few of the barriers preventing surgeons from being more honest with their patients, there is a supporting body of evidence that patients cite poor communication and lack of transparency as primary drivers to file a lawsuit after experiencing a complication.[149,150,151,152]

Plastic surgeons performing these procedures should be familiar with the incidence and risk factors for these complications to provide better preoperative patient education and set more realistic patient expectations. Perioperative patient optimization with evidence-based safety recommendations is also critical to minimize these acute complications. In the unfortunate scenario that such a complication occurs, plastic surgeons should be able to diagnose and manage the complication with confidence but, most importantly, be prepared to support their patients through this process.

Key Points

- Moderate to large hematomas should be drained acutely to avoid negative long-term sequela including compromise of the aesthetic result, capsular contracture, compromise of skin flaps and nipple areolar complex (NAC), infection, and delayed wound healing.
- Judicious use of drains can help to reduce the incidence of seromas, particularly in cases involving extensive capsular revision or use of acellular dermal matrix. Untreated seromas can lead to negative long-term sequelae.
- Existing data suggests that use of perioperative antibiotics can reduce the risk of implant-associated infections. Intraoperative pocket irrigation with antibiotic fluid may also help to reduce infection rates. The data on postoperative antibiotics is less well defined, and no standard recommendations regarding them exist.
- NAC necrosis is a devastating complication. Its incidence can be reduced with careful attention to meticulous surgical technique as well as careful preoperative planning, taking into consideration the anatomy of the blood supply to the NAC as well as previous surgery. Patient factors such as smoking, obesity, and diabetes may also increase this risk.
- Sequential compression devices should be applied to reduce the risk of deep venous thrombosis, and the Caprini score should be used to identify patients at high risk who would benefit from chemoprophylaxis.

References

[1] The Aesthetic Society (American Society for Aesthetic Plastic Surgery; ASAPS). Cosmetic (Aesthetic) Surgery National Data Bank Statistics. 2018. URL: https://www.surgery.org/sites/default/files/ASAPS-Stats2018_0.pdf. Accessed July 16, 2019

[2] Kaoutzanis C, Winocour J, Gupta V, et al. Incidence and risk factors for major hematomas in aesthetic surgery: analysis of 129,007 patients. Aesthet Surg J. 2017; 37(10):1175–1185

[3] Richard P, Huesler R, Banic A, Erni D, Plock JA. Perioperative risk factors for haematoma after breast augmentation. J Plast Surg Hand Surg. 2013; 47(2): 130–134

[4] Basile FV, Basile AR, Basile VV. Use of selective serotonin reuptake inhibitors antidepressants and bleeding risk in breast cosmetic surgery. Aesthetic Plast Surg. 2013; 37(3):561–566

[5] Gupta V, Yeslev M, Winocour J, et al. Aesthetic breast surgery and concomitant procedures: incidence and risk factors for major complications in 73,608 cases. Aesthet Surg J. 2017; 37(5):515–527

[6] Collins JB, Verheyden CN. Incidence of breast hematoma after placement of breast prostheses. Plast Reconstr Surg. 2012; 129(3):413e–420e

[7] Gabriel SE, Woods JE, O'Fallon WM, Beard CM, Kurland LT, Melton LJ, III. Complications leading to surgery after breast implantation. N Engl J Med. 1997; 336(10):677–682

[8] Khavanin N, Jordan SW, Rambachan A, Kim JYS. A systematic review of single-stage augmentation-mastopexy. Plast Reconstr Surg. 2014; 134(5):922–931
[9] Hvilsom GB, Hölmich LR, Henriksen TF, Lipworth L, McLaughlin JK, Friis S. Local complications after cosmetic breast augmentation: results from the Danish Registry for Plastic Surgery of the breast. Plast Reconstr Surg. 2009; 124(3):919–925
[10] Araco A, Gravante G, Araco F, Delogu D, Cervelli V, Walgenbach K. A retrospective analysis of 3,000 primary aesthetic breast augmentations: postoperative complications and associated factors. Aesthetic Plast Surg. 2007; 31 (5):532–539
[11] Codner MA, Mejia JD, Locke MB, et al. A 15-year experience with primary breast augmentation. Plast Reconstr Surg. 2011; 127(3):1300–1310
[12] Carpelan A, Kauhanen S, Mattila K, Jahkola T, Tukiainen E. Reduction mammaplasty as an outpatient procedure: a retrospective analysis of outcome and success rate. Scand J Surg. 2015; 104(2):96–102
[13] Stevens WG, Gear AJL, Stoker DA, et al. Outpatient reduction mammaplasty: an eleven-year experience. Aesthet Surg J. 2008; 28(2):171–179
[14] Handel N, Jensen JA, Black Q, Waisman JR, Silverstein MJ. The fate of breast implants: a critical analysis of complications and outcomes. Plast Reconstr Surg. 1995; 96(7):1521–1533
[15] Stevens WG, Nahabedian MY, Calobrace MB, et al. Risk factor analysis for capsular contracture: a 5-year Sientra study analysis using round, smooth, and textured implants for breast augmentation. Plast Reconstr Surg. 2013; 132(5):1115–1123
[16] Pittet B, Montandon D, Pittet D. Infection in breast implants. Lancet Infect Dis. 2005; 5(2):94–106
[17] Bengtson B, Brody GS, Brown MH, et al. Late Periprosthetic Fluid Collection after Breast Implant Working Group. Managing late periprosthetic fluid collections (seroma) in patients with breast implants: a consensus panel recommendation and review of the literature. Plast Reconstr Surg. 2011; 128 (1):1–7
[18] Khan SM, Smeulders MJC, Van der Horst CM. Wound drainage after plastic and reconstructive surgery of the breast. Cochrane Database Syst Rev. 2015 (10):CD007258
[19] Nathan B, Singh S. Postoperative compression after breast augmentation. Aesthetic Plast Surg. 2001; 25(4):290–291
[20] Grotting JC, Hanemann MS Jr. Reoperative aesthetic breast surgery. In: Scuderi N, Toth BA, eds. International Textbook of Aesthetic Surgery. 1st ed. Berlin: Springer; 2016:295–312
[21] Hall-Findlay EJ, Shestak KC. Breast reduction. Plast Reconstr Surg. 2015; 136 (4):531e–544e
[22] Hanemann MS, Jr, Grotting JC. Evaluation of preoperative risk factors and complication rates in cosmetic breast surgery. Ann Plast Surg. 2010; 64(5): 537–540
[23] Davis GM, Ringler SL, Short K, Sherrick D, Bengtson BP. Reduction mammaplasty: long-term efficacy, morbidity, and patient satisfaction. Plast Reconstr Surg. 1995; 96(5):1106–1110
[24] Hammond DC. Short scar periareolar inferior pedicle reduction (SPAIR) mammaplasty. Plast Reconstr Surg. 1999; 103(3):890–901, discussion–902
[25] Lassus C. A 30-year experience with vertical mammaplasty. Plast Reconstr Surg. 1996; 97(2):373–380
[26] Lejour M. Vertical mammaplasty: early complications after 250 personal consecutive cases. Plast Reconstr Surg. 1999; 104(3):764–770
[27] LeRoy J, Given KS. Wound infection in breast augmentation: the role of prophylactic perioperative antibiotics. Aesthetic Plast Surg. 1991; 15(4):303–305
[28] Menke H, Eisenmann-Klein M, Olbrisch RR, Exner K. Continuous quality management of breast hypertrophy by the German Association of Plastic Surgeons: a preliminary report. Ann Plast Surg. 2001; 46(6):594–598, discussion 598–600
[29] Serletti JM, Davenport MS, Herrera HR, Caldwell EH. Efficacy of prophylactic antibiotics in reduction mammoplasty. Ann Plast Surg. 1994; 33(5):476–480
[30] O'Grady KF, Thoma A, Dal Cin A. A comparison of complication rates in large and small inferior pedicle reduction mammaplasty. Plast Reconstr Surg. 2005; 115(3):736–742
[31] Fischer JP, Cleveland EC, Shang EK, Nelson JA, Serletti JM. Complications following reduction mammaplasty: a review of 3538 cases from the 2005–2010 NSQIP data sets. Aesthet Surg J. 2014; 34(1):66–73
[32] Keramidas E. Zero breast implant infection rate and 0.05% hematoma rate following 1720 silicone implant placements for primary breast augmentation: surgical technique or surgeon luck? Aesthetic Plast Surg. 2009; 33(1): 123–124
[33] Kompatscher P, von Planta A, Spicher I, et al. Comparison of the incidence and predicted risk of early surgical site infections after breast reduction. Aesthetic Plast Surg. 2003; 27(4):308–314
[34] Kaoutzanis C, Gupta V, Winocour J, Shack B, Grotting JC, Higdon K. Incidence and risk factors for major surgical site infections in aesthetic surgery: analysis of 129,007 patients. Aesthet Surg J. 2017; 37(1):89–99
[35] Shermak MA, Chang D, Buretta K, Mithani S, Mallalieu J, Manahan M. Increasing age impairs outcomes in breast reduction surgery. Plast Reconstr Surg. 2011; 128(6):1182–1187
[36] Brand KG. Infection of mammary prostheses: a survey and the question of prevention. Ann Plast Surg. 1993; 30(4):289–295
[37] Beer GM, Spicher I, Cierpka KA, Meyer VE. Benefits and pitfalls of vertical scar breast reduction. Br J Plast Surg. 2004; 57(1):12–19
[38] Culver DH, Horan TC, Gaynes RP, et al. National Nosocomial Infections Surveillance System. Surgical wound infection rates by wound class, operative procedure, and patient risk index. Am J Med. 1991; 91 3B:152S–157S
[39] Elward AM, McAndrews JM, Young VL. Methicillin-sensitive and methicillin-resistant Staphylococcus aureus: preventing surgical site infections following plastic surgery. Aesthet Surg J. 2009; 29(3):232–244
[40] Harel M. Late postoperative infection in a breast reduction case. Plast Reconstr Surg. 1998; 102(5):1775
[41] Tobin G, Shaw RC, Goodpasture HC. Toxic shock syndrome following breast and nasal surgery. Plast Reconstr Surg. 1987; 80(1):111–114
[42] Wharton M, Chorba TL, Vogt RL, Morse DL, Buehler JW. Case definitions for public health surveillance. MMWR Recomm Rep. 1990; 39 RR-13:1–43
[43] Stevens DL, Bisno AL, Chambers HF, et al. Infectious Diseases Society of America. Practice guidelines for the diagnosis and management of skin and soft tissue infections: 2014 update by the Infectious Diseases Society of America. Clin Infect Dis. 2014; 59(2):e10–e52
[44] Macadam SA, Mehling BM, Fanning A, et al. Nontuberculous mycobacterial breast implant infections. Plast Reconstr Surg. 2007; 119(1):337–344
[45] Pajkos A, Deva AK, Vickery K, Cope C, Chang L, Cossart YE. Detection of subclinical infection in significant breast implant capsules. Plast Reconstr Surg. 2003; 111(5):1605–1611
[46] Wolfe JM, Moore DF. Isolation of Mycobacterium thermoresistibile following augmentation mammaplasty. J Clin Microbiol. 1992; 30(4):1036–1038
[47] Bernardi C, Saccomanno F. Late Klebsiella pneumoniae infection following breast augmentation: case report. Aesthetic Plast Surg. 1998; 22(3):222–224
[48] Clegg HW, Bertagnoll P, Hightower AW, Baine WB. Mammaplasty-associated mycobacterial infection: a survey of plastic surgeons. Plast Reconstr Surg. 1983; 72(2):165–169
[49] Heistein JB, Mangino JE, Ruberg RL, Bergese JJ. A prosthetic breast implant infected with Mycobacterium fortuitum. Ann Plast Surg. 2000; 44(3):330–333
[50] Juang YC, Wang LS, Chen CH, Lin CY. Mycobacterium fortuitum mastitis following augmentation mammaplasty: report of a case. Taiwan Yi Xue Hui Za Zhi. 1989; 88(3):278–281
[51] Lalani T, Zenn MR, Sexton DJ. Breast implant infections. UpToDate. URL: https://www.uptodate.com/contents/breast-implant-infections. Updated November 1, 2018. Accessed July 16, 2019
[52] Classen DC, Evans RS, Pestotnik SL, Horn SD, Menlove RL, Burke JP. The timing of prophylactic administration of antibiotics and the risk of surgical-wound infection. N Engl J Med. 1992; 326(5):281–286
[53] McDonald M, Grabsch E, Marshall C, Forbes A. Single- versus multiple-dose antimicrobial prophylaxis for major surgery: a systematic review. Aust N Z J Surg. 1998; 68(6):388–396
[54] Steinberg JP, Braun BI, Hellinger WC, et al. Trial to Reduce Antimicrobial Prophylaxis Errors (TRAPE) Study Group. Timing of antimicrobial prophylaxis and the risk of surgical site infections: results from the Trial to Reduce Antimicrobial Prophylaxis Errors. Ann Surg. 2009; 250(1):10–16
[55] Stone HH, Haney BB, Kolb LD, Geheber CE, Hooper CA. Prophylactic and preventive antibiotic therapy: timing, duration and economics. Ann Surg. 1979; 189(6):691–699
[56] Ganske I, Hoyler M, Fox SE, Morris DJ, Lin SJ, Slavin SA. Delayed hypersensitivity reaction to acellular dermal matrix in breast reconstruction: the red breast syndrome? Ann Plast Surg. 2014; 73 Suppl 2:S139–S143
[57] Pittman TA, Fan KL, Knapp A, Frantz S, Spear SL. Comparison of different acellular dermal matrices in breast reconstruction: the 50/50 Study. Plast Reconstr Surg. 2017; 139(3):521–528
[58] Bobrow BJ, Pollack CV, Jr, Gamble S, Seligson RA. Incision and drainage of cutaneous abscesses is not associated with bacteremia in afebrile adults. Ann Emerg Med. 1997; 29(3):404–408

[59] de Mestral C, Nathens AB. Prevention, diagnosis, and management of surgical site infections: relevant considerations for critical care medicine. Crit Care Clin. 2013; 29(4):887–894

[60] Chun JK, Schulman MR. The infected breast prosthesis after mastectomy reconstruction: successful salvage of nine implants in eight consecutive patients. Plast Reconstr Surg. 2007; 120(3):581–589

[61] Courtiss EH, Goldwyn RM, Anastasi GW. The fate of breast implants with infections around them. Plast Reconstr Surg. 1979; 63(6):812–816

[62] Spear SL, Howard MA, Boehmler JH, Ducic I, Low M, Abbruzzesse MR. The infected or exposed breast implant: management and treatment strategies. Plast Reconstr Surg. 2004; 113(6):1634–1644

[63] Spear SL, Seruya M. Management of the infected or exposed breast prosthesis: a single surgeon's 15-year experience with 69 patients. Plast Reconstr Surg. 2010; 125(4):1074–1084

[64] Kendrick AS, Chase CW. Salvage of an infected breast tissue expander with an implant sizer and negative pressure wound management. Plast Reconstr Surg. 2008; 121(3):138e–139e

[65] Wilkinson TS, Swartz BE, Toranto IR. Resolution of late-developing periprosthetic breast infections without prosthesis removal. Aesthetic Plast Surg. 1985; 9(2):79–85

[66] Lyle WG, Outlaw K, Krizek TJ, Koss N, Payne WG, Robson MC. Prophylactic antibiotics in plastic surgery: trends of use over 25 years of an evolving specialty. Aesthet Surg J. 2003; 23(3):177–183

[67] Krizek TJ, Gottlieb LJ, Koss N, Robson MC. The use of prophylactic antibacterials in plastic surgery: a 1980s update. Plast Reconstr Surg. 1985; 76(6): 953–963

[68] Krizek TJ, Koss N, Robson MC. The current use of prophylactic antibiotics in plastic and reconstructive surgery. Plast Reconstr Surg. 1975; 55(1):21–32

[69] Ariyan S, Martin J, Lal A, et al. Antibiotic prophylaxis for preventing surgical-site infection in plastic surgery: an evidence-based consensus conference statement from the American Association of Plastic Surgeons. Plast Reconstr Surg. 2015; 135(6):1723–1739

[70] Adams WP, Jr, Conner WC, Barton FE, Jr, Rohrich RJ. Optimizing breast pocket irrigation: an in vitro study and clinical implications. Plast Reconstr Surg. 2000; 105(1):334–338, discussion 339–-343

[71] Adams WP, Jr, Rios JL, Smith SJ. Enhancing patient outcomes in aesthetic and reconstructive breast surgery using triple antibiotic breast irrigation: six-year prospective clinical study. Plast Reconstr Surg. 2006; 118(7) Suppl: 46S–52S

[72] Araco A, Gravante G, Araco F, Delogu D, Cervelli V, Walgenbach K. Infections of breast implants in aesthetic breast augmentations: a single-center review of 3,002 patients. Aesthetic Plast Surg. 2007; 31(4):325–329

[73] Abrahamian FM, Snyder EW. Community-associated methicillin-resistant Staphylococcus aureus: incidence, clinical presentation, and treatment decisions. Curr Infect Dis Rep. 2007; 9(5):391–397

[74] McConeghy KW, Mikolich DJ, LaPlante KL. Agents for the decolonization of methicillin-resistant Staphylococcus aureus. Pharmacotherapy. 2009; 29(3): 263–280

[75] Perl TM, Cullen JJ, Wenzel RP, et al. Mupirocin And The Risk Of Staphylococcus Aureus Study Team. Intranasal mupirocin to prevent postoperative Staphylococcus aureus infections. N Engl J Med. 2002; 346(24):1871–1877

[76] Dupeyron C, Campillo B, Bordes M, Faubert E, Richardet J-P, Mangeney N. A clinical trial of mupirocin in the eradication of methicillin-resistant Staphylococcus aureus nasal carriage in a digestive disease unit. J Hosp Infect. 2002; 52(4):281–287

[77] Ellis MW, Griffith ME, Dooley DP, et al. Targeted intranasal mupirocin to prevent colonization and infection by community-associated methicillin-resistant Staphylococcus aureus strains in soldiers: a cluster randomized controlled trial. Antimicrob Agents Chemother. 2007; 51(10):3591–3598

[78] Cunningham BL, Gear AJL, Kerrigan CL, Collins ED. Analysis of breast reduction complications derived from the BRAVO study. Plast Reconstr Surg. 2005; 115(6):1597–1604

[79] Saleem L, John JR. Unfavourable results following reduction mammoplasty. Indian J Plast Surg. 2013; 46(2):401–407

[80] Hanwright PJ, Hirsch EM, Seth AK, et al. A multi-institutional perspective of complication rates for elective nonreconstructive breast surgery: an analysis of NSQIP data from 2006 to 2010. Aesthet Surg J. 2013; 33(3):378–386

[81] `Hansen J, Chang S. Overview of breast reduction. UpToDate. URL: https://www.uptodate.com/contents/overview-of-breast-reduction. Updated April 30, 2019. Accessed July 16, 2019

[82] Mandrekas AD, Zambacos GJ, Anastasopoulos A, Hapsas DA. Reduction mammaplasty with the inferior pedicle technique: early and late complications in 371 patients. Br J Plast Surg. 1996; 49(7):442–446

[83] Shah R, Al-Ajam Y, Stott D, Kang N. Obesity in mammaplasty: a study of complications following breast reduction. J Plast Reconstr Aesthet Surg. 2011; 64(4):508–514

[84] Nahabedian M, Gutowski KA. Complications of reconstructive and aesthetic breast surgery. UpToDate. URL: https://www.uptodate.com/complications-of-reconstructive-and-aesthetic-breast-surgery. Updated October 10, 2017. Accessed July 16, 2019

[85] Agarwal S, Ettinger RE, Kung TA, Kozlow JH, Brown DL. Cohort study of immediate implant exchange during acute infection in the setting of breast reconstruction. J Plast Reconstr Aesthet Surg. 2017; 70(7):865–870

[86] Dabbah A, Lehman JA, Jr, Parker MG, Tantri D, Wagner DS. Reduction mammaplasty: an outcome analysis. Ann Plast Surg. 1995; 35(4):337–341

[87] DeFazio MV, Fan KL, Avashia YJ, et al. Inferior pedicle breast reduction: a retrospective review of technical modifications influencing patient safety, operative efficiency, and postoperative outcomes. Am J Surg. 2012; 204(5):e7–e14

[88] van Deventer PV, Page BJ, Graewe FR. The safety of pedicles in breast reduction and mastopexy procedures. Aesthetic Plast Surg. 2008; 32(2):307–312

[89] Handel N, Yegiyants S. Managing necrosis of the nipple areolar complex following reduction mammaplasty and mastopexy. Clin Plast Surg. 2016; 43 (2):415–423

[90] le Roux CM, Pan W-R, Matousek SA, Ashton MW. Preventing venous congestion of the nipple-areola complex: an anatomical guide to preserving essential venous drainage networks. Plast Reconstr Surg. 2011; 127(3):1073–1079

[91] Gravante G, Araco A, Sorge R, et al. Postoperative wound infections after breast reductions: the role of smoking and the amount of tissue removed. Aesthetic Plast Surg. 2008; 32(1):25–31

[92] Handel N. Secondary mastopexy in the augmented patient: a recipe for disaster. Plast Reconstr Surg. 2006; 118(7) Suppl:152S–163S, discussion 164S–165S, 166S–-167S

[93] Murray JD, Jones GE, Elwood ET, Whitty LA, Garcia C. Fluorescent intraoperative tissue angiography with indocyanine green: evaluation of nipple-areola vascularity during breast reduction surgery. Plast Reconstr Surg. 2010; 126(1):33e–34e

[94] Singer R, Krant SM. Intravenous fluorescein for evaluating the dusky nipple-areola during reduction mammaplasty. Plast Reconstr Surg. 1981; 67(4): 534–535

[95] Pannucci CJ, Nelson JA, Chung CU, et al. Medicinal leeches for surgically uncorrectable venous congestion after free flap breast reconstruction. Microsurgery. 2014; 34(7):522–526

[96] Friedman HI, Fitzmaurice M, Lefaivre JF, Vecchiolla T, Clarke D, Clarke D. An evidence-based appraisal of the use of hyperbaric oxygen on flaps and grafts. Plast Reconstr Surg. 2006; 117(7) Suppl:175S–190S, discussion 191S–-192S

[97] Becker H. The use of intradermal tattoo to enhance the final result of nipple-areola reconstruction. Plast Reconstr Surg. 1986; 77(4):673–676

[98] Spear SL, Convit R, Little JW, III. Intradermal tattoo as an adjunct to nipple-areola reconstruction. Plast Reconstr Surg. 1989; 83(5):907–911

[99] Green RA, Dowden RV. Mondor's disease in plastic surgery patients. Ann Plast Surg. 1988; 20(3):231–235

[100] Khan UD. Incidence of Mondor disease in breast augmentation: a retrospective study of 2052 breasts using inframammary incision. Plast Reconstr Surg. 2008; 122(2):88e–89e

[101] Pignatti M, Loschi P, Pedrazzi P, Marietta M. Mondor's disease after implant-based breast reconstruction. Report of three cases and review of the literature. J Plast Reconstr Aesthet Surg. 2014; 67(11):e275–e277

[102] Viana GAP, Okano FM. Superficial thrombophlebitis (Mondor's disease) after breast augmentation surgery. Indian J Plast Surg. 2008; 41(2):219–221

[103] Heit JA, Silverstein MD, Mohr DN, Petterson TM, O'Fallon WM, Melton LJ, III. Predictors of survival after deep vein thrombosis and pulmonary embolism: a population-based, cohort study. Arch Intern Med. 1999; 159(5):445–453

[104] Kearon C. Natural history of venous thromboembolism. Circulation. 2003; 107(23) Suppl 1:I22–I30

[105] Pannucci CJ. Evidence-based recipes for venous thromboembolism prophylaxis: a practical safety guide. Plast Reconstr Surg. 2017; 139(2):520e–532e

[106] Winocour J, Gupta V, Kaoutzanis C, et al. Venous thromboembolism in the cosmetic patient: analysis of 129,007 patients. Aesthet Surg J. 2017; 37(3): 337–349

[107] Alderman AK, Collins ED, Streu R, et al. Benchmarking outcomes in plastic surgery: national complication rates for abdominoplasty and breast augmentation. Plast Reconstr Surg. 2009; 124(6):2127–2133

[108] Mlodinow AS, Khavanin N, Ver Halen JP, Rambachan A, Gutowski KA, Kim JYS. Increased anaesthesia duration increases venous thromboembolism risk in plastic surgery: A 6-year analysis of over 19,000 cases using the NSQIP dataset. J Plast Surg Hand Surg. 2015; 49(4):191–197
[109] Arnold DM, Kahn SR, Shrier I. Missed opportunities for prevention of venous thromboembolism: an evaluation of the use of thromboprophylaxis guidelines. Chest. 2001; 120(6):1964–1971
[110] Kim JYS, Khavanin N, Rambachan A, et al. Surgical duration and risk of venous thromboembolism. JAMA Surg. 2015; 150(2):110–117
[111] Wakefield TW, McLafferty RB, Lohr JM, Caprini JA, Gillespie DL, Passman MA, Executive Committee of the American Venous Forum. Call to action to prevent venous thromboembolism. J Vasc Surg. 2009; 49(6):1620–1623
[112] Joint Commission. Surgical Care Improvement Project (SCIP) Measure Information Form (Version 2.1c). Joint Commission; 2006. URL: https://www.jointcommission.org/assets/1/18/2zn_SCIP-VTE-2_1c.pdf. Accessed July 17, 2019
[113] Office of the Surgeon General; National Heart, Lung and Blood Institute. The Surgeon General's Call to Action to Prevent Deep Vein Thrombosis and Pulmonary Embolism. Rockville, MD: Office of the Surgeon General; 2008
[114] Pannucci CJ, Shanks A, Moote MJ, et al. Identifying patients at high risk for venous thromboembolism requiring treatment after outpatient surgery. Ann Surg. 2012; 255(6):1093–1099
[115] Gould MK, Garcia DA, Wren SM, et al. Prevention of VTE in nonorthopedic surgical patients: Antithrombotic Therapy and Prevention of Thrombosis, 9th ed: American College of Chest Physicians Evidence-Based Clinical Practice Guidelines. Chest. 2012; 141(2 Suppl):e227S–e277S
[116] Caprini JA. Thrombosis risk assessment as a guide to quality patient care. Dis Mon. 2005; 51(2–3):70–78
[117] Rogers SO, Jr, Kilaru RK, Hosokawa P, Henderson WG, Zinner MJ, Khuri SF. Multivariable predictors of postoperative venous thromboembolic events after general and vascular surgery: results from the patient safety in surgery study. J Am Coll Surg. 2007; 204(6):1211–1221
[118] Davison SP, Venturi ML, Attinger CE, Baker SB, Spear SL. Prevention of venous thromboembolism in the plastic surgery patient. Plast Reconstr Surg. 2004; 114(3):43E–51E
[119] Pannucci CJ, Laird S, Dimick JB, Campbell DA, Henke PK. A validated risk model to predict 90-day VTE events in postsurgical patients. Chest. 2014; 145(3):567–573
[120] Bahl V, Hu HM, Henke PK, Wakefield TW, Campbell DA, Jr, Caprini JA. A validation study of a retrospective venous thromboembolism risk scoring method. Ann Surg. 2010; 251(2):344–350
[121] Stroud W, Whitworth JM, Miklic M, et al. Validation of a venous thromboembolism risk assessment model in gynecologic oncology. Gynecol Oncol. 2014; 134(1):160–163
[122] Shuman AG, Hu HM, Pannucci CJ, Jackson CR, Bradford CR, Bahl V. Stratifying the risk of venous thromboembolism in otolaryngology. Otolaryngol Head Neck Surg. 2012; 146(5):719–724
[123] Pannucci CJ, Barta RJ, Portschy PR, et al. Assessment of postoperative venous thromboembolism risk in plastic surgery patients using the 2005 and 2010 Caprini Risk score. Plast Reconstr Surg. 2012; 130(2):343–353
[124] Swanson E. The case against chemoprophylaxis for venous thromboembolism prevention and the rationale for SAFE anesthesia. Plast Reconstr Surg Glob Open. 2014; 2(6):e160
[125] Bitar G, Mullis W, Jacobs W, et al. Safety and efficacy of office-based surgery with monitored anesthesia care/sedation in 4778 consecutive plastic surgery procedures. Plast Reconstr Surg. 2003; 111(1):150–156, discussion 157–158
[126] Ersek RA. Dissociative anesthesia for safety's sake: ketamine and diazepam—a 35-year personal experience. Plast Reconstr Surg. 2004; 113(7):1955–1959
[127] Ersek RA. General anesthesia gases are a common denominator in cases of thromboembolism. Aesthet Surg J. 2009; 29(4):340–341
[128] Pannucci CJ, MacDonald JK, Ariyan S, et al. Benefits and risks of prophylaxis for deep venous thrombosis and pulmonary embolus in plastic surgery: a systematic review and meta-analysis of controlled trials and consensus conference. Plast Reconstr Surg. 2016; 137(2):709–730
[129] Pannucci CJ, Dreszer G, Wachtman CF, et al. Postoperative enoxaparin prevents symptomatic venous thromboembolism in high-risk plastic surgery patients. Plast Reconstr Surg. 2011; 128(5):1093–1103
[130] Ho KM, Tan JA. Stratified meta-analysis of intermittent pneumatic compression of the lower limbs to prevent venous thromboembolism in hospitalized patients. Circulation. 2013; 128(9):1003–1020
[131] Murphy RX, Jr, Alderman A, Gutowski K, et al. Evidence-based practices for thromboembolism prevention: summary of the ASPS Venous Thromboembolism Task Force Report. Plast Reconstr Surg. 2012; 130(1):168e–175e
[132] Pannucci CJ, Kovach SJ, Cuker A. Microsurgery and the hypercoagulable state: a hematologist's perspective. Plast Reconstr Surg. 2015; 136(4):545e–552e
[133] Pannucci CJ, Wachtman CF, Dreszer G, et al. The effect of postoperative enoxaparin on risk for reoperative hematoma. Plast Reconstr Surg. 2012; 129(1):160–168
[134] Leonardi MJ, McGory ML, Ko CY. The rate of bleeding complications after pharmacologic deep venous thrombosis prophylaxis: a systematic review of 33 randomized controlled trials. Arch Surg. 2006; 141(8):790–797, discussion 797–799
[135] Moser KM, Fedullo PF, LitteJohn JK, Crawford R. Frequent asymptomatic pulmonary embolism in patients with deep venous thrombosis. JAMA. 1994; 271(3):223–225
[136] Meignan M, Rosso J, Gauthier H, et al. Systematic lung scans reveal a high frequency of silent pulmonary embolism in patients with proximal deep venous thrombosis. Arch Intern Med. 2000; 160(2):159–164
[137] Sandler DA, Martin JF. Autopsy proven pulmonary embolism in hospital patients: are we detecting enough deep vein thrombosis? J R Soc Med. 1989; 82(4):203–205
[138] Bounameaux H, de Moerloose P, Perrier A, Reber G. Plasma measurement of D-dimer as diagnostic aid in suspected venous thromboembolism: an overview. Thromb Haemost. 1994; 71(1):1–6
[139] Wells PS, Anderson DR, Bormanis J, et al. Application of a diagnostic clinical model for the management of hospitalized patients with suspected deep-vein thrombosis. Thromb Haemost. 1999; 81(4):493–497
[140] Lennox AF, Delis KT, Serunkuma S, Zarka ZA, Daskalopoulou SE, Nicolaides AN. Combination of a clinical risk assessment score and rapid whole blood D-dimer testing in the diagnosis of deep vein thrombosis in symptomatic patients. J Vasc Surg. 1999; 30(5):794–803
[141] Aschwanden M, Labs KH, Jeanneret C, Gehrig A, Jaeger KA. The value of rapid D-dimer testing combined with structured clinical evaluation for the diagnosis of deep vein thrombosis. J Vasc Surg. 1999; 30(5):929–935
[142] Goodacre S, Sampson F, Thomas S, van Beek E, Sutton A. Systematic review and meta-analysis of the diagnostic accuracy of ultrasonography for deep vein thrombosis. BMC Med Imaging. 2005; 5:6
[143] Bernardi E, Camporese G, Büller HR, et al. Erasmus Study Group. Serial 2-point ultrasonography plus D-dimer vs whole-leg color-coded Doppler ultrasonography for diagnosing suspected symptomatic deep vein thrombosis: a randomized controlled trial. JAMA. 2008; 300(14):1653–1659
[144] Kearon C, Bauer K. Clinical presentation and diagnosis of the nonpregnant adult with suspected deep vein thrombosis of the lower extremity. UpToDate. URL: https://www.uptodate.com/contents/clinical-presentation-and-diagnosis-of-the-nonpregnant-adult-with-suspected-deep-vein-thrombosis-of-the-lower-extremity. Updated November 30, 2017. Accessed July 16, 2019
[145] Osborn JM, Stevenson TR. Pneumothorax as a complication of breast augmentation. Plast Reconstr Surg. 2005; 116(4):1122–1126, discussion 1127–1128
[146] Keyes GR, Singer R, Iverson RE, et al. Analysis of outpatient surgery center safety using an Internet-based quality improvement and peer review program. Plast Reconstr Surg. 2004; 113(6):1760–1770
[147] Vera-Merchancano R, Hernández-Palazón J, Fuentes-García D, Fernández-Rodríguez LE. Intraoperative bilateral tension pneumothorax in a patient undergoing breast augmentation surgery with general anesthesia. J Plast Reconstr Aesthet Surg. 2014; 67(6):e165–e166
[148] Bintcliffe OJ, Hallifax RJ, Edey A, et al. Spontaneous pneumothorax: time to rethink management? Lancet Respir Med. 2015; 3(7):578–588
[149] Witman AB, Park DM, Hardin SB. How do patients want physicians to handle mistakes? A survey of internal medicine patients in an academic setting. Arch Intern Med. 1996; 156(22):2565–2569
[150] Mazor KM, Simon SR, Yood RA, et al. Health plan members' views about disclosure of medical errors. Ann Intern Med. 2004; 140(6):409–418
[151] Gallagher TH, Waterman AD, Ebers AG, Fraser VJ, Levinson W. Patients' and physicians' attitudes regarding the disclosure of medical errors. JAMA. 2003; 289(8):1001–1007
[152] Burroughs TE, Waterman AD, Gallagher TH, et al. Patients' concerns about medical errors during hospitalization. Jt Comm J Qual Patient Saf. 2007; 33(1):5–14

14 Management of Acute Complications of Aesthetic Breast Surgery Part II—Malpositions and Rippling

Alexandra Bucknor, Munique Maia, Sumner A. Slavin, Bernard T. Lee, and Samuel J. Lin

Summary

Implant malposition, inframammary fold asymmetry/deformity, and implant rippling remain an important driving factor in patient dissatisfaction after breast augmentation. Knowledge of how to approach both the patient and operative management is of the utmost importance. With adequate preoperative planning and careful management of patient expectations, these complications may be addressed with satisfactory results. In this chapter, we detail the underlying etiology and describe various operative approaches for managing this group of complications.

Keywords: implant malposition, symmastia, rippling, patient expectations, augmentation, inframammary fold

14.1 Introduction

14.1.1 Definitions

Implant and Inframammary Fold Malposition

Implant malposition, in which a breast implant is incorrectly positioned, is the second most common complication arising after breast augmentation, second to capsular contracture (discussed in Chapters 13 and 15).

Implant malposition may manifest in different ways, and in some cases, the displacement may occur in more than one direction. Medial malposition may cause confluence of the breasts in the midline, known as symmastia. The term *symmastia* was coined by Spence et al in 1984, combining the Greek *syn* (together) with *mastos* (breast) to describe a "presternal blending" of the breasts.[1] Symmastia more commonly occurs with the placement of large implants, overdissection of the pocket medially, and use of the subglandular plane (▶ Fig. 14.1).[2] Superior malposition leads to a "high-riding" implant, or "Snoopy nose" deformity (▶ Fig. 14.2). Snoopy nose deformity, also called double bubble type A or waterfall deformity, occurs when the implant is positioned cephalad to the glandular tissue. Inferior malposition may lead to the "double-bubble" effect, where the breast tissue is seen to lie superior to the implant (▶ Fig. 14.3). Lateral malposition (telemastia) is also observed and can create a wide separation between breasts.

Inframammary fold (IMF) malposition manifests as one that does not maintain symmetry with the contralateral breast or when the implant migrates inferior to the proposed pocket. This is demonstrated in Case 1 in the Case Series at the end of this chapter.

Implant Rippling

Implant rippling occurs where there is loss of the normal smooth curvature of the breast and, instead, wrinkles or ridges in the implant are transmitted to the skin. This is demonstrated in Case 2 in the Case Series at the end of this chapter.

14.1.2 Importance of These Complications

In the event of any of the complications in the preceding subsection occurring, patients may present for revision surgery with high expectations, given the emotionally charged nature of the operative journey they have likely endured.[3] Moreover, previous work has shown that breast augmentation is one of the procedures most commonly associated with aesthetic malpractice claims.[4] Undertaking revisionary breast surgery can be challenging and complex, even for the most experienced surgeons. In this chapter we outline the pathophysiology and etiology of implant malposition, including symmastia, implant lateralization and inframammary fold malposition, and rippling, in addition to discussing operative approaches to managing these findings.

14.1.3 Etiology of Implant Malposition

Implant malpositions may be multifactorial. However, as described by Brown et al, they can usually be ascribed to one or more of five categories: "patient factors, procedure selection, implant selection, surgical technique, and postoperative management."[5] An understanding of these is crucial in determining the management strategy employed.

Patient Factors

Thin skin envelope and thin soft tissue overlying the implant are among the most frequently noted causes of implant malposition. This may be related to quality of the native tissue or to postoperative tissue atrophy.[6] A combination of poor-quality tissue and stretching over time can cause implant malposition, especially laterally and inferiorly. Small-breasted women of slight stature may fall into this category. It is recommended that the measured pinch-thickness of the upper breast pole coverage should be at least 2 cm for subglandular placement to be safe; otherwise deeper or dual-plane placement may be warranted to avoid implant rippling or palpability.

The Snoopy nose breast may occur in women with preexisting ptosis. Ptosis of the glandular breast tissue relative to the implant and superior bulge caused by the implant are noted. The unsatisfactory look is further worsened by the ptotic appearance of the nipple areolar complex (NAC). Moreover, chest wall asymmetries and aberrant chest wall contouring, such as that present in pectus excavatum, may displace an implant. Vigorous contraction of the pectoralis major muscle in athletic individuals may lead to superolateral malposition. These factors must be observed or circumnavigated in any attempt at revision surgery.

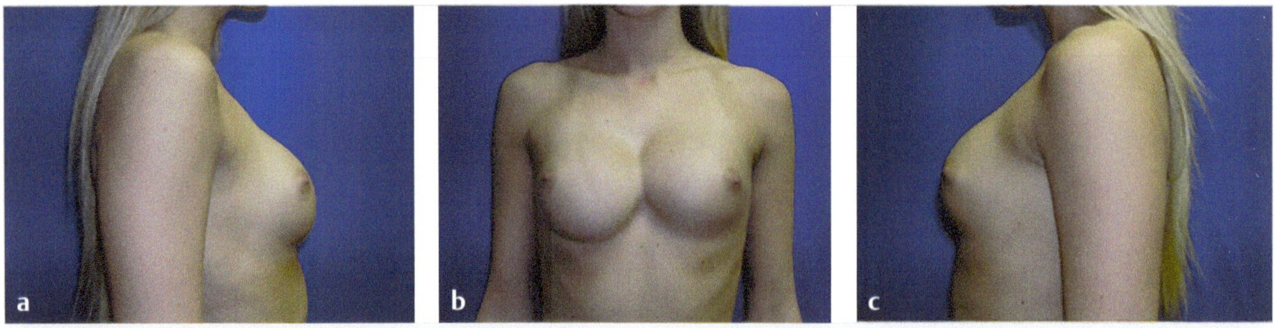

Fig. 14.1 (a–c) 21-year-old woman who had transaxillary augmentation with saline implants. Medial implant malposition, also known as symmastia, is shown. Lateral position of the nipple areolar complex is also observed.

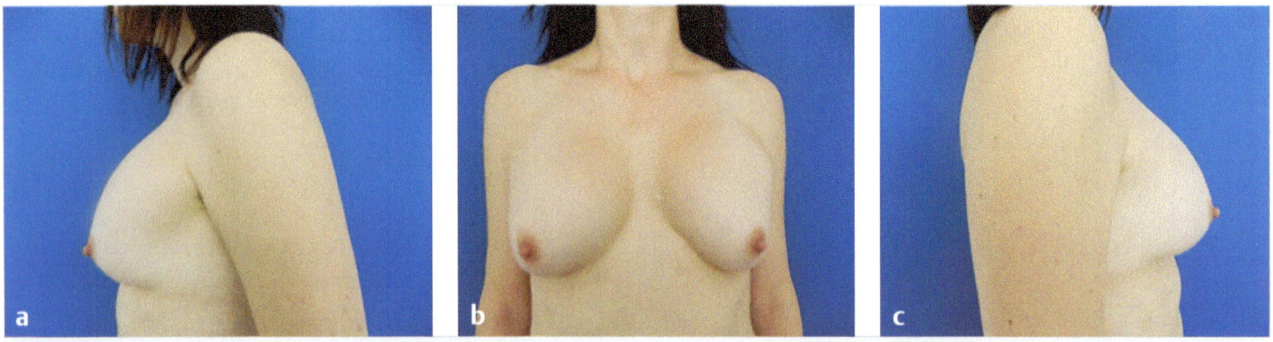

Fig. 14.2 (a–c) 48 year-old woman presented with bilateral capsular contractures 15 years after transaxillary breast augmentation with saline implants. Capsular contracture led to breast implant superior malposition, causing a Snoopy nose deformity. Here, you can also see the shortened nipple-to-inframammary fold distance.

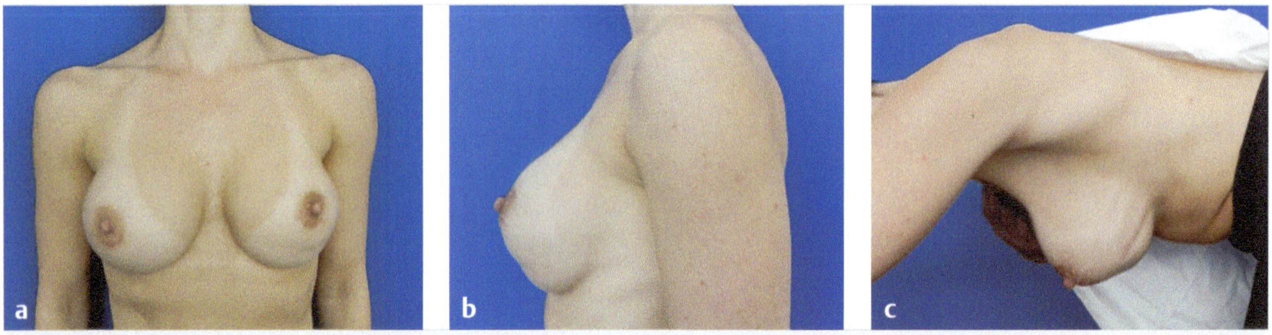

Fig. 14.3 (a–c) 35-year-old woman presented with complaints of left breast pain on the lower pole. She had a history of bilateral breast augmentation with saline implants 10 years prior (350 mL was placed on the right and 290 mL on the left). Anterior and lateral standing views highlight the inferior malposition of the implant on the left breast.

Patients who present with tuberous breast deformity are at high risk of developing double-bubble deformity and high-riding implant.

Procedure Selection and Surgical Technique

The contribution of procedure selection and surgical techniqe to implant malposition primarily consists of the plane in which the implant was placed and the incisions used to approach the augmentation. For example, subglandular implant placement may more often predispose to medial displacement, because of lack of pectoralis support in that region. In contrast, subpectoral placement may lead to lateral displacement as a result of strong overlying muscle contraction. Symmastia can also occur in the subpectoral plane if the pectoralis major muscle is detached from the chest wall too aggressively. As discussed, implant malposition can be caused by technical error. Therefore, precise pocket dissection is important to avoid these complications.

Disruption of the native IMF may be more likely with inframammary incisions, leading to inferior malposition. Excessive IMF dissection may lead to caudal displacement of the implant with respect to the breast mound, creating a second, parallel IMF inferior to the native IMF and breast mound; this is known as the "double-bubble" deformity, as previously mentioned.[7] This may be unprecedented, when overdissection occurs in the context of hematoma evacuation; thus, it is important to minimize the risk of postoperative complications that may necessitate dissection. Meticulous hemostasis and minimization of surgical tissue trauma are essential. Where postoperative accumulation of fluid arises, early detection and prompt drainage are essential to avoid creation of a larger implant pocket.

Other situations may be anticipated, but tricky to avoid. For example, in women with particularly constricted breast bases, it may be necessary to lower the IMF in order to bring the NAC superiorly to a more central position. However, without particular attention to release of the tight IMF, it may often persist and form a second crease superior to the new IMF.

Another commonly encountered scenario is that of the patient who would have benefited from a combined augmentation–mastopexy but instead has an augmentation with a large implant. In this case, poor procedure selection may lead to the aforementioned complications.

Implant Selection

One of the most important considerations is that of implant size. While patients may desire large implants relative to their frame, it is important to respect the natural breast footprint. Rapid tissue expansion may also lead to stretching and thinning of the skin and overlying soft tissue, removing the supportive envelope required to maintain implant position. Horizontal displacement, vertical displacement, or a combination of these may result. Where vertical displacement occurs, a phenomenon known as "bottoming out" may be observed, where the nipple-to-IMF distance increases.

The surface of the implant is also important. Textured implants may lower capsular contracture rates and reduce the rate of implant migration. It has been suggested that this may be due to greater tissue integration or disruption of collagen deposition. However, textured implants have thicker shells and may be prone to traction rippling. This may be in part due to the heightened tissue integration.

Finally, but no less crucially, the choice of implant composition must be considered carefully. Because of concerns regarding the safety of silicone implants given recent reports of textured silicone-associated anaplastic large cell lymphoma (ALCL), saline implants represent a safer alternative. However, saline implants, despite the advantages of their lowered contracture rates and relative safety in the event of leakage, are more likely to exhibit rippling. Moreover, implants that are not filled adequately are also more prone to rippling.

Finally, capsular contracture is an important cause of implant malposition, as seen in ▶ Fig. 14.2.

Postoperative Management

Adequate patient education, particularly regarding use of supportive clothing, is essential. Timely follow-up is important to enable early identification and treatment of complications that may predispose to implant malposition (such as infection, hematoma, and seroma development).

14.2 Management

14.2.1 Preoperative Evaluation

Having considered which category or categories of complication may apply to your patient, now you must consider how to move forward and address the issue. When faced with any breast augmentation revision surgery, a surgeon must return to basic principles: history and physical examination, in addition to elucidating patient expectations and setting appropriate goals.

History

This section covers three main themes: the operative course, the patient's personal and breast-specific health, and the patient's concerns and expectations.

It is important to elucidate the patient's operative course up until the time of presentation. The first task is to note when the primary augmentation took place and what the specific indication was. Previous operation notes are useful in determining details about the implant itself, including composition, surface, shape, size, and fill. The use of adjunctive materials such as acellular dermal matrices (ADMs) must be noted. Ascertaining the location of the implant pocket is crucial, as is determination of the incisions used to access the pocket.

In taking the patient's personal history, the surgeon asks questions to evaluate the patient's general health, looking for risk factors that may affect any revisionary surgery undertaken. This includes wound healing problems, smoking, or steroid use. The surgeon ascertains any factors that may have influenced the development of implant malposition; for example, did the patient undergo massive weight loss or become pregnant?

In addition, it is important to characterize the patient expectations. What is she most dissatisfied by? This may include asymmetry, overall quality of life, and ill-fitting clothes. What does she hope to achieve? This is important, as it will not always be possible—or sensible—to attempt to correct all concerns.

Physical Examination

During the physical examination, the surgeon seeks to understand further the cause of the malposition. The breast soft tissues are examined. Comprehensive palpation to exclude abnormal masses of the breast and axilla is also performed. Any pre-existing asymmetry is noted and highlighted to the patient. Adequacy of soft tissue coverage should be determined, such as by using the pinch test. Degree of ptosis is ascertained, in addition to nipple position on the breast mound. Measurements include sternal notch-to-nipple distance, nipple-to-IMF distance, and breast width. Abnormalities of the relevant musculoskeletal anatomy, known or unknown, must be identified, such as chest contour abnormalities and the quality of the pectoralis major muscle.

Chasan and Francis outline three important preoperative considerations.[8] First, the preoperative exam includes supine photographs in the preoperative panel as well as upright images. This is to facilitate assessment of lateral displacement of the breasts. Second, capsulorrhaphy is simulated digitally and the areola-to-breast mound relationship evaluated. This is to confirm that the relationship remains acceptable and that the NAC does not need repositioning. Third, to the plane in which the implant lies must be clarified.

In addition to standard and supine views as proposed by Chasan and Francis, the authors find that views with the patient bending forward are helping in revealing certain deformities.

14.2.2 Operative Planning and Execution

As per Brown's paper, the variety of approaches can be broadly classified into two groups: adjustment of the original implant pocket and creation of a new pocket.[5]

The patient is marked preoperatively in the standing position. Where possible, the authors endeavor to reopen the breast pocket via the original incision. However, the surgeon must be able to access and correct the problem area directly, and if this is not possible with the original incision, then a new incision is chosen. In the authors' practice, several surgeons prefer the periareolar incision. This incision gives easy access to all quadrants of the breast, and in the authors' experience, correction of the IMF malposition appears to be easier with this incision than when using the IMF incision.

Adjustment of the Existing Pocket

For adjustment of the existing pocket to be an appropriate option for the patient, the implant capsule should be of sufficient thickness but must not be contracted. There should be sufficient soft tissue coverage, and the relationships between the soft tissue and the implant should be within acceptable parameters. In adjusting the existing pocket, the authors consider the need for capsulodesis, strip capsulectomy, or capsulorrhaphy. Thermal capsulorrhaphy is a variant of capsulorrhaphy employed by some surgeons, in which the capsule is cauterized prior to closure in an attempt to obliterate dead space due to heat-induced capsule thickening and contracture.[9] Combinations of these may be required; for example, a capsulotomy may be performed in a location opposite the capsulorrhaphy ("mirror image" capsulotomy) to reduce tension. Capsular flaps may be further used to strengthen capsulorrhaphy. These techniques may also be used in conjunction with ADMs, which can add extra tissue support and also provide additional tissue coverage.

Creation of a New Pocket

In cases where the main issue is skin rippling, significant malposition, or contracture, it may be advisable to change the plane in which the implant lies. For that purpose, a new pocket can be created to fit the desired implant dimensions. A subglandular implant is most commonly relocated to the subpectoral or subfascial plane. The subpectoral implant can be exchanged for a subfascial or subglandular pocket. However, site exchange in subpectoral implants frequently occurs in the context of a paucity of soft tissue coverage; Maxwell and Gabriel also describe the use of a neopectoral pocket, where the anterior implant capsule is preserved and the implant is placed in a pocket "deep to the pectoralis major but superficial to the anterior capsule."[10] This is ideal for use in subpectoral site exchange in the context of volume-depleted breasts. When concerns arose about the use of silicone implants, many surgeons made use of larger saline implants, placing them subpectorally to provide adequate coverage.[10] Revision surgery in this context often requires maintenance of pectoralis cover to address the volume deficit.

The dual-plane technique as described by Tebbets may be appropriate in certain cases, including patients with inadequate tissue for a submuscular to subglandular exchange and those with bottoming out of the implant, or as an alternative to capsulectomy/capsulotomy in superior malposition.[11] The superior aspect of the implant maintains pectoralis coverage, while the lower pole is repositioned to lie deep to the lower pole breast tissue.

The implant capsule itself can be used to create a more appropriately sized implant pocket with reinforced walls in order to address the issue of periprosthetic tissue inadequacy. However, malposition may recur as the reinforcing capsular flaps can relax with time. This has led to a shift in practice toward the use of ADMs, which have been shown to enable more precise control of the implant pocket and position. This technique can be particularly beneficial for reinforcing the inferolateral and inferomedial aspects.

Careful tissue handling is mandatory, together with proactive hemostasis. In this way, the risk of postoperative hematoma, seroma, and inflammation is limited. The surgeon must be wary of repeating previous mistakes, including avoiding excessive pocket dissection or incomplete pectoralis release where applicable.

Finally, the authors account for soft tissue quality in their approach. Often a mastopexy must be done with the revision in certain cases where ptosis is present.

Use of Acellular Dermal Matrices

In the population of women undergoing breast augmentation, who are frequently of thin stature, paucity of skin and soft tissue coverage can be a problem. This contributes to the development of visible surface irregularities. Deformities and deficiencies such as these may be addressed using ADMs, frequently used in conjunction with the aforementioned techniques. Ayeni et al described the use of a single, thick or "ultra-thick" sheet of ADM placed directly onto the capsule in an onlay fashion if no capsulotomy or capsulectomy is being carried out.[12] Here, a parachute technique helps with correct placement. The use of ADMs may help to reduce tension on suture lines, maintain implant position, and define the IMF. This may also be helpful in patients with musculoskeletal contour abnormalities, acting as a stabilizer against implant migration.

Similarly, implant malposition can be corrected by placing ADM over the capsulorrhaphy, taking care to secure it in such a way that avoids tension over the repair, changing the implant position from subglandular to subpectoral, and then fixing the ADM to the rib perichondrium, serratus anterior, and pectoralis.

In the case of symmastia, given that medial soft tissue deficiency is the usual culprit, reinforcement of the midline is necessary. Medial capsulorrhaphy with superimposed ADM secured to both the capsule and chest wall can be very effective. Few tacking sutures are required. With subpectoral implants, the posterior capsule may be "rolled up" up after dissection from the ribs, to provide additional purchase for the tacking sutures.

Fat Grafting

Fat grafting has been the subject of much controversy over the years; however, it can yield many benefits in the management of contour deformities. Indeed, fat grafting can be used for minor rippling to improve the soft tissue coverage.

14.3 Case Series

14.3.1 Case 1

A 37-year-old woman had a history of two previous augmentation mammoplasties. These were done through areolar incisions and involved placement of saline implants of 310 mL on the right and 330 mL on the left. The patient noted that there were some issues with positioning of the implant in the area of the inframammary crease. At the end of the first operation, she thought that the right implant was higher than the left and then had a second operation to have this corrected. At the time of the consultation, she reported that the right breast was lower than the left, and she was unhappy about the result. ▶ Fig. 14.4 shows the right breast implant with inferior malposition, as well as double-bubble deformity and IMF malposition.

Intraoperatively, the capsule was inspected and was seen to have extension below the IMF and extension laterally and superolaterally. Furthermore, there was scar tissue medially, preventing the implant from occupying an optimal position in the medial and inferomedial aspects.

Reconstruction of the IMF was then carried out with capsulorrhaphies using 3–0 Vicryl sutures (Ethicon, Bridgewater, MA). Additional sutures were placed inferomedially and laterally to create a satisfactory pocket with proper placement of the implant. Following that, strips of AlloDerm ADM (BioHorizons, Birmingham, AL) were placed in the pocket to provide an additional layer of tissue and to decrease rippling and wrinkling that had been present preoperatively. The AlloDerm was secured with 3–0 Vicryl sutures.

The patient was inspected and seen to have a marked improvement in appearance with restoration of the IMF contour to a normal location. Postoperative pictures show correction of the double-bubble deformity and IMF malposition (▶ Fig. 14.5).

14.3.2 Case 2

A 47-year-old woman presented 10 years after breast augmentation. She noted rippling and wrinkling, particularly in the lateral aspects, and lateral migration when lying down, particularly on the right. ▶ Fig. 14.6 and ▶ Fig. 14.7 show severe bilateral rippling and lateral malposition (right breast worse than left). The importance of alternative views is shown, as the rippling is exaggerated by bending forward and there is exaggeration of the displacement in the supine position.

In view of her severe rippling and wrinkling, treatment consisted of exchange of saline for silicone implants and capsulorrhaphies reinforced with AlloDerm, as previously described for Case 1. Postoperative pictures are shown in ▶ Fig. 14.8.

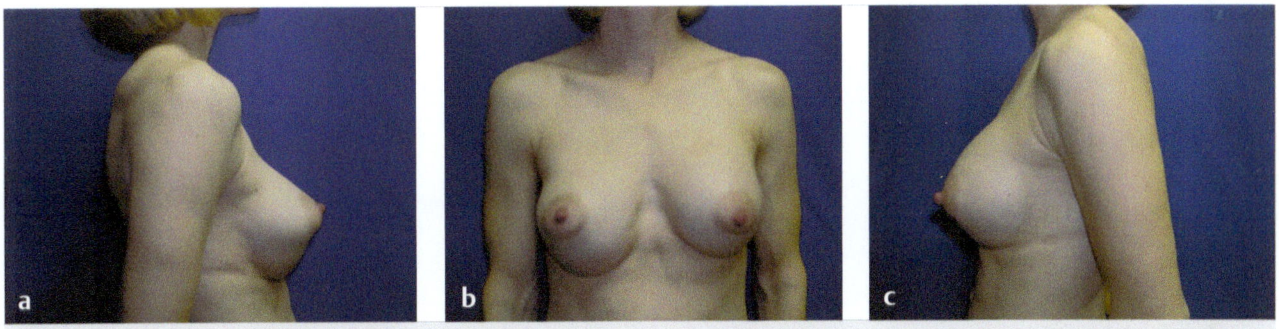

Fig. 14.4 (a–c) Case 1. A 37-year-old woman with history of two previous augmentation mammaplasties. Preoperative photos demonstrate inframammary fold malposition in standing anterior and lateral views.

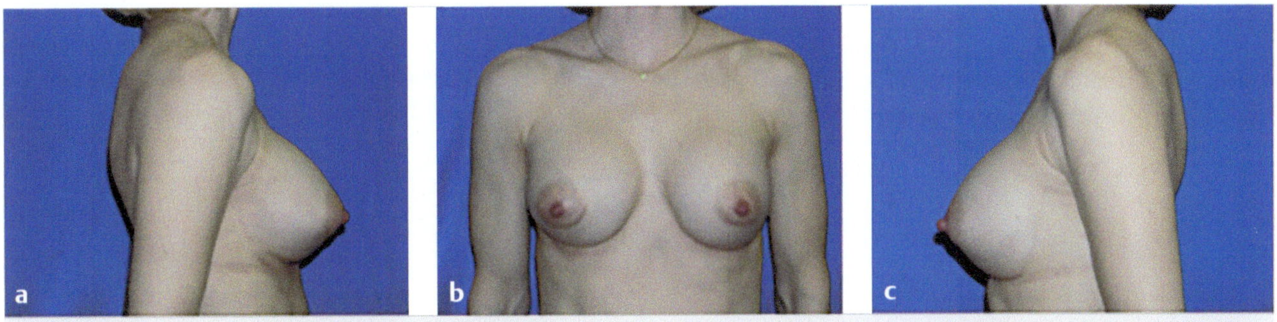

Fig. 14.5 (a–c) Case 1. A 37-year-old woman with history of two previous augmentation mammaplasties. Postoperative anterior and lateral standing photos show improvement of the inframammary fold malposition.

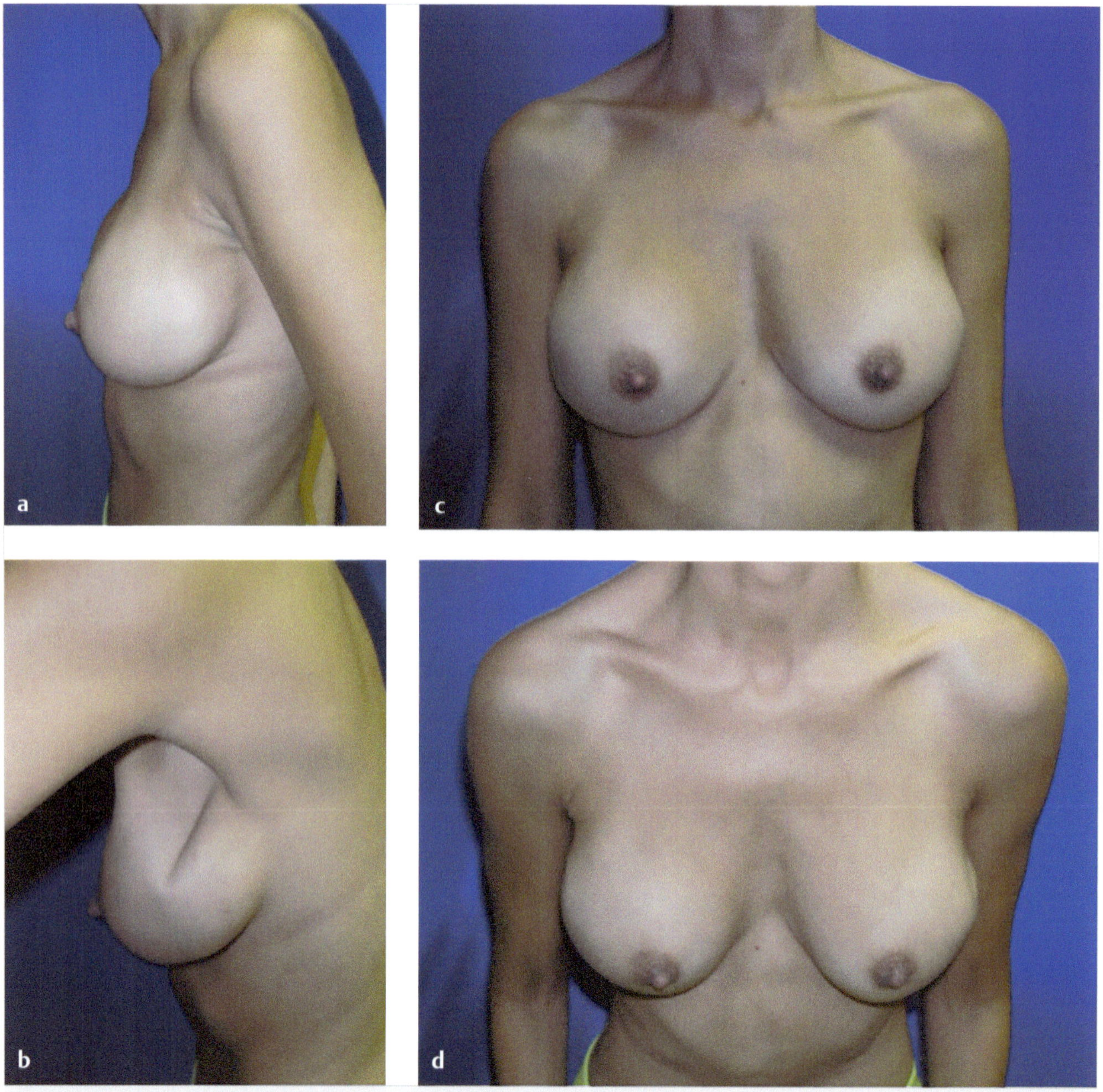

Fig. 14.6 Case 2. A 47-year-old woman who presented with rippling 10 years after breast augmentation. Preoperative photos shown: **(a,b)** lateral standing and bending forward, **(c,d)** anterior standing and bending forward. In both, the rippling is exaggerated by bending forward.

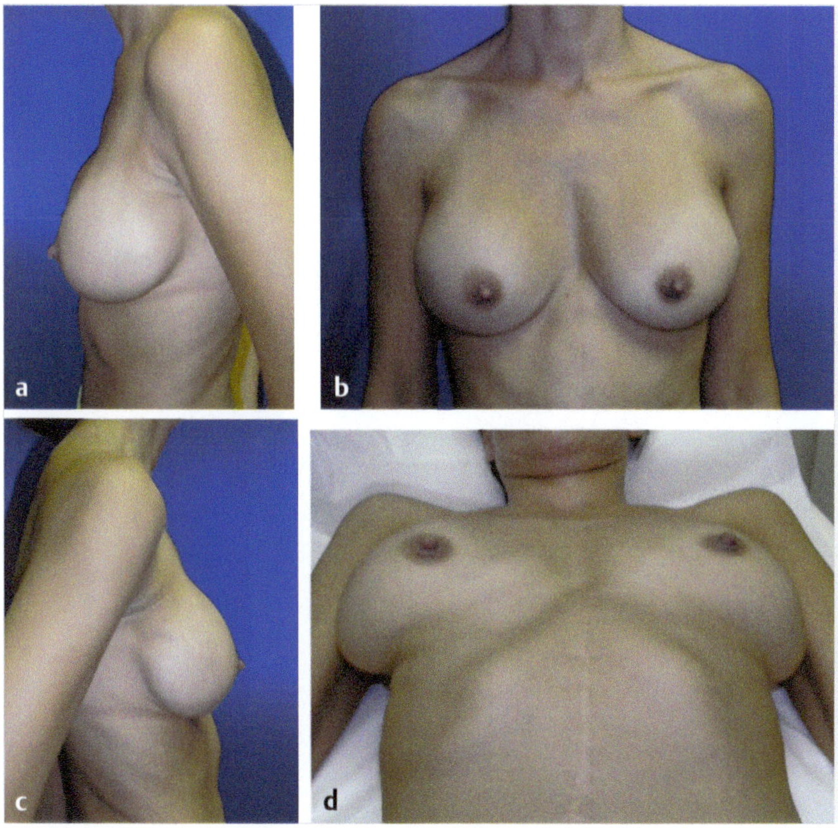

Fig. 14.7 Case 2. A 47-year-old woman who presented with rippling 10 years after breast augmentation. Preoperative photos shown: **(a,c)** lateral, **(b)** anterior, and **(d)** supine. Lateral displacement is demonstrated on supine positioning.

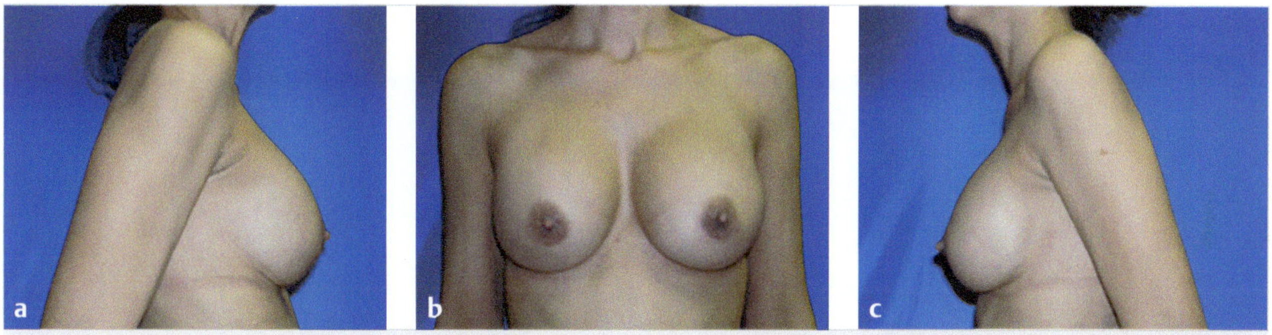

Fig. 14.8 Case 2. A 47-year-old woman who presented with rippling 10 years after breast augmentation. Postoperative photos shown: **(a,c)** lateral and **(b)** anterior views.

14.4 Conclusion

The management of secondary breast deformity in the augmented patient can be very challenging; understanding the etiology and exacerbating factors can help to set realistic revision surgery goals with patients. Preoperative planning and careful choice of management strategy can optimize outcomes.

Key Points

- Several factors contribute to implant malposition after primary breast augmentation. These factors include patient characteristics, implant selection, procedure selection, surgical technique, and postoperative management.
- It is important to recognize which factors are the primary causes of a particular implant malposition in planning correction of the deformity.
- Preoperative photos in multiple views are essential in preoperative planning.
- In patients with rippling, it may be advantageous to change the existing pocket, implant size, or implant type and also consider fat grafting as an adjunct.
- The adjustment of an existing pocket and the creation of a new pocket are both viable choices and must be weighed based on patient factors.
- Acellular dermal matrix has become an invaluable tool in reinforcing the inframammary fold and also capsulorrhaphy.

References

[1] Spence RJ, Feldman JJ, Ryan JJ. Symmastia: the problem of medial confluence of the breasts. Plast Reconstr Surg. 1984; 73(2):261–269

[2] Peters W. Iatrogenic disorders following breast surgery. In: Neligan P, Grotting JC, eds. Plastic Surgery, Vol. 5: Breast. 3rd ed. New York, NY: Elsevier Saunders; 2013:115–116

[3] Pozner JN, White JB, Newman MI. Use of porcine acellular dermal matrix in revisionary cosmetic breast augmentation. Aesthet Surg J. 2013; 33(5):681–690

[4] Gorney M. Ten years' experience in aesthetic surgery malpractice claims. Aesthet Surg J. 2001; 21(6):569–571

[5] Brown MH, Somogyi RB, Aggarwal S. Secondary breast augmentation. Plast Reconstr Surg. 2016; 138(1):119e–135e

[6] Maxwell GP, Gabriel A. Acellular dermal matrix for reoperative breast augmentation. Plast Reconstr Surg. 2014; 134(5):932–938

[7] Ricci JA, Driscoll DN. Removing the ambiguity from the double bubble. Plast Reconstr Surg. 2015; 136(6):864e–865e

[8] Chasan PE, Francis CS. Capsulorrhaphy for revisionary breast surgery. Aesthet Surg J. 2008; 28(1):63–69

[9] Harris R, Raphael P, Harris SW. Thermal capsulorrhaphy: a modified technique for breast pocket revision. Aesthet Surg J. 2014; 34(7):1041–1049

[10] Maxwell GP, Gabriel A. The neopectoral pocket in revisionary breast surgery. Aesthet Surg J. 2008; 28(4):463–467

[11] Tebbets JB. Dual plane breast augmentation: optimizing implant soft-tissue-relationships in a wide range of breast types. PRS. 2001; 107(5):1255–1272

[12] Ayeni OA, Ibrahim AMS, Lin SJ, Slavin SA. Acellular dermal matrices in breast surgery: tips and pearls. Clin Plast Surg. 2012; 39(2):177–186

15 Capsular Contracture and Biofilms—Etiology, Prevention, and Treatment

Pratik Rastogi and Anand K. Deva

Summary
The development of clinically apparent peri-implant capsular contracture can be a challenging problem, both for the patient as well as for the surgeon. In this chapter, the classification, pathogenesis, prevention, and treatment options will be discussed.

Keywords: capsular contracture, biofilm, extracellular polysaccharide (EPS) matrix, implant texturing, capsulectomy, capsulotomy, acellular dermal matrix

15.1 Introduction

Capsular contracture (CC) is a common but unpredictable complication following aesthetic and reconstructive breast prosthesis implantation. The reported rates of CC vary widely, ranging from 0.5% to 59%.[1,2] The heterogeneity of reported studies (implant type, surgical technique, and follow up period) precludes an accurate estimate of overall incidence. Nonetheless, CC is one of the commonest indications for reoperation in aesthetic breast surgery.[3] Moreover, revisional surgery is technically challenging, with poorer patient satisfaction.[4] This chapter aims to review the pathogenesis of CC formation with a focus on the subclinical infection theory, biofilm formation, and the implications of implant texturing and planes. The evidence for current nonoperative and operative strategies for CC will also be evaluated.

15.2 Classification

Although various classification tools have been proposed to score the severity of CCs, the Baker and Spear's modified Baker grading systems are the most widely used scales.[5,6] These classifications are simple grading systems that recognize clinical features such as implant visibility and firmness.

15.3 Pathogenesis

Several hypotheses have been proposed to account for the pathogenesis of capsular formation in prosthetic breast surgery (▶ Fig. 15.1).

15.3.1 Biofilm and Subclinical Infection Theory

Most bacterial species in nature exist in two different forms: free-floating *planktonic* form or as a sessile *biofilm*.[7] The preliminary stage of biofilm formation begins with the reversible attachment of planktonic cells to a surface, mediated by pili, flagellae, and van der Waals forces.[7,8] The bacterial secretion of extracellular polysaccharide (EPS) matrix, the hallmark of biofilm formation, contributes to irreversible adhesion of the microbes to the underlying implant surface. Following attachment, bacteria proliferate and continue to synthesize EPS matrix, resulting in the formation of highly structured microcolonies.[7,9] These microcolonies vary in pH, oxygen concentration, nutrient availability, and cell density. Sustained growth and differentiation of the microcolonies culminate in the formation of a mature biofilm community. Dispersion of biofilm cells through active or passive detachment may contribute to local extension over the implant surface.[7,8]

The biofilm architecture contributes to host resistance and survival advantages.[7,8] The EPS matrix serves as a diffusion block and mechanical barrier to antimicrobials and immune cells; the reduced metabolic activity of sessile bacteria increases antimicrobial tolerance; and the microarchitecture allows transfer of antimicrobial resistance genes carried on mobile genetic elements (plasmids).[7,8] The host immune response to the presence of bacterial biofilms and their associated antigens induces a prolonged and sustained inflammatory response. Although the recruitment of proinflammatory cells (macrophages and lymphocytes) and proteases aids in dislodging biofilms, they also damage normal tissue. The recruitment of macrophages and myofibroblasts within the chronic inflammatory milieu contributes to capsule formation.[8] Studies suggest that myofibroblast-driven centrifugal forces directly contribute to contracture formation around a prosthesis.[10,11]

Although biofilms are typically polymicrobial, a few species are overrepresented. *Staphylococcus epidermidis,* a normal constituent of skin and endogenous breast microflora, is the most frequently identified organism on breast implants removed because of CC.[12,13,14,15,16] Other bacterial species implicated in the formation of breast implant biofilms include *Propionibacterium acnes, Staphylococcus aureus, Bacillus, Escherichia coli, Mycobacterium* species, *Corynebacterium,* and *Lactobacillus.*[7,12,13,14,15] Potential microbial sources include contaminated implants, contaminated saline, poor surgical technique, and mammary duct disturbance, particularly with periareolar surgical approaches. The mammary ducts host bacterial colonies in more than 90% of cases.[17] Predisposing factors for late colonization include secondary seeding from bacteremia (e.g., dental source).[14] Rieger et al recently demonstrated a clear correlation between the degree of CC and the presence of bacterial biofilms on implant surfaces.[13] Interestingly, a recent study has confirmed high levels of bacteria in breast implant–associated anaplastic large cell lymphoma (ALCL) specimens, with a gram-negative shift in the microbiome as compared to the more traditional biofilm species detected in CC cases.[18]. The gram-negative profile has been implicated in the malignant transformation,[18] a distinction from the inflammation and fibrosis pattern observed in CC alone.

15.3.2 Implant Texturing

Two systematic reviews [19,20] have confirmed the protective effect of surface implant texturing on the rate of CC. These

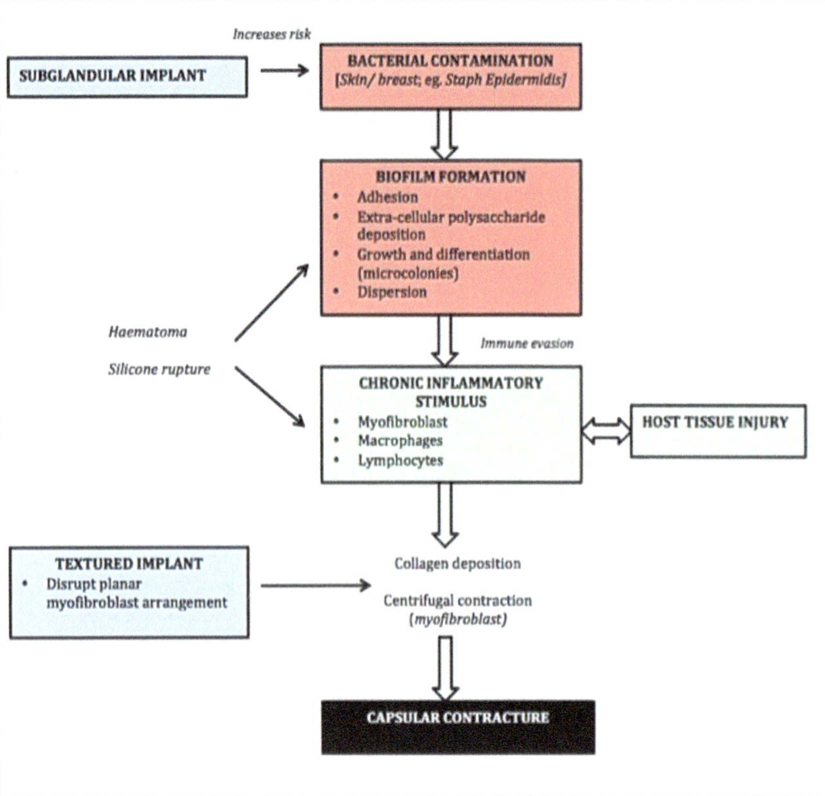

Fig. 15.1 Pathogenesis of capsular contracture. For simplicity, the complex interaction between textured implants and biofilm formation has been excluded.

studies collectively reported a greater incidence of CC in smooth implants (5–7 times) over a three-year follow-up period.[19,20] Brandt and colleagues[21,22] have theorized that smooth-surfaced implants experience increased contracture rates because they predispose to a planar arrangement of fibroblasts with organized collagen deposition and bridging synovial epithelium around implants, favoring CC formation. By contrast, as textured implants typically have grooves larger than the diameter of a fibroblast, the surface texturing causes the cells to anchor in deep and random patterns, disrupting any planar arrangement or centrifugal moment.[7,23]

The relationship between implant texturing and biofilm development is complex. Several in vitro studies have reported higher rates of biofilm formation in textured implants compared to smooth implants, given their greater surface area and enhanced bacterial adhesion on rough surfaces.[7,24,25,26] Contrastingly, Jacombs et al reported no significant difference in the rate of biofilm formation between smooth surface implants and textured surface implants following deliberate inoculation with human *S. epidermidis* in a porcine model.[26] The authors suggested that a threshold of biofilm load exists, which, once crossed, leads to significant potentiation of capsule formation, regardless of implant texturing. Despite this, the recent implication of textured implants and biofilms in the causation of ALCL warrants discussion. Loch-Wilkinson et al[27] proposed that the contamination of textured implants with biofilm leads to chronic antigen stimulation in genetically susceptible hosts, prompting the proliferation of mutant T cells into malignant clones.

15.3.3 Implant Position and Incision Choice

A recent meta-analysis demonstrated significantly higher rates of CC with periareolar (7.2%) incisions as compared to combined nonperiareolar approaches (inframammary and transaxillary; 3.1%).[28] Periareolar incisions increase the risk of transection of large end ducts, leading to implant contamination with intraductal material and subsequent biofilm formation. Arguably, the release of bacterially colonized material may continue until the transected ducts have healed and scarred. The impact of transaxillary approaches on CC formation has been variably reported. Previous criticisms of hematoma formation from blind transaxillary pocket dissection have been largely addressed through endoscopic assistance. Tebbetts reported a decrease in CC from 4.2% to 1.3% after adopting an endoscopic transaxillary technique.[29]

Moreover, implant pocket location also appears to have an impact on development of CC. Recent meta-analyses have reported that subpectoral implant placement is associated with a lower incidence of CC, as compared to subglandular implants.[19,20] It is hypothesised that this results from reduced exposure to endogenous glandular bacteria.

15.3.4 Other Factors

Postoperative hematoma formation, silicone breast implant ruptures, and radiation therapy preceding or following reconstruction with implants have all been in varying degrees implicated with the development of CC.[30,31,32,33]

15.4 Prevention

On the basis of increasing evidence supporting the subclinical infection theory and biofilm formation as a significant cause of CC, Deva et al[34] proposed a "14-point plan" to reduce the risk of prosthetic contamination at the time of implantation. These steps represent a codification of evidence to support bacterial mitigation strategies at the time of implant deployment. Since publication of the plan, an increasing number of surgeons and breast registries have supported the integration of these steps into their clinical practice. Many of the principles of the 14-point plan,[34] shown in Box 15.1 (p. 189), rely simply upon meticulous operative planning and aseptic surgical technique. However, the use of drainage tubes and pocket irrigation warrants a closer evaluation of existing scientific evidence.

Box 15.1 The 14-Point Checklist

1. Use intravenous antibiotic prophylaxis at the time of anesthetic induction.
2. Avoid periareolar incisions.
3. Use nipple shields to prevent spillage of bacteria into the pocket.
4. Perform careful atraumatic dissection to minimize devascularized tissue.
5. Perform careful hemostasis.
6. Avoid dissection into the breast parenchyma. The use of a dual-plane, subfascial pocket has anatomic advantages.
7. Perform pocket irrigation with triple antibiotic solution or povidone-iodine.
8. Use an introduction sleeve (Keller funnel, cut-off glove, povidone-iodine-impregnated drapes) to minimize skin contact with implant.
9. Use new instruments and drapes, and change surgical gloves prior to handling the implant.
10. Minimize the time of implant opening.
11. Minimize repositioning and replacement of the implant.
12. Use a layered closure.
13. Avoid using a drainage tube, which can be a potential site of entry for bacteria.
14. Use antibiotic prophylaxis to cover subsequent procedures that breach skin or mucosa.

15.4.1 Pocket Irrigation

Burkhardt and colleagues championed the use of povidone-iodine for breast pocket irrigation as a means of preventing subclinical pocket infection.[35,36,37] Following in vitro studies, Adams et al reported that pocket irrigation with triple antibiotic solution (cefazolin, gentamicin, bacitracin) with or without povidone-iodine was associated with low CC rates in primary aesthetic breast augmentation and implant-based breast reconstruction.[38,39] A systematic evaluation of routine antibiotic pocket irrigation is difficult, as most existing studies have a high risk of bias as well as significant clinical and methodological heterogeneity. Two recent studies, however, have shown a 10-fold reduction in capsular contracture following use of either antiseptic or antibiotic irrigation.[40,41]

15.4.2 Drainage Tubes

The theoretical argument for use of drainage tubes is to reduce the risk of hematoma formation, which may stimulate local inflammatory reactions and serve as a culture medium for microorganisms. Despite this rationale, closed suction drains provide a direct portal of entry for bacteria into the surgical site, increasing the risk of infection, biofilm formation, and CC.[2,42,43] Dower demonstrated biofilm bacterial contamination of drains as early as 2 hours postoperatively.[43] Araco et al reported a five-fold increase in the risk of developing an acute infection when drains were used, in a retrospective review of breast augmentation cases.[2] Similarly, Henriksen et al reported that use of drains increased CC by at least twofold.[42]

15.5 Management

15.5.1 Nonsurgical

No scientific consensus exists regarding the use of nonsurgical modalities in the management of established CC.

Leukotriene Receptor Antagonists

Leukotriene receptor antagonists (zafirlukast and montelukast) can reduce the severity of CC by modulating the inflammatory response to implant placement. Several clinical studies have demonstrated a reduction in Baker grading of CC with administration of zafirlukast (20 mg twice daily) for a period of 3–6 months.[44,45,46] Another study conducted by Mazzocchi et al demonstrated that mammary compliance declined following cessation of zafirlukast, suggesting that the long-term effect of the drug is contingent on persistent dosing.[47] Dosing must be counterbalanced against drug side effects (hepatic).[31] In regard to contracture prevention, a recent study conducted by Bresnick ($n = 1{,}122$ primary breast augmentation cases) reported that prophylactic use of zafirlukast (20 mg twice daily) for 3 months postoperatively was associated with significantly reduced CC rates compared with untreated patients (2.2% versus 5%) at 1 year of follow-up.[48] No statistical significant difference in CC rates was observed with prophylactic administration of montelukast. It is hypothesised that zafirlukast inhibits cysteinyl leukotrienes (LTC_4, LTD_4, LTE_4), suppressing their effects on macrophages and myofibroblasts.[48] Montelukast has a narrower spectrum of action (it does not inhibit LTC_4 or LTE_4), which may account for its reduced efficacy.[48]

Corticosteroids

Many papers have reported the use of corticosteroid injections (triamcinolone acetonide) in the management of established CC.[49,50,51,52] A study conducted by Sconfienza et al demonstrated that ultrasound-guided injection of 40 mg of triamcinolone acetonide in the peri-implant area of breasts with Baker grade IV CC was effective in reducing capsular thickness and patient discomfort, even in patients who had undergone adjuvant chemoradiotherapy.[52] Anecdotally, the risk profile of corticosteroid injections, such as soft tissue atrophy, discoloration, implant perforation, and infection, means that they are not routinely utilized by most surgeons.[53]

Other Modalities

Other studies have reported benefits of oral vitamin E supplementation[54,55] and ultrasound therapy[56,57] for management of established CC. Most of these studies reflect local institution-related practice, and limited clinical evidence exists to support their routine use.

15.5.2 Surgical

Revision breast surgery in augmentation mammaplasty presents particular challenges. In addition to CC, the thinned soft tissue interface and scarred breast envelope may contribute to ptosis and implant malposition. For most surgeons, the management principles of established CC involve a combination of capsulectomy, site change, and implant exchange in either an immediate or a staged approach.

Capsulectomy versus Capsulotomy

A systematic review conducted by Wan and Rohrich[4] reported that capsulectomy was associated with variable contracture recurrence rates (0–53%), similar to those observed with open capsulotomy (0–54%). Additionally, conflicting scientific evidence exists regarding the benefits of total versus partial capsulectomy.[4,58,59] Proponents for total capsulectomy argue that contracted capsules are colonized with biofilm and should be excised as completely as possible. Critics, however, argue that biofilms are only one aspect in CC formation, with negative bacterial cultures seen in up to 33% of contracted capsules.[4,12,14] Consequently, they argue that open capsulotomy alone may be effective in disrupting myofibroblast tension around the prosthesis. Given the inadequate scientific evidence, Box 15.2 (p. 190) highlights key principles in the surgical decision making for capsule management.[4,58,59,60,61,62]

Box 15.2 Management Principles for Capsulectomy (Partial versus Total) and Capsulotomy

1. Total capsulectomy may be attempted in the subglandular plane (provided adequate breast tissue exists). If the overlying gland is significantly atrophic, an anterior capsulectomy may compromise skin or cause distortion. In these cases, posterior capsulectomy alone may be performed.
2. Anterior capsulectomy is recommended in the subpectoral plane to avoid chest wall injury.
3. Thick, calcific, or granulomatous capsules should be excised to minimize breast distortion and prevent interference with future mammography.
4. In cases where capsulectomy (total/ partial) would excessively damage surrounding tissue (particularly with atrophic gland or pectoralis major), open capsulotomy (with or without radial scoring) is appropriate.

Change of Implant Site or Plane

Most surgeons strongly advocate change of implant site or plane at the time of revisional surgery to limit new periprosthetic scar formation and inflammation. Wan and Rohrich[4] reported that site change procedures (with limited or no capsulectomy) were associated with lower CC recurrence rates (0–12%) compared with no site change (0–54%). The vast majority of the studies included in the review used a neo-pocket as their method of pocket conversion, which is not representative of plane change in the traditional sense. Nonetheless, most surgeons agree that subglandular contractures are best treated with conversion to the subpectoral pocket or dual-plane technique.[4] Equally, most advocate staying in the submuscular plane to manage subpectoral contractures as well, with neo-pocket formation or limited capsulectomy.[4,63,64] Conversion to a subglandular plane is rarely preferred, as the overlying tissue is often inadequate and the plane naturally subjects the implant to a higher endogenous bacterial load.[4,19,20]

Implant Exchange

Most surgeons strongly advocate for implant exchange in revisional surgery. Wan and Rohrich[4] reported that implant exchange (with or without pocket change) was associated with lower CC recurrence rates (0–26%) compared to studies in which no implant exchange was performed (0–54%).

Acellular Dermal Matrices

Current literature suggests a potential role for acellular dermal matrices (ADMs) as a reinforcement in regions of atrophic breast tissue or at the site of the capsulectomy, where it acts an antigen-free barrier between the implant and breast tissue.[4,65,66,67,68,69]. The barrier is believed to dampen the host-foreign body immune response and reduce the risk of capsule formation. Basu et al[69] demonstrated significantly reduced chronic inflammatory changes, giant cell infiltrate, and capsule fibrosis in integrated ADM compared to implant capsules in a histopathologic study. Moreover, in their systematic review, Wan and Rohrich[4] reported that ADM was associated with consistently lower CC recurrence rates (0–7%), with a mean follow-up of 3 years. However, the short follow-up period and the confounding bias of concomitant site change or capsulectomy procedures in these studies mean that the true benefits of ADM placement are difficult to define exclusively. Consequently, indications for ADM use in revisional contracture management are evolving.

15.6 Conclusion

The role of biofilm formation and the subclinical infection theory in the pathogenesis of CC is well established. In genetically susceptible individuals who are preconditioned to a gram-negative microbiome, the chronic inflammation associated with biofilms may promote clonal proliferation of mutated T cells, implicated in the pathobiology of ALCL. Nonetheless, the sine qua non of CC prevention is meticulous aseptic technique and surgical planning (incision, implant type, and plane) as espoused by the 14 point plan.[34] Although nonoperative strategies such as leukotriene receptor antagonists (specifically zafirlukast) have being studied, their use is adjunctive in established CC at best. Revisional surgery in the management of CC is challenging. Surgical approaches have traditionally involved a combination of capsulectomy (partial/ total) and change of implant plane, pocket, or both as well as implant exchange. This recognizes the importance of biofilm eradication and the site change principle to limit periprosthetic scar tissue and inflammation. Although ADM use has potentially demonstrated some reduction in short-term CC rates, its current indications are evolving.

Key Points

- The host immune response to the presence of bacterial biofilms and their associated antigens induces a prolonged and sustained inflammatory response. Although the recruitment of proinflammatory cells (macrophages and lymphocytes) and proteases aids in dislodging biofilms, they also damage normal tissue. The recruitment of macrophages and myofibroblasts, within the chronic inflammatory milieu, contributes to capsule formation.
- Subpectoral implant placement is associated with a lower incidence of capsular contraction (CC) as compared to subglandular implants.
- Postoperative hematoma formation, silicone breast implant ruptures, and radiation therapy preceding or following reconstruction with implants have all been in varying degrees implicated with the development of CC.
- Management of CC include both nonsurgical (leukotriene receptor antagonists) and surgical options (capsulotomy, capsulectomy, implant exchange, change of implant size or plane, and use of acellular dermal matrix).

15.7 Disclosures

Prof. Deva is a consultant to Allergan, Mentor (Johnson & Johnson), and KCI. He has previously coordinated industry-sponsored research for these companies relating to both biofilms and breast prostheses. Dr. Rastogi has no affiliations or financial interests to disclose.

References

[1] Malata CM, Feldberg L, Coleman DJ, Foo IT, Sharpe DT. Textured or smooth implants for breast augmentation? Three year follow-up of a prospective randomised controlled trial. Br J Plast Surg. 1997; 50(2):99–105

[2] Araco A, Gravante G, Araco F, Delogu D, Cervelli V, Walgenbach K. A retrospective analysis of 3,000 primary aesthetic breast augmentations: postoperative complications and associated factors. Aesthetic Plast Surg. 2007; 31(5): 532–539

[3] Gabriel SE, Woods JE, O'Fallon WM, Beard CM, Kurland LT, Melton LJ, III. Complications leading to surgery after breast implantation. N Engl J Med. 1997; 336(10):677–682

[4] Wan D, Rohrich RJ. Revisiting the management of capsular contracture in breast augmentation: a systematic review. Plast Reconstr Surg. 2016; 137(3): 826–841

[5] Spear SL, Baker JL, Jr. Classification of capsular contracture after prosthetic breast reconstruction. Plast Reconstr Surg. 1995; 96(5):1119–1123, discussion–1124

[6] Baker J. Augmentation mammoplasty. In: Owsley JQ Jr, Peterson RA, eds. Symposium on Aesthetic Surgery of the Breast: Proceedings of the Symposium of the Educational Foundation of the American Society of Plastic and Reconstructive Surgeons, Inc., and the American Society for Aesthetic Plastic Surgery, Inc., held at Scottsdale, Arizona, November 23-26, 1975. St. Louis, MO: CV Mosby; 1978: 253–263

[7] Ajdic D, Zoghbi Y, Gerth D, Panthaki ZJ, Thaller S. The relationship of bacterial biofilms and capsular contracture in breast implants. Aesthet Surg J. 2016; 36 (3):297–309

[8] Clinton A, Carter T. Chronic wound biofilms: pathogenesis and potential therapies. Lab Med. 2015; 46(4):277–284

[9] López D, Vlamakis H, Kolter R. Biofilms. Cold Spring Harb Perspect Biol. 2010; 2(7):a000398

[10] Hwang K, Sim HB, Huan F, Kim DJ. Myofibroblasts and capsular tissue tension in breast capsular contracture. Aesthetic Plast Surg. 2010; 34(6):716–721

[11] Baker JL, Jr, Chandler ML, LeVier RR. Occurrence and activity of myofibroblasts in human capsular tissue surrounding mammary implants. Plast Reconstr Surg. 1981; 68(6):905–912

[12] Pajkos A, Deva AK, Vickery K, Cope C, Chang L, Cossart YE. Detection of subclinical infection in significant breast implant capsules. Plast Reconstr Surg. 2003; 111(5):1605–1611

[13] Rieger UM, Mesina J, Kalbermatten DF, et al. Bacterial biofilms and capsular contracture in patients with breast implants. Br J Surg. 2013; 100(6):768–774

[14] Schreml S, Heine N, Eisenmann-Klein M, Prantl L. Bacterial colonization is of major relevance for high-grade capsular contracture after augmentation mammaplasty. Ann Plast Surg. 2007; 59(2):126–130

[15] Virden CP, Dobke MK, Stein P, Parsons CL, Frank DH. Subclinical infection of the silicone breast implant surface as a possible cause of capsular contracture. Aesthetic Plast Surg. 1992; 16(2):173–179

[16] Galdiero M, Larocca F, Iovene MR, et al. Microbial evaluation in capsular contracture of breast implants. Plast Reconstr Surg. 2018; 141(1):23–30

[17] Mladick RA. Significance of Staphylococcus epidermidis causing subclinical infection. Plast Reconstr Surg. 2005; 115(5):1426–1427, author reply 1427–-1428

[18] Hu H, Johani K, Almatroudi A, et al. Bacterial biofilm infection detected in breast implant-associated anaplastic large-cell lymphoma. Plast Reconstr Surg. 2016; 137(6):1659–1669

[19] Wong CH, Samuel M, Tan BK, Song C. Capsular contracture in subglandular breast augmentation with textured versus smooth breast implants: a systematic review. Plast Reconstr Surg. 2006; 118(5):1224–1236

[20] Barnsley GP, Sigurdson LJ, Barnsley SE. Textured surface breast implants in the prevention of capsular contracture among breast augmentation patients: a meta-analysis of randomized controlled trials. Plast Reconstr Surg. 2006; 117(7):2182–2190

[21] Barr S, Hill E, Bayat A. Current implant surface technology: an examination of their nanostructure and their influence on fibroblast alignment and biocompatibility. Eplasty. 2009; 9:e22

[22] Brandt B, Breiting V, Christensen L, Nielsen M, Thomsen JL. Five years experience of breast augmentation using silicone gel prostheses with emphasis on capsule shrinkage. Scand J Plast Reconstr Surg. 1984; 18(3):311–316

[23] den Braber ET, de Ruijter JE, Smits HT, Ginsel LA, von Recum AF, Jansen JA. Effect of parallel surface microgrooves and surface energy on cell growth. J Biomed Mater Res. 1995; 29(4):511–518

[24] Myint AA, Lee W, Mun S, Ahn CH, Lee S, Yoon J. Influence of membrane surface properties on the behavior of initial bacterial adhesion and biofilm development onto nanofiltration membranes. Biofouling. 2010; 26(3):313–321

[25] Teughels W, Van Assche N, Sliepen I, Quirynen M. Effect of material characteristics and/or surface topography on biofilm development. Clin Oral Implants Res. 2006; 17 Suppl 2:68–81

[26] Jacombs A, Tahir S, Hu H, et al. In vitro and in vivo investigation of the influence of implant surface on the formation of bacterial biofilm in mammary implants. Plast Reconstr Surg. 2014; 133(4):471e–480e

[27] Loch-Wilkinson A, Beath KJ, Knight RJW, et al. Breast implant-associated anaplastic large cell lymphoma in Australia and New Zealand: high-surface-area textured implants are associated with increased risk. Plast Reconstr Surg. 2017; 140(4):645–654

[28] Li S, Chen L, Liu W, Mu D, Luan J. Capsular contracture rate after breast augmentation with periareolar versus other two (inframammary and transaxillary) incisions: a meta-analysis. Aesthetic Plast Surg. 2018; 42(1):32–37

[29] Tebbetts JB. Axillary endoscopic breast augmentation: processes derived from a 28-year experience to optimize outcomes. Plast Reconstr Surg. 2006; 118 (7) Suppl:53S–80S

[30] Embrey M, Adams EE, Cunningham B, Peters W, Young VL, Carlo GL. A review of the literature on the etiology of capsular contracture and a pilot study to determine the outcome of capsular contracture interventions. Aesthetic Plast Surg. 1999; 23(3):197–206

[31] Chong SJ, Deva AK. Understanding the etiology and prevention of capsular contracture: translating science into practice. Clin Plast Surg. 2015; 42(4):427–436

[32] Hölmich LR, Lipworth L, McLaughlin JK, Friis S. Breast implant rupture and connective tissue disease: a review of the literature. Plast Reconstr Surg. 2007; 120(7) Suppl 1:62S–69S

[33] McCarthy CM, Pusic AL, Disa JJ, McCormick BL, Montgomery LL, Cordeiro PG. Unilateral postoperative chest wall radiotherapy in bilateral tissue expander/implant reconstruction patients: a prospective outcomes analysis. Plast Reconstr Surg. 2005; 116(6):1642–1647
[34] Deva AK, Adams WP, Jr, Vickery K. The role of bacterial biofilms in device-associated infection. Plast Reconstr Surg. 2013; 132(5):1319–1328
[35] Burkhardt BR, Demas CP. The effect of Siltex texturing and povidone-iodine irrigation on capsular contracture around saline inflatable breast implants. Plast Reconstr Surg. 1994; 93(1):123–128, discussion 129––130
[36] Burkhardt BR, Eades E. The effect of Biocell texturing and povidone-iodine irrigation on capsular contracture around saline-inflatable breast implants. Plast Reconstr Surg. 1995; 96(6):1317–1325
[37] Burkhardt BR, Fried M, Schnur PL, Tofield JJ. Capsules, infection, and intraluminal antibiotics. Plast Reconstr Surg. 1981; 68(1):43–49
[38] Adams WP, Jr, Conner WC, Barton FE, Jr, Rohrich RJ. Optimizing breast pocket irrigation: an in vitro study and clinical implications. Plast Reconstr Surg. 2000; 105(1):334–338, discussion 339––343
[39] Adams WP, Jr, Rios JL, Smith SJ. Enhancing patient outcomes in aesthetic and reconstructive breast surgery using triple antibiotic breast irrigation: six-year prospective clinical study. Plast Reconstr Surg. 2006; 118(7) Suppl:46S–52S
[40] Blount AL, Martin MD, Lineberry KD, Kettaneh N, Alfonso DR. Capsular contracture rate in a low-risk population after primary augmentation mammaplasty. Aesthet Surg J. 2013; 33(4):516–521
[41] Giordano S, Peltoniemi H, Lilius P, Salmi A. Povidone-iodine combined with antibiotic topical irrigation to reduce capsular contracture in cosmetic breast augmentation: a comparative study. Aesthet Surg J. 2013; 33(5):675–680
[42] Henriksen TF, Fryzek JP, Hölmich LR, et al. Surgical intervention and capsular contracture after breast augmentation: a prospective study of risk factors. Ann Plast Surg. 2005; 54(4):343–351
[43] Dower R, Turner ML. Pilot study of timing of biofilm formation on closed suction wound drains. Plast Reconstr Surg. 2012; 130(5):1141–1146
[44] Scuderi N, Mazzocchi M, Fioramonti P, Bistoni G. The effects of zafirlukast on capsular contracture: preliminary report. Aesthetic Plast Surg. 2006; 30(5): 513–520
[45] Scuderi N, Mazzocchi M, Rubino C. Effects of zafirlukast on capsular contracture: controlled study measuring the mammary compliance. Int J Immunopathol Pharmacol. 2007; 20(3):577–584
[46] Reid RR, Greve SD, Casas LA. The effect of zafirlukast (Accolate) on early capsular contracture in the primary augmentation patient: a pilot study. Aesthet Surg J. 2005; 25(1):26–30
[47] Mazzocchi M, Dessy LA, Alfano C, Scuderi N. Effects of zafirlukast on capsular contracture: long-term results. Int J Immunopathol Pharmacol. 2012; 25(4): 935–944
[48] Bresnick SD. Prophylactic leukotriene therapy for the reduction of capsular contracture in primary silicone breast augmentation: experience with over 1100 cases. Plast Reconstr Surg. 2017; 139(2):379e–385e
[49] Caffee HH. Intracapsular injection of triamcinolone for intractable capsule contracture. Plast Reconstr Surg. 1994; 94(6):824–828
[50] Caffee HH. Capsule injection for the prevention of contracture. Plast Reconstr Surg. 2002; 110(5):1325–1328
[51] Caffee HH, Rotatori DS. Intracapsular injection of triamcinolone for prevention of contracture. Plast Reconstr Surg. 1993; 92(6):1073–1077
[52] Sconfienza LM, Murolo C, Callegari S, et al. Ultrasound-guided percutaneous injection of triamcinolone acetonide for treating capsular contracture in patients with augmented and reconstructed breast. Eur Radiol. 2011; 21(3):575–581
[53] Bachour Y, Verweij SP, Gibbs S, et al. The aetiopathogenesis of capsular contracture: A systematic review of the literature. J Plast Reconstr Aesthet Surg. 2018; 71(3):307–317
[54] Cook M, Johnson N, Zegzula HD, Schray M, Glissmeyer M, Sorenson L. Prophylactic use of pentoxifylline (Trental) and vitamin E to prevent capsular contracture after implant reconstruction in patients requiring adjuvant radiation. Am J Surg. 2016; 211(5):854–859
[55] Baker JL, Jr. The effectiveness of alpha-tocopherol (vitamin E) in reducing the incidence of spherical contracture around breast implants. Plast Reconstr Surg. 1981; 68(5):696–699
[56] Planas J. Prophylactic use of external ultrasound for breast implant capsular contracture. Aesthet Surg J. 2002; 22(2):205–207
[57] Planas J, Cervelli V, Planas G. Five-year experience on ultrasonic treatment of breast contractures. Aesthetic Plast Surg. 2001; 25(2):89–93
[58] Collis N, Sharpe DT. Recurrence of subglandular breast implant capsular contracture: anterior versus total capsulectomy. Plast Reconstr Surg. 2000; 106 (4):792–797
[59] Costagliola M, Atiyeh BS, Rampillon F. An innovative procedure for the treatment of primary and recurrent capsular contracture (CC) following breast augmentation. Aesthet Surg J. 2013; 33(7):1008–1017
[60] Lee HK, Jin US, Lee YH. Subpectoral and precapsular implant repositioning technique: correction of capsular contracture and implant malposition. Aesthetic Plast Surg. 2011; 35(6):1126–1132
[61] Spear SL, Carter ME, Ganz JC. The correction of capsular contracture by conversion to "dual-plane" positioning: technique and outcomes. Plast Reconstr Surg. 2006; 118(7) Suppl:103S–113S, discussion–114S
[62] Barbosa MV, Nahas FX, Ferreira LM. Capsulectomy: a mandatory procedure in the presence of capsular calcification. Plast Reconstr Surg. 2006; 117(5): 1654–1655
[63] Adams WP, Jr, Mallucci P. Breast augmentation. Plast Reconstr Surg. 2012; 130(4):597e–611e
[64] Rohrich RJ, Parker TH, III. Aesthetic management of the breast after explantation: evaluation and mastopexy options. Plast Reconstr Surg. 2007; 120(1): 312–315
[65] Hartzell TL, Taghinia AH, Chang J, Lin SJ, Slavin SA. The use of human acellular dermal matrix for the correction of secondary deformities after breast augmentation: results and costs. Plast Reconstr Surg. 2010; 126(5):1711–1720
[66] Hester TR, Jr, Ghazi BH, Moyer HR, Nahai FR, Wilton M, Stokes L. Use of dermal matrix to prevent capsular contracture in aesthetic breast surgery. Plast Reconstr Surg. 2012; 130(5) Suppl 2:126S–136S
[67] Maxwell GP, Gabriel A. Non-cross-linked porcine acellular dermal matrix in revision breast surgery: long-term outcomes and safety with neopectoral pockets. Aesthet Surg J. 2014; 34(4):551–559
[68] Maxwell GP, Gabriel A. Efficacy of acellular dermal matrices in revisionary aesthetic breast surgery: a 6-year experience. Aesthet Surg J. 2013; 33(3): 389–399
[69] Basu CB, Leong M, Hicks MJ. Acellular cadaveric dermis decreases the inflammatory response in capsule formation in reconstructive breast surgery. Plast Reconstr Surg. 2010; 126(6):1842–1847

16 Breast Implant–Associated Anaplastic Large Cell Lymphoma

Mark W. Clemens and Berry Fairchild

Summary

Breast implant-associated anaplastic large cell lymphoma (BIA-ALCL) is a rare peripheral T cell lymphoma that can develop after placement of a textured breast implant for either cosmetic or reconstructive purposes. BIA-ALCL most commonly follows an indolent course, with excellent prognosis when treated surgically in early-stage disease. On the other hand, disseminated cancer and deaths from BIA-ALCL have been reported, highlighting the importance of appropriate surveillance, early diagnosis, and prevention of progression to advanced disease through adequate treatment. Most commonly, BIA-ALCL presents approximately one decade after implant placement with capsule-confined disease, seroma, or less frequently as a mass adjacent to the implant. Standardized treatment regimens include surgical intervention with implant removal and total capsulectomy, which is the cornerstone of disease management. This chapter will review the clinical features, diagnosis, treatment, and prognosis of BIA-ALCL.

Keywords: breast implant-associated ALCL, anaplastic large cell lymphoma (ALCL), non-Hodgkin's lymphoma, CD30, late seroma

16.1 Introduction

Approximately 313,735 breast implants were placed in 2018 in the United States for cosmetic or reconstructive purposes, with more than 10 million women having breast implants worldwide.[1] The first case of breast implant–associated anaplastic large-cell lymphoma (BIA-ALCL) was reported in 1997.[2] Starting in 2011, the U.S. Food and Drug Administration (FDA) has published safety communications cautioning women with breast implants about the risk of BIA-ALCL.[3] Although BIA-ALCL commonly follows an indolent course and has an excellent prognosis when treated surgically, disseminated cancer and deaths from BIA-ALCL have been reported.[4] BIA-ALCL most commonly presents with localized disease, as a seroma (80%) or mass (40%) adjacent to an implant. Early diagnosis followed by appropriate surgical treatment prevents progression to advanced disease.[5] The purpose of this chapter is to review the clinical features, diagnosis, treatment, and prognosis of BIA-ALCL.

16.2 Classification

Lymphoma is a cancer of the immune system. Lymphoma develops from B or T lymphocytes, natural killer cells, or plasma cells and includes Hodgkin's lymphoma (10%), non-Hodgkin's lymphoma (NHL), multiple myeloma, and immunoproliferative diseases.[6,7] It is the most common malignancy of the blood, affecting up to one in 50 in the general population.[8] ALCL is a type of NHL characterized by large anaplastic lymphoid cells that express the cell surface protein CD30,[9] which is a marker for activated T cells, occurring normally on approximately 1–5% of circulating lymphocytes.

Peripheral T cell lymphomas comprise less than 15% of all adult lymphomas. Anaplastic large cell lymphoma (ALCL), a subset of peripheral T cell lymphoma, comprise less than 2% of all lymphomas. The 2016 revisions of the World Health Organization (WHO) classification of lymphoid neoplasms recognize three distinct lymphoma forms of ALCL: anaplastic lymphoma kinase (ALK)-positive systemic ALCL, ALK-negative systemic ALCL, and breast implant–associated ALCL (BIA-ALCL). Primary cutaneous ALCL (PC-ALCL) is recognized as a lymphoproliferative disorder. ALK expression is a result of the t(2;5) translocation involving chromosomes 2p23 and 5q35, creating an oncogenic fusion protein of the ALK gene and nucleophosmin gene.[10] BIA-ALCL does not express the ALK translocation and therefore is ALK-negative in all reported cases.

ALCL subtypes display variable degrees of clinical aggressiveness. Systemic ALCL typically follows a very aggressive course, rapidly evolving when left untreated. Most patients with systemic ALCL present with disseminated stage III or IV disease, commonly with systemic symptoms (B symptoms) and extranodal disease (40–60%). ALK positivity indicates a better prognosis.[11] BIA-ALCL does not express ALK.[12]

PC-ALCL tends to be clinically indolent and has excellent prognosis, with disease specific survival rates of 85% at 5–10 years.[13] Systemic spread is uncommon (approximately 5%); however, when present, the prognosis of PC-ALCL appears to be unchanged and favorable.[13,14,15] BIA-ALCL is classified as a lymphoma by the WHO despite less aggressive behavior. In early-stage disease confined to an effusion, BIA-ALCL is most similar to a lymphoproliferative disorder and likely becomes infiltrative in later stages with increasing mutational burden.

16.3 Pathogenesis

No clear etiology of chronic immune stimulation has been identified in BIA-ALCL. Proposed theories describing the pathogenesis of BIA-ALCL include chronic inflammatory response to particulate matter, presence of subclinical biofilm, induction after mechanical abrasion, and genetic predisposition. Deva, Prince, and colleagues propose a "unifying theory" that four primary factors provide impetus for inflammation, contributing to the malignant degeneration of ALCL: gram-negative bacterial biofilm, high surface area texturing, sufficient time of exposure, and host susceptibility by genetic predisposition.

16.3.1 Bacterial Biofilms and Inflammatory Response

Scientific observations support the biofilm hypothesis that textured implants harbor significantly higher levels of gram-negative bacteria, which correlate with lymphocyte activation.[16]

Bizjak et al proposed that in BIA-ALCL, chronic activation of local and systemic immune systems may cause neoplastic transformation. Polyclonal activation of T cells may result in monoclonal T cell expansion in a genetically at-risk host, ultimately leading to lymphoma.[17] In the context of chronic inflammation, host genetic factors influence the likelihood of malignant transformation.[18]

Deva and colleagues have shown that bacteria are significantly more likely to attach to textured implants. Textured implants develop a higher load of bacterial biofilm, and once a threshold biofilm is reached on both smooth and textured implants, propensity toward capsular contracture is potentiated.[19] Bacterial biofilm of patients with BIA-ALCL shows a microbiome with a predominance of gram-negative rods and the bacteria *Ralstonia pickettii*, in contrast to the microbiome in nontumor capsules, which is *Staphylococcus* spp. predominant.[20,21]

A link between bacterial biofilm and T cell hyperplasia has been demonstrated in both pigs and humans. Chronic biofilm infection of mammary prosthesis is associated with a T cell–predominant lymphocytic infiltration and bacterial load around an implant. In pigs, increased numbers of T cell–predominant lymphocytes were seen in textured implant capsules compared with smooth implant capsules.[22] Bacteria can be related to capsular contracture. Preliminary studies suggest that BIA-ALCL cells may be derived from Th1/Th17 cells in capsular tissues and seromas. Th1/Th17 are antigen-driven memory T cells, supporting the hypothesis that BIA-ALCL results from chronic bacterial antigen stimulation. BIA-ALCL displays a diffuse CD30 expression on the cell surface.[23] Investigations regarding whether select biomarkers (JunB, SATB1) will identify nonmalignant precursors of BIA-ALCL are pending.[24]

16.3.2 Texturing

Reported cases of BIA-ALCL almost exclusively involve textured implants.[25] As of September 30, 2018, the FDA had received 457 unique medical device reports of BIA-ALCL, with surface characteristics available for 334; of those, 310 (92.8%) were textured implants. Twenty-eight cases of BIA-ALCL following smooth implant reported to the FDA had either minimal or no clinical history and were therefore unreliable.[26,27] Out of 173 consecutive BIA-ALCL patients, all patients with known implant characteristics had a history of textured implants.[21]

Lista and colleagues reviewed adverse sequelae associated with textured implants including malrotation, capsular contracture, and late seroma and identified no cases of BIA-ALCL in 440 patients reviewed over 9 years,[28] but this sample size was inadequate to evaluate BIA-ALCL appropriately. The proposed incidence of BIA-ALCL ranges from 1 in 1,000 to 1 in 30,000 women with breast implants (see Epidemiology section), necessitating a larger sample population. While not intended to be an epidemiologic study, the prospective CA/CARE Trial reported by McGuire et al represents the largest prospective series ever reported on textured implants. This study revealed six cases of BIA-ALCL in 17,656 women, equating to an incidence of 1 in 2,943 women with textured Biocell breast implants (95% confidence interval: 1,350–8,000).[29]

Tribology is the observed effect of friction between two objects. Orthopedic implants have been hypothesized to increase carcinogenicity via tribology.[30] Brody suggests that the etiology of BIA-ALCL is likely multifactorial and that the textured surface may act as the inciting stimulus for BIA-ALCL mutation.[12] No investigation with relation to implants in BIA-ALCL has yet been reported.

16.3.3 Genetic Predisposition

Genetic predisposition may help explain the rarity of this condition. Blombery et al identified acquired activating mutations in *JAK1* and *STAT3* in two cases of BIA-ALCL, with a germline *JAK3* variant as a possible contributor to disease development. The aberrancy in the JAK1/STAT3 pathway supports the inflammatory model of pathogenesis and suggests that similar fundamental driving genetic lesions exist between BIA-ALCL and systemic ALK-negative ALCL despite clinical differences.[18] DiNapoli confirmed that mutations in JAK-STAT pathway genes occur in BIA-ALCL, identified *SOCS1* mutation for the first time in this disease, and identified *TP53* and *DNMT3A* mutations as additional somatic events.[31]

16.4 Epidemiology

BIA-ALCL is a rare disease with unknown exact incidence, most commonly presenting one decade after implant placement. The median age of onset of BIA-ALCL is 50 years old.[32] There is a very low absolute risk of developing BIA-ALCL, with a high relative risk in women with textured breast implants compared with the general population. An 18-fold higher rate of developing BIA-ALCL in the setting of breast implants has been reported.[33] Epidemiologic studies that fail to show an association between breast implants and lymphoma are limited by sample size and length of follow-up.[34,35,36]

One hundred thirty-nine case reports of BIA-ALCL were individually reported between 1997 and 2016, with a significant increase in reporting in 2011, reflecting increased physician awareness of the disease after the FDA safety communication.[37] As stated earlier, the FDA's Manufacturer and User Facility Device Experience (MAUDE) database contains 457 unique reports of BIA-ALCL through September 30, 2018.[27] Worldwide, 573 adverse event reports of BIA-ALCL had been reported to government authorities as of October 17, 2019.[38]

Cosmetic and reconstructive implants appear to be equally associated with BIA-ALCL risk. Risk has not been linked to implant type (saline versus silicone). However, BIA-ALCL has been reported almost exclusively with textured implants.[39] Comparing the number of textured implants sold to cases of BIA-ALCL, a lifetime prevalence of 1 in 30,000 is estimated, which is 67.6 times higher than primary ALCL in the general population.[40] In Australia, the Therapeutic Goods Administration estimated a BIA-ALCL disease risk between 1 in 1,000 and 1 in 10,000 women with textured breast implants.[41] The risk discrepancy between the United States and Australia may be due to discrepancy in physician reporting or geographic predisposition, and requires further investigation. Interestingly, the U. S. CA/CARE Trial, the largest published prospective textured implant study to date, reports a BIA-ALCL prevalence within the Australian estimated range (1 in 2,943 women with biocell implants).[29]

16.5 Disease Characteristics

Onset of BIA-ALCL ranges from 2 to 28 years after breast implantation, most commonly occurring between 7 and 10 years. Unilateral disease is much more common than bilateral disease, which occurs rarely, in approximately 4.9% of patients.[42]

BIA-ALCL initially arises as an effusion adjacent to an implant and then infiltrates into the luminal surface of the scar capsule.[43] Approximately 60–80% of patients present with a seroma surrounding the implant; 17–40% present with a mass. The presence of capsular contracture is both rare (8–10%) and possibly nonspecific for BIA-ALCL.[44]

16.6 Diagnosis

16.6.1 Symptoms

Standardized diagnosis and management guidelines for BIA-ALCL have been developed by the National Comprehensive Cancer Network (NCCN) (▶ Fig. 16.1). The finding of seroma presenting more than 1 year after placement of breast implants should raise concern and prompt investigation for BIA-ALCL.[45] Physical exam should include inspection and palpation of bilateral breast, axillae, neck and chest wall. The most common presentation of BIA-ALCL is a periprosthetic fluid collection or mass. Other symptoms include breast enlargement, skin rash, capsular contracture, and lymphadenopathy.[46]

16.6.2 Imaging and Diagnostic Tests

Ultrasound, the preferred initial imaging modality to investigate BIA-ALCL, can be used to define the extent of a fluid collection (sensitivity 84%, specificity 75%), identify masses (sensitivity 46%, specificity 100%), and evaluate enlarged regional lymph nodes. Magnetic resonance imaging (MRI) or positron emission tomography (PET) can be used if ultrasound is indeterminate. While a small volume of periprosthetic fluid may be normal, seromas should be investigated with fine needle aspiration (FNA). FNA can be performed under ultrasound guidance in a clinic setting or by interventional radiology. Seroma fluid should be aspirated for analysis, along with samples of the capsule and any suspicious masses, and should be sent for cytology. Immunohistochemistry and flow cytometry for T cell markers, specifically CD30 immunohistochemistry, is necessary to establish the diagnosis of BIA-ALCL.[46]

16.6.3 Pathology

Due to the rarity of the disease, communication with the pathologist is imperative and should include explicit directions to rule out BIA-ALCL. Pathologic examination should include cytologic examination of seroma fluid with cell block cytology, flow cytometry, and CD30 immunohistochemistry. Cell block cytology demonstrates anaplastic large cells, and flow cytometry demonstrates a single T cell clonally expanded population.[47,48]

If lymphoma diagnosis is indeterminate, additional hematopathologist consultation at a center with experience in this disease

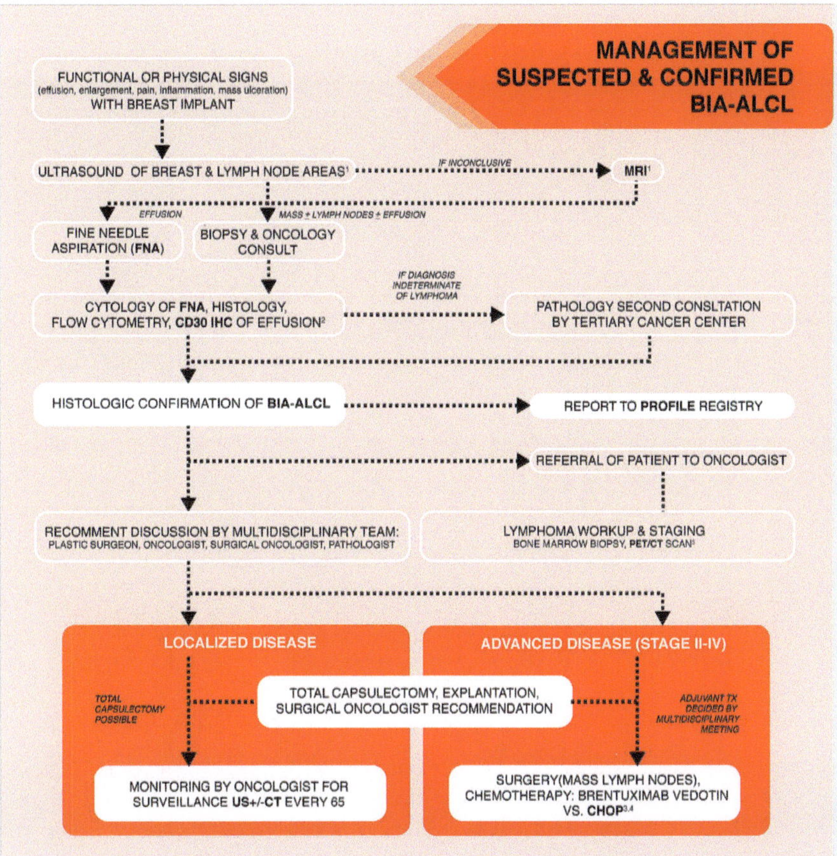

Fig. 16.1 Algorithm for diagnosis and treatment of breast implant–associated anaplastic large cell lymphoma following National Comprehensive Cancer Network (NCCN) guidelines. (Adapted from Clemens MW, Butler CE. ASPS/PSF efforts on BIA-ALCL. Plast Surg News 2015;26(7), 2015.)

should be pursued. If the pathology is negative, referral to a plastic surgeon for benign seroma management is suitable. When pathology is positive, referral to a lymphoma oncologist and surgical oncologist with complete workup and staging is indicated.

16.7 Staging

16.7.1 Staging Tests

Following pathologic confirmation of BIA-ALCL, a multidisciplinary team approach should be used. Routine lab tests include complete blood count (CBC), comprehensive metabolic panel (CMP), lactate dehydrogenase (LDH), hepatitis B, and pregnancy test. PET scan is the preferred modality to evaluate for systemic spread to regional lymph nodes and organ involvement in pathologically confirmed cases.[49] Staging is determined from a combination of imaging and pathologic findings at time of surgery and serves to distinguish localized from disseminated disease.

16.7.2 Staging Systems

The two staging systems used for BIA-ALCL are the Ann Arbor staging system and the MD Anderson (MDA) BIA-ALCL tumor–node–metastasis (TNM) staging system. The Lugano revision to the Ann Arbor staging system is a lymphoma staging, with Stage IE disease limited to a single extranodal site (i.e., breast or capsule) and Stage IIE defining spread to local lymph nodes.[50] Using this system, most patients are classified as having early-stage disease (83–84% Stage IE, 10–16% Stage IIE, versus only 0–7% with Stage IV disease).[40,44]

The MDA BIA-ALCL TNM staging system is modeled after the American Joint Committee on Cancer (AJCC) TNM system for staging solid tumors (▸ Fig. 16.2, ▸ Table 16.1). This TNM

Table 16.1 MD Anderson solid tumor TNM staging for breast implant–associated ALCL

TNM or Stage Designation	Description
T: tumor extent	
T1	Confined to effusion or a layer on luminal side of capsule
T2	Early capsule infiltration
T3	Cell aggregates or sheets infiltrating the capsule
T4	Lymphoma infiltrates beyond the capsule
N: lymph node	
N0	No lymph node involvement
N1	One regional lymph node (+)
N2	Multiple regional lymph nodes (+)
M: metastasis	
M0	No distant spread
M1	Spread to other organs/distant sites
Stage	
IA	T1N0M0
IB	T2N0M0
IC	T3N0M0
IIA	T4N0M0
IIB	T1–3N1M0
III	T4N1–2M0
IV	TanyNanyM1

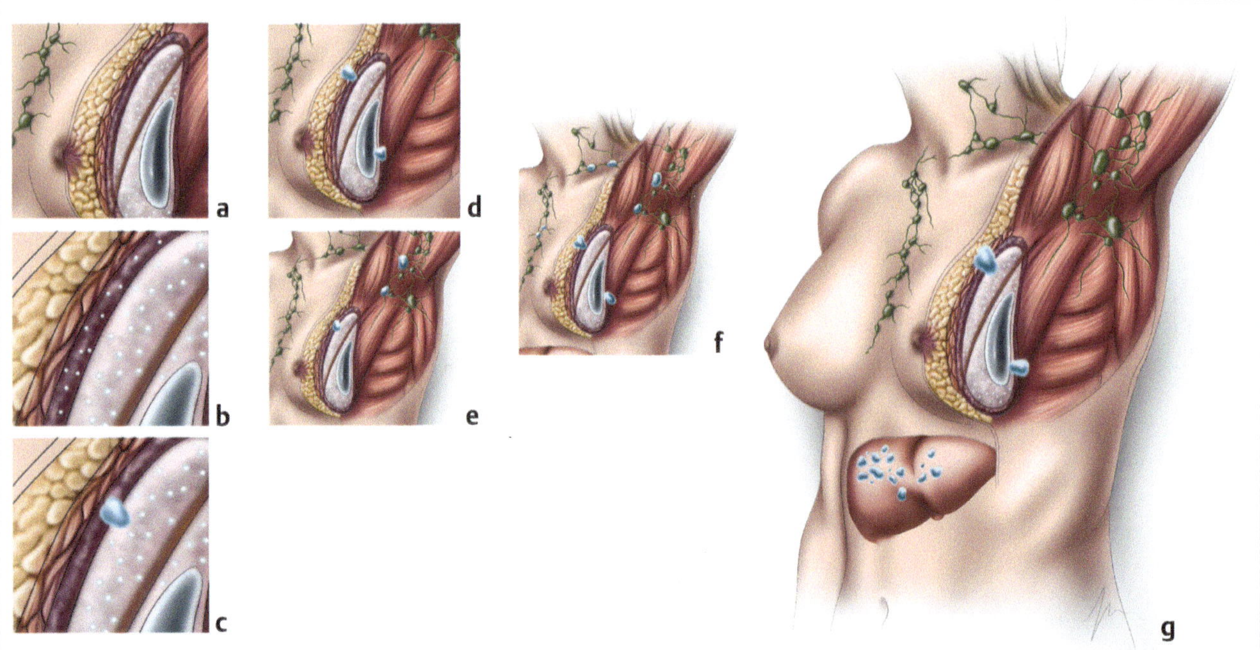

Fig. 16.2 (a-g) Clinical and pathologic staging of BIA-ALCL follows the MD Anderson Solid Tumor Staging System, modeled after the American Joint Committee on Cancer (AJCC) TNM (tumor–lymph node–metastasis) stages. (Adapted from Clemens MW, Medeiros LJ, Butler CE, et al. Complete surgical excision is essential for patients with breast implant-associated anaplastic large cell lymphoma. J Clin Oncol 2016;34(2):160–168.)

staging system may be more appropriate for patients who have BIA-ALCL, as this disease is more similar to other solid tumors than other lymphomas. Additionally, the MDA TNM staging system has been shown to be more accurate in predicting overall survival than the Ann Arbor lymphoma staging system.[51]

16.8 Treatment

16.8.1 Surgical Treatment

Treatment follows the established standardized guidelines, formulated on best available evidence-based approach by the NCCN.[45] All patients with BIA-ALCL should undergo surgical resection of the implant, total capsulectomy, and resection of any associated masses with negative margins. Oncologic technique should be employed, including specimen orientation, placement of clips in the resection cavity, and use of different instruments on each implant. In cases of bilateral implants, the contralateral implant and capsule should be removed to lessen the risk of recurrence or second contralateral disease.[44] There is no role for sentinel lymph node biopsy, as implants can drain into multiple lymph node basins. Excisional biopsies should be performed for clinically or radiographically enlarged lymph nodes, as 14% of such nodes are pathologically involved.[40]

Complete surgical resection provides definitive therapy and is curative in the majority (> 85%) of patients. BIA-ALCL has an estimated median overall survival of 13 years after complete surgical excision. Event-free survival was shown to be significantly higher with complete surgery (96%) than with limited surgery (40%) and adjuvant therapy (chemotherapy 76%, radiation 82%).

16.8.2 Chemotherapy

Optimal management of disseminated, persistent, or recurrent disease is less clear. For patients with localized disease (Ann Arbor stage IE, MDA TNM stage IA–IIA), no adjuvant chemotherapy or radiation is necessary. In patients with unresectable chest wall invasion or regional lymph node involvement (Ann Arbor stage IIE, MDA TNM stage IIB though IV), adjunctive chemotherapy is recommended.[45] Patients who fail surgical therapy alone or who have proven disseminated disease should be managed similarly as de novo ALK-negative systemic ALCL. Anthracycline-based regimens (CHOP: cyclophosphamide, doxorubicin, vincristine, and prednisone) are used as first-line therapy in advanced BIA-ALCL.[45] However, 32% of patients treated with systemic chemotherapy alone experienced disease recurrence, suggesting this treatment may be insufficient.[44]

16.8.3 Brentuximab Vedotin

Brentuximab vedotin is an anti-CD30 antibody–drug conjugate with a potential role in the treatment of BIA-ALCL. CD30 is an ideal pharmacologic target, highly expressed on malignant cells with limited expression in normal tissues. Phase I studies using brentuximab vedotin as a primary treatment of systemic ALCL display excellent response and manageable toxicity.[52,53] One case report demonstrated complete remission using brentuximab vedotin in the context of refractory disease for the treatment of BIA-ALCL.[54] No recurrences have been reported after treatment with brentuximab. NCCN guidelines allow for the administration of brentuximab vedotin as first-line therapy in place of an anthracycline-based regimen. Further research is needed to delineate its exact role.

16.8.4 Radiation

In one review of 60 patients, addition of radiation provided no significant benefit compared with surgical treatment alone.[40] There is no evidence to support routine radiation use for BIA-ALCL. Therefore, it is not recommended in cases of complete remission after appropriate surgical treatment. Radiation therapy has been used in locoregionally advanced, unresectable cases and is recommended by the NCCN for local residual or unresectable disease.[55]

16.8.5 Treatment Comparison

Treatment with complete surgical excision has shown better overall survival and event-free survival than treatment with partial capsulectomy, systemic chemotherapy, or radiation.[56] One review of 87 patients with BIA-ALCL compared different treatment regimens: surgery alone (40%), surgery and radiation (9%), surgery and chemotherapy (19%), surgery, chemotherapy, and radiation (30%), and chemotherapy alone (2%). ▶ Fig. 16.3 shows the survival curves according to treatment approaches and TNM staging.[44] ▶ Fig. 16.4 and ▶ Fig. 16.5 demonstrate pathologic confirmation and a patient treated with curative surgery, respectively.

16.8.6 Reconstruction

Replacement with textured implant is not recommended following definitive treatment for BIA-ALCL. Several patients have undergone immediate or delayed smooth implant replacement after BIA-ALCL treatment at the authors' institution, and while this appears to be an acceptable option, these patients are currently undergoing surveillance. No recurrences or progression of disease have been reported; however, long-term data on this population is not yet available.

16.8.7 Follow-Up

Patients should maintain clinical follow-up every 6 months for the 2 years following definitive treatment of BIA-ALCL, as recommended by multidisciplinary consensus reports.[57] Annual ultrasounds may be continued for at least 2 years, with the addition of chest/abdominal/pelvic computed tomography (CT) scans with contrast or PET scan every 6 months as clinically indicated.

16.9 Prognosis

Insufficient data regarding prognosis of BIA-ALCL is available. In general, with complete surgical resection, BIA-ALCL is an indolent disease with good prognosis. However, the presence of a mass lesion, extracapsular extension, or bilateral disease are indicators of worse prognosis. One retrospective review of 60 patients with BIA-ALCL showed a higher rate of complete remission in patients without a mass (93% of 42 patients) than in those with a mass present (72% of 18 patients).[40]

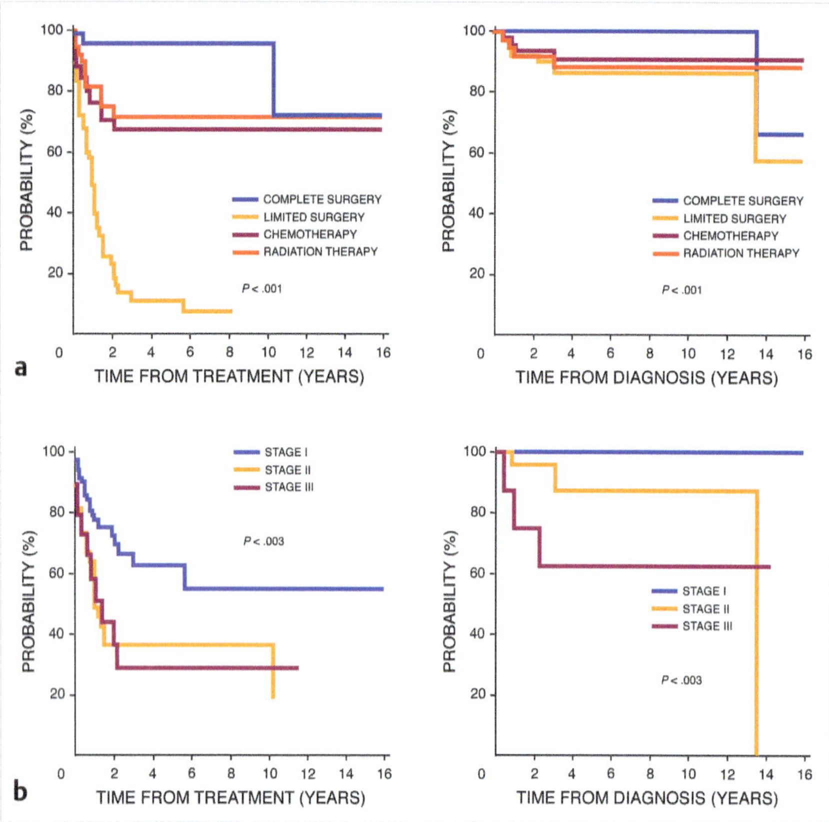

Fig. 16.3 Survival curves according to **(a)** treatment approach and **(b)** MD Anderson solid tumor staging. Event-free survival is shown at left, overall survival at right. (Adapted from Clemens MW, Medeiros LJ, Butler CE, et al. Complete surgical excision is essential for patients with breast implant-associated anaplastic large cell lymphoma. J Clin Oncol 2016;34(2):160–168.)

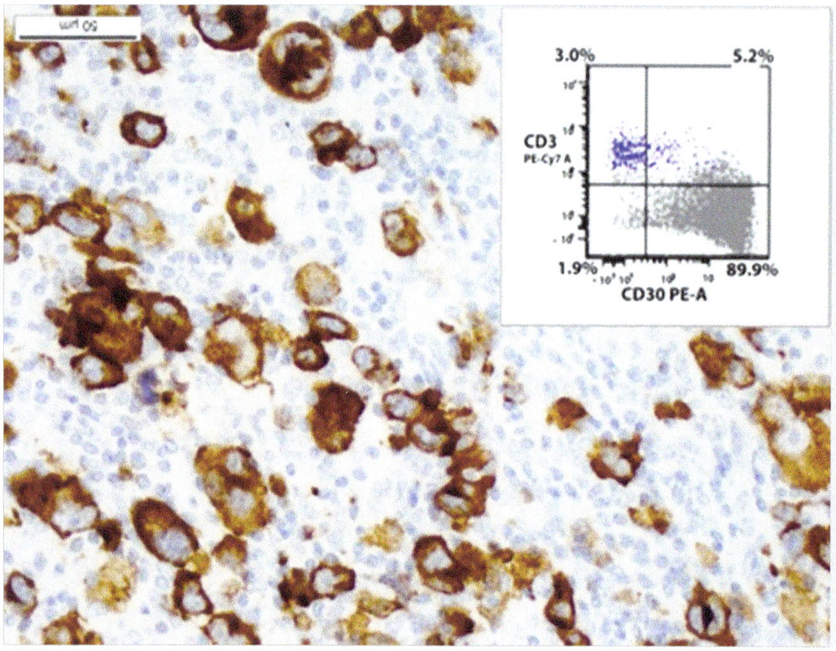

Fig. 16.4 A malignant effusion in a BIA-ALCL patient demonstrates large pleomorphic anaplastic cells with prominent horseshoe-shaped nuclei, and nuclear folding and strong diffuse CD30 reactivity by immunohistochemistry (CD30 immunohistochemistry with hematoxylin counterstain). Inset demonstrates a single T-cell clone on flow cytometry. Positive cytology, CD30 expression, and clonality demonstrated here are required for diagnosis.

While the majority of patients with BIA-ALCL have a relatively indolent clinical course, reports of death attributable to disease highlight the importance of timely diagnosis and appropriate surgical treatment. A case from our institution illustrates this. A 38-year-old woman who received bilateral breast augmentation with silicone implants for cosmesis in 1987 noticed a palpable mass in the left breast 9 years later. Subsequent FNA of the mass confirmed the diagnosis of BIA-ALCL (Lugano stage IE, MDA TNM stage IIA). There was no cutaneous involvement or systemic disease present at time of diagnosis. For cosmetic reasons, the patient refused surgery to remove her breast implants. She underwent CHOP chemotherapy followed by regional

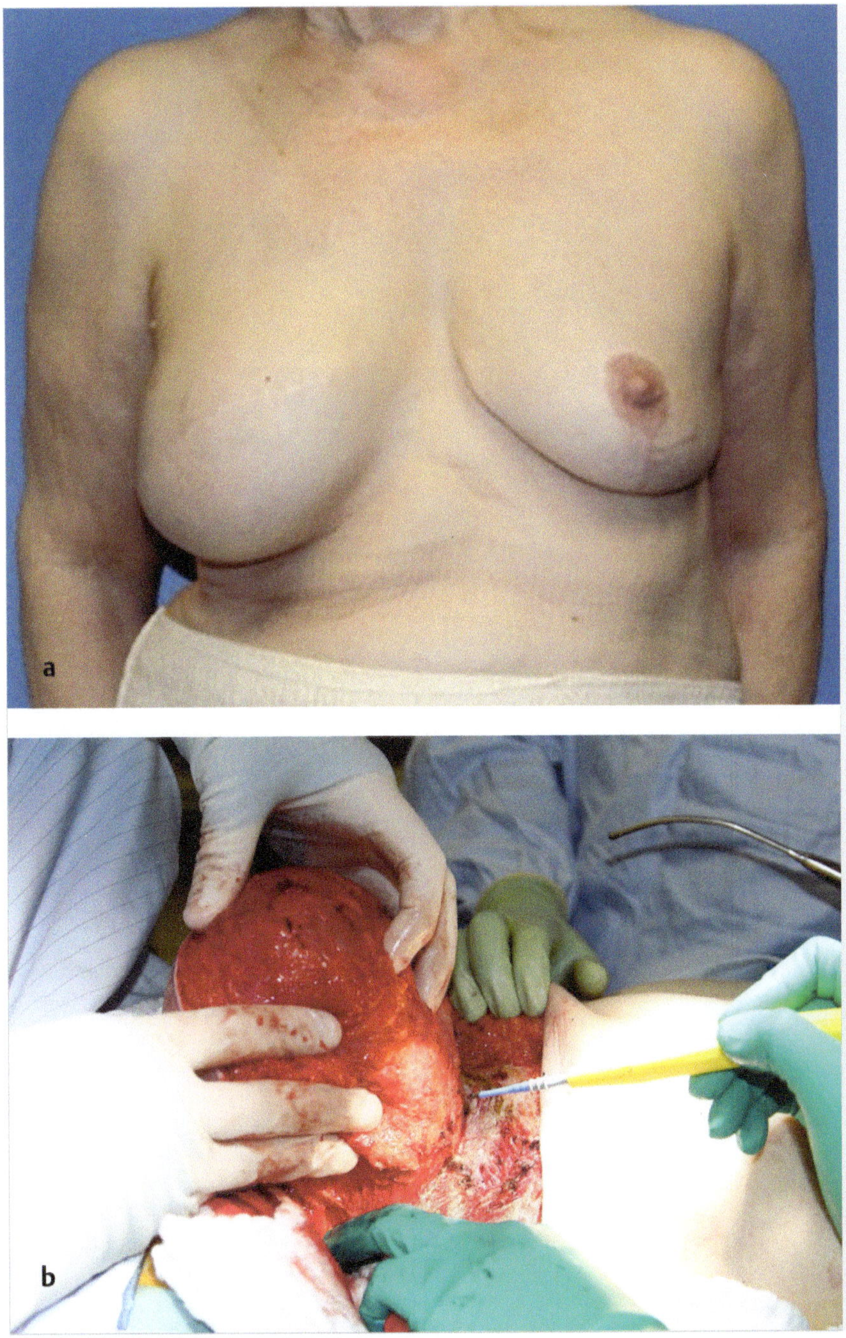

Fig. 16.5 A 77-year-old woman underwent postmastectomy prosthetic reconstruction for breast cancer in 2003. **(a)** Eleven years after implantation, she developed rapid swelling of the right breast, manifested as marked breast asymmetry. BIA-ALCL was diagnosed on fine needle aspiration. **(b)** Patient then received a total capsulectomy and implant removal.

radiation. The patient experienced recurrence of disease within 4 months of adjunctive treatment. Her disease rapidly progressed to involve the central nervous system, with meningeal disease and subsequent death.

This case emphasizes that the presence of a mass in BIA-ALCL is associated with a worse prognosis and that exclusion of adequate surgical treatment may change the disease course and outcome drastically. Surgery may be the difference between an indolent and potentially fatal disease. To date, 16 disease-related deaths have been reported worldwide, with the majority demonstrating significant delay in diagnosis or no surgical intervention.

16.10 Medical-Legal Considerations

16.10.1 Informed Consent

Package insert warnings regarding the existence of BIA-ALCL were added in the United States and Canada after the FDA made recommendations to implant manufacturers in 2011. The issue of informed consent becomes progressively apparent as awareness and understanding of the disease increases. Risk disclosure serves to respect patient autonomy and carries lasting consequences for both surgeon and patient. Informed consent should include both common (> 1 percent of procedures) and rare (< 1 percent of procedures), but serious, adverse events.[58] Inclusion of BIA-ALCL in consent for breast implant placement should increase as awareness of the disease increases. Informed consent examples have been developed by the American Society of Plastic Surgeons (ASPS) and are available on plasticsurgery.org.[59]

16.10.2 Screening

Sampling and pathologic review of effusions including CD30 immunohistochemistry are important to evaluate for malignancy and should be performed promptly when clinical concern for BIA-ALCL is present. Complications related to cosmetic breast implants may not be covered by insurance; therefore, patients may be less likely to undergo BIA-ALCL screening. A similar issue arises with regard to screening for breast implant rupture. In 2006, the FDA recommended that all women with silicone breast implants undergo MRI 3 years after implant placement to evaluate for failure (rupture). Lack of insurance coverage for this screening test decreased compliance.[60] This knowledge underscores the importance of physician involvement and identification of those needing BIA-ALCL screening.

16.10.3 Counseling Women with Breast Implants

In 2017 the FDA released an updated safety communication cautioning women with breast implants about BIA-ALCL.[1] Included are the following recommendations for counseling women with breast implants: they should get routine mammography, perform regular self-breast exams, and see a physician if changes occur. Women with breast implants may have an increased risk of developing BIA-ALCL in the capsule around the implant. BIA-ALCL most frequently occurs with textured implants and most typically presents with late seroma, but it may present with capsular contracture or masses. Screening and prophylactic implant removal are not recommended in asymptomatic individuals.[61]

16.10.4 PROFILE Registry

The FDA recommends that histologic confirmation of BIA-ALCL be reported to the PROFILE (Patient Registry and Outcomes for Breast Implants and Anaplastic Large Cell Lymphoma Etiology and Epidemiology) registry of the ASPS, a prospective registry and repository for BIA-ALCL data. As of December 2017, 184 unique cases had been reported. As part of a global network of plastic surgery societies, ASPS was aware of 489 unique cases worldwide and 16 disease-related deaths at that time. Using a registry of confirmed cases may help determine the exact role of breast implants in disease development, help elucidate the impact of genetic predisposition, and ascertain patient or implant modifiable risk factors.

16.11 Conclusion

BIA-ALCL is a rare CD-30-positive, ALK-negative peripheral T cell lymphoma associated with placement of breast implants for reconstruction or cosmesis. BIA-ALCL cases with reliable surgical histories are uniformly associated with textured implants. On average, the disease presents, about a decade after implant placement, with seroma or, less commonly, a mass adjacent to the implant. Periprosthetic effusions arising in a delayed fashion should be aspirated and screened for CD30. Surgery plays a pivotal role in the management of BIA-ALCL, heavily influencing outcomes. Understanding the biology of BIA-ALCL allows more targeted and effective therapies. NCCN guidelines include the most recent important advances in our understanding of the disease and should guide diagnostic approaches and therapeutic strategies. Improved physician awareness is imperative to optimize the management of patients with BIA-ALCL.

Key Points

- Breast implant–associated anaplastic large cell lymphoma (BIA-ALCL) is a relatively rare occurrence.
- Anaplastic lymphoma kinase is import in defining types of ALCL: anaplastic lymphoma kinase (ALK)-positive systemic ALCL, ALK-negative systemic ALCL, and BIA- ALCL. BIA-ALCL does not express the ALK translocation and therefore is ALK-negative in all reported cases.
- No clear etiology of chronic immune stimulation has been identified in BIA-ALCL. Proposed theories describing the pathogenesis of BIA-ALCL include chronic inflammatory response to particulate matter, presence of subclinical biofilm, induction after mechanical abrasion, and genetic predisposition.
- The biofilm hypothesis states that textured implants harbor significantly higher levels of gram-negative bacteria and *Ralstonia pickettii*, which correlate with lymphocyte activation.
- The onset of BIA-ALCL ranges from 2 to 28 years after breast implantation, most commonly occurring between 7 and 10 years.
- BIA-ALCL most commonly presents with localized disease, as a seroma (80%) or mass (40%) adjacent to an implant.
- Ultrasound is the preferred initial imaging modality to investigate BIA-ALCL. Seroma or mass should be evaluated with fine-needle aspiration (FNA) and sent for cytology testing for CD30 immunohistochemistry.
- Positron emission tomography (PET) scan is the preferred modality to evaluate for systemic spread to regional lymph nodes and organ involvement in pathologically confirmed cases.
- Surgical resection of the implant, total capsulectomy, and resection of any associated masses with negative margins are definitive therapy and curative in the majority (> 85%) of patients. The contralateral implant and capsule should be removed to lessen the risk of recurrence or second contralateral disease.
- CHOP (cyclophosphamide, doxorubicin, vincristine, and prednisone) is used as first-line chemotherapy in advanced BIA-ALCL. Brentuximab vedotin is an anti-CD30 antibody–drug conjugate with a potential role in the treatment of BIA-ALCL.
- There is no evidence to support routine radiation use for BIA-ALCL.

- Surveillance after definitive treatment includes annual ultrasounds for at least 2 years with the addition of chest/abdominal/pelvic computed tomography (CT) scans with contrast or PET scan every 6 months as clinically indicated.

References

[1] 2018 Plastic Surgery Statistics Report. American Society of Plastic Surgeons. URL: https://www.plasticsurgery.org/documents/News/Statistics/2018/plastic-surgery-statistics-full-report-2018.pdf. Accessed March 9th, 2020

[2] Keech JA, Jr, Creech BJ. Anaplastic T-cell lymphoma in proximity to a saline-filled breast implant. Plast Reconstr Surg. 1997; 100(2):554–555

[3] US Food and Drug Administration. Breast implant-associated anaplastic large-cell lymphoma (BIA-ALCL). URL: https://www.fda.gov/medical-devices/breast-implants/breast-implant-associated-anaplastic-large-cell-lymphoma-bia-alcl. Updated April 2, 2019. Accessed July 18, 2019

[4] Carty MJ, Pribaz JJ, Antin JH, et al. A patient death attributable to implant-related primary anaplastic large cell lymphoma of the breast. Plast Reconstr Surg. 2011; 128(3):112e–118e

[5] Kim B, Roth C, Young VL, et al. Anaplastic large cell lymphoma and breast implants: results from a structured expert consultation process. Plast Reconstr Surg. 2011; 128(3):629–639

[6] Clemens MW, Miranda RN. Coming of age: breast implant-associated anaplastic large cell lymphoma after 18 years of investigation. Clin Plast Surg. 2015; 42(4):605–613

[7] LaCasce AS, Ng AK. Hodgkin Lymphoma: Epidemiology and Risk Factors. UpToDate. URL: https://www.uptodate.com/contents/hodgkin-lymphoma-epidemiology-and-risk-factors Updated May 22, 2019. Accessed July 18, 2019

[8] National Cancer Institute. Adult Non-Hodgkin Lymphoma Treatment (PDQ®)–Patient Version. URL: https://www.cancer.gov/types/lymphoma/patient/adult-nhl-treatment-pdq. Updated June 14, 2019. Accessed July 18, 2019

[9] Stein H, Mason DY, Gerdes J, et al. The expression of the Hodgkin's disease associated antigen Ki-1 in reactive and neoplastic lymphoid tissue: evidence that Reed-Sternberg cells and histiocytic malignancies are derived from activated lymphoid cells. Blood. 1985; 66(4):848–858

[10] Morris SW, Kirstein MN, Valentine MB, et al. Fusion of a kinase gene, ALK, to a nucleolar protein gene, NPM, in non-Hodgkin's lymphoma. Science. 1994; 263(5151):1281–1284

[11] Jacobsen E. Anaplastic large-cell lymphoma, T-/null-cell type. Oncologist. 2006; 11(7):831–840

[12] Swerdlow SH, Campo E, Pileri SA, et al. The 2016 revision of the World Health Organization classification of lymphoid neoplasms. Blood. 2016; 127(20): 2375–2390

[13] Bekkenk MW, Geelen FA, van Voorst Vader PC, et al. Primary and secondary cutaneous CD30(+) lymphoproliferative disorders: a report from the Dutch Cutaneous Lymphoma Group on the long-term follow-up data of 219 patients and guidelines for diagnosis and treatment. Blood. 2000; 95(12):3653–3661

[14] Willemze R, Jaffe ES, Burg G, et al. WHO-EORTC classification for cutaneous lymphomas. Blood. 2005; 105(10):3768–3785

[15] Kim B, Roth C, Chung KC, et al. Anaplastic large cell lymphoma and breast implants: a systematic review. Plast Reconstr Surg. 2011; 127(6):2141–2150

[16] Deva AK. Reply: Chronic biofilm infection in breast implants is associated with an increased T-cell lymphocytic infiltrate: implications for breast implant-associated lymphoma. Plast Reconstr Surg. 2015; 135(6):1059e–1060e

[17] Bizjak M, Selmi C, Praprotnik S, et al. Silicone implants and lymphoma: The role of inflammation. J Autoimmun. 2015; 65:64–73

[18] Blombery P, Thompson ER, Jones K, et al. Whole exome sequencing reveals activating JAK1 and STAT3 mutations in breast implant-associated anaplastic large cell lymphoma anaplastic large cell lymphoma. Haematologica. 2016; 101(9):e387–e390

[19] Jacombs A, Tahir S, Hu H, et al. In vitro and in vivo investigation of the influence of implant surface on the formation of bacterial biofilm in mammary implants. Plast Reconstr Surg. 2014; 133(4):471e–480e

[20] Hu H, Jacombs A, Vickery K, Merten SL, Pennington DG, Deva AK. Chronic biofilm infection in breast implants is associated with an increased T-cell lymphocytic infiltrate: implications for breast implant-associated lymphoma. Plast Reconstr Surg. 2015; 135(2):319–329

[21] Brody GS, Deapen D, Taylor CR, et al. Anaplastic large cell lymphoma occurring in women with breast implants: analysis of 173 cases. Plast Reconstr Surg. 2015; 135(3):695–705

[22] Orofino N, Guidotti F, Cattaneo D, et al. Marked eosinophilia as initial presentation of breast implant-associated anaplastic large cell lymphoma. Leuk Lymphoma. 2016; 57(11):2712–2715

[23] Clemens MW, Miranda RN. Commentary on: CD30+T cells in late seroma may not be diagnostic of breast implant-associated anaplastic large cell lymphoma. Aesthet Surg J. 2017; 37(7):776–778

[24] Kadin ME, Deva A, Xu H, et al. Biomarkers provide clues to early events in the pathogenesis of breast implant-associated anaplastic large cell lymphoma. Aesthet Surg J. 2016; 36(7):773–781

[25] Doren EL, Miranda RN, Selber JC, et al. U.S. epidemiology of breast implant-associated anaplastic large cell lymphoma. Plast Reconstr Surg. 2017; 139(5): 1042–1050

[26] Srinivasa DR, Miranda RN, Kaura A, et al. Global adverse event reports of breast implant-associated ALCL: an international review of 40 government authority databases. Plast Reconstr Surg. 2017; 139(5):1029–1039

[27] US Food and Drug Administration. Medical Device Reports of Breast Implant-Associated Anaplastic Large Cell Lymphoma. URL: https://www.fda.gov/medical-devices/breast-implants/medical-device-reports-breast-implant-associated-anaplastic-large-cell-lymphoma. Updated April 2, 2019. Accessed on July 18, 2019

[28] Lista F, Tutino R, Khan A, Ahmad J. Subglandular breast augmentation with textured, anatomic, cohesive silicone implants: a review of 440 consecutive patients. Plast Reconstr Surg. 2013; 132(2):295–303

[29] McGuire P, Reisman NR, Murphy DK. Risk factor analysis for capsular contracture, malposition, and late seroma in subjects receiving Natrelle 410 form-stable silicone breast implants. Plast Reconstr Surg. 2017; 139(1):1–9

[30] Dunstan E, Sanghrajka AP, Tilley S, et al. Metal ion levels after metal-on-metal proximal femoral replacements: a 30-year follow-up. J Bone Joint Surg Br. 2005; 87(5):628–631

[31] Di Napoli A. Targeted next generation sequencing of breast implant-associated anaplastic large cell lymphomareveals mutations in JAK/STAT signalling pathway genes, TP53 and DNMT3A. Br J Haematol. 2016

[32] Lazzeri D, Agostini T, Bocci G, et al. ALK-1-negative anaplastic large cell lymphoma associated with breast implants: a new clinical entity. Clin Breast Cancer. 2011; 11(5):283–296

[33] de Jong D, Vasmel WL, de Boer JP, et al. Anaplastic large-cell lymphoma in women with breast implants. JAMA. 2008; 300(17):2030–2035

[34] Vase MØ, Friis S, Bautz A, Bendix K, Sørensen HT, d'Amore F. Breast implants and anaplastic large-cell lymphoma: a Danish population-based cohort study. Cancer Epidemiol Biomarkers Prev. 2013; 22(11):2126–2129

[35] Largent J, Oefelein M, Kaplan HM, Okerson T, Boyle P. Risk of lymphoma in women with breast implants: analysis of clinical studies. Eur J Cancer Prev. 2012; 21(3):274–280

[36] Brinton LA. The relationship of silicone breast implants and cancer at other sites. Plast Reconstr Surg. 2007; 120(7) Suppl 1:94S–102S

[37] Clemens MW, Jacobsen E. Breast Implant Associated Anaplastic Large Cell Lymphoma. UpToDate. URL: https://www.uptodate.com/contents/breast-implant-associated-anaplastic-large-cell-lymphoma Updated Feb. 19, 2019. Accessed July 18, 2019

[38] Groth AK, Graf R. Breast Implant-Associated Anaplastic Large Cell Lymphoma (BIA-ALCL) and the Textured Breast Implant Crisis. Aesthetic Plast Surg. 2020; 44(1):1–12

[39] Miranda RN, Aladily TN, Prince HM, et al. Breast implant-associated anaplastic large-cell lymphoma: long-term follow-up of 60 patients. J Clin Oncol. 2014; 32(2):114–120

[40] Doren EL, Miranda RN, Selber JC, et al. U.S. epidemiology of breast implant-associated anaplastic large cell lymphoma. Plast Reconstr Surg. 2017; 139(5): 1042–1050

[41] Australian Government, Department of Health: Therapeutic Goods Administration. Breast Implants and Anaplastic Large Cell Lymphoma: Update—TGA's review of textured breast implants and preliminary outcomes. URL: https://www.tga.gov.au/alert/breast-implants-and-anaplastic-large-cell-lymphoma. Updated July 11, 2019. Accessed July 18, 2019

[42] Bautista-Quach MA, Nademanee A, Weisenburger DD, Chen W, Kim YS. Implant-associated primary anaplastic large-cell lymphoma with simultaneous involvement of bilateral breast capsules. Clin Breast Cancer. 2013; 13(6):492–495

[43] Clemens MW, Medeiros LJ, Butler CE, et al. Complete surgical excision is essential for the management of patients with breast implant-associated anaplastic large-cell lymphoma. J Clin Oncol. 2016; 34(2):160–168

[44] Clemens MW, Horwitz SM. NCCN consensus guidelines for the diagnosis and management of breast implant-associated anaplastic large cell lymphoma. Aesthet Surg J. 2017; 37(3):285–289

[45] National Comprehensive Cancer Network. Clinical Practice Guidelines in Oncology (NCCN Guidelines) for Non-Hodgkin's Lymphomas. URL: https://www.nccn.org/professionals/physician_gls/f_guidelines.asp#nhl. Published 2017. Accessed August 3, 2017
[46] Jaffe ES, Ashar BS, Clemens MW, et al. Best Practices Guideline for the Pathologic Diagnosis of Breast Implant-Associated Anaplastic Large-Cell Lymphoma. J Clin Oncol. 2020
[47] George EV, Pharm J, Houston C, et al. Breast implant-associated ALK-negative anaplastic large cell lymphoma: a case report and discussion of possible pathogenesis. Int J Clin Exp Pathol. 2013; 6(8):1631–1642
[48] Wu D, Allen CT, Fromm JR. Flow cytometry of ALK-negative anaplastic large cell lymphoma of breast implant-associated effusion and capsular tissue. Cytometry B Clin Cytom. 2015; 88(1):58–63
[49] Adrada BE, Miranda RN, Rauch GM, et al. Breast implant-associated anaplastic large cell lymphoma: sensitivity, specificity, and findings of imaging studies in 44 patients. Breast Cancer Res Treat. 2014; 147(1):1–14
[50] Cheson BD, Fisher RI, Barrington SF, et al. Alliance, Australasian Leukaemia and Lymphoma Group, Eastern Cooperative Oncology Group, European Mantle Cell Lymphoma Consortium, Italian Lymphoma Foundation, European Organisation for Research, Treatment of Cancer/Dutch Hemato-Oncology Group, Grupo Español de Médula Ósea, German High-Grade Lymphoma Study Group, German Hodgkin's Study Group, Japanese Lymphorra Study Group, Lymphoma Study Association, NCIC Clinical Trials Group, Nordic Lymphoma Study Group, Southwest Oncology Group, United Kingdom National Cancer Research Institute. Recommendations for initial evaluation, staging, and response assessment of Hodgkin and non-Hodgkin lymphoma: the Lugano classification. J Clin Oncol. 2014; 32(27):3059–3068
[51] Clemens MW, Jacobsen ED, Horwitz SM. 2019 NCCN Consensus Guidelines on the Diagnosis and Treatment of Breast Implant-Associated Anaplastic Large Cell Lymphoma (BIA-ALCL). Aesthetic Surgery Journal. 2019; 39 (Suppl_1):S3–S13
[52] Vaklavas C, Forero-Torres A. Safety and efficacy of brentuximab vedotin in patients with Hodgkin lymphoma or systemic anaplastic large cell lymphoma. Ther Adv Hematol. 2012; 3(4):209–225
[53] Zinzani PL, Sasse S, Radford J, Gautam A, Bonthapally V. Brentuximab vedotin in relapsed/refractory Hodgkin lymphoma: An updated review of published data from the named patient program. Crit Rev Oncol Hematol. 2016; 104: 65–70
[54] Bartlett NL, Chen R, Fanale MA, et al. Retreatment with brentuximab vedotin in patients with CD30-positive hematologic malignancies. J Hematol Oncol. 2014; 7:24
[55] Estes CF, Zhang D, Reyes R, Korentager R, McGinness M, Lominska C. Locally advanced breast implant-associated anaplastic large-cell lymphoma: a case report of successful treatment with radiation and chemotherapy. Front Oncol. 2015; 5:26
[56] Clemens MW, Medeiros LJ, Butler CE, et al. Complete surgical excision is essential for the management of patients with breast implant-associated anaplastic large-cell lymphoma. J Clin Oncol. 2016; 34(2):160–168
[57] Kim B, Predmore ZS, Mattke S, van Busum K, Gidengil CA. Breast implant-associated anaplastic large cell lymphoma: updated results from a structured expert consultation process. Plast Reconstr Surg Glob Open. 2015; 3(1):e296
[58] Slovic P. Perception of risk. Science. 1987; 236(4799):280–285
[59] American Society of Plastic Surgeons. 2018 Informed Consent Kit—Breast, Body, Hand. URL: https://www1.plasticsurgery.org/shopping/product.aspx?id=27073&cat=7&to=shopasps Published 2018. Accessed July 18, 2019
[60] Chung KC, Malay S, Shauver MJ, Kim HM. Economic analysis of screening strategies for rupture of silicone gel breast implants. Plast Reconstr Surg. 2012; 130(1):225–237
[61] Aladily TN, Medeiros LJ, Amin MB, et al. Anaplastic large cell lymphoma associated with breast implants: a report of 13 cases. Am J Surg Pathol. 2012; 36 (7):1000–1008

17 Managing and Mitigating Risk in Aesthetic Breast Surgery

Michele Ann Manahan and Neal R. Reisman

Summary
This chapter is a brief introduction to medical and legal risks in aesthetic breast surgery, which have many components and are very complex. The chapter will address general essential aspects of medical legal risk mitigation, including comprehensive informed consent process recommendations. Additionally, practice management strategies to develop and sustain a successful cosmetic breast surgery practice are presented, such as revisional policy considerations. Specific circumstances to be considered, including augmentation mastopexy, anaplastic large cell lymphoma, capsulectomy/capsulorraphy, breast reduction, and fat injections, will also be highlighted.

Keywords: patient selection, informed consent, revision policy, practice management, augmentation mastopexy, capsular surgery, anaplastic large cell lymphoma, breast reduction, fat injections

17.1 Preoperative Considerations

17.1.1 Preoperative Consultation

A keyword in risk management is "foreseeability." Foreseeable risks should be determined individually for each patient and addressed with prospective patients as well as taken into consideration for treatment plans. The mitigation of foreseeable risk should, in fact, be considered a guiding principle for the bulk of clinical care.

17.1.2 Patient Selection

Avoiding risk begins with patient selection, and patient selection begins with thorough patient consultation, including conversation as well as physical examination. The informed consent process begins with exactly that: a process in which prospective patients explain their goals and expectations. This is then assessed through the physician's frame of reference, incorporating the history and physical examination findings. The ongoing interactions and dialogue between surgeon and patient refine these expectations and goals in an attempt to match the procedure most "foreseeable" in achieving those goals.

Some prospective patients are significantly unrealistic and convey unobtainable goals. Others may be unaware of or unable to express their true intentions. The keys are recognizing these observations and attempting to educate the patient about safe, reliable, and predictable goals. Some patients learn from prior consultations not to divulge their true intent for fear of being dismissed. While never guaranteed, direct emphasis on respect and honesty may help patients to disclose their true beliefs.

The ongoing process of complete informed consent, in contrast to the limited act of signing an "informed consent document," should continue over a period of time during which these dialogues occur to assess these necessary goals honestly. It is generally unwise to see a prospective patient one time and attempt to accomplish, assess, and disclose the informed consent process. Time must remain for questions and answers as well as contemplation to expose goals and expectations fully and to render a determination as to whether these are achievable.

Gorney and Martello have emphasized the importance of the intersection of patient deformity and patient concern, which can be very helpful in assessing patients' expectations. Prospective patients who have a notable deformity associated with a mindset of "Anything you can do, Doc, would be wonderful" are most acceptable from a patient selection standpoint. Conversely, the patient with a minimal, barely visible deformity associated with the mindset of "I cannot live, work, or enjoy any relationships until this is erased" is a poor candidate for surgery. Those in the middle of the spectrum present the biggest challenges for physicians to assess.[1]

17.1.3 Informed Consent

As just highlighted, informed consent is a *process* involving complete engagement of physician and patient, not merely the signing of pages that purport to reflect this process. Some prospective patients have seen many doctors and yet do not complete an acceptable process of informed consent. Completion of the informed consent documentation signifies that a balance between desiring an outcome and accepting the risks, timing, costs, and commitment to the procedure has been achieved. Specific legal standards apply to designation of appropriate informed consent. The options for standards applying to informed consent are (1) what a reasonable patient needs to know to make an informed decision or (2) what a reasonable physician feels needs to be explained for a patient to make an informed decision. States vary regarding which of these standards is used, and it is important to understand your state's medical practices law and what standard of informed consent is used.[2]

17.1.4 Patient Education

The process of informed consent is an important one, and the better understanding the patient achieves, the better choices are made. The burden of completion lies upon the physician. Effective education is a powerful tool in this endeavor. There are nine recognized learning styles described by Dr. Howard Garner. Three have achieved importance in understanding this process. It behooves the surgeon and his or her team to utilize these three in a discussion.

The first is *visual* learning. Many patients need to see results, photographs, schematics, or some demonstrative drawing to which they can relate. There are videotapes, booklets, and other sources supplying this information for the many procedures involved in aesthetic breast surgery. One must be cautious about using photographs (either of past results or computer-modified preoperative images) that create or imply a warranty that such result is what the prospective patient will achieve. Likewise, patients often bring in pictures from magazines and the Internet that may be helpful in determining their expectations, but these should not be made part of the medical record.

The second common learning style is *auditory*. Many patients would rather listen to a detailed story as an explanation about the procedure than look at images. This can often be combined with the third common learning style, *kinesthetic*. This establishes a personalized story or example to which the prospective patient can directly relate.

Consider the example of a prospective breast augmentation patient. Use of preoperative and postoperative photographs, diagrams of breast anatomy to demonstrate potential planes, videotapes of patient testimonials or even portions of the procedure, and booklets about the perioperative experience certainly provide visual information to the patient. The office team may explain in detail how decisions are made and how the surgery is accomplished as well as what to expect. The physician may employ the kinesthetic aspect by discussing with the prospective patient, for example, her thoughts and experiences during a prior pregnancy when her breasts enlarged to a DD cup size. This patient possesses her own built-in, personalized understanding of how her DD cup size was related to her current goals. The highest prospective patient retention and retention of information likely occurs when all three learning styles are seamlessly incorporated in the informed consent process.[3,4,5]

17.2 Practice Management Pitfalls

17.2.1 Team Approach and Responsibilities

The responsibility of informed consent lies finally with the operating surgeon. It is essential that the entire office team be consistent in messaging, and office staff may provide additional levels of information beyond the physician-patient conversation throughout this process. Surgeons often delegate education to patient coordinators, physician extenders, and nursing personnel, which may be appropriate, but this cannot replace the surgeon's primary and ultimate responsibility toward ensuring the adequacy of informed consent.

17.2.2 Documentation

The attempted complete documentation of the informed consent process can be onerous. Even with maximum effort, the medical record could never reflect the entirety of the patient–physician interaction. However, when conflict arises, the contemporaneously completed medical record can be a powerful protection.

17.2.3 Electronic Record

The digital age may provide assistance as well as potential problems as the record is created. The surgeon might remember lengthy discussions addressing risks, hazards, and choices while the record indicates 12 minutes spent in the exam room, implying brief visits in a hurried environment, causing concern should litigation arise. In addition, many digital electronic health records utilize "smart" text that is created by default and may or may not be correct. The busy surgeon may not take the appropriate amount of time to correct misstatements, thus creating an inappropriate record and implying slipshod practices or care. Given the quantity burden of automatic alerts meant to provide protections against medical mistakes, providers have been shown to be prone to overriding them, increasing their liability. Additionally, issues of concurrent or overlapping surgery may be demonstrated through review of time stamps and other information readily available in the medical record.[5,6,7,8,9]

17.2.4 Revisional Policies

Formally documented, discussed, and signed policies related to responsibilities for costs incurred with the initial surgery as well as for revision surgery, should it be necessary, are likely to be as important as clinical and informed consent documentation. Many approaches exist. One should consider whether the patient or the practice will bear the financial burden of unexpected laboratory and imaging testing (including pathologic review of breast tissue), inpatient admission, or other medical care should complications occur. This raises the question of how one might define a complication. Does an acceptable result but dissatisfied patient qualify? How unacceptable does the result need to be? If further operative procedures are considered, will professional fees be waived? Will the patient or the practice bear the facility and anesthesia fees? Will the patient be obligated to return to the practice for a discount? Who might pay for necessary care at another facility? One also might be able to include social media comment control when offering revision services, potentially waiving a surgical fee for a specific period of time in exchange for limiting social media comments.

17.3 Intraoperative Considerations

"Who, What, When, Where, Why, and How" represent important considerations related to operative considerations in aesthetic breast surgery. Patient scrutiny of the operative process is on the rise. Expectations for the experience of care are changing. Greater emphasis is now placed on *who* participates and *how who* does *what*. Those surgeons in academic practices must explain trainee competence, assistance, and involvement in care, while those surgeons in private practice must be prepared to do the same with physician extenders. Patients may expect to be aware of, for example, physician assistants or residents performing unsupervised incision closure.[10,11] Surgeons should also carefully consider *where* procedures are performed. It is important to understand accreditation for ambulatory surgery centers and accepted standards for types of patients treated and types of procedures performed in office space, ambulatory surgery centers, and hospital facilities.[12,13] Differences between hospital outpatient department and ambulatory surgery center fee structures may also be important for both the patient's and the surgeon's finances. The *when* and the *why* should be confirmed on the day of surgery. The preoperative preparation dictates the surgical planning, but confirmation of absence of change in clinical condition or expectation of outcome and arrangement of appropriate postoperative care and environment must occur just prior to the start of the procedure.

17.4 Postoperative Considerations

The proverb "There's many a slip 'twixt the cup and the lip" clearly applies to postoperative care in plastic surgery. Careful preoperative counseling and preparation (and documentation of such) regarding expected postoperative dressing, garment, and incision management, activity restrictions, time frames for changes, warning signs and symptoms of complications, and routine and urgent follow-up plans minimize patient questions and caregiver concerns and may even prevent complications. Tools to facilitate these processes exist in the form of printed instructions available from many sources.

17.5 Specific Risks Related to Breast Surgery

17.5.1 Tobacco Cessation

Smoking deserves a special precaution for breast reductions, breast lifts, and implant-based surgery. It is well accepted that nicotine use interferes with blood supply and can certainly negatively affect many aspects of breast surgery, promoting wounds, infections, and capsular contracture. In addition, many smokers cough with anesthesia, further creating possible difficulties in the early recovering period. Cardiovascular risk is also increased.[14,15,16]

Understanding how difficult it is to stop smoking should cause concern in the patient who too readily volunteers that she has quit. Many patients fail to disclose their continued smoking habit or getting secondhand smoke from another. The additional consent documents outlining the severity of complications related to smoking may be argued not to be enough to warrant proceeding. One could argue that a patient cannot consent to a negligent surgery, and the surgeon has a duty to protect the patient—sometimes from herself. Cotinine is a urine test that measures the presence of nicotine metabolites in the patient. It may be wise to establish this test before surgery and be cautious of proceeding if it is positive. This, however, remains an area of debate in plastic surgery.[17,18]

17.5.2 Breast Implants

There are a number of important considerations when implants are used. Liability can be noted when improper implant choices are made. Patients must be prepared for long term follow-up and maintenance procedures. Silicone consequences and anaplastic large cell lymphoma must be documented to be understood by the patients.

Implant Size and Profile

Dimensional planning, at least including chest measurements, may demonstrate quantifiable effort to assist the patient in development of proper choices of implants. Two common occurrences are noted when reviewing litigation cases. The first is choosing a high-profile implant with its inherent larger volume, leading to stretch deformity and malposition or ptosis. Critics may fault undesirable volume and blame the surgeon for undesirable results. The high-profile implant choice certainly has a place and should be associated with documentation in the medical record supporting that choice. There is a significant difference between a 500 mL moderate-profile and a 500-mL high-profile implant. The second is used in an attempt to position the breast higher on the chest. Patients with a longer chest height often seek a higher rest position with more cleavage, which can rarely be achieved. The higher-profile, larger implant choice may initially seem to achieve the goal, but because of its additional weight, the soft tissues stretch and it soon fails. As a result of the negligent implant choice, the plaintiff requires a mastopexy with its inherent scarring and still have a lower breast position on the chest, which would all have been avoided with proper implant selection. Understanding breast shape, size, and the relative influence of components of these on surgical options and outcomes may improve predictability of and satisfaction with results.[19,20,21]

The consultation associated with implant selection should be directly with the prospective patient and include a private discussion without other family or friend "stakeholders." There are many stories of a partner controlling the discussion, resulting in an inappropriately large choice. After surgery the boyfriend is gone, and now the practice has to interact with an unhappy patient. It has been said that "You earn your living from whom you operate on, but you earn your reputation from whom you don't."

Materials Management

It is wise to corroborate selected implant choices prior to administration of anesthesia and to ensure that implants will be in the operating facility prior to the day of surgery. It is prudent to order not only one size of implant but an appropriate range of sizes.

Implant Characteristics

Choices of implant shape, material, and shell may all translate into specific potential incurred liabilities. Patients must be aware of silicone-associated complications such as lymphadenopathy and granulomata, which may persist despite implant removal. Financing of implant imaging, such as magnetic resonance imaging (MRI) for silicone implant surveillance, should also be addressed preoperatively. Keeping up-to-date with U.S. Food and Drug Administration (FDA) recommendations for use of breast implants and maintaining proper required documentation associated with use of silicone implants is beneficial.[22]

Breast Implant–Associated Anaplastic Large Cell Lymphoma

In 2016, the World Health Organization officially recognized breast implant–associated anaplastic large cell lymphoma (BIA-ALCL) as a distinct disease from other ALCL entities, and it is known that deaths have occurred from this (see also Chapter 16). The presentation most commonly includes delayed seroma but may also include mass. Suggestions include heightened awareness of this rare but dangerous disease and familiarity with current recommendations for diagnosis (including aspiration of peri-implant fluid for CD30-positive and ALK-negative T lymphocytes), imaging workup, treatment (multidisciplinary care and complete bilateral capsulectomy with bilateral implant removal and consideration of adjuvant therapies). Current plastic surgery literature supports inclusion of specific discussions regarding BIA-ALCL in the informed consent process.[23,24]

Specimen Management

Preoperative financial disclosures become particularly important when ALCL is being considered, as costs for cytology and fluid evaluation may be expensive. One should also consider preoperatively the level of comfort with breast tissue specimen disposal versus pathologic examination, which will increase costs. Patients should be aware preoperatively of these choices and plans.

17.5.3 Mastopexy

Mastopexy creates additional risks and concerns, whether performed alone or in conjunction with implant placement. The smoking concern is real and suggests strict compliance with not performing a mastopexy in a smoker. Further considerations with mastopexy involve continued laxity and stretch attendant on skin type. The dialogue should include predictions for continued bottoming and shape changes over time if skin quality is poor. Scars will stretch despite best care as the patient's genetic propensity will triumph. Relapse may not be as significant as initially seen, but it will occur. It is wise to have a specific, written revision policy to address recurrent stretch and expected changes, covering a future time period of years. This may include patient compliance with visits and recommended care in addition to a clear financial disclosure of future costs and over what period of time.

17.5.4 Autologous Fat Grafting

Fat injections where appropriate can assist in creating fullness in areas where an implant might not. This tool may also be used for augmentation without prosthetic material. As a newer technique with a history of concerns over imaging, as well as recent FDA interest in defining the meaning of and appropriate use of fat grafting, one should continue to follow developing practice standards carefully in this field. One might also expect that over time, certain fat harvest or processing techniques that are currently debated may show themselves to be better or worse than others. One could imagine that use of outdated techniques, which may have been acceptable only a short time before in a rapidly changing field, would predispose to liability.[25,26,27,28,29]

17.5.5 Reduction Mammaplasty

Technique

Many of the procedure-specific concerns pertinent to mastopexy apply equally to reduction mammaplasty including smoking, scarring, planning for skin type, and relapse. Additionally, expected shape changes and changes to areola size should be addressed preoperatively. The potential for nipple graft or nipple loss must be addressed. Patient expectation for breast position changes that are not a component of this type of surgery must be elucidated and addressed. The surgeon should consider whether removal of lateral chest wall tissue beyond the anatomic margins of the breast will routinely be included in the reduction approach. If not, this may be specifically discussed with the patient in advance to avoid postoperative concern over imbalance and irregular contour between breast and lateral chest. Additionally, the difficulty of quantifying breast size and managing acceptance of postoperative results related to this must be addressed with patients in forthright ways.[30,31]

Insurance Coverage

Patient goals in reduction mammaplasty range from those equivalent to aesthetic mastopexy to acceptance of possible deformity or dysfunction, particularly of the nipple, to an attempt to reduce symptomatic burden associated with gigantomastia. Insurance criteria for payment vary and may include preoperative conservative therapy requirements as well as intraoperative minimums for resected weight. The surgeon must be aware of existing insurance contract details and allowances for patient billing if payment is denied by insurance. These details must be declared to the patient in advance of final creation of the surgical plan.[30,31]

17.6 Conclusions

Overall, aesthetic breast surgery covers a wide range of procedures, which may be performed on a vast spectrum of patients with an even wider variety of expectations. Forethought and careful preparation, in concert with careful optimization of the patient–physician relationship through thorough and ongoing communication, fortified with careful, supportive documentation, will increase the "foreseeability" of the experience for all involved. With careful preparation, aesthetic breast surgery may become a reliable source of practice growth and a pillar of practice maintenance.

Key Points

- Avoiding foreseeable risks should be the basis of all clinical practice.
- Avoiding risks begins with patient selection; patients with significantly unrealistic expectations or who have minor deformities rather than enormous concerns are red flags.
- Informed consent is an ongoing process involving complete engagement of both physician and patient.
- Better understanding achieved by the patient aids in the informed consent process and leads to better decision making in the end.
- Patients demonstrate a variety of learning styles, including auditory, visual, and kinesthetic. These should all be utilized in educating a patient.
- A careful discussion of the "who, what, when, where, why and how" of a procedure should be discussed in detail preoperatively.

- Formally documented, discussed, and signed policies related to responsibilities for costs incurred with the initial surgery as well as of revision surgery should be documented.
- Careful preoperative counseling and preparation regarding expected postoperative care is essential for patient satisfaction.

References

[1] Gorney M, Martello J. Patient selection criteria. Clin Plast Surg. 1999; 26(1): 37–40, vi

[2] Raab EL. The parameters of informed consent. Trans Am Ophthalmol Soc. 2004; 102:225–230, discussion 230--232

[3] Leeb D, Bowers DG, Jr, Lynch JB. Observations on the myth of "informed consent.". Plast Reconstr Surg. 1976; 58(3):280–282

[4] Godwin Y. Do they listen? A review of information retained by patients following consent for reduction mammoplasty. Br J Plast Surg. 2000; 53(2): 121–125

[5] Hong P, Makdessian AS, Ellis DA, Taylor SM. Informed consent in rhinoplasty: prospective randomized study of risk recall in patients who are given written disclosure of risks versus traditional oral discussion groups. J Otolaryngol Head Neck Surg. 2009; 38(3):369–374

[6] Troxel DB. Analysis of EHR contributing factors in medical professional liability claims. Mich Med. 2015; 114(3):16–17

[7] Kreimer S. Avoiding an EHR-related malpractice suit. Med Econ. 2015; 92 (20):66–69

[8] Greenberg M, Ridgely MS. Clinical decision support and malpractice risk. JAMA. 2011; 306(1):90–91

[9] van der Sijs H, Aarts J, Vulto A, Berg M. Overriding of drug safety alerts in computerized physician order entry. J Am Med Inform Assoc. 2006; 13(2): 138–147

[10] Abelson J, Saltzman J, Kowalczyk L, Allen S. Clash in the name of care. The Boston Globe. October 25, 2015. URL: https://apps.bostonglobe.com/spotlight/clash-in-the-name-of-care/story/. Accessed July 19, 2019

[11] Mello MM, Livingston EH. Managing the risks of concurrent surgeries. JAMA. 2016; 315(15):1563–1564

[12] Haeck PC, Swanson JA, Iverson RE, et al. ASPS Patient Safety Committee. Evidence-based patient safety advisory: patient selection and procedures in ambulatory surgery. Plast Reconstr Surg. 2009; 124(4) Suppl:6S–27S

[13] American Society of Plastic Surgeons. Pathways to preventing adverse events in ambulatory surgery. Arlington Heights, IL: ASPS; 2011. URL: https://www.plasticsurgery.org/Documents/Health-Policy/Patient-Safety/patient-safety-2011-adverse-events-ambulatory-surgery.pdf Accessed July 19, 2019

[14] Manahan MA, Buretta KJ, Chang D, Mithani SK, Mallalieu J, Shermak MA. An outcomes analysis of 2142 breast reduction procedures. Ann Plast Surg. 2015; 74(3):289–292

[15] Blount AL, Martin MD, Lineberry KD, Kettaneh N, Alfonso DR. Capsular contracture rate in a low-risk population after primary augmentation mammaplasty. Aesthet Surg J. 2013; 33(4):516–521

[16] Nolan MB, Warner DO. Perioperative tobacco use treatments: putting them into practice. BMJ. 2017; 358:j3340

[17] Warner DO. Tobacco dependence in surgical patients. Curr Opin Anaesthesiol. 2007; 20(3):279–283

[18] Saboye J. Plastic reconstructive and esthetic surgery and tobacco, a legal approach. Ann Chir Plast Esthet. 2015; 60(1):e67–e70

[19] Hidalgo DA, Sinno S. Current trends and controversies in breast augmentation. Plast Reconstr Surg. 2016; 137(4):1142–1150

[20] Brown T. Patient expectations after breast augmentation: the imperative to audit your sizing system. Aesthetic Plast Surg. 2013; 37(6):1134–1139

[21] Hall-Findlay EJ. The three breast dimensions: analysis and effecting change. Plast Reconstr Surg. 2010; 125(6):1632–1642

[22] U.S. Food and Drug Administration. Breast Implants. URL: https://www.fda.gov/medical-devices/implants-and-prosthetics/breast-implants/ Updated April 2, 2019. Accessed July 19, 2019

[23] American Society of Plastic Surgeons. BIA-ALCL Physician Resources. URL: https://www.plasticsurgery.org/for-medical-professionals/health-policy/bia-alcl-physician-resources Updated July 12, 2019. Accessed July 19, 2019

[24] Clemens MW, Miranda RN, Butler CE. Breast implant informed consent should include the risk of anaplastic large cell lymphoma. Plast Reconstr Surg. 2016; 137(4):1117–1122

[25] Pinell-White XA, Etra J, Newell M, Tuscano D, Shin K, Losken A. Radiographic implications of fat grafting to the reconstructed breast. Breast J. 2015; 21(5): 520–525

[26] Khouri RK, Eisenmann-Klein M, Cardoso E, et al. Brava and autologous fat transfer is a safe and effective breast augmentation alternative: results of a 6-year, 81-patient, prospective multicenter study. Plast Reconstr Surg. 2012; 129(5):1173–1187

[27] Rubin JP, Coon D, Zuley M, et al. Mammographic changes after fat transfer to the breast compared with changes after breast reduction: a blinded study. Plast Reconstr Surg. 2012; 129(5):1029–1038

[28] Regulatory considerations for human cells, tissues, and cellular tissue-based products: Minimal manipulation and homologous use. https://www.fda.gov/regulatory-information/search-fda-guidance-documents/regulatory-considerations-human-cells-tissues-and-cellular-and-tissue-based-products-minimal. Accessed March 2, 2020

[29] Shim YH, Zhang RH. Literature review to optimize the autologous fat transplantation procedure and recent technologies to improve graft viability and overall outcome: a systematic and retrospective analytic approach. Aesthetic Plast Surg. 2017; 41(4):815–831

[30] Reisman NR. Medicolegal issues in breast reduction. Clin Plast Surg. 2016; 43 (2):441–444

[31] Frey JD, Koltz PF, Bell DE, Langstein HN. The complex insurance reimbursement landscape in reduction mammaplasty: how does the American plastic surgeon navigate it? Ann Plast Surg. 2014; 72(1):23–29

Part V

Easing the Transition to Technological Adoption

V

18 Evaluation and Surgical Management of Gynecomastia

R. Brannon Claytor and Joseph R. Spaniol

Summary

Gynecomastia is very common, with an incidence of up to 50–70% in the general population, and is thus one of the most common reasons for men to seek help from a plastic surgeon. The surgeon must be adept at the evaluation, workup, and surgical management of the disease. Given recent advances in technology, plastic surgeons have more in their armamentarium than ever before. This chapter reviews the disease process and recent evidence to modify the workup, and present a "reconstructive ladder" approach to gynecomastia, which will help the reader assimilate the new technologies into a more cohesive methodology.

Keywords: gynecomastia, pseudogynecomastia, male feminization, cryolipolysis, ultrasound-assisted liposuction, radiofrequency-assisted liposuction

18.1 Definitions and Epidemiology

Gynecomastia is defined as a benign proliferation of glandular tissue of the male breast. Pseudogynecomastia, often seen in obese men, refers to fat deposition without glandular proliferation. Gynecomastia is a relatively common entity, with a reported prevalence between one-third and two-thirds of the male population,[1,2] and occurs transiently in most infant males, 14–65% of adolescent males, and 57–72% of men aged 50–80 years.[3,4,5,6] It is most commonly bilateral, and it persists beyond 12 months in about 10–20% of males, at which time fibrosis occurs and regression is unlikely.[1,7,8,9] Gynecomastia can be quite anguishing and has been shown to disturb the mental and social health of adolescent and adult males.[10,11,12,13]

18.2 Etiology

Imbalances between estrogens, which stimulate mammary gland growth, and androgens, which inhibit it, are responsible for the pathologic changes that occur in gynecomastia. These imbalances can result from a multitude of systemic conditions (Box 18.1 (p.210)) and medications. It is important to note that many historical references identifying drugs as contributing to gynecomastia were based on poor-quality evidence, though medications have been found culpable in up to 25% of cases. A recent systematic review of drug-induced gynecomastia elucidates which medications are supported by the best data and clearest pathophysiology as causing gynecomastia.[14] These medications are summarized in ▶ Table 18.1.

Box 18.1 Pathologic Classification of Gynecomastia

- Increased serum estrogen
  - Increased endogenous production
    - Leydig or Sertoli cell tumors
    - Eutopic or ectopic human chorionic gonadotropin–secreting tumors
    - Adrenocortical tumors
  - Higher aromatization
    - Aging
    - Obesity
    - Hyperthyroidism
    - Liver disease
    - Familial or sporadic aromatase excess syndrome
    - Klinefelter's syndrome
    - Testicular tumors
    - Refeeding after starvation
  - Exogenous sources
    - Topical estrogen creams
    - Oral estrogen ingestion
  - Displacement of estrogen from sex hormone–binding globulin
    - Medications such as spironolactone and ketoconazole
  - Decreased estrogen metabolism
    - Cirrhosis
- Decreased testosterone synthesis
  - Primary gonadal failure
    - Trauma
    - Radiation
    - Drugs
    - Klinefelter's syndrome
    - Congenital anorchia
  - Secondary hypogonadism
    - Hypothalamic diseases
    - Pituitary failure
    - Kallmann's syndrome
  - Decreased androgen action
    - Androgen receptor defect
    - Antiandrogen drugs
- Miscellaneous
  - Chronic renal failure
  - Liver disease
  - Human immunodeficiency virus (HIV)
  - Chronic illness
  - Enhanced breast tissue sensitivity
  - Environmental agents
    - Embalming agents
    - Lavender and tea tree oils
    - Phenothrin in delousing agents

From Beck Do, Rios JL. Gynecomastia. In: Janis JE. Essentials of Plastic Surgery. 2nd ed. New York, NY: Thieme Medical Publishers; 2014; 573–579

Table 18.1 Evidence for specific drugs historically considered associated with gynecomastia

Drugs with good quality of evidence for association with gynecomastia	Drugs with fair quality of evidence for association with gynecomastia	Drugs with poor quality of evidence for association with gynecomastia
Spironolactone	Risperidone	Antipsychotics
Cimetidine	Verapamil	Antidepressants
Ketoconazole	Nifedipine	Benzodiazepines
hGH	Omeprazole	Anticonvulsants
Estrogens	Efavirenz	Calcium channel blockers
Antiandrogens (flutamide, bicalcutamide, cyproterone acetate)	Alkylating agents	ACE inhibiors
GnRH analogs (goserelin, leuprorelin)	Anabolic steroids	Antiarrhythmics
5-alpha-reductase inhibitors (finasteride, dutasteride)	Alcohol	Antilipidemics
	Opioids (heroin, methadone)	Antacids
		Prokinetics
		Anti-TB medications
		Antibiotics
		HIV medications (stavudine, indinavir, saquinavir)

Abbreviations: ACE, angiotensin-converting enzyme; GnRH: gonadotrophin-releasing hormone; hGH: human growth hormone; HIV: human immunodeficiency virus; TB: tuberculosis.
Data from Deepinder F, Braunstein GD. Drug-induced gynecomastia: an evidence-based review. Expert Opin Drug Saf 2012;11:779–795

18.3 Pathology

On histologic review, gynecomastia is initially described as "florid," characterized by hyperplasia of ductal epithelium, and increased inflammatory cells, subareolar fat, and blood vessels. This process typically either regresses within the first year or transitions to the "fibrous" state, noted for a predominance of stromal fibrosis with minimal ductal proliferation.

18.3.1 Diagnosis

A careful history must be obtained, focusing on the age of onset of breast enlargement, symptoms of discomfort or tenderness, recreational drug and alcohol use, and the effect that chest feminization has had on the patient's psychological and social well-being. A review of systems should focus on symptoms from systemic pathologies that contribute to gynecomastia including thyroid, liver, kidney, and adrenal disease, in addition to any malignancies. Physical exam should assess the amount of glandular versus adipose tissue, ptosis, skin access, masses. Abnormal findings on testicular, thyroid, or liver exam should prompt workup specific to that organ system. Overall feminizing characteristics should also raise concern for an underlying endocrinologic derangement. Routine endocrinology workup is not necessary, as a recent study evaluating the utility of endocrinologic referral in the workup of gynecomastia found that only 7.6% of patients had secondary gynecomastia. Referral led to expensive blood tests, which were positive in only 1.7% of cases. The authors concluded that a referral to endocrinology should be considered if an endocrine disorder is suspected on initial evaluation.[8] Findings suggestive of such a disorder include galactorrhea, abnormal testicular examination, features of Klinefelter's syndrome (small, firm testes, gynecomastia, above-average height, long limbs, and abdominal obesity), visual disturbances, and rapid gynecomastia progression.[15] Men with Klinefelter's syndrome are not candidates for liposuction, as they have a 58-fold increase in breast cancer risk and thus should be managed with excisional procedures.[16]

Finally, a primary goal at the initial evaluation is to screen for characteristics consistent with breast cancer. Tissue in gynecomastia is soft, firm, or elastic, but generally not hard. The area affected arises beneath and extends radially from below the nipple areolar complex (NAC) and is bilateral in most cases. Breast carcinoma, on the other hand, is more typically firm in nature, often outside the NAC, and is most commonly unilateral. Also, skin dimpling, nipple retraction, nipple bleeding, and nipple discharge are factors associated more commonly with breast cancer and should prompt investigation, starting with a diagnostic mammogram and biopsies as indicated.[1]

18.3.2 Staging

Simon, Hoffman, and Kahn originally divided gynecomastia into four grades: grade 1 (small enlargement, no skin excess); grade 2a (moderate enlargement, no skin excess); grade 2b (moderate enlargement with extra skin); grade 3 (marked enlargement with extra skin). The authors recommended skin resection in grades 2b and 3.[17] Rohrich et al later submitted a revised classification scheme after the advent of ultrasound-assisted liposuction: grade I: minimal hypertrophy (< 250 g of breast tissue) without ptosis; grade II: moderate hypertrophy (250–500 g of breast tissue) without ptosis; grade III: severe hypertrophy (> 500 g breast tissue) with grade I ptosis; grade IV: severe hypertrophy with grade II or III ptosis.[18] Assessing the stage of the disease is helpful in planning nonoperative and surgical management.

18.4 Management

Gynecomastia that persists beyond 12 months in general has progressed to the fibrous state just described and is unlikely to regress.[1,17,18] Prior to that time, a trial of observation is appropriate. If there is a component of pseudogynecomastia, an attempt at weight loss should also be considered, and if the gynecomastia is found to be medication-induced, stopping the offending agent for a period of time is prudent. The surgical treatments for gynecomastia increase in their level of invasiveness with increasing stage of gynecomastia. ▶ Fig. 18.1 illustrates a stepwise approach to gynecomastia similar to the reconstructive ladder, in which options are evaluated beginning with the simplest and progressing up the ladder to the more complex.

If there is absence of or a very minimal component of glandular hypertrophy in Grade I or II pseudogynecomastia (no skin excess), cryolipolysis (Coolsculpting, ZELTIQ Aesthetics, Pleasanton, CA) can achieve marked improvement.[19] However, most patients will require two sessions, and thus, patient education and managing expectations are key when considering cryolipolysis in pseudogynecomastia. In patients with pseudogynecomastia but with more significant volume (i.e., Grade II or III), liposuction is a better option than cryolipolysis, as liposuction allows for removal of greater volume in one session. The addition of a basket-type cannula may allow more aggressive

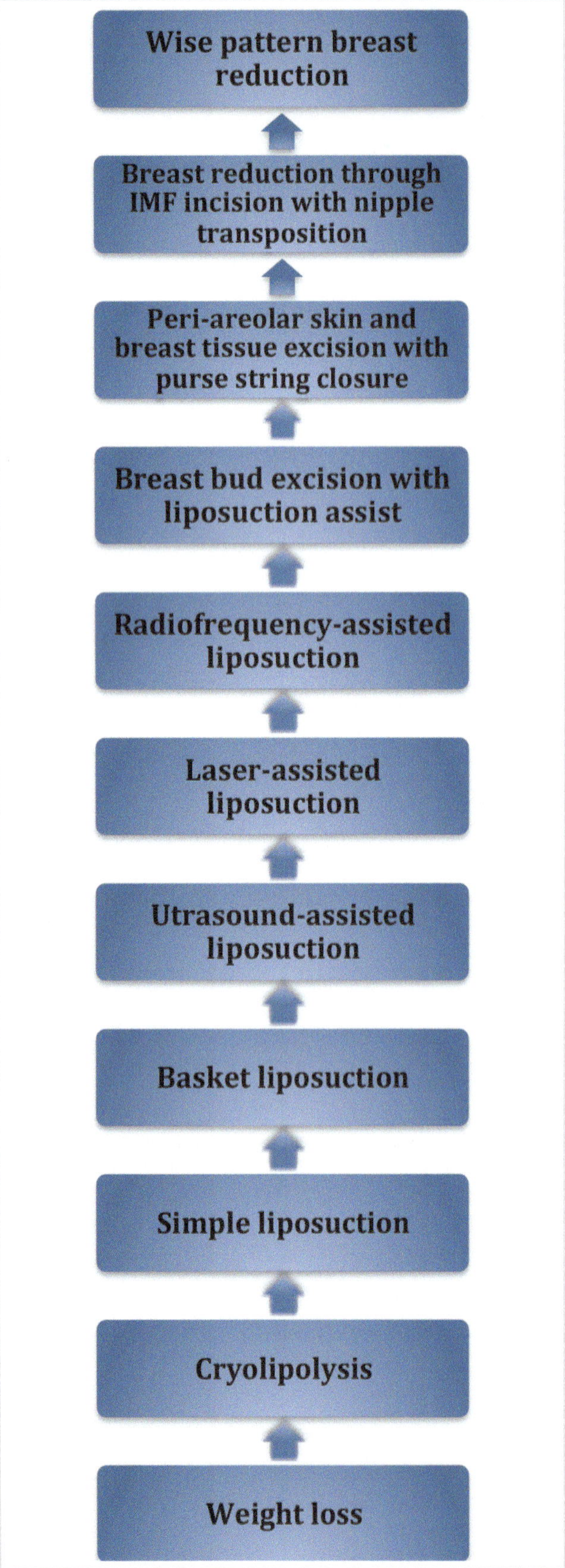

Fig. 18.1 The "reconstructive ladder" approach to gynecomastia.

resection of the subareolar dense, fibrous, glandular tissue in patients with more of a glandular component.

Ultrasound-assisted liposuction (VASER, Solta, Bothell, WA), initially introduced for gynecomastia in the mid 1990s, has gained popularity in many centers due to several advantages.[18,20] Compared to traditional liposuction, ultrasound-assisted liposuction has been shown to be associated with lower intraoperative conversion to open excision, improved postoperative pain scores and bruising, smoother breast contour, improved skin retraction, and release of more triglycerides per mL of hemoglobin loss.[18,21,22] Even in Grade IV gynecomastia (> 500 g breast tissue with grade II or III ptosis), Rohrich and colleagues reported that less than half (43%) required further surgery.[18] Since that study, their group has found that with the addition of a pull-through excision of the glandular tissue through a stab incision at the lateral inframammary fold (IMF), almost no patients require further surgery.[23]

Laser-assisted lipolysis (LAL) for gynecomastia, in addition to decreasing breast volume, provides significant dermal tightening and has yielded very good results.[24,25] Laser light energy is converted to thermal energy in fat cells, causing them to rupture. Coagulation effects of the laser decrease bleeding complications and stimulate collagen formation in the dermis.[26] In a study of 28 patients, Trelles and colleagues described their method of approach.[27] Initial fibrotic attachments are broken down in cases where the breast is more conical and firm. This is then followed by insertion of a 980-nm wavelength diode laser, with delivery of 8–12 kJ of total average accumulated energy per breast, depending on the breast size. The cannula is first passed in a deep plane, then by a quicker movement in a more superficial plane, aiming for equal disbursement of energy to the dermis. During the laser use, the skin is cooled using an external air flow device, and skin temperature is monitored using an infrared thermometer. Traditional liposuction is then carried out. SmartLipo, a 1064-nm Nd:YAG laser (Cynosure, Langen, Germany), has shown significant improvement in gynecomastia. The thermal treatment can induce skin tightening in addition to more effective tissue separation with liposuctioning following the prescribed amount of energy deployed to break up the dense gynecomastia tissue.[28]

Similar to laser-assisted lipolysis, radiofrequency-assisted liposuction (RFAL) also offers the benefit of liposuction with additional soft tissue contraction.[29] RFAL also distributes energy over a greater volume of tissue than LAL, also allowing for contracture of soft tissues, but over a more uniform area, and possibly a lower risk of focal burns.[30,31] RFAL has shown promising results for some patients with gynecomastia in one study in Europe.[32]

If there is a substantial glandular component that cannot be treated effectively with the techniques just described, a small, crescent-shaped incision at the inferior border of the NAC can be utilized to remove the underlying gland with adjunctive liposuction.[33] Keeping the glandular incision at the edge of the NAC renders the resultant scar practically invisible, and most patients will be satisfied with this. Sometimes a crescent-shaped incision is insufficient to resect enough skin. In such cases, with moderate skin excess, a complete periareolar eccentric skin resection with purse string closure is useful to remove excess skin and correct ptosis while continuing to hide the scar at the edge of the NAC.[34,35]

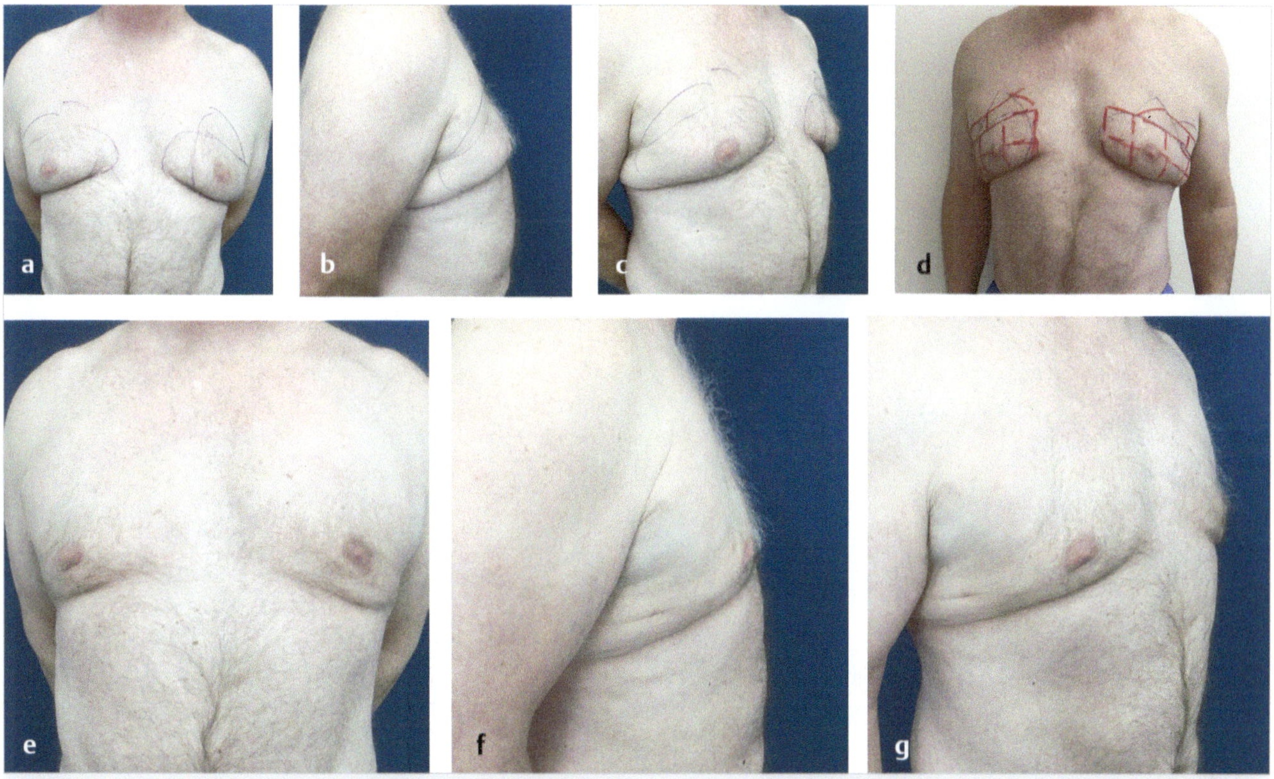

Fig. 18.2 (a–c) This 57-year-old man, BMI 28.7, presented with gynecomastia. **(d)** Preoperative markings at time of surgery are the number of squares for treatment area. These aid in the surgical planning for the treatment and the amount of energy needed. Patient underwent laser-assisted liposuction with 10 kJ of energy per breast. He also had 250 mL of fat removed from each breast, totaling 500 mL. **(e–g)** show post-op photos taken at 6 months.

If skin excess is severe, a reduction through an incision at the IMF may be required.[36,37] The NAC is preserved on a de-epithelialized dermoglandular pedicle and delivered to its new location. The new nipple location is placed at the junction of the fifth rib and the lateral border of the pectoralis major muscle, or at 0.33 times the distance from the sternal notch to the pubis.[38,39] Finally, in extreme cases, a breast reduction through a Wise-pattern incision may be necessary (Chapter 12, Reduction Mammaplasty). However, in the senior author's experience, Wise-pattern reductions or other techniques that produce vertical scars on the chest are not ideal and should be avoided.

18.5 Outcomes

The biggest complications are asymmetry and unsatisfactory results, particularly when the patient still feels that he has more tissue than he desires. Another challenge can be change in nipple sensation and even change in nipple color. Men are very sensitive to nipple stimulation, and this may become altered following surgery.[40] Changes in neural connections to the nipple may result in less pilar erectile changes with stimulation. The most frequent postoperative complication with male gynecomastia surgery is hematoma formation. This may result from the more aggressive nature of the liposuction needed to break up the dense attachments of male breast tissue or the increased vascular nature of male breast tissue. Occasionally, contour irregularities can result after liposuction for gynecomastia.

The surgical treatment of gynecomastia is the third most common aesthetic surgical procedure for men, with almost 25,000 procedures performed in 2018, representing a 48% increase since 2014.[41] Examples of laser-assisted liposuction are shown in ▶ Fig. 18.2, ▶ Fig. 18.3, and ▶ Fig. 18.4. Men are, overall, extremely satisfied with the results, reporting significant improvements in general health, quality of life, functional capacity, and mental health, and 96% endorse a male breast reduction procedure as "worth it."[13,42,43] It is only through a diligent history and physical, shared decision making, management of expectations, and a command of the spectrum of surgical options available that such excellent results are possible.

Key Points

- Gynecomastia remains one of the most common reasons men seek help from a plastic surgeon.
- A focused history and physical including a testicular exam should be done; however, most cases are idiopathic.
- Many historical references that identified various drugs as contributing to gynecomastia were based on poor-quality evidence. Some have more evidence to support that claim than others.
- Relatively recent advances in technology include cryolipolysis, ultrasound-assisted liposuction, laser-assisted lipolysis, and radiofrequency-assisted liposuction.

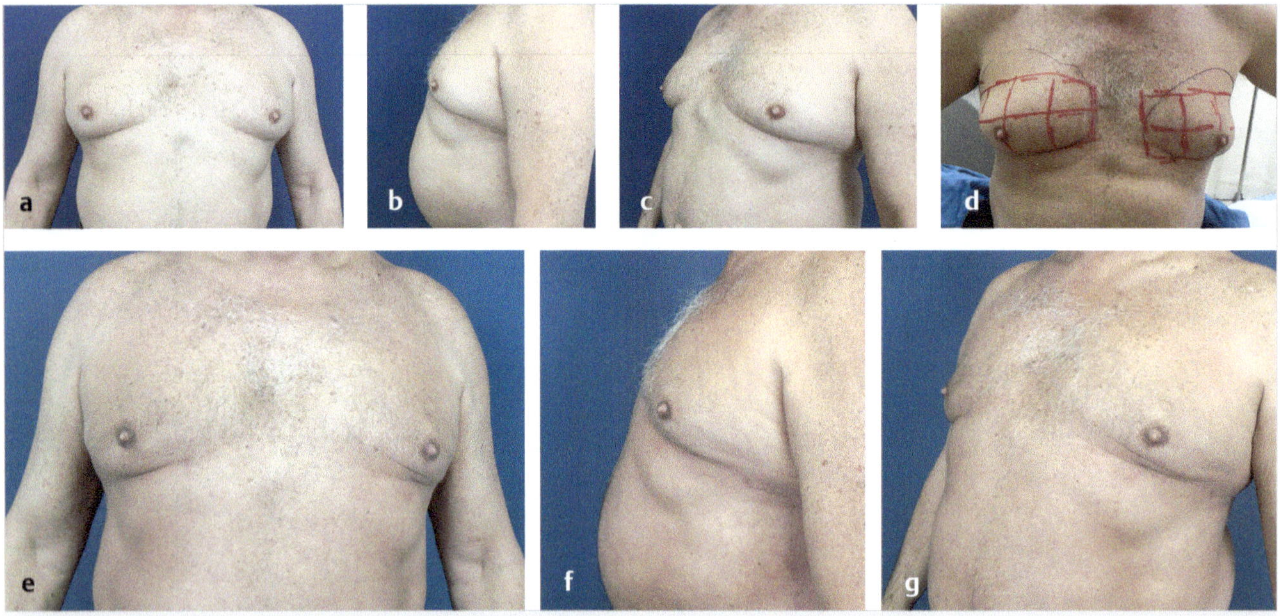

Fig. 18.3 (a–c) This 69-year-old man, BMI 29.1, presented with gynecomastia. **(d)** Preoperative markings for treatment with laser-assisted liposuction, applying 10 kJ per side. He had 225 mL of fat removed from the left side and 275 mL fat from the right side. **(e–g)** Postoperative photos taken at 6 weeks.

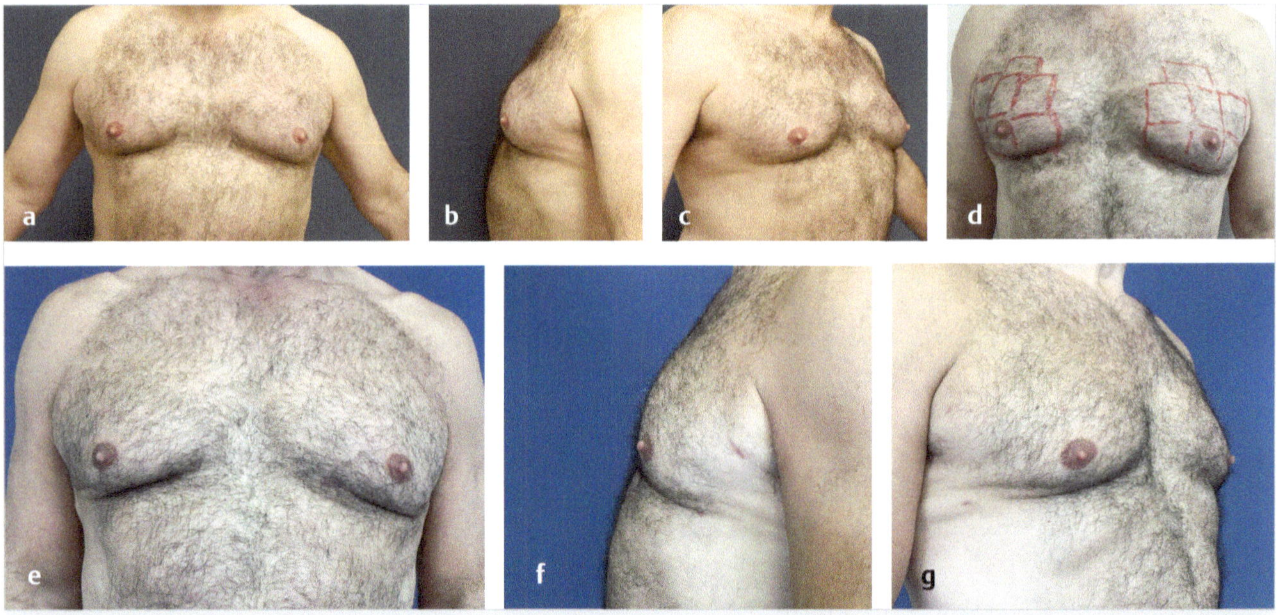

Fig. 18.4 (a–c) This 57 year-old man presented with gynecomastia. **(d)** Preoperative markings for treatment with laser-assisted liposuction, applying 10 kJ per side in addition to 250 mL of liposuction per side. **(e–g)** Postoperative photos.

- The best approach to the individual patient requires a working knowledge of traditional surgical modalities with the ability to draw from these newer technologies.
- Patients are, overall, extremely satisfied with their results, reporting significant improvements in general health, quality of life, functional capacity, and mental health.

References

[1] Braunstein GD. Clinical practice. Gynecomastia. N Engl J Med. 2007; 357(12): 1229–1237
[2] Georgiadis E, Papandreou L, Evangelopoulou C, et al. Incidence of gynaecomastia in 954 young males and its relationship to somatometric parameters. Ann Hum Biol. 1994; 21(6):579–587
[3] Biro FM, Lucky AW, Huster GA, Morrison JA. Hormonal studies and physical maturation in adolescent gynecomastia. J Pediatr. 1990; 116(3):450–455
[4] Nuttall FQ. Gynecomastia as a physical finding in normal men. J Clin Endocrinol Metab. 1979; 48(2):338–340
[5] Niewoehner CB, Nuttal FQ. Gynecomastia in a hospitalized male population. Am J Med. 1984; 77(4):633–638
[6] Johnson RE, Murad MH. Gynecomastia: pathophysiology, evaluation, and management. Mayo Clin Proc. 2009; 84(11):1010–1015
[7] Karp NS. Gynecomastia. In: Thorne CH, Chung CK, Gosain AK, et al, eds. Grabb and Smith's Plastic Surgery. 7th ed. Philadelphia, PA: Lippincott Williams & Wilkins; 2014:615–619
[8] Kumanov P, Deepinder F, Robeva R, Tomova A, Li J, Agarwal A. Relationship of adolescent gynecomastia with varicocele and somatometric parameters: a cross-sectional study in 6200 healthy boys. J Adolesc Health. 2007; 41(2):126–131
[9] Malhotra AK, Amed S, Bucevska M, Bush KL, Arneja JS. Do adolescents with gynecomastia require routine evaluation by endocrinology? Plast Reconstr Surg. 2018; 142(1):9e–16e
[10] Nuzzi LC, Cerrato FE, Erickson CR, et al. Psychosocial impact of adolescent gynecomastia: a prospective case-control study. Plast Reconstr Surg. 2013; 131 (4):890–896
[11] Kinsella C, Jr, Landfair A, Rottgers SA, et al. The psychological burden of idiopathic adolescent gynecomastia. Plast Reconstr Surg. 2012; 129(1):1–7
[12] Colombo-Benkmann M, Buse B, Stern J, Herfarth C. Indications for and results of surgical therapy for male gynecomastia. Am J Surg. 1999; 178(1):60–63
[13] Davanço RA, Sabino Neto M, Garcia EB, Matsuoka PK, Huijsmans JP, Ferreira LM. Quality of life in the surgical treatment of gynecomastia. Aesthetic Plast Surg. 2009; 33(4):514–517
[14] Deepinder F, Braunstein GD. Drug-induced gynecomastia: an evidence-based review. Expert Opin Drug Saf. 2012; 11(5):779–795
[15] Chang S, Skakkebæk A, Gravholt CH. Klinefelter Syndrome and medical treatment: hypogonadism and beyond. Hormones (Athens). 2015; 14(4):531–548
[16] Swerdlow AJ, Schoemaker MJ, Higgins CD, Wright AF, Jacobs PA, UK Clinical Cytogenetics Group. Cancer incidence and mortality in men with Klinefelter syndrome: a cohort study. J Natl Cancer Inst. 2005; 97(16):1204–1210
[17] Simon BE, Hoffman S, Kahn S. Classification and surgical correction of gynecomastia. Plast Reconstr Surg. 1973; 51(1):48–52
[18] Rohrich RJ, Ha RY, Kenkel JM, Adams WP, Jr. Classification and management of gynecomastia: defining the role of ultrasound-assisted liposuction. Plast Reconstr Surg. 2003; 111(2):909–923, discussion 924--925
[19] Munavalli GS, Panchaprateep R. Cryolipolysis for targeted fat reduction and improved appearance of the enlarged male breast. Dermatol Surg. 2015; 41 (9):1043–1051
[20] Hammond DC, Arnold JF, Simon AM, Capraro PA. Combined use of ultrasonic liposuction with the pull-through technique for the treatment of gynecomastia. Plast Reconstr Surg. 2003; 112(3):891–895, discussion 896--897
[21] Kenkel JM, Robinson JB, Jr, Beran SJ, et al. The tissue effects of ultrasound-assisted lipoplasty. Plast Reconstr Surg. 1998; 102(1):213–220
[22] Hodgson ELB, Fruhstorfer BH, Malata CM. Ultrasonic liposuction in the treatment of gynecomastia. Plast Reconstr Surg. 2005; 116(2):646–653, discussion 654--655
[23] Bailey SH, Guenther D, Constantine F, Rohrich RJ. Gynecomastia management: an evolution and refinement of technique at UT Southwestern Medical Center. Plast Reconstr Surg Glob Open. 2016; 4(6):e734
[24] Wolfenson M, Hochman B, Ferreira L. Laser lipolysis: skin tightening using a diode laser. Plast Reconstr Surg. 2015; 135(5):1378–1380
[25] Matarasso A. Discussion: laser lipolysis: skin tightening in lipoplasty using a diode laser. Plast Reconstr Surg. 2015; 135(5):1378–1380
[26] Goldman A. Submental Nd:YAG laser-assisted liposuction. Lasers Surg Med. 2006; 38(3):181–184
[27] Trelles MA, Mordon SR, Bonanad E, et al. Laser-assisted lipolysis in the treatment of gynecomastia: a prospective study in 28 patients. Lasers Med Sci. 2013; 28(2):375–382
[28] Schafer JB. White paper: Smartlipo improves male gynecomastia outcomes with minimal scarring. In: Smartlipo TriPlex: Better Science. Better Results. A Smartlipo Compendium. Langen, Germany: Cynosure; 2011:34–37
[29] Chia CT, Theodorou SJ, Hoyos AE, Pitman GH. Radiofrequency-assisted liposuction compared with aggressive superficial, subdermal liposuction of the arms: a bilateral quantitative comparison. Plast Reconstr Surg Glob Open. 2015; 3(7):e459
[30] Paul M, Blugerman G, Kreindel M, Mulholland RS. Three-dimensional radiofrequency tissue tightening: a proposed mechanism and applications for body contouring. Aesthetic Plast Surg. 2011; 35(1):87–95
[31] Paul M, Mulholland RS. A new approach for adipose tissue treatment and body contouring using radiofrequency-assisted liposuction. Aesthetic Plast Surg. 2009; 33(5):687–694
[32] Blugerman G, Schalvezon D, Mulholland RS, Soto JA, Siguen M. Gynecomastia treatment using radiofrequency-assisted liposuction (RFAL). Eur J Plast Surg. 2013; 36(4):231–236
[33] Webster JP. Mastectomy for gynecomastia through a semicircular intra-areolar incision. Ann Surg. 1946; 124:557–575
[34] Martin AE, Olinger TA, Yu JC. Surgical correction of gynecomastia: a geometric approach. Plast Reconstr Surg. 2015; 135(5):1392–1394
[35] Cederna PS. Correction of gynecomastia. In: Guyuron B, Eriksson E, Persing JA, et al, eds. Plastic Surgery: Indications and Practice, 1st ed. St. Louis, MO: Saunders; 2009:727–736
[36] Davidson BA. Concentric circle operation for massive gynecomastia to excise the redundant skin. Plast Reconstr Surg. 1979; 63(3):350–354
[37] Wray RC, Jr, Hoopes JE, Davis GM. Correction of extreme gynaecomastia. Br J Plast Surg. 1974; 27(1):39–41
[38] Toy JW, Rubin JP. Contouring of the arms, breast, upper trunk, and male chest in the massive weight loss patient. In: Neligan PC, Grotting JC, eds. Plastic Surgery, Vol. 5: Breast. 3rd ed. New York, NY: Saunders; 2012:573–581
[39] Murphy TP, Ehrlichman RJ, Seckel BR. Nipple placement in simple mastectomy with free nipple grafting for severe gynecomastia. Plast Reconstr Surg. 1994; 94(6):818–823
[40] Nahabedian MY. Breast deformities and mastopexy. Plast Reconstr Surg. 2011; 127(4):91e–102e
[41] American Society for Aesthetic Plastic Surgery. Cosmetic (Aesthetic) Surgery National Data Bank Statistics 2018. URL: https://surgery.org/sites/default/files/ASAPS-Stats2018.pdf. Published 2018. Accessed July 21, 2019
[42] RealPatientRatings.com. Male Breast Reduction. URL: https://www.realpatientratings.com/male-breast-reduction?asaps. Updated 2019. Accessed July 21, 2019
[43] Hardy N. Everything You Need to Know about Gynecomastia Surgery. URL: https://www.realself.com/gynecomastia-surgery. Updated January 6, 2019. Accessed July 21, 2019

19 Aesthetics of the Male Breast

Douglas S. Steinbrech and John T. Stranix

Summary

Pectoral augmentation with a silicone implant is an excellent way to get patients the chest they want. This chapter reviews the anatomy and the technical details of a procedure that any aesthetic surgeon who performs routine breast augmentation on women should be quite comfortable performing on men. Additional information is given about BodyBanking fat grafting to enhance a more natural contour and about pectopexy for patients who may require a chest lift.

Keywords: silicone implant, chest enhancement, pectoral enhancement, pectoralis major, pectoralis minor, BodyBanking fat grafting, Pectopexy, eccentric periareolar pectopexy

19.1 Introduction

Men's chest reshaping with implants was first described in 1965 for reconstruction of chest wall deformities related to pectus excavatum.[1] The use of pectoral implants in chest wall deformities such as pectus excavatum,[2,3,4] Poland syndrome,[5] and pectoralis major rupture have constituted the majority of literature to date.[6] Early procedures involved subcutaneous implant placement through a presternal incision and were plagued with complications related to implant exposure and seroma formation. The recent use of subpectoral pocket dissection through an axillary incision has significantly improved outcomes.[7,8]

The first-generation pectoral implants were constructed using a papier-mâché moulage as a model to create a customized silicone form.[2,3] In the early 1990s, prefabricated pectoral implants for male patients became available.[7,8] These implants contained a cohesive silicone gel within a textured seven-layer capsule. The design was rectangular in shape with rounded borders and a lateral axillary extension.

A better understanding of male chest aesthetic anatomy, improved implant design, and refinements in surgical technique have enabled pectoral implants to evolve from a primarily reconstructive procedure into a powerful tool for cosmetic male chest enhancement[9,10,11,12] (Adams B, personal communication). Various sizes, shapes, and projections are now available for use (▸ Fig. 19.1).

19.2 Physical Evaluation

19.2.1 The Ideal Candidate

The ideal candidate for male chest implants has the following characteristics:

- Realistic expectations and goals.
- Compliant with instruction.
- Lean; very little body fat.
- Symmetric chest anatomy.
- Good skin quality.
- Attractive preoperative shape ("pretty in, pretty out").

Despite all of these desired features, pectoral implant placement can be very helpful in other situations where the circumstances are less ideal. For instance, implants may be used in concert with other modalities such as liposuction or BodyBanking (developed by the senior author) with fat grafting to the superomedial area of the chest, which can improve the contour in older patients who would benefit from a composite implant/fat strategy for better upper pole volume with a more natural appearance. Also, an eccentric "Easter-egg" periareolar skin excision, or pectopexy, can help in older patients to lift the lower poles. Finally, employing technology such as BodyTite (Inmode, Lake Forest, CA), utilizing radiofrequency energy, may help to tighten the lower chest skin in patients who refuse a periareolar incision.

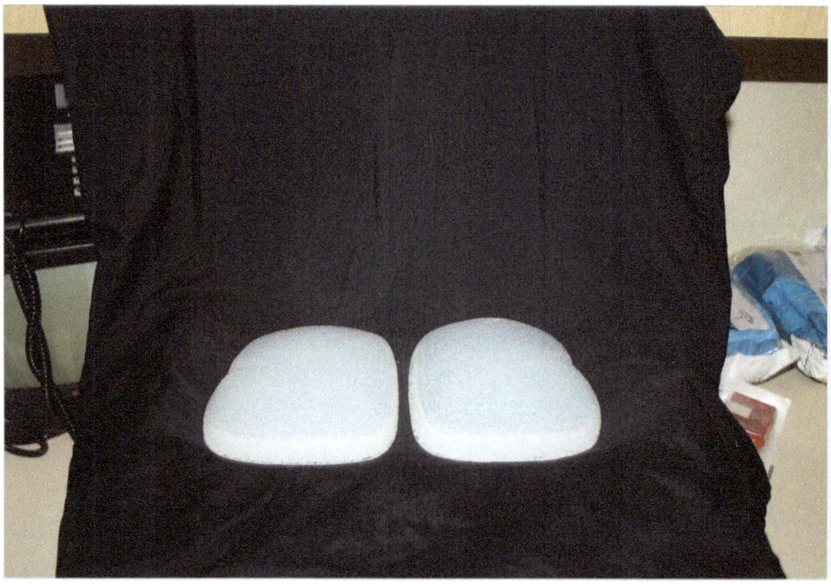

Fig. 19.1 An example of a pectoral implant made from semisolid silicone material. The product may be custom-trimmed for the specific needs of the patient's anatomy.

19.2.2 Implant Goals

The goals of an implant are as follows:

- A natural-appearing result.
- Central cleavage.
- Undetectable implant borders or "step-offs."
- Aesthetic ally congruent with the other muscle groups.
- Chest wall harmony.

19.2.3 Physical Exam

The preoperative physical exam includes the following steps:

- The quality of skin and subcutaneous tissue is examined for laxity and fatty deposits.
- The pectoralis muscle is evaluated at rest and in flexed position while standing. Clavicular, sternal, and costal attachments are defined.
- The width is measured from sternum to anterior axillary line along the lower pole.
- The height is measured from the clavicle to the lower border in the midclavicular line.
- The shoulders, rib cage, sternum, scapula, and spine are evaluated for skeletal abnormalities such as scoliosis, pectus excavatum/carnitum, or Poland syndrome.
- Any asymmetry is noted and pointed out to the patient at the time of examination.

19.3 Anatomy

The aesthetics of the male chest are largely defined by the shape and development of the pectoralis major muscles. A muscular male chest exhibits superior fullness with a transition to a firm inferior chest at the level of the inframammary fold (IMF) and medially over the central sternum. The lateral edge of the pectoralis muscle extends upward from the linea semilunaris to the anterior axillary line.

The pectoralis major is divided into clavicular and sternocostal heads. The clavicular head originates from the anterior border of the medial half of the clavicle, while the sternocostal head originates from the anterior surface of the sternum, the superior six costal cartilages, and the aponeurosis of the anterior rectus sheath and external oblique muscle. The fibers converge to insert on the anteromedial proximal humerus along the lateral lip of the bicipital groove. The pectoral branch of the thoracoacromial artery and perforating vessels from the internal mammary artery provide blood supply to the pectoralis major.

The lower two-thirds of the pectoralis major muscle are innervated by the medial pectoral nerve, which is closely associated with the lateral thoracic vessels. The medial pectoral nerve is at risk for injury during lateral subpectoral dissection, as it passes through or around the pectoralis minor muscle to enter the pectoralis major along the inferolateral border. The lateral pectoral nerve travels more superiorly with the thoracoacromial vessels and innervates the upper third of the pectoralis major muscle. This nerve may also be damaged during more superior subpectoral dissection.

The pectoralis minor is a thin triangular muscle beneath the pectoralis major. It arises from the superolateral surfaces of ribs 3 through 5 and inserts onto the medial border of the coracoid process of the scapula. Arterial supply is derived from the pectoral branch of the thoracoacromial artery, and the medial pectoral nerve provides innervation. The muscle is covered anteriorly by the clavipectoral fascia and divides the axillary lymph nodes according to their position relative to the muscle: level 1, lateral; level 2, deep; and level 3, medial.

The axillary region is directly below the shoulder joint and contains the axillary artery and vein, brachial plexus, and lymph nodes. The anterior boundary consists of the lower border of the lateral pectoralis major, which forms the anterior axillary fold, and is separated from the overlying subcutaneous tissue by the clavipectoral fascia. The posterior boundary is formed by the latissimus dorsi and teres major muscles, which form the posterior axillary fold.

19.4 Solid Silicone Implant

19.4.1 Preoperative Markings

The markings are performed with the patient standing fully upright and the surgeon sitting. The chest anatomy is precisely delineated, with particular attention to any asymmetry present. Abducting the patient's arm and then raising it over his head helps to define the lateral pectoral border clearly and define the axillary skin crease for incision marking. Repeated flexing of the pectoralis muscle with the arm down also assists in delineation of borders for precise markings. In addition to noting any anatomic differences between sides and incorporating them into the operative plan, asymmetries should be pointed out to the patient and clearly documented. Preoperative photographs are especially helpful to illustrate the asymmetry for the patient. While the implant size, shape, and pocket position should be adjusted to correct asymmetry as well as possible, preoperative identification is paramount to achieving aesthetic success and for managing patient expectations.

With the arm abducted 90°, the access incision is marked along a natural crease in the hair-bearing area of the axilla. Typically this incision is 3 to 4 cm long to allow insertion of a gently folded implant. Returning the arms to the patient's sides, the infrapectoral fold (IPF) is marked out. The patient is then instructed to flex his pectoral muscles to delineate the medial orgin of the pectoralis major on the sternum to determine how far medially to make the implant pocket. At this point, areas for BodyBanking augmentation are also delineated (▶ Fig. 19.2).

The inferior edge of the implant pocket is marked so that it lies under the inferior aspect of the areola. Accordingly, the areas of release to create the implant pocket are marked out. It is important to ensure that the implant is not too large laterally, as it may rub against the arm and cause discomfort. Any areas of BodyBanking fat grafting medially would be marked out now. BodyBanking with grafted fat will allow more volume centrally, creating desired enhanced cleavage for a superior result. It also may be used superiorly to blend the implant to the clavicle to prevent a superior implant step-off with subclavicular hollowing—the unnatural stigmata of a rookie pectoral augmentation.

After all areas of interest have been marked and highlighted, the surgeon should stand up and step a few feet back to assess the overall symmetry. While it is important to be exacting in delineation of anatomic boundaries, minor unilateral variation is typically present, and it is paramount that each side of the chest

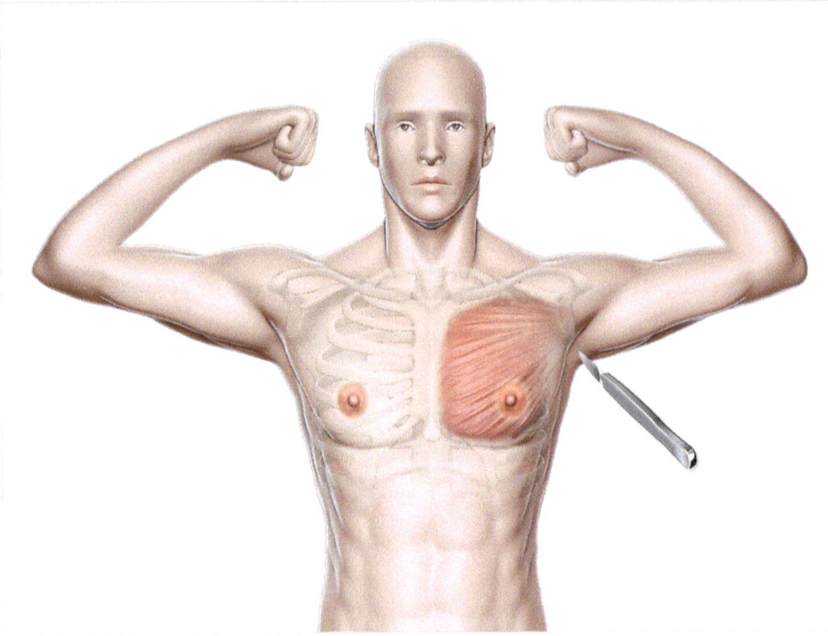

Fig. 19.2 Standard pre-operative measuring. The diagram shows a 4- to 6-cm incision placed in the natural axillary crease. The vertical and horizontal measurements are documented. The zone of the pocket is marked out for precise pocket dissection.

matches the other. Precise markings translate to operative success and help to avoid patient dissatisfaction postoperatively.

19.4.2 Positioning

The patient is placed is a supine position on the operating table. Sequential compression boots are applied to the legs, antibiotic prophylaxis is given, and general anesthesia is administered. The arms are abducted to 90° and secured to arm boards. The antiseptic surgical prep is widely applied from the neck to the umbilicus, extending down to the table bilaterally; the axilla is prepped last. The operative field is then draped in a sterile fashion with exposure of the entire chest, bilateral axilla, and epigastric area. Antimicrobial drape (Ioban, 3 M, St. Paul, MN) may be additionally placed over the surgical field to secure drapes in place and minimize risk of contamination.

19.4.3 Steps for Augmentation with Pectoral Implant

To minimize intravenous and inhalational anesthesia requirements and improve hemostasis, the axillary incision, lateral chest subcutaneous tissue, and pectoralis muscle are injected with 2% lidocaine with 1:100,000 epinephrine. After a wait of 5 to 7 minutes for the vasoconstrictive effect, the axillary incision is made (▸ Fig. 19.3). Using a combination of dissecting scissors and cautery, a relatively superficial subcutaneous tunnel is developed toward the lateral border of the pectoralis major muscle. Meticulous hemostasis is maintained, and care must be taken to avoid deeper axillary contents.

After the lateral border of the pectoralis major is defined, blunt finger dissection is performed under the edge of the pectoralis major to develop an intermuscular plane between the pectoralis major and minor (▸ Fig. 19.4). A lighted retractor is inserted, and hemostasis is again checked. Using an Agris-Dingman dissector, blunt intermuscular dissection is performed to open the potential space under the pectoralis major. The intermuscular plane is relatively bloodless.

An endoscope is then used to visualize the medial and inferior insertions of the pectoralis muscle. These insertions are selectively released with cautery under direct endoscopic visualization to obtain the appropriate pocket size required for the implant. Once the surgeon is satisfied with endoscopic release, an Agris-Dingman is reinserted to confirm that the pocket dissection matches the preoperatively marked area for placement. The lighted retractor and endoscope are then used again to confirm hemostasis, and the pocket is irrigated with triple-antibiotic solution.

At this point, surgical gloves are changed for a "no-touch" technique. The implant is opened and bathed in triple-antibiotic solution. Both implants are custom trimmed at this time. An 8-mm corner is trimmed in the superolateral corner of the implant for orientation. Clean, unused implant retractors are inserted into the axillary incision under the pectoralis major muscle, and the implant is gently folded and inserted in proper orientation with care taken to avoid fracturing of the implant. Following insertion, the Agris-Dingman is inserted to check for folds in the implant, which are corrected as needed, without causing further dissection that would result in undue bleeding late in the game (▸ Fig. 19.5).

Once the procedure has been completed on the contralateral side, the patient is sat upright on the operating table to confirm appropriate and symmetric implant orientation, projection, and height. When the surgeon is satisfied with the appearance of the chest wall, bilateral 10-mm drains may be placed directly superficial to the implant if there is any question about hemostasis. (Note that the lead author rarely uses drains for pectoral augmentation at this point, feeling that long-term use of drains may cause endogenous atrophy of important periaxillary lymphatic drainage systems, resulting in a rebound seroma once the drain is removed.) It is important to avoid any drain contact with the chest wall skin during placement to minimize the risk of contamination (▸ Fig. 19.6).

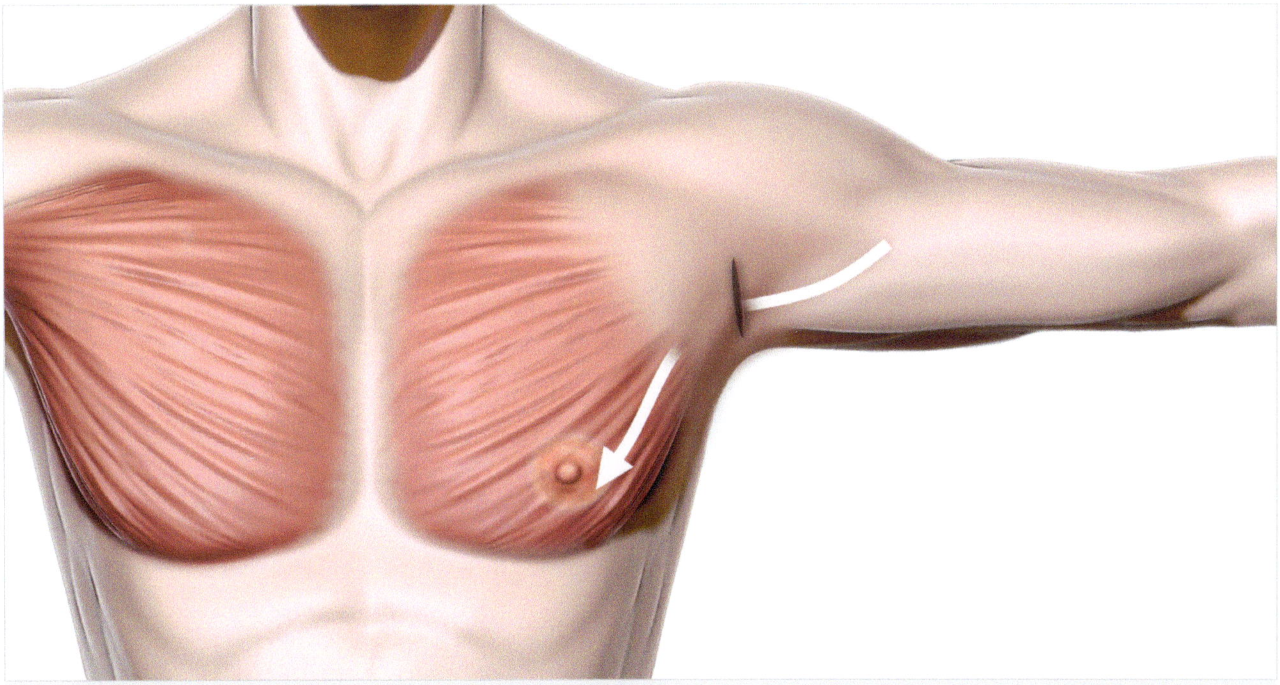

Fig. 19.3 The patient on the table with arm at 120° for better access to the lateral chest pocket. The am may be secured under sterile drapes with an arm strap. The incision is hidden in the natural skin crease of the axilla.

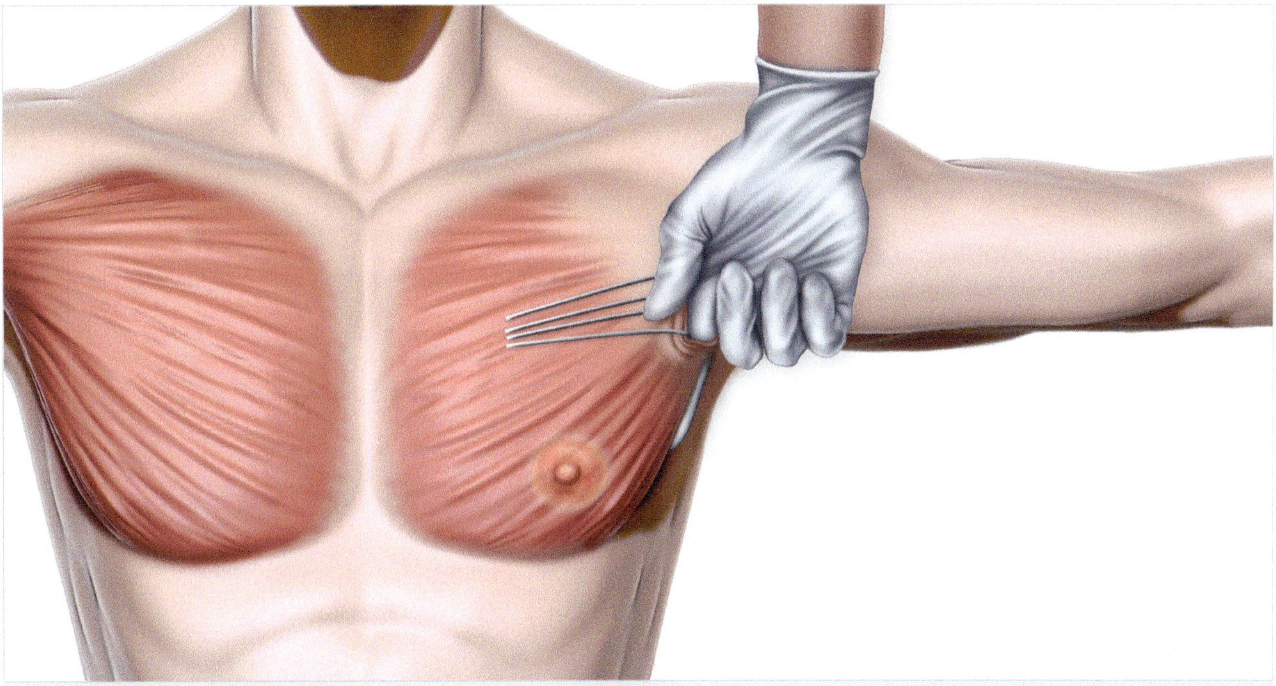

Fig. 19.4 Blunt finger dissection. With the assistant supplying retraction, gentle blunt finger dissection allows the surgeon to gain access to the intermuscular plane between the pectoralis major and minor. This will be the pocket for the endoscopically assisted dissection.

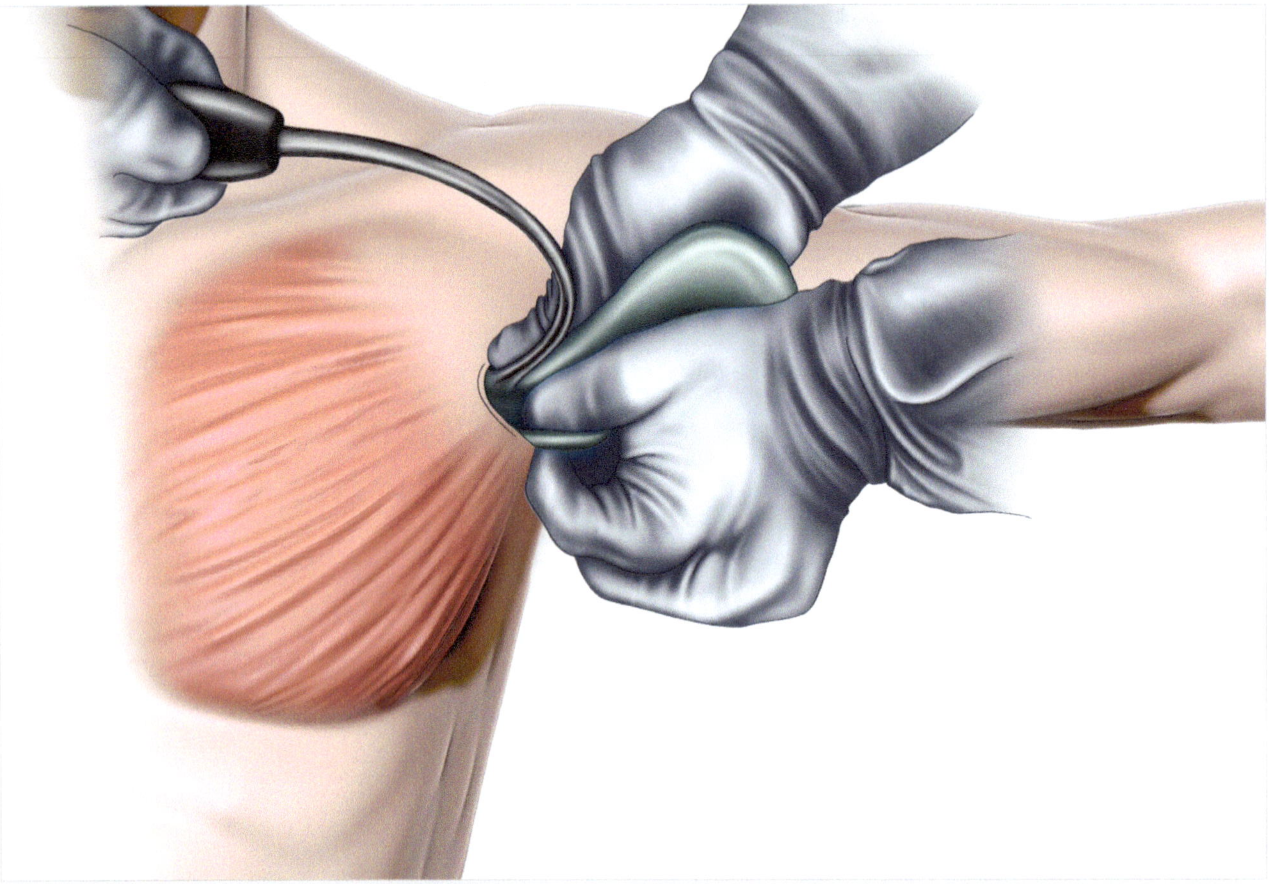

Fig. 19.5 Insertion of gently folded silicone pectoral implant. Once the endoscope has confirmed a precise pocket dissection, the surgeon uses a "restricted-touch" technique with changed glove to maneuver the implant into position.

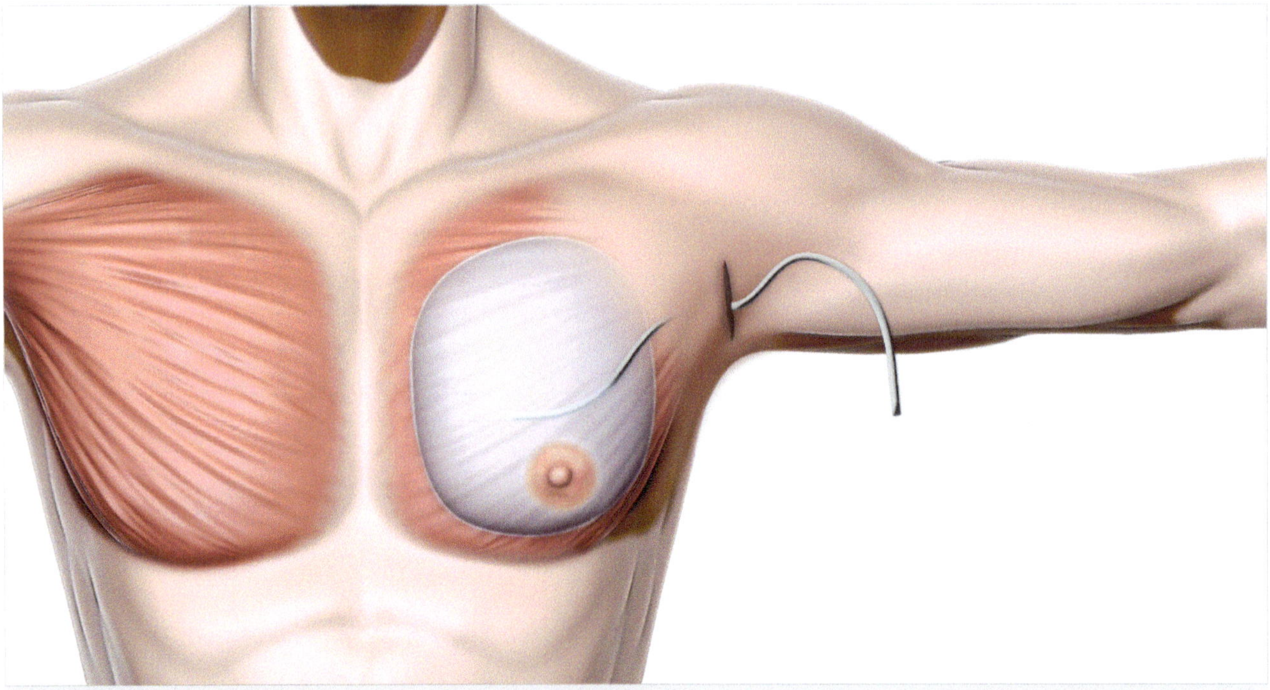

Fig. 19.6 If there is any question about hemostasis, 10-mm drains may be placed, avoiding any contact between the drain and the chest wall skin.

The lighted retractor is again used to check for hemostasis within the axillary tunnel. The lateral pectoral border is reapproximated with the chest wall with interrupted 2–0 Vicryl (Ethicon, Bridgewater, MA) sutures to prevent lateral implant displacement. The deep subcutaneous layer is closed with interrupted 2–0 Vicryl, and a running subcutaneous 3–0 Monocryl (Ethicon) is used for skin closure. If a drain is used, it should be secured with 3–0 nylon and connected to a closed suction bulb.

Any BodyBanking fat grafting can be performed with a long curved 2-mm cannula via a 2-mm incision in the axillary area (away from the primary pectoralis incision). To prevent passive fat egression, entry nick incisions may be made 4 cm inferior to the medial area to be grafted. All of these nick incisions should be closed with 5–0 plain gut suture.

19.4.4 Postoperative Dressing

The incisions are dressed with Mastisol (Ferndale Laboratories, Ferndale, MI) and two layers of 1-in (25-mm) Steri-Strips (3 M, St. Paul, MN), first along the length of the incisions and then crossing perpendicular strips on top. Dry gauze is secured over the incisions with paper tape. The 2-inch 3 M foam panels are placed lateral to the implant to form external lateral compression buttresses. Also, a central cleavage booster roll is placed to prevent central fat migration. The compression vest is secured.

19.5 Postoperative Care

The patient is seen in the office the following day for evaluation of implant positioning. Education is again provided, with particular emphasis on the importance of compliance with compression vest wear and activity limitations. Specific limitations to address are no pushing/pulling and no lifting anything heavier than 5–10 lb (2.25–9 kg) for the first week; no overhead work, and no working out for 1 month. At the 1-week postoperative visit, the buttresses are removed and slow range-of-motion exercises are initiated. Drains, if used, are left in place until the outputs are below 25 mL/day (typically 2 to 3 weeks). The compression vest must be worn at all times for 6 weeks. Postoperative photos are obtained 3 months after implant placement.

19.6 Management of Complications

Seromas are the most common complication and typically present as new-onset tense, relatively painless swelling, and the treatment of choice is percutaneous aspiration. This is best prevented by minimizing axillary lymphatic disruption intraoperatively, insisting on good patient compliance with compression vests, and minimizing dead space on implant placement. Superficial infections often respond to oral antibiotic therapy covering skin flora; however, deep-space infections would require implant removal. Postoperative asymmetry may occur as a result of either implant malposition or rotation. This may be avoided by thorough identification of pre-existing chest wall asymmetry and avoiding overdissection of the implant pocket. Wound dehiscence and implant exposure are potential complications that are often related to excessive tension on skin due to poor closure technique or excessively large implant size. Nerve injury and capsular contracture are other potential complications following pectoral implant placement; however, these are rare in our experience and have not resulted in long-term disability.

19.7 Case Examples

19.7.1 Case 1: Ectomorphic Body Type

This is a 27-year-old, 6-ft 0-in (183-cm), 163-lb (74-kg) ectomorphic man who underwent endoscopic intermuscular pectoral implantation with a 185-mL silicone implant (▶ Fig. 19.7). In this case, great care must be taken to shave the implant superiorly for a natural contour. Postoperative results at 13 months demonstrate appropriate subtle volume increase which is natural-appearing, has great definition, and complements without overpowering the balance of the other upper body muscle groups.

19.7.2 Case 2: Meso-Ectomophic Body Type

This is a 29-year-old, 5-ft 11-in (180-cm), 165-lb (75-kg) meso-ectomophic man who underwent endoscopic intermuscular pectoral implantation with a 185-mL silicone implant (▶ Fig. 19.8). BodyBanking of fat was performed superiorly to give a softer superior contour up to the clavicle, preventing an artificial step-off with a visible implantlike appearance. BodyBanking was also utilized medially to give greater central defining cleavage that the implant cannot achieve because of the limitations of the medial pectoral insertions on the sternum. Postoperative results at 23 months demonstrate increased volume with a natural contour and no visible incision.

19.7.3 Case 3: Ecto-Mesomorphic Body Type

This is a 36-year-old, 5-ft 10in (178-cm), 215-lb (97.5-kg) ecto-mesomophic man who underwent endoscopic intermuscular pectoral implantation with a 285-mL silicone implant (▶ Fig. 19.9). Postoperative results at 16 months demonstrate increased volume with a natural contour and no visible incision.

19.7.4 Case 4: The Heavyweight Mesomorphic Bodybuilder

This is a 46-year-old, 5-ft 8-in (173-cm), 205-lb (93-kg) heavyweight, mesomophic male bodybuilder who underwent endoscopic intermuscular pectoral implantation with a 385-mL silicone implant (▶ Fig. 19.10). Interestingly, mesomorphic bodybuilders find it difficult to build their chests compared to other muscle groups. In this case, there was no need to shave the implant, as the patient already had a significant amount of muscular coverage and he desired more aggressive projection. Postoperative results at 7 months demonstrate excellent volume increase with a more pronounced upper fullness.

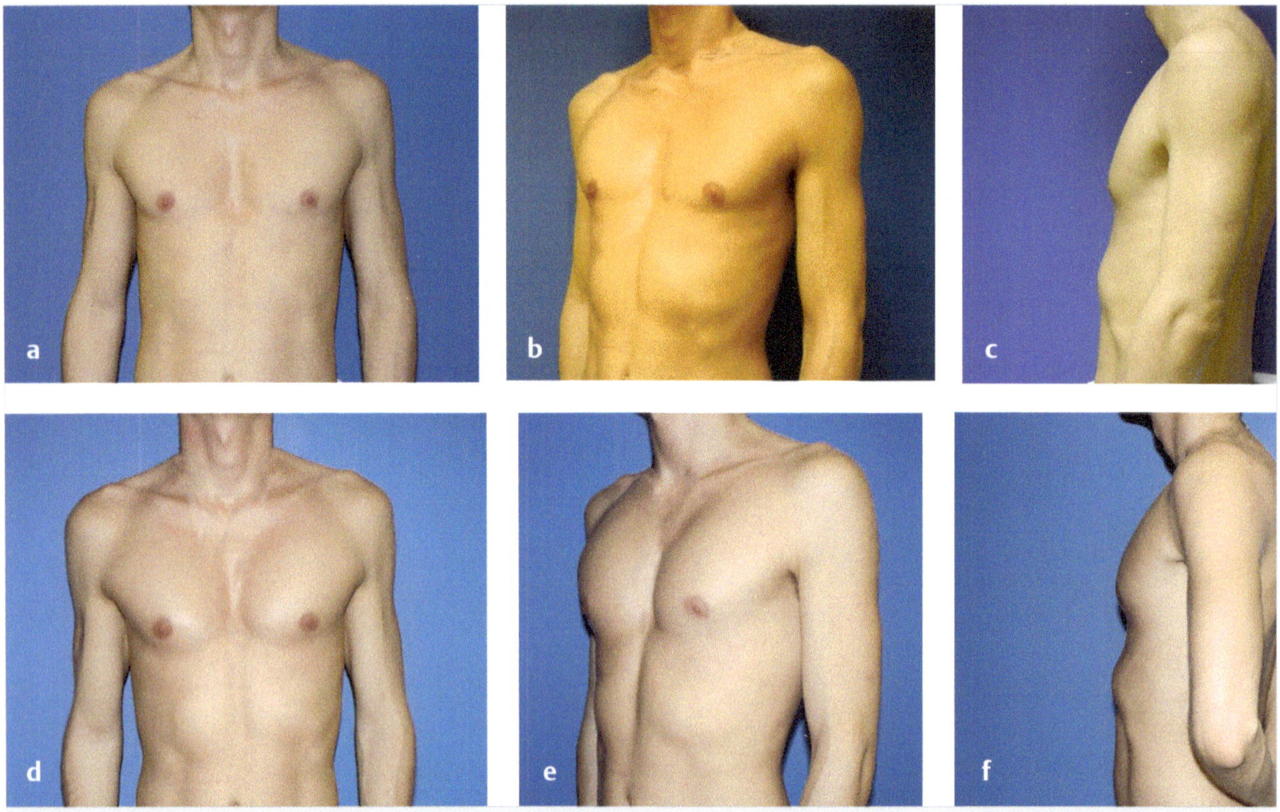

Fig. 19.7 Pectoral enhancement in an ectomorphic man. **(a–c)** Preoperative views. **(d–f)** Postoperative views.

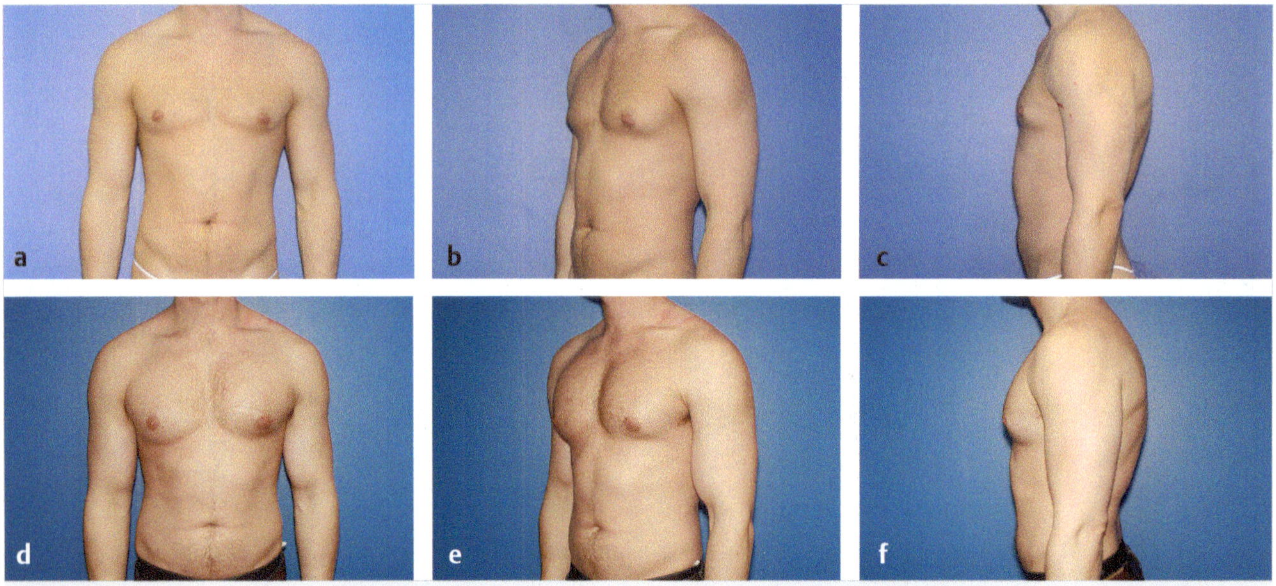

Fig. 19.8 Pectoral enhancement in meso-ectomorphic man. **(a–c)** Preoperative views. **(d–f)** Postoperative views.

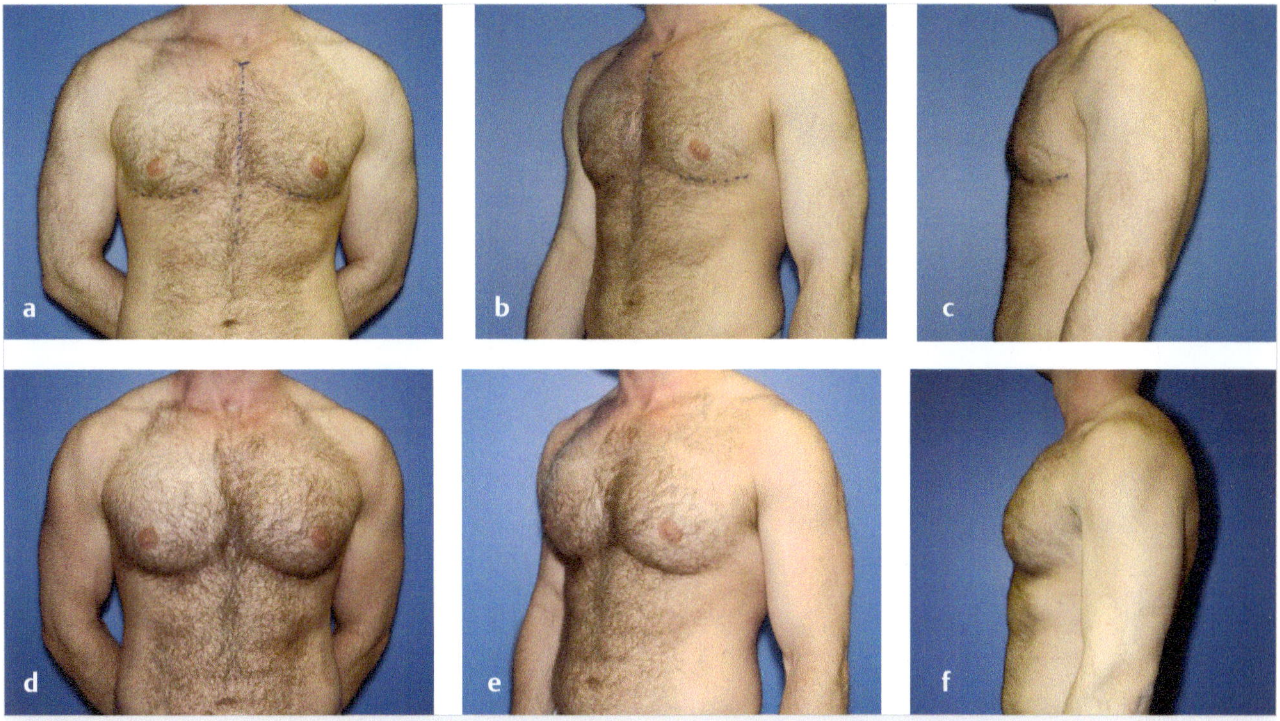

Fig. 19.9 Pectoral enhancement in ecto-mesomorphic man. **(a–c)** Preoperative views. **(d–f)** Postoperative views.

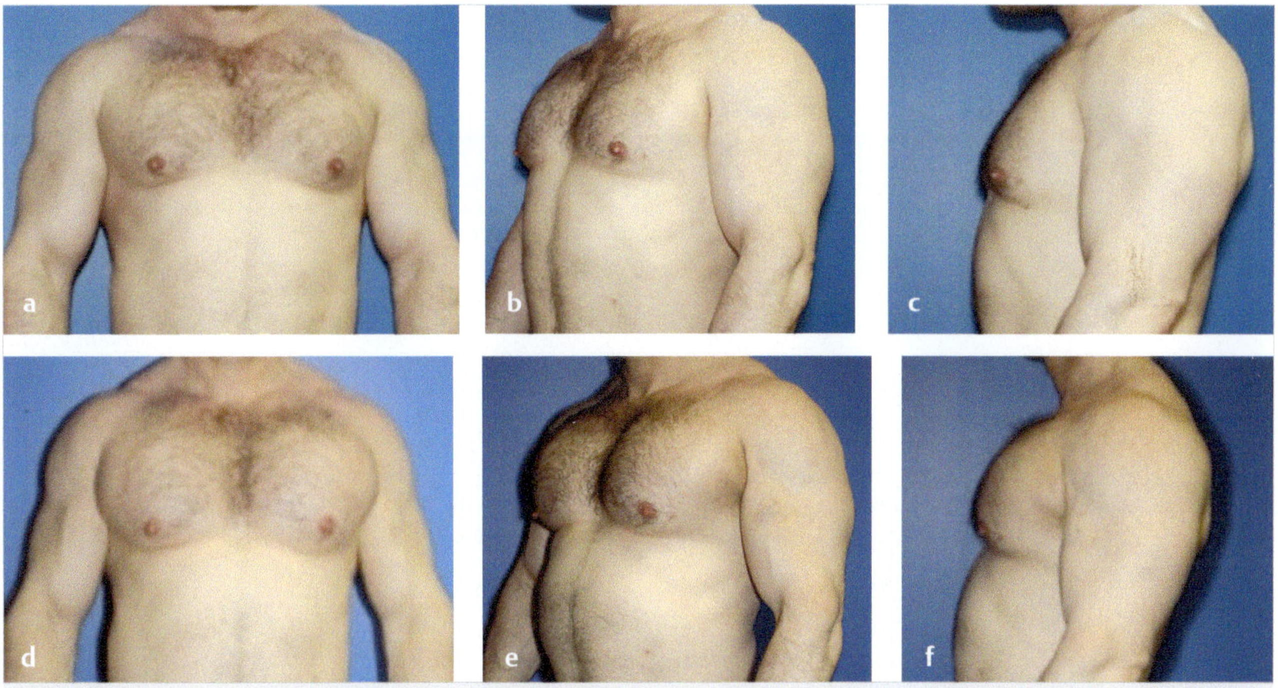

Fig. 19.10 Pectoral enhancement in heavyweight mesomorphic bodybuilder. **(a–c)** Preoperative views. **(d–f)** Postoperative views.

Box 19.1 Pearls and Pitfalls

Pearls
- Aim for a tapered, square-shaped implant to give adequate upper volume without a step-off.
- Implant may have to be shaved or tapered laterally and/or superiorly to avoid step-off.
- Follow careful patient selection.
- Implant placement may be combined with biceps and shoulder implantation through the same incision.
- Utilize the power of BodyBanking composite fat grafting for enhanced result in size, shape, and symmetry.
- Have postop garment drapes sterile prior to procedure.

Pitfalls
- Do not begin with large implants/tissue ratio if not well-initiated about implantation techniques.
- Avoid an uncooperative patient.
- Ensure that the patient wears compression.
- Ensure that the patient avoids chest exercises for 3 months.
- Encourage the patient to have pets stay with friends during early healing.
- If performing composite fat grafting, do not place fat contiguous to the implant.

19.8 Steps for Pectoral Augmentation

See also the Pearls and Pitfalls listed in Box 19.1.

19.8.1 Equipment

- Lighted retractor
- Endoscope; implant retractor (Video 19.1)
- MuscleGel implant
- Ioban antimicrobial drape

19.8.2 Sutures

- 2–0 Vicryl suture
- 3–0 Vicryl suture
- 3–0 Monocryl suture
- 4–0 nylon suture drain stitch

19.8.3 Preoperative Markings

1. Patient should be standing, doctor sitting.
2. Carefully evaluate any asymmetry; tell patient; document it in writing and with photo.
3. Correct asymmetry by pocket position or implant size and shape.
4. Always mark midline of body first.
5. Mark incision in natural crease of axilla: 3–4 cm for a folded implant to be inserted.
6. Mark the IPF (infrapectoral fold).
7. Flex to mark insertion of pectoralis major on sternum to determine how far medially to make pocket.
8. Mark out BodyBanking area of composite fat augmentation.
9. Mark out periareolar eccentric “Easter egg” purse string pectopexy if needed.
10. Mark inferior edge of implant over lower area of areola.
11. Mark out medial and inferior areas to be released.
12. Make sure implant not too large laterally, lest it rub against arm.

19.8.4 Positioning

1. Secure arms at 90°.
2. Place sequential compression boots and sterile drapes over the legs.
3. Perform supine prep from neck to umbilicus to back, including axilla last.

19.8.5 Steps for Pectoral Augmentation

1. Inject area with 2% lidocaine with 1:100,000 epinephrine to incision, lateral chest, and subcutaneously and sub pectoralis major muscle.
2. Make axillary incision with hemostasis.
3. Perform subcutaneous tunneling, spreading with scissors and electrocautery, avoiding axillary contents.
4. Use finger dissection to get under pectoralis major muscle.
5. Use lighted retractor to check for hemostasis.
6. Perform blunt gentle dissection with Agris-Dingman to open potential intermuscular space.
7. Use camera to take endoscopic view for selective medial and inferior parasternal insertion release.
8. Irrigate with triple-antibiotic solution.
9. Cut a 5-mm corner in the superiolateral corner of the MuscleGel implant for orientation.
10. Change of gloves for “no-touch” technique.
11. Insert implant carefully to avoid fracture of the implant.
12. Check for folds of the implant with the Agris-Dingman.
13. Sit patient after both implants are placed to confirm orientation.
14. Place 10-mm drain superficial to implant, avoiding the chest wall.
15. Use lighted retractor to check for bleeding in the axillary tunnel.
16. Reapproximate lateral pectoral border to chest wall with 2–0 Vicryl.
17. Reapproximate deep subcutaneous layer with 2–0 Vicryl.
18. Close skin with running 3–0 Monocryl.
19. Use 3–0 nylon drain stitch if drain is required.

19.8.6 Postoperative Dressing

- Mastisol and 1-in linear and crossing Steri-Strips
- Gauze and paper tape
- Ace bandage and compression vest

19.8.7 Postoperative Care

1. Check day 1 to educate patient about implant positioning
2. Week 1 postop visit
3. Drain removal 2–3 weeks depending on < 25 mL/day
4. Compression vest for 4 weeks
5. After 1 week, slow range-of-motion

6. No workout for 1 month
7. Postoperative photos at 3 months

Key Points

- Patient selection is critical. Avoid patients who have unrealistic expectations or who may be noncompliant.
- The goals for pectoral augmentation are to create a natural appearing result with minimal "step-offs" and with congruency with other muscle groups.
- Preoperative markings are critical for ideal positioning of the implant as well as identifying areas for fat grafting.
- Carefult pocket dissection with attention to preoperative markings will optimize outcomes.
- Adjunctive techniques such as periareolar skin excision, pectopexy, or radiofrequency energy for skin tightening can be utilized in certain patients.

References

[1] Murray JF. Correction of pectus excavatum by synthetic subcutaneous implant. Presented at the Annual Meeting of the American Society of Plastic and Reconstructive Surgery. Philadelphia, PA, October 1965
[2] Marks MW, Argenta LC, Lee DC. Silicone implant correction of pectus excavatum: indications and refinement in technique. Plast Reconstr Surg. 1984; 74 (1):52–58
[3] Sørensen JL. Subcutaneous silicone implants in pectus excavatum. Scand J Plast Reconstr Surg Hand Surg. 1988; 22(2):173–176
[4] Snel BJ, Spronk CA, Werker PM, van der Lei B. Pectus excavatum reconstruction with silicone implants: long-term results and a review of the english-language literature. Ann Plast Surg. 2009; 62(2):205–209
[5] Marks MW, Argenta LC, Izenberg PH, Mes LG. Management of the chest-wall deformity in male patients with Poland's syndrome. Plast Reconstr Surg. 1991; 87(4):674–678, discussion 679––681
[6] Hodgkinson DJ. Chest wall implants: their use for pectus excavatum, pectoralis muscle tears, Poland's syndrome, and muscular insufficiency. Aesthetic Plast Surg. 1997; 21(1):7–15
[7] Aiache AE. Male chest correction. Pectoral implants and gynecomastia. Clin Plast Surg. 1991; 18(4):823–828
[8] Novack BH. Alloplastic implants for men. Clin Plast Surg. 1991; 18(4):829–855
[9] Horn G. A new concept in male chest reshaping: anatomical pectoral implants and liposculpture. Aesthetic Plast Surg. 2002; 26(1):23–25
[10] Pereira LH, Sabatovich O, Santana KP, Picanço R. Pectoral muscle implant: approach and procedure. Aesthetic Plast Surg. 2006; 30(4):412–416
[11] Benito-Ruiz J, Raigosa JM, Manzano-Surroca M, Salvador L. Male chest enhancement: pectoral implants. Aesthetic Plast Surg. 2008; 32(1):101–104
[12] Flores-Lima G, Eppley BL. Body contouring with solid silicone implants. Aesthetic Plast Surg. 2009; 33(2):140–146

Part VI

Other Aesthetic Breast Surgery Topics

VI

20 Evaluation and Treatment of Congenital Breast Deformities

Raja Mohan, Akash Chandawarkar, and Justin Sacks

Summary

Congenital deformities of the breast are quite commonly encountered by plastic surgeons because anatomic abnormalities associated with these conditions affect the appearance of the breasts. Each deformity or condition is unique in terms of etiology, workup, and treatment method. Each deformity can be classified under one of the subtypes of congenital deformities of the breast, including hyperplastic conditions, hypoplastic conditions, and deformational conditions. All of these conditions pose reconstructive challenges for plastic surgeons aiming to achieve symmetry and restore the natural anatomy that was hindered during the developmental process. This chapter provides a review of the most common conditions and summarizes the treatment methods for each one.

Keywords: breast embryology, congenital deformities, tuberous breast, Poland syndrome, inverted nipple

20.1 Introduction and Embryology

Congenital breast defects usually can be traced to abnormal development. Therefore, an understanding of normal breast development is critical and can help the plastic surgeon identify appropriate treatments and management of potentially associated conditions.

The breast is a modified sweat gland whose development begins in the fourth to sixth week of gestation.[1,2] Strips of thickened ectoderm appear bilaterally on the ventral surface extending from the axillae to the groin, known as mammary ridges or milk lines (▸ Fig. 20.1). By the seventh to eighth week of gestation, the 15–20 buds within each of the paired mammary ridges begin to involute and undergo apoptosis, with the exception of a single pair of buds (primary mammary buds) that persist at the fourth to fifth intercostal space.[1,2,3] At 8 weeks, the primary bud epithelial tissue begins to invest the underlying mesoderm, known as the disk stage.[4] The underlying mesenchymal connective tissue eventually develops into the superfascial system and Cooper's suspensory ligaments.[3] Between 8 and 14 weeks, the epithelial tissue continues to grow deeper, completing the globular and cone stages, thereby beginning to form buds, which branch into primitive breast alveoli.[4] At 16 weeks, 15–25 epithelial branches are formed, while concurrently differentiation of sweat and sebaceous glands begins. At the start of the third trimester, lactiferous ducts and branches begin to form as small lumina develop within the mammary buds in response to placental sex hormones that initiate the canalization of the epithelial branches.[3,4] The canalization stage continues into childhood. The convergence of these lactiferous ducts is a shallow pit that eventually becomes the nipple. The areola begins developing at 5 months.

At birth, male and female breasts are indistinguishable, with 15–20 mammary lobules that drain into ampullae via the main lactiferous ducts.[1] After birth, the nipple starts to protrude from the areola, and further branching and terminal duct development continues until 2 years of age. Breast development is then suspended until thelarche. In North America, puberty generally starts between 8 and 12 years, during which hypothalamic release of gonadotropin-releasing hormone (GnRH) begins a hormonal cascade that resumes breast development. Increased GnRH stimulates release of the pituitary hormones follicle-stimulating hormone (FSH) and luteinizing hormone (LH),

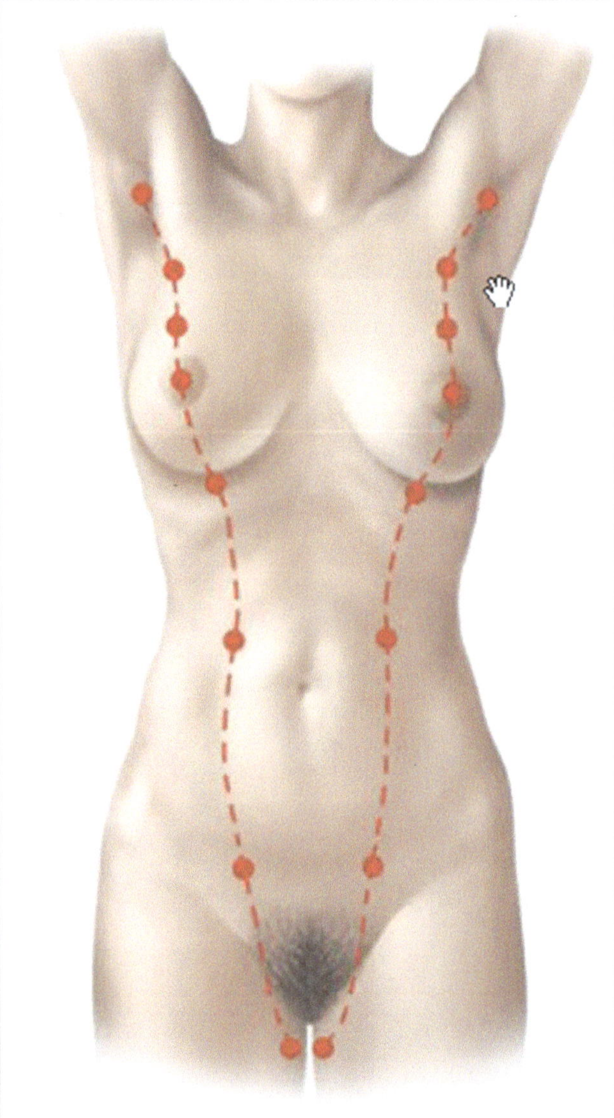

Fig. 20.1 Demonstration of bilateral milk lines that extend from the axillae to the groin. These are common sites of polythelia and polymastia presentation. (Reproduced from Gilroy AM, MacPherson BR, Schuenke M, Schulte E, Schumacher U, eds. Atlas of Anatomy. 3rd ed. Stuttgart, Germany: Thieme Medical Publishers; 2016.)

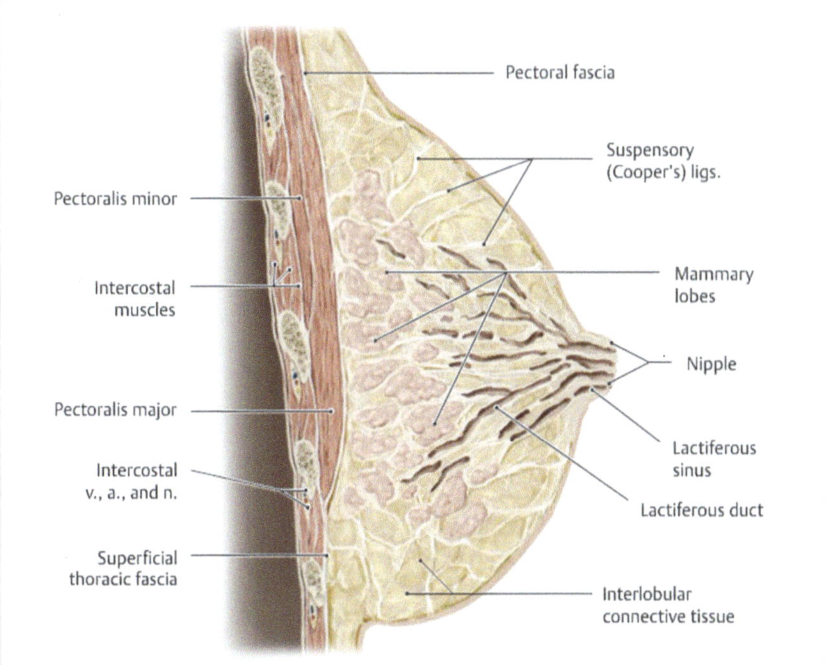

Fig. 20.2 Anatomic structures of the female breast. (Reproduced from Gilroy AM, MacPherson BR, Schuenke M, Schulte E, Schumacher U, eds. Atlas of Anatomy. 3rd ed. Stuttgart, Germany: Thieme Medical Publishers; 2016.)

Table 20.1 Tanner stage classification

Tanner stage	Event
I (preadolescent)	Papilla elevation above level of chest wall
II (breast budding)	Breast and papilla elevation, increased areola diameter
III	Ongoing enlargement of breasts and areolae
IV	Elevation of areola and papilla above breast mound
V	Elevation of papilla with regression of areola

which induces maturation of ovarian follicles. These follicles release systemic progestin and estrogen, which in turn induce proliferation of mammary ductal epithelium, surrounding stroma, collecting ducts, terminal lobules, and breast buds (▶ Fig. 20.2). Volume increases with concomitant vascular and connective tissue proliferation.[1] Overall breast development is commonly described by the Tanner stages (▶ Table 20.1).[5]

20.2 Hyperplastic Conditions

20.2.1 Polythelia

Polythelia, or supernumerary nipples, is the most common encountered anomaly of the pediatric breast.[4,6] The incidence of the condition has been reported to vary from 0.22% to 5.6%.[7] Males and females are generally affected equally,[6,7] and there are some reported differences in incidence between ethnic groups.[2] Cases tend to be sporadic, although reports of familial cases have been reported.[4,6] The etiology is failure of the mammary ridge to regress, although the cause of failure remains unknown.[4] There have been reports of associations with other ectodermal abnormalities, particularly urologic.[2,4,6]

Given the pathophysiology, supernumerary nipples are found at birth anywhere along the milk line (▶ Fig. 20.1). However, other locations have been reported, suggesting an alternative etiology for the condition.[3,7] Most cases are unilateral, without right- or left-side preference, and usually occur in the area below the breast and above the lower abdominal skin.[3,7] Polythelia is usually recognized at birth and often initially confused with nevi or other skin lesions. The nipple can vary from having partial to complete areola, with some even with fully elevated breast tissue.[4]

Polythelia can generally be observed. Elective treatment for irritation or cosmetic purposes can be accomplished with simple elliptical excision. Pigmented lesions are exceptions and should be treated with early prepubertal excision and histopathologic workup, as cancerous degeneration has been reported.[6,7] If the decision for excision is after the onset of puberty in females, glandular growth may warrant a wider excision.[6] If the supernumerary nipple to be excised is on the breast itself, magnetic resonance imaging (MRI) can confirm which nipple areolar complex (NAC) is associated with glandular and ductal tissue. Elliptical excision of the nonassociated nipple proceeds with a subsequent modified Benelli mastopexy to transpose the true NAC into the skin defect.[6] Additional workup, including physical exam, urinalysis, and renal ultrasound, should be undertaken to rule out any associated renal anomalies.[4]

20.2.2 Polymastia

Polymastia, sometimes referred to as ectopic breast, is a congenital condition of extra-anatomic breast tissue. It has a lower incidence than polythelia,[7] occurring in 0.1–1.0% of all live births.[3] The etiology is similar to that of polythelia, likely due to failure of the mammary ridge to regress in utero.[4] There is a female predominance,[2] and generally cases are sporadic in nature. However, familial inheritance has been reported. Polymastia can also be associated with chromosomal abnormalities and other anomalies of the thoracic or urogenital system.[3,6,7]

Table 20.2 Kajava classification of polythelia

Kajava classification	Breast tissue	Areola	Nipple
1. Complete breast	Present	Present	Present
2. Supernumerary breast	Present	Absent	Present
3. Supernumerary breast	Present	Present	Absent
4. Ectopic breast	Present	Absent	Absent
5. Pseudomamma	Absent (fatty tissue present)	Present	Present
6. Polythelia	Absent	Present/ Absent	Present
7. Polythelia areolae	Absent	Present	Absent
8. Polythelia pilosa (patch of hair only)	Absent	Absent	Absent

Unlike polythelia, polymastia often goes unnoticed until puberty, when the glandular tissue responds to hormonal influences.[4,6] Pregnancy and lactation involve similar hormonal changes that can also trigger latent polymastia. This condition also generally occurs along the milk line, most commonly in the axilla (▶ Fig. 20.1).[3,4] In fact, it is often mistaken for lymphadenopathy or a lipoma. The ectopic breast tissue most commonly manifests as a scanty amount of tissue with a small NAC, but presentation can vary widely.[2,4] Because breast tissue responds to systemic signaling, accessory breast tissue is subject to the same physiologic changes and disease processes as normal breast tissue.[2,4]

Resection is generally considered for cosmetic reasons as well as for pathologic risk reduction. Timing of resection generally occurs after breast development has completed to avoid continued growth of retained tissue. Type of resection depends on size and location.[7] If there is a third distinct breast mount, simple mastectomy with avoidance of inframammary fold (IMF) disruption and soft tissue envelope of the remaining breast is warranted. If the ectopic tissue is adjoined to the normal breast, tissue-sparing techniques with skin de-epithelialization and accessory nipple excision can be performed. Because of high complication rates of resection in the axilla, liposuction can be useful for reduction of fatty components of the accessory tissue and definition of the planes between the accessory tissue and underlying axilla.[2] Follow-up is warranted for continued cancer surveillance of any possible residual tissue.[6] The common etiology of polythelia and polymastia brings about a wide variety of presentations. These are organized by the Kajava classification system (▶ Table 20.2).

20.2.3 Virginal Hypertrophy or Mammary Hyperplasia

Mammary hyperplasia or virginal hypertrophy is a rare condition of unknown etiology.[3,4,5] It is thought that the glandular tissue is hyperresponsive to normal levels of hormones, causing rapid and disproportionate breast growth. Notably, the fatty and fibrous elements of the breast tissue are increased rather than the glandular component.[3] Despite the proposed hormonal etiology, there is no association with obesity or increased risk of breast cancer.[3,4] This condition is typically sporadic; however, one case of hereditary pattern has been reported.[4]

Mammary hyperplasia usually presents shortly after puberty, approximately between the ages of 11 and 16. If it presents before puberty, cases are usually bilateral. Virginal or postpubertal presentation can be unilateral or bilateral.[6] Patients generally have normal endocrine studies and otherwise normal growth of the remainder of the body.[6] Growth occurs rapidly and is disproportionate to the rest of the body.[4] Sternal notch-to-nipple distance can increase several centimeters per month. Onset of symptoms can occur over the course of a few months. The rapidity of expansion causes skin changes such as striae, thin skin, and dilated veins. The breast is dense and tender on physical exam. Patients usually present with significant discomfort due to the weight of the breast, and this can cause significant psychological stress.

The goals of treatment are volume reduction, symmetry, and anatomically correct NAC.[6] Timing of definitive surgery is usually delayed until the end of puberty, after breast growth has been static for approximately 1 year, to avoid revisions.[3,6] However, if patients are highly symptomatic, earlier surgical treatment is warranted. Standard treatment is breast reduction; however, regrowth after reduction can occur. Antiestrogenic medical adjuncts (such as medroxyprogesterone acetate, dydrogesterone, tamoxifen, and bromocriptine [if pregnant]) play a significant role in decreasing the rates of regrowth after reduction.[4] Recalcitrant regrowth may require revisional surgery (or mastectomy for extreme cases) with free nipple grafts or nipple areolar reconstruction.[4] Counseling with a psychiatrist or psychologist is recommended in the treatment plan, especially to ensure that patients can accept the risks of surgery including potential scarring, diminished nipple sensitivity, and reduced ability to breastfeed.[3]

20.3 Hypoplastic Conditions

20.3.1 Asymmetry

Breast asymmetry is a generic term that refers to the variable hypoplasia of one or both breasts. It occurs frequently (as high as 80% in patients presenting to a single plastic surgery clinic desiring augmentation or reduction mammaplasty) and has a large variety of presentation on a continuum from minor to more than an entire size difference between breasts.[3,8]

Because the goal of treatment is symmetry, treatment is optimally performed after full development to allow for planning.[2] For mild asymmetries, augmentation of the smaller breast, with or without reduction or mastopexy of the larger breast, can help achieve symmetry (▶ Fig. 20.3, ▶ Fig. 20.4). For more severe asymmetries, staged reconstruction with tissue expansion and overinflation can allow for breast ptosis and a larger skin envelope before the permanent implant is inserted.[3] Lipofilling can help adjust for small asymmetries or revisions.[2] If both breasts are hypoplastic, differential augmentation of both breasts may be required.[6] It is important to note that differential physiologic changes can occur to each reconstructed breast with aging, weight gain, or pregnancy, which may require additional procedures.[3]

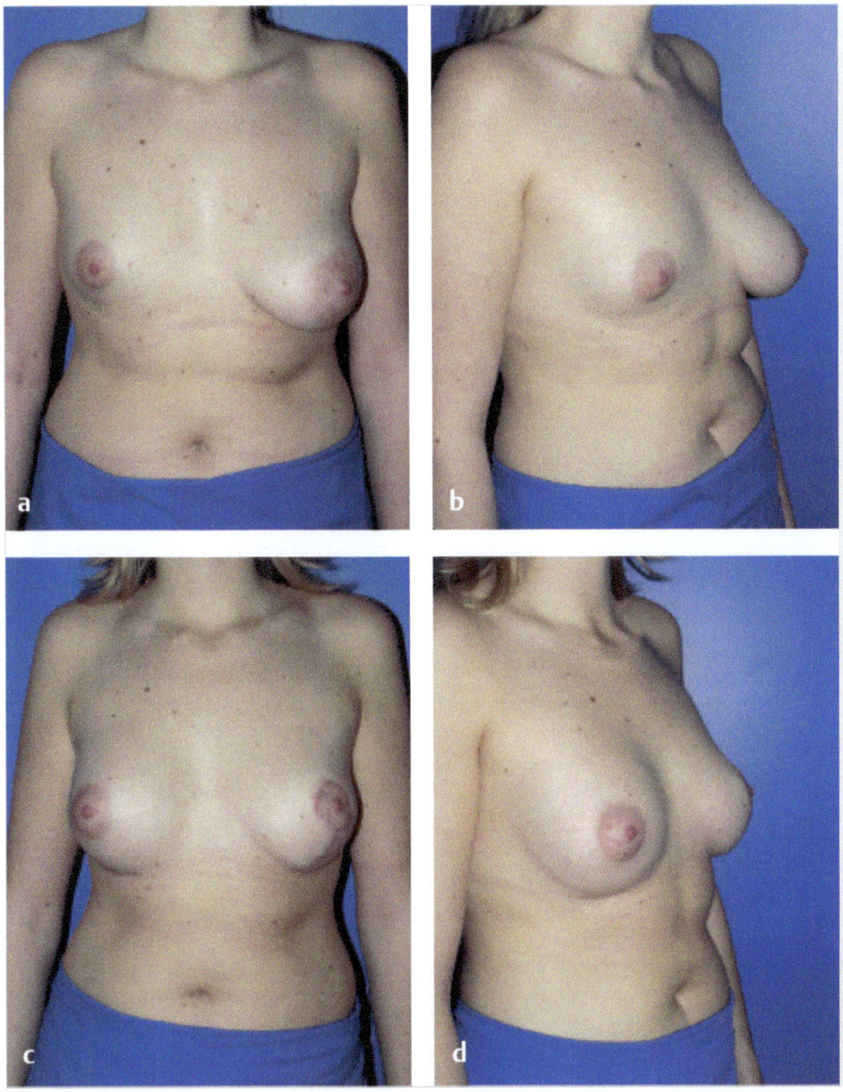

Fig. 20.3 Patient aged 23 with asymmetric breasts. **(a,b)** Preoperative photographs showing right-sided hypoplasia with respect to the normal appearance of the left breast. **(c,d)** Postoperative photographs after right-sided augmentation and Lejour mastopexy on the left. (Reproduced from Gabka CJ, Bohmert H, Blondeel PN. Plastic and Reconstructive Surgery of the Breast. Stuttgart, Germany: Thieme Medical Publishers; 2009.)

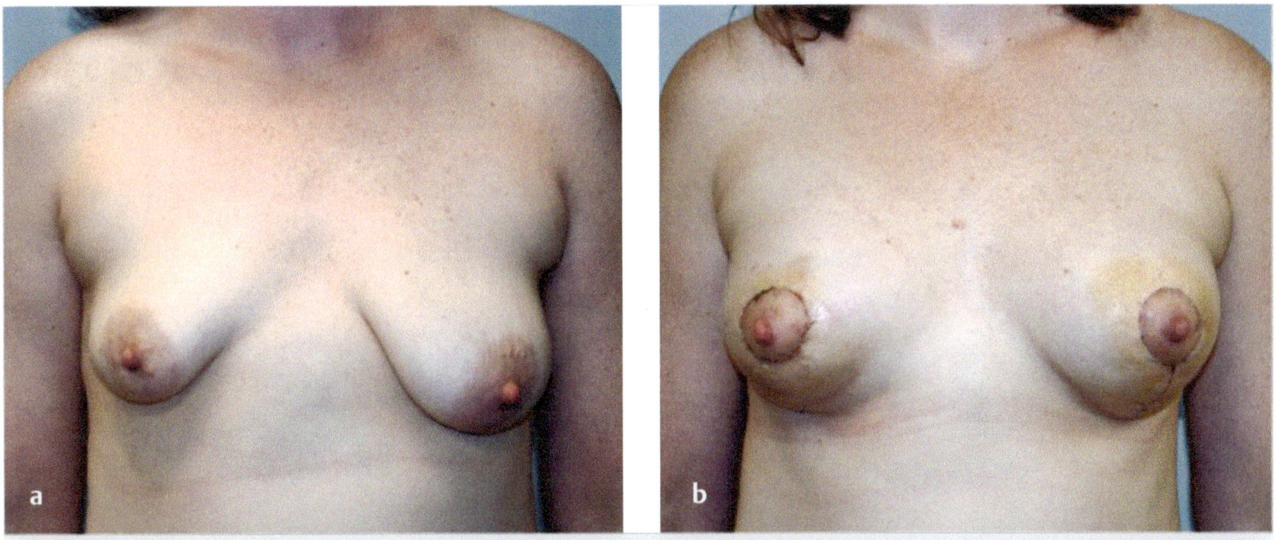

Fig. 20.4 **(a)** Patient aged 36 with breast asymmetry. She underwent an asymmetrical breast augmentation with overlying mastopexy. A 325-mL implant was placed on the right with periareolar mastopexy, and a 250-mL implant was placed on the left side with a vertical mastopexy. **(b)** Postoperative photograph. (Reproduced from Nahai F. Art of Aesthetic Surgery: Principles and Techniques, 2nd ed. New York: Thieme Medical Publishers; 2010.)

Table 20.3 Elsahy classification of asymmetric breasts

Elsahy asymmetry classification	Definition
Type I	Unilateral micromastia
Type II	Unilateral macromastia
Type III	Micro- and macromastia
Type IV	Bilateral asymmetric micromastia
Type V	Bilateral asymmetric macromastia

Elsahy's classification system for asymmetry is shown in ▶ Table 20.3.[9] The most common types of asymmetry in one study were found to be type IV (bilateral asymmetric micromastia) followed by type V (bilateral asymmetric macromastia).[8] Classification of patients to a particular asymmetry category can assist with preoperative surgical planning.

20.3.2 Athelia

Athelia consists of the absence of the NAC, with or without associated amastia (absence of breast tissue). The true incidence is unknown.[4] The etiology is thought to be an abnormality of mammary ridge involution. Studies have implicated parathyroid-related hormone deficiency in the lack of proliferation of mesenchyme that forms the NAC.[10] There is almost uniform association with syndromes or clusters of anomalies, including[2,4]

- Syndromes and symptom complexes: Poland syndrome, choanal atresia–athelia syndrome, Al Awadi/Raas-Rothschild syndrome, scalp–ear–nipple (SEN) syndrome.
- Anomalies: dermoid cysts, ectodermal dysplasia.

Presentation can be unilateral or bilateral and is usually noted at birth. At that time, treatment options should focus on a thorough workup for associated abnormalities. Nipple reconstruction is usually deferred until puberty.[4] In females with isolated athelia, reconstruction is performed after the completion of breast development for location and symmetry purposes. Female cases of athelia associated with amastia have delayed nipple reconstruction after breast reconstruction is completed. For males, nipple reconstruction can begin at puberty; however, there is a paucity of landmarks if the athelia is bilateral to determine the appropriate anatomic location. Studies by Beer provide the following equations for anatomical nipple location[11]:

- Distance A (mid-sternal line to nipple) = 2.4 cm + (0.09 × circumference of thorax).
- Distance B (sternal notch to intersection with A) = 1.2 cm + (0.28 × sternum length) + (0.1 × circumference of thorax).

When the appropriate timing and location for NAC reconstruction is determined, reconstruction can proceed with similar techniques to those performed after mastectomy.[4] Options include traditional tattooing, local tissue flaps, and skin grafts based on patient preference.

20.3.3 Amastia

Amastia, or the absence of breast tissue, is a rare condition that can have significant impact on self-esteem and health-related quality of life.[5] Amastia is a congenital ectodermal defect that results in the mammary ridge completely disappearing or failing to develop in the first place.[2] This can occur sporadically, familially, or via exposure to teratogenic drugs during the first trimester (e.g., dehydroepiandrosterone, methimazole/carbimazole).[12] This condition most commonly presents unilaterally as a variant of Poland syndrome,[3,6,7,12] which is discussed elsewhere in this chapter. Bilateral amastia can present concomitantly with other anomalies related to ectodermal defects including cleft palate, pectoral muscle or upper-limb deformities, urologic abnormalities, or epidermal abnormalities.[2,6,7,13] Amastia may be a part of other syndromes, such as acral–renal–ectodermal dysplasia–lipoatrophic diabetes (AREDYLD) syndrome,[12] so a full body workup is warranted upon diagnosis of amastia.

Treatment of amastia follows principles of postoncologic breast reconstruction, but specific attention should be paid to timing as well as placement of the IMF and nipple given the lack of anatomic landmarks.[7] Tissue expanders with final autologous or prosthetic reconstruction should be planned. The timing of tissue expansion can follow the development of the unaffected side (if unilateral) or with comparisons to the patient's peers (if bilateral).[3] Final reconstruction should be undertaken after the patient reaches full maturity. If autologous reconstruction is chosen, flaps such as the deep inferior epigastric perforator flap, transverse upper gracilis flap, gluteal flap, or latissimus dorsi flap should be considered.[6] It is important to be wary of possible aberrancies in blood supply due to associated abnormalities in planning of autologous reconstruction.[6] If unilateral prosthetic reconstruction is planned, especially at an early stage, patients will require lifelong follow-up due to breast changes over time. Patients should be advised that revisional surgery might be warranted in the future for symmetry purposes.[3]

20.3.4 Amazia

There are relatively few reports of amazia, a condition characterized by absence of glandular breast tissue with a normal NAC.[13] The condition is the result of atrophy of the entire mammary ridge between 7 and 10 weeks of gestation with a concomitant improper regression of the accessory nipple along the milk line. There have been reports of bilateral amazia with bilateral choanal atresia and midface hypoplasia.

As a part of the surgical treatment plan, psychological evaluation and follow-up are important since many patients notice their development is abnormal and unlike their peers'. Because this condition can be confused with a normal variant, definitive diagnosis with imaging is needed to confirm the complete lack of breast tissue.[13] In patients with sufficient and good skin quality, augmentation mammaplasty can be performed using methods similar to a cosmetic breast augmentation. Patients with deficiency of skin may require reconstruction using expander–implant-based reconstruction or autologous tissue. The common treatment methods for breast reconstruction of a mastectomy defect can be applied in these cases.

20.3.5 Tuberous Breast Deformity

Tuberous breast deformities are a common complaint for patients desiring breast surgery, but the exact incidence is unknown.[4] Tuberous breast deformity equates to a congenital breast deformity with herniated breast protruding through a constricting fascial ring beneath the areola. Patients typically have an enlarged NAC with deficiency of glandular volume of the breast in different quadrants. It is bilateral in 89% of cases, and volumetric asymmetry of > 100 g is present in two-thirds of patients.[3]

The most common abnormalities present in a tuberous breast deformity are as follows[2,6]:

- Hypoplastic breast with deficient base diameter.
- Herniation of breast tissue into areola.
- Deficient skin envelope.
- IMF malposition (typically too high or absent).

There are various hypotheses on how this condition originates, including the following:

1. The lower pole fascia tightly adheres the dermis to the muscle, thereby restricting lower pole breast expansion and forcing expansion toward the NAC.[1,6]
2. A constriction at the breast base causes deficiency of breast tissue in the vertical and horizontal dimensions.[1,3,5]

There are two types of classification systems in the literature describing the stages and extent of the tuberous breast deformity (▶ Table 19.4, ▶ Table 19.5).[14,16]

There are various treatment methods depending on the type and severity of the defect. The general principles involve addressing any components of abnormal anatomy present[7]:

- Release constricted base.
- Lower IMF and set appropriate nipple-to-IMF length.
- Reduce areolar size.
- Correct herniated breast tissue.
- Correct any asymmetry.
- Augment if needed for volume.
- Address in one or two stages depending on the type of deformity.

Herniation of breast tissue through the NAC requires the release of any constriction ring present as well as the reduction of NAC size.[6] Radial scoring of the constricted base of the breast allows glandular tissue to distribute and fill the breast quadrants.[3,4] If the IMF is absent or high, this needs to be lowered, and local tissue can be recruited (Ryan flap) if needed.

Volume can be added with either autologous tissue, an alloplastic implant, or autologous fat grafting. One method to determine the new position of the IMF is to multiply the implant height by 0.55, since 55% of the glandular volume is located in the lower pole of the breast.[17] Anatomic implants are better suited for patients with tuberous breast deformities, since most of the volume is needed in the lower pole. If the patient desires to be a much larger size, staging the augmentation may produce a more predictable result. The implant can be placed in a subglandular or submuscular pocket using an inframammary or periareolar incision. Patients in need of areolar reduction or ptosis repair may require a circumareolar or vertical pattern mastopexy (▶ Fig. 20.5).

More severe tuberous breast deformities may necessitate the use of a tissue expander or autologous flap to address constrictions, lack of glandular volume, and skin deficiencies.[4] Any skin deficiency most likely will require multiple stages to address the deformity.

Complications with any implant-based procedure include infection, hematoma, capsular contracture, implant failure, asymmetry, and wound dehiscence.[2] Even despite correction, a short nipple-to-IMF (N-IMF) distance and large NAC may persist, requiring further revision.

Table 19.4 Heimburg classification of tuberous breast deformity

Heimburg classification	Definition
Type I	Hypoplasia of lower medial quadrant
Type II	Hypoplasia of lower medial and lateral quadrants; sufficient subareolar skin
Type III	Hypoplasia of lower lateral and medial quadrants; deficiency of subareolar skin
Type IV	Severe breast constriction; minimal breast base

20.4 Deformational Conditions

20.4.1 Inverted Nipple

An inverted nipple is reported to be present in 2% of the general population, and there is a positive family history in 50% of patients with this condition.[2] Very often this condition goes unnoticed, but some patients do desire correction because of difficulties with breastfeeding or for concerns associated with cosmesis. It is due to tethering of the breast ducts as well as the development of fibrous bands posterior to the nipple in gestation.[2]

Many surgical treatment methods have been described for inverted nipples that persist into adolescence and adulthood. Some involve tightening the areolar edges circumferentially using suture techniques or using adjacent flaps to augment the nipple base. A short circumareolar incision can be made in order to allow release of the tight bands that cause inversion.[2]

Complications of procedures include the loss of nipple sensation, recurrence, and inability to breastfeed. Inability to breastfeed occurs secondary to the division of the breast ducts during repair of the inverted nipple. Some techniques have been described that involve meticulous dissection of release of fibrous bands while leaving breast ducts intact.[18]

20.4.2 Poland Syndrome

Poland syndrome occurs in 1 in 7,000 to 10,000 people worldwide. It generally affects men more than women (3:1 ratio), with the right side of the body being affected more commonly. Familial forms of the disease have been described involving a mutation of an autosomal dominant gene. One proposed theory for the etiology of the complex is an interruption of the blood supply to the upper limb secondary to hypoplasia of the subclavian artery.[3,7] As a result, the pectoralis major muscle does not develop, and ipsilateral hand anomalies are possible.[4]

Table 19.5 Grolleau classification of tuberous breast deformity

Grolleau classification	Definition
Type I	Lower medial quadrant deficiency
Type II	Lower lateral and medial quadrant deficiencies
Type III	Deficiencies of all four quadrants

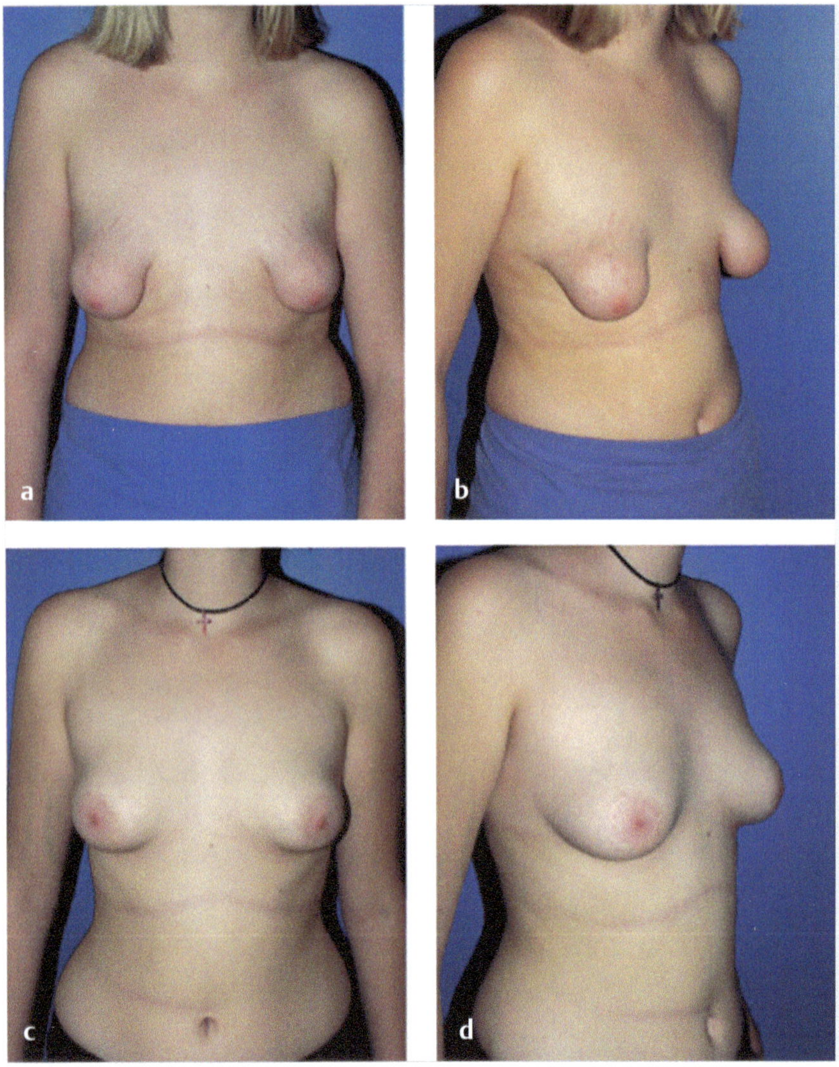

Fig. 20.5 Patient aged 24 with bilateral tuberous breast deformity. **(a,b)** Preoperative photographs. **(c,d)** Postoperative photographs taken 9 months after periareolar correction. (Reproduced from Gabka CJ, Bohmert H, Blondeel PN. Plastic and Reconstructive Surgery of the Breast. Stuttgart, Germany: Thieme Medical Publishers; 2009.)

Anatomic abnormalities and components of the complex include the following[2,4,7]:

- Hypoplasia of breast and NAC (present in 33%).
- Absence of pectoralis major (costosternal) and pectoralis minor muscles.
- Scarcity of subcutaneous tissue.
- Deficiencies involving other neighboring thoracic muscles (latissimus dorsi, external oblique, serratus anterior).
- Deformity of costal cartilages II–IV (possible decrease in pulmonary vital capacity).
- Alopecia of axillary and mammary regions.
- Ipsilateral brachysyndactyly (present in up to 56%).
- Renal anomalies.

Treatment for this syndrome involves not only addressing the cosmetic deformity and lack of breast tissue but also evaluating for other abnormalities such as chest wall depression and paradoxical movement of the chest wall. Treatment proceeds when contralateral breast development has completed in order to obtain symmetry.[6]

With regard to treatment, the most appropriate reconstruction is determined by evaluation of the chest wall, pectoralis muscle, and soft tissue volume. In the rare patient with an unstable chest wall, bone grafts may be required to stablilize the chest wall. The pectoralis deficiency can be addressed in several ways. In cases of partial absence of the muscle in which the anterior axillary fold is defined, the primary focus is on soft tissue augmentation with either autologous tissue flaps or prosthesis. The type of soft tissue augmentation should take into account the contralateral breast shape and volume. Patients requiring glandular volume with an adequate skin envelope can undergo augmentation mammaplasty. Lipofilling using autologous fat grafting is another option for mild deformities. Patients who have not completed puberty, have deficient skin volume, or have asymmetry can undergo staged reconstruction with a tissue expander followed by placement of a permanent implant (▸ Fig. 20.6). In cases of total absence of the pectoralis muscle, an ipsilateral neurotized latissimus dorsi myocutaneous flap can be performed with subsequent soft tissue augmentation with autologous perforator flap or prosthesis. Patients with more severe deformities may require autologous flap reconstruction with the possible use of an implant for further projection and volume (▸ Fig. 20.7). One commonly used option is an ipsilateral latissimus dorsi flap, which can also be neurotized to

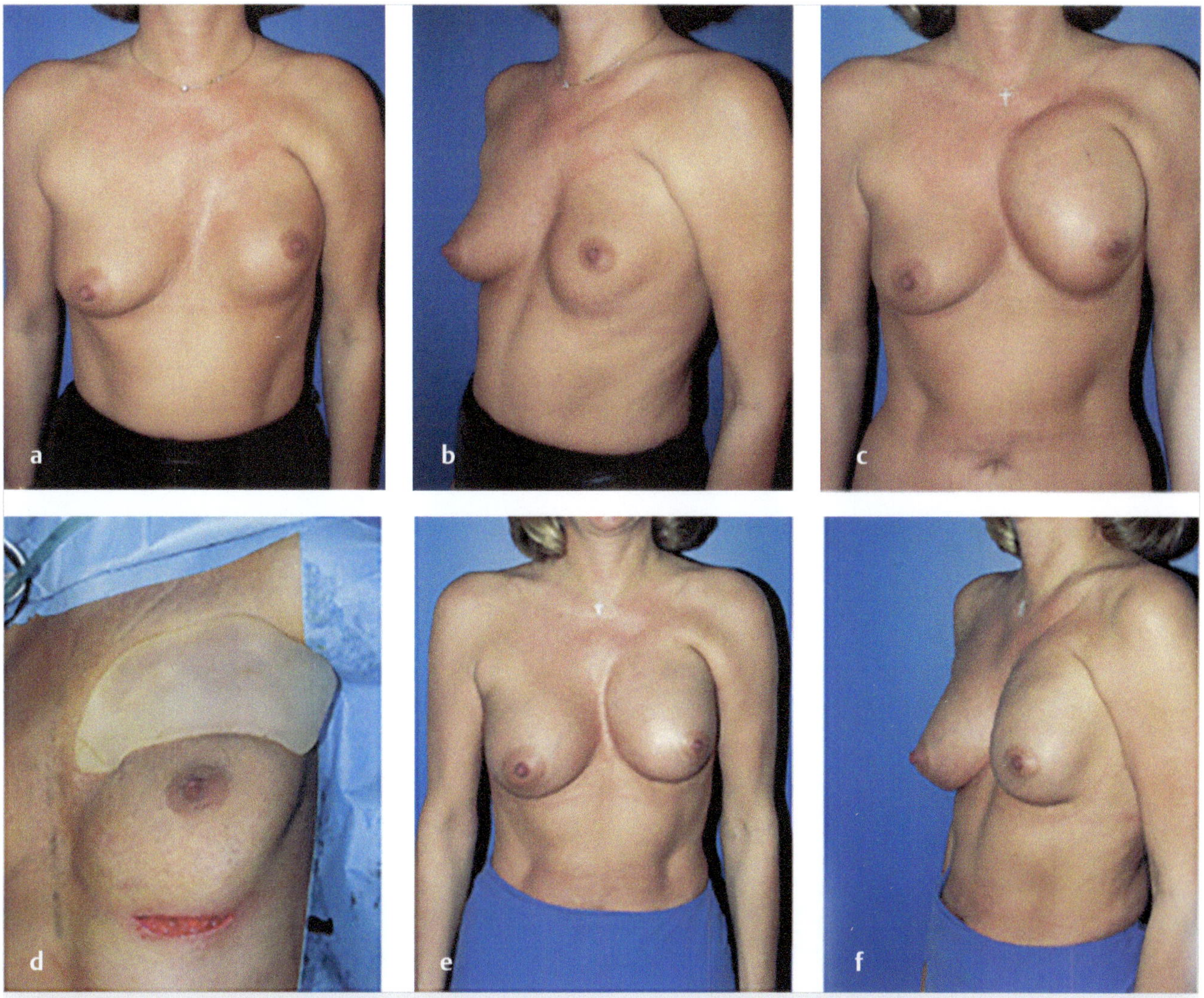

Fig. 20.6 (a–f) Patient aged 48 with severe Poland syndrome who underwent staged expander–implant-based reconstruction of her pectus deformity. (Reproduced from Gabka CJ, Bohmert H, Blondeel PN. Plastic and Reconstructive Surgery of the Breast. Stuttgart, Germany: Thieme Medical Publishers; 2009.)

provide a dynamic transfer (▶ Fig. 20.8). The position of the NAC may need to be lowered, and in such cases tissue expansion prior to soft tissue reconstruction may be performed to expand the area of the chest wall preferentially to effect the necessary movement of the NAC.

Severe malformations of the chest wall may require more extensive reconstruction with autologous flaps, prosthetic mesh, and/or bony reconstruction using split rib grafts. The goal of chest wall reconstruction is to provide a stable bony framework, and any instability can be reconstructed with split rib grafts to bridge bony gaps.[7] Any local flap option may have aberrant or compromised vasculature, requiring preoperative imaging before any reconstruction is pursued.[4]

20.5 Conclusion

Congenital deformities of the breast include a wide range of conditions and deformities that can be classified into one of three categories: hyperplastic, hypoplastic, and deformational. Each condition has its own proposed etiology and set of anatomic abnormalities. Some are associated with medical conditions affecting other organ systems. Any congenital deformity of the breast requires a thorough workup to rule out any other comorbid conditions. The treatment methods for these conditions stem from the general principles used in aesthetic and reconstructive plastic surgery of the breast. The goal with each treatment is to achieve symmetry and create a naturally

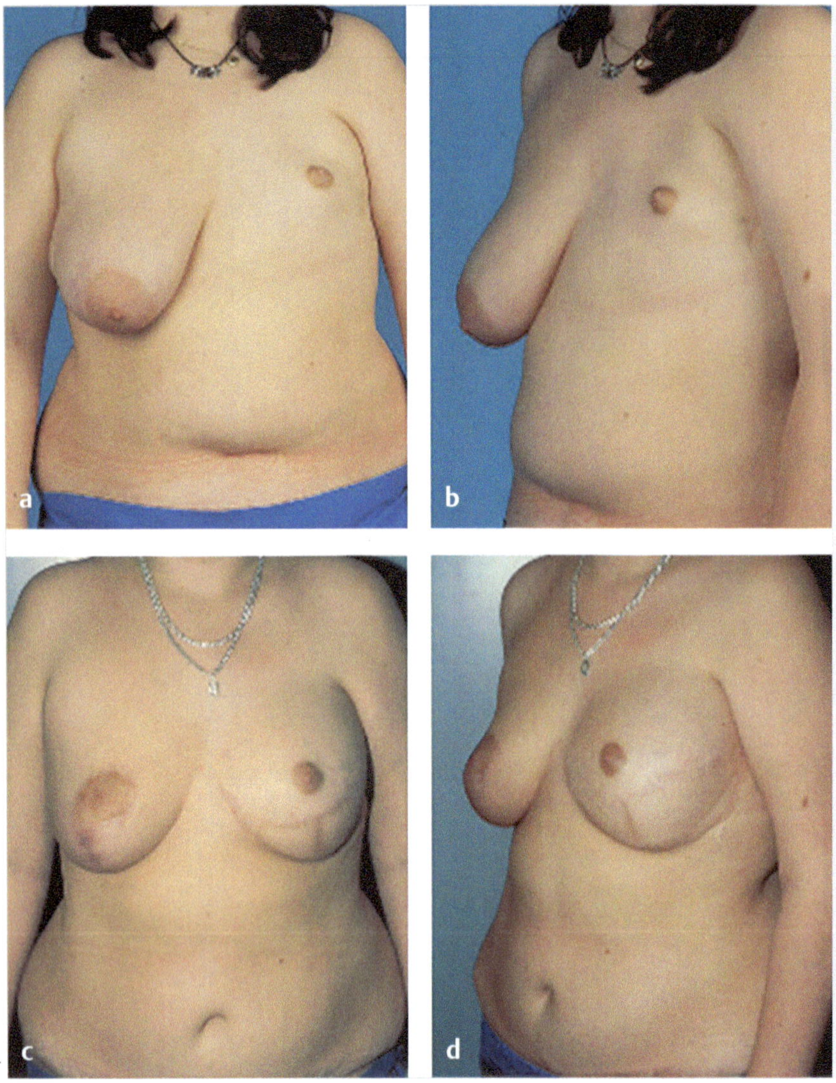

Fig. 20.7 (a–d) Patient with severe Poland syndrome who underwent a transverse rectus abdominis myocutaneous (TRAM) flap to reconstruct defect. (Reproduced from Gabka CJ, Bohmert H, Blondeel PN. Plastic and Reconstructive Surgery of the Breast. Stuttgart, Germany: Thieme Medical Publishers; 2009.)

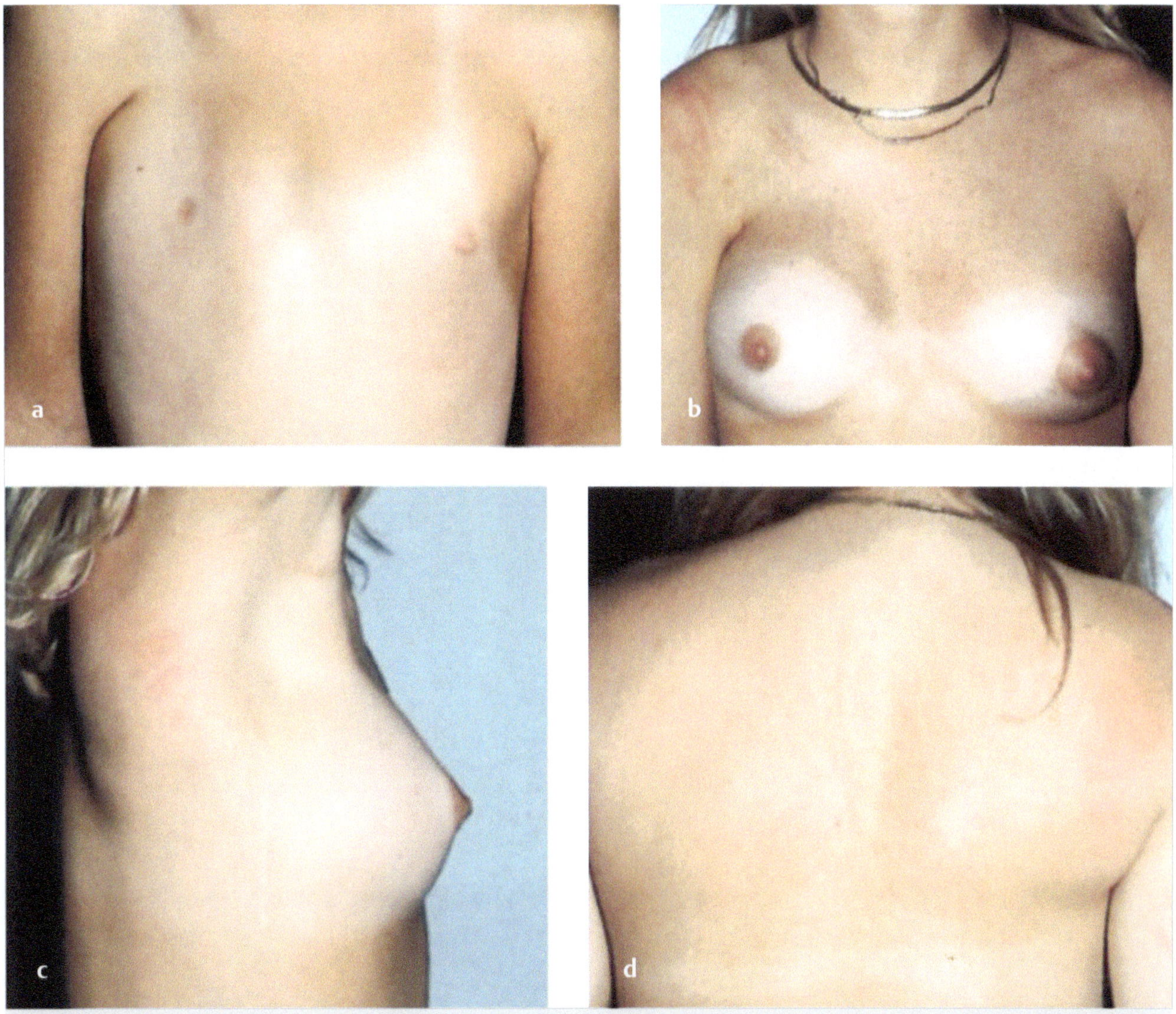

Fig. 20.8 (a–d) Patient aged 9 with Poland syndrome who had nipple malposition. She underwent a latissimus dorsi flap to the affected side and an asymmetric bilateral augmentation mammaplasty seven years later. (Reproduced from Nahai F. Art of Aesthetic Surgery: Principles and Techniques, 2nd ed. New York: Thieme Medical Publishers; 2010.)

appearing breast. The key for any plastic surgeon is first to diagnose the condition and understand what is *normal* before formulating a treatment plan. This chapter serves as a review of the most common congenital conditions any plastic surgeon may encounter in clinical practice.

Key Points

- Polythelia is a common condition that can be observed or managed with excision.
- Mammary hyperplasia is a hormonally mediated condition that sometimes requires surgical intervention with reduction techniques.
- Amastia, athelia, and amazia are all rare conditions requiring reconstructive techniques to address the type of breast tissue that is missing.
- Patients with tuberous breast deformity may present requesting a breast augmentation, but the procedure to address the various deformities requires more than adding volume.
- Poland syndrome is a condition that may require the use of autologous tissue or expander-implant-based reconstruction for correction.

References

[1] Lemaine V, Simmons PS. The adolescent female: Breast and reproductive embryology and anatomy. Clin Anat. 2013; 26(1):22–28

[2] Kulkarni D, Dixon JM. Congenital abnormalities of the breast. Womens Health (Lond). 2012; 8(1):75–86, quiz 87––88

[3] Pryor LS, Lehman JA, Jr, Workman MC. Disorders of the female breast in the pediatric age group. Plast Reconstr Surg. 2009; 124(1) Suppl:50e–60e

[4] Latham K, Fernandez S, Iteld L, Panthaki Z, Armstrong MB, Thaller S. Pediatric breast deformity. J Craniofac Surg. 2006; 17(3):454–467

[5] Tanner JM, Whitehouse RH. Clinical longitudinal standards for height, weight, height velocity, weight velocity, and stages of puberty. Arch Dis Child. 1976; 51(3):170–179
[6] Sadove AM, van Aalst JA. Congenital and acquired pediatric breast anomalies: a review of 20 years' experience. Plast Reconstr Surg. 2005; 115(4):1039–1050
[7] Caouette-Laberge L, Borsuk D. Congenital anomalies of the breast. Semin Plast Surg. 2013; 27(1):36–41
[8] DeLuca-Pytell DM, Piazza RC, Holding JC, Snyder N, Hunsicker LM, Phillips LG. The incidence of tuberous breast deformity in asymmetric and symmetric mammaplasty patients. Plast Reconstr Surg. 2005; 116(7):1894–1899, discussion 1900–1901
[9] Elsahy NI. Correction of asymmetries of the breasts. Plast Reconstr Surg. 1976; 57(6):700–703
[10] Pellegrini JR, Wagner RF, Jr. Polythelia and associated conditions. Am Fam Physician. 1983; 28(3):129–132
[11] Beer GM, Budi S, Seifert B, Morgenthaler W, Infanger M, Meyer VE. Configuration and localization of the nipple-areola complex in men. Plast Reconstr Surg. 2001; 108(7):1947–1952, discussion–1953
[12] Patil LG, Shivanna NH, Benakappa N, Ravindranath H, Bhat R. Congenital amastia. Indian J Pediatr. 2013; 80(10):870–871
[13] Dreifuss SE, Macisaac ZM, Grunwaldt LJ. Bilateral congenital amazia: a case report and systematic review of the literature. J Plast Reconstr Aesthet Surg. 2014; 67(1):27–33
[14] Grolleau JL, Lanfrey E, Lavigne B, Chavoin JP, Costagliola M. Breast base anomalies: treatment strategy for tuberous breasts, minor deformities, and asymmetry. Plast Reconstr Surg. 1999; 104(7):2040–2048
[15] Mandrekas AD, Zambacos GJ. Aesthetic reconstruction of the tuberous breast deformity. Plast Reconstr Surg. 2004; 113(7):2231–2232
[16] von Heimburg D. Refined version of the tuberous breast classification. Plast Reconstr Surg. 2000; 105(6):2269–2270
[17] Mallucci P, Branford OA. Design for natural breast augmentation: the ICE principle. Plast Reconstr Surg. 2016; 137(6):1728–1737
[18] Gould DJ, Nadeau MH, Macias LH, Stevens WG. Inverted nipple repair revisited: a 7-year experience. Aesthet Surg J. 2015; 35(2):156–164

21 Transgender Breast Surgery

Paul R. Weiss and Loren S. Schechter

Summary
Many individuals with gender dysphoria seek surgical therapy to help alleviate their symptoms and allow them to become the persons they know themselves to be. Breast augmentation or mastectomy/chest reconstruction is often requested by transgender and gender-diverse individuals. While previously considered "cosmetic" in nature, these procedures have been shown to have significant therapeutic benefits and are often deemed medically necessary by patients, health care providers, and insurance companies. This chapter reviews indications, surgical techniques, and other considerations in providing care for transgender and gender-diverse individuals.

Keywords: transgender, gender-diverse, gender dysphoria, augmentation mammoplasty, mastectomy/chest reconstruction

21.1 Introduction

Gender dysphoria is a condition where an individual's assigned gender at birth causes significant distress or impairment. Many transgender and gender-diverse individuals who suffer from gender dysphoria seek surgical therapy to alleviate their symptoms. Breast or chest surgery, specifically either augmentation mammaplasty or mastectomy/chest reconstruction, are commonly requested procedures in the transgender and gender-diverse population. The overall goal of such procedures is to relieve or alleviate symptoms of gender dysphoria and allow individuals to live as the people they know themselves to be. Individual goals vary between patients. In some individuals, breast or chest surgery may be the only procedure requested, while in others, such surgery is one of many steps in their transition. From a technical perspective, the goals of surgery include a successful cosmetic and functional result with minimal complications. While breast and chest/reconstruction surgery were formerly considered "cosmetic," they have increasingly been recognized as therapeutic and medically necessary procedures.

In caring for the transgender or gender-diverse individual, the surgeon functions as part of the multidisciplinary healthcare team. This team may include mental health professionals, primary care providers, and endocrinologists. As a team member, the operating surgeon should understand the diagnosis that has led to the recommendation for surgery; medical comorbidities that may impact the surgical outcome; the effects of hormonal therapy (when applicable) on the patient's health; and factors that may predict the patient's ultimate satisfaction with the surgical result.[1] Furthermore, the surgeon should help coordinate the patient's postoperative care to ensure continuity.

Surgeons caring for transgender and gender-diverse individuals should be familiar with the World Professional Association for Transgender Health (WPATH)'s Standards of Care (SOC).[2] These guidelines provide a flexible framework to help provide care to transgender and gender-diverse individuals. While procedures such as augmentation mammaplasty and chest surgery are not as invasive as genital surgery, the surgeon should take care in order to ensure that individuals pursuing such surgery are appropriate candidates.

The SOC recommend that individuals who request breast or chest surgery have one referral letter from a mental health provider. Mental health providers can come from a variety of disciplines (psychology, psychiatry, social work, nursing, family practice, etc.) and should have specific training and experience in caring for transgender and gender-diverse individuals. In addition to mental health evaluation, input from a patient's primary care doctor or, in some cases, endocrinologist is useful in confirming that an individual is medically fit for surgery. The surgeon should, when needed, communicate directly with members of the healthcare team, especially if there are any questions regarding a patient's appropriateness for surgery. The SOC recommend the following criterion for individuals who desire breast or chest surgery[2]:

1. Persistent, well-documented gender dysphoria.
2. Capacity to make a fully informed decision and to consent to treatment.
3. Age of majority in a given country (if younger, additional recommendations apply).
4. Reasonably good control of any significant medical or mental health concerns that may be present.

Hormone therapy is not a prerequisite for mastectomy/chest reconstruction surgery or augmentation mammaplasty. However, some insurance plans may require hormone therapy to preauthorize surgery. In the authors' experience, it is uncommon for individuals requesting augmentation mammaplasty to achieve sufficient breast growth with hormonal therapy alone. However, 12 months of feminizing hormone therapy prior to augmentation mammaplasty may help to maximize breast growth and achieve a more stable result following surgery.

In appropriate surgical candidates, an in-person consultation should be obtained. During the consultation, the surgeon should discuss the surgical techniques, the advantages and disadvantages of the techniques, the limitations of the procedure, and the risks and possible complications of the various techniques.[2] Furthermore, the surgeon should discuss the individual's expectations from surgery and review the postoperative care. Patients who have unrealistic expectations are at risk for disappointment with their final results.

If an individual decides to proceed with surgery, written documentation of informed consent should be included in the patient's chart.

21.2 Augmentation Mammaplasty in Trans Women

21.2.1 Breast Development and Hormone Therapy

Breast development in prenatal life is independent of sex hormones and is, therefore, the same in males and females.[3] During embryonic development, breast buds composed of networks of tubules develop from the ectoderm. In females, these tubules will eventually become mature milk ducts. Until puberty, the tubule networks of the breast buds remain quiet. At puberty, male and female breast development diverges. In females, estrogen and progestins, in conjunction with growth hormone and insulin-like growth factor 1 (IGF-1), result in growth and maturation of the tubules into the ductal system of the breasts. Estrogens are generally believed to induce breast proliferation, whereas progestins result in differentiation.[4] Progestins are not thought to have a significant role in breast volume.[5] In contrast, in puberty of males, androgens (testosterone and dihydrotestosterone) increase about 10-fold higher compared to females, and estrogen is about 10-fold lower compared to females. The high levels of androgens strongly inhibit the action of estrogen in the breast at puberty, resulting in lack of breast development in men.

In trans women, some breast growth occurs with suppression of androgens and supplementation with estrogens. Androgen blockade can be achieved with antiandrogens. In the United States, spironolactone is the most commonly used antiandrogen, whereas in Europe, cytoproterone acetate is extensively used. One major difference between the agents is that cytoproterone also has progestogenic properties in addition to its antiandrogenic effects. Cytoproterone is not approved for use in the United States due to concerns of hepatotoxicity. Some centers use gonadotropin-releasing hormone (GnRH) analogs to suppress androgen production, but cost limits use of these agents. Alternatively, orchiectomy is an effective way to reduce androgen levels.

Breast size typically begins to increase 2–3 months after the start of hormone therapy. Initially, breast buds begin to form and breast growth progresses over 2 years.[4,6] Because growth takes place over a period of time, the SOC recommend hormone therapy for at least 1 year prior to breast augmentation.[2] However, response to hormone therapy varies among individuals, and breast and nipple development in trans women is rarely as complete as it is in cis women. Additionally, in some individuals, hormone therapy results in primarily subareolar breast hypertrophy with scant breast development elsewhere in the breast. As such, it is not uncommon for breast augmentation to be undertaken prior to 1 year of hormone use.

Few studies have addressed the optimal hormone regimen to maximize breast growth in trans women. While studies have demonstrated the effectiveness of various hormone therapies, reported data are observational and subjective.[7,8,9,10] The majority of available literature does not suggest that estrogen type or dose affects final breast size in trans women.[4] In addition, current data do not provide evidence that progestins enhance breast growth.[4] Some authors suggest that younger age, tissue sensitivity, and body weight may impact breast size.[11,12,13,14,15] Furthermore, shoulder width may play a role in perceived breast size and adequacy of growth.[16] Overall, literature suggests that 60–70% of trans women seek surgical breast augmentation because final breast size with hormone therapy is unsatisfactory.[4]

Patients should be counseled on the degree of breast growth they may expect from hormone therapy and appropriate options should they desire larger breasts. Unfortunately, some trans women have resorted to "pumping," an illegal and dangerous practice of injecting liquid silicone into breast tissue to enhance breast size. Serious complications of pumping range from local inflammatory reactions to pulmonary embolism and death.[17] Still, because it is an inexpensive alternative compared to approved treatments, the potentially deadly practice continues.[18]

21.2.2 Augmentation Mammaplasty

Many trans women who experience inadequate breast growth with hormone therapy continue to wear external prostheses or padded bras. As such, augmentation mammaplasty may be requested. Breast augmentation can be performed at the same time as vaginoplasty; this can help decrease surgery time and cost in individuals who desire both procedures. In a retrospective survey of 107 trans women, Kanhai et al reported that 80% of participants had mammaplasty and vaginoplasty simultaneously.[19] However, all patients in this series underwent vaginoplasty. The percent of patients undergoing both procedures at the same time is likely far lower and varies between clinical practices. In some regions, shortages of trained surgeons and limited third-party coverage may reduce access to vaginoplasty procedures.

Anatomic differences between the male and female chest are relevant as to implant selection, incision choice, and pocket location.[20] The chest and sternum of cis men are not only wider than the chest of cis women, but the pectoralis major muscle is usually more robust. Furthermore, the areola of cis men is both smaller and more lateral compared to the areola of cis women. In general, in trans women, the skin envelope is tighter (particularly below the nipple areola), the distance between the nipple and inframammary fold (IMF) is less, and there is less breast ptosis (▶ Fig. 21.1).[21]

Anatomic characteristics may require lowering the IMF by release of the sternal attachments along the rib and release of the lower sternal attachments of the pectoralis major muscle (▶ Fig. 21.2). In releasing the sternal attachments of the pectoralis muscle, the overlying pectoralis fascia is left intact. These maneuvers may assist with implant positioning relative to the position of the nipple areolar complex (NAC) and also help to prevent lateral implant displacement. Due to the wider chest wall diameter and, consequently, wider inter-nipple distance in trans women, a wide inter-breast width is common, even with the selection of larger implants.

The implants may be placed in either a subglandular or a subpectoral pocket. This decision depends on clinical characteristics, including the degree of breast growth in response to hormonal therapy. Subglandular implants may be more palpable and may have higher rates of capsular contracture due to less soft tissue coverage overlying the implant, although opinions vary about whether submuscular placement reduces capsular contracture. However, subpectoral implants may be more prone to displacement and animation deformities due to the activity of the overlying pectoralis major muscle. The subpectoral position is preferred for thin individuals, while the subglandular position may be chosen for bodybuilders. Overall, the subpectoral position remains the most common pocket location, but the subglandular position may be appropriate for obese individuals or individuals with adequate soft tissue coverage.

In terms of incisions, transaxillary, periareolar, or IMF approaches may be used. The choice of incision is tailored to

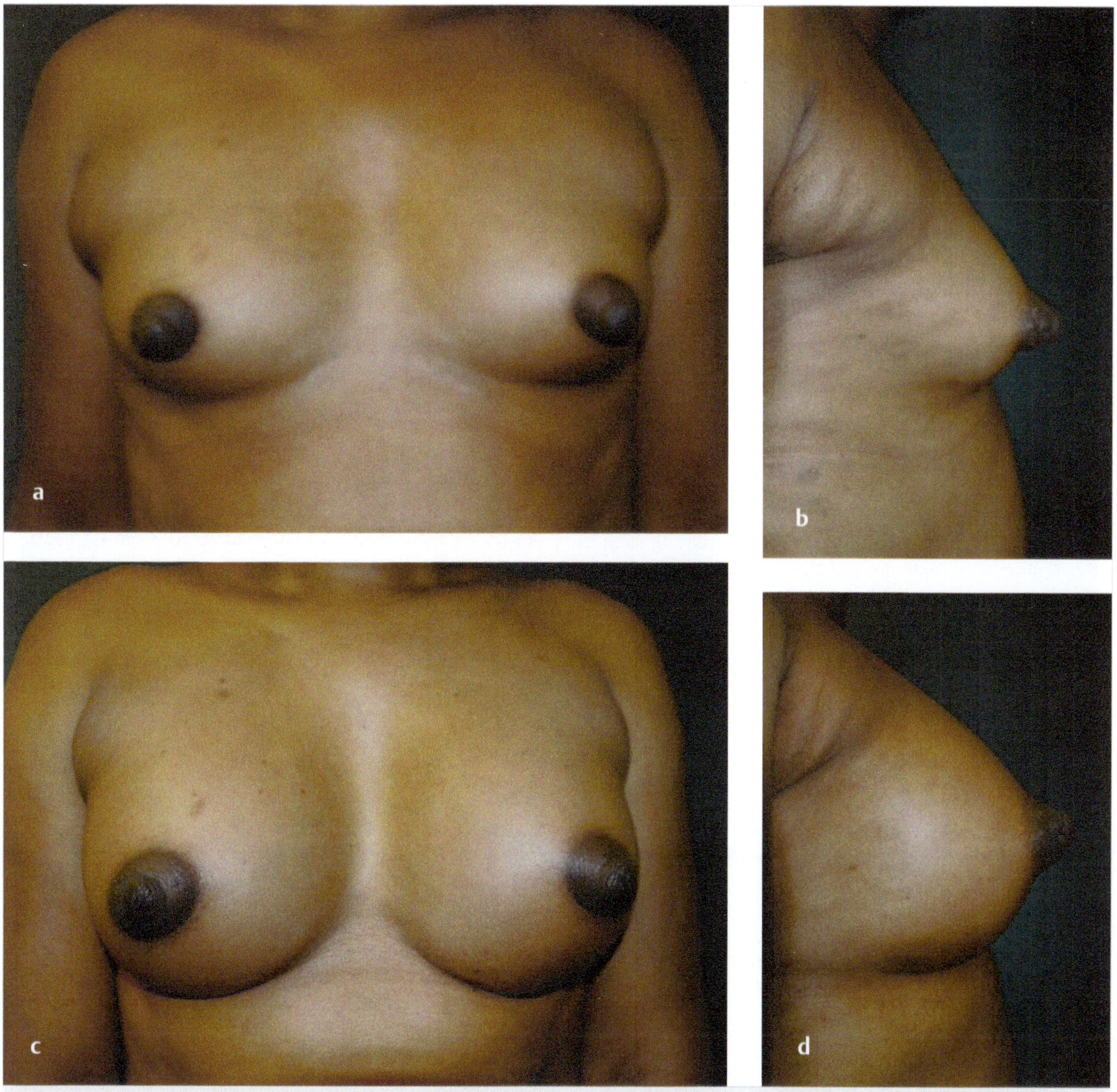

Fig. 21.1 (a,b) Pre- and **(c,d)** postoperative pictures of breast augmentation with smooth silicone gel submuscular.

the requests and the anatomy of the individual. Due to the smaller size of the areola in trans women compared to cis women, and the use of larger implants, an IMF approach is most commonly chosen. Transaxillary incisions are sometimes used, whereas periareolar incisions are infrequently utilized. With the increased use of form-stable implants, larger incisions are often required, also favoring an IMF approach.

Implant selection is based upon patient preference and may also vary with surgeon preference. Most commonly, silicone implants (either round or form-stable) are utilized. Implant choice may be based upon base diameter, desired size, and nipple-to-IMF distance. The form-stable implants may assist with decreasing upper pole fullness, although long-term data is not yet available. With both devices, adjustment of the IMF may be required. Since the writing of this chapter, form stable implants are no longer used due to concerns associated with ALCL.

Selection of the final implant may be assisted with the use of intraoperative sizers. Additionally, secure fascial closure is important to maintain the position of the IMF.

Many trans women prefer larger implants. Kanhai et al reported that the average size of implants in trans women nearly doubled in their practice from 165 mL in 1979 to 287 mL in 1996.[20] In a long-term follow-up study of 107 patients, the authors reported that 25% of patients were unhappy with their mammaplasty.[19] A breast that was too small was the most common reason for dissatisfaction. Further augmentation was reported in 19% of these patients.

In order to decrease the risk of venous thromboembolism, hormones are discontinued 2 weeks prior to surgery, and either fractionated or unfractionated heparin is administered subcutaneously upon induction of anesthesia. Following surgery, a compression bra is worn for 3 weeks. The individual is also

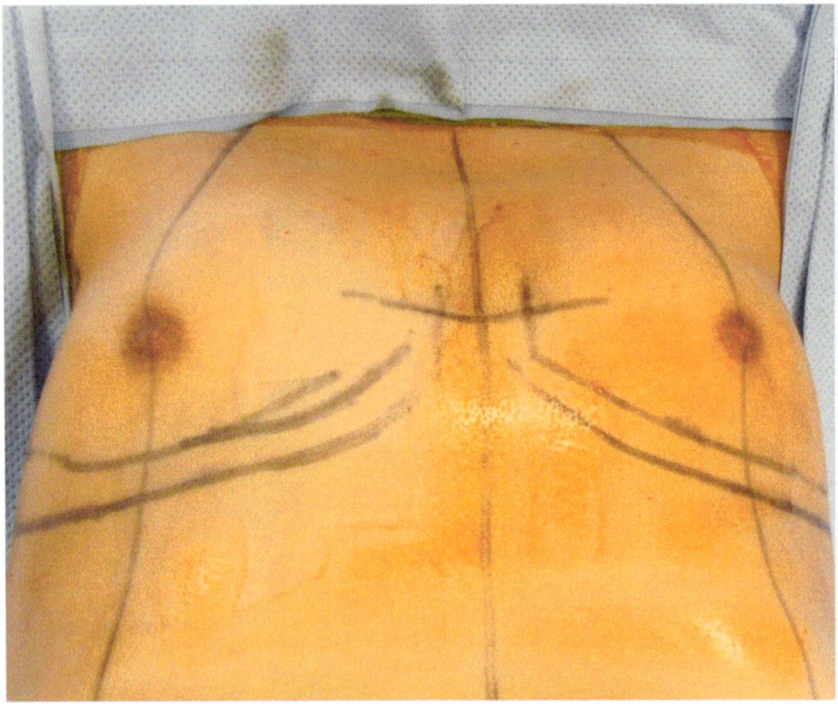

Fig. 21.2 Preoperative markings to lower the inframammary crease.

instructed to limit upper body exercise for the first several weeks following surgery, so as to decrease the risk of implant displacement. Gentle breast massage is instituted approximately 7–10 days following surgery.

21.2.3 Third-Party Payer Coverage

While there has been significant progress in third-party coverage for gender-confirming procedures, many, but not all, insurance providers continue to consider breast augmentation a "cosmetic" procedure. As such, they may deny insurance benefits. However, the SOC point out that in some individuals, a "cosmetic" procedure can have a radical and permanent effect on their quality of life.[2] In fact, research has suggested that gains in breast satisfaction, psychosocial well-being, and sexual well-being after breast augmentation in transgender individuals are statistically significant and clinically meaningful.[22] Because insurance benefits vary, benefits should be reviewed on a case-by-case basis to determine whether augmentation mammaplasty is covered.

21.3 Mastectomy/Chest Reconstruction in Trans Men

21.3.1 Hormone Therapy

Although hormone therapy is not a prerequisite for mastectomy/chest reconstruction surgery in trans men, many individuals desire testosterone therapy for masculinization. Several formulations of testosterone are available, but it is most commonly administered intramuscularly or topically. Dosage should be titrated to reach plasma concentrations of an adult male. Testosterone binds to androgen receptors throughout the body and can suppress ovarian production of estrogen and progesterone. Because testosterone is converted peripherally to estradiol by the aromatase enzyme, estradiol will often remain measurable in trans men.

Testosterone therapy does not cause significant change in breast appearance aside from the growth of chest hair. However, on a microscopic level, some changes have been observed. Evaluation of surgically removed breast tissue from 100 trans men who had received testosterone therapy for at least 6 months showed decreased glandular tissue and increased fibrous connective tissue in 93% of the pathologic samples.[23] In addition, there was mild lobular atrophy and severe lobular atrophy in 86% and 7% of the tissues samples, respectively. Two fibroadenomas, 34 fibrocystic lesions, and no carcinomas were reported.

21.3.2 Breast Binding

Trans men often use breast binding as a means to hide breast tissue. Breast binding involves using tight material to hold the breasts flat against the torso to hide them more easily beneath clothing. Little is known about the long-term health effects, if any, of breast binding. However, breast binding over several years can decrease skin elasticity and quality, and, as a result, can affect the surgical technique and aesthetic results from mastectomy and chest reconstruction.

21.3.3 Mastectomy/Chest Reconstruction

Chest-wall contouring is an important surgical step for many trans men. For some transgender and gender-diverse individuals, chest surgery is the only desired surgery while in others, chest surgery is one step in transitioning. The goals of chest

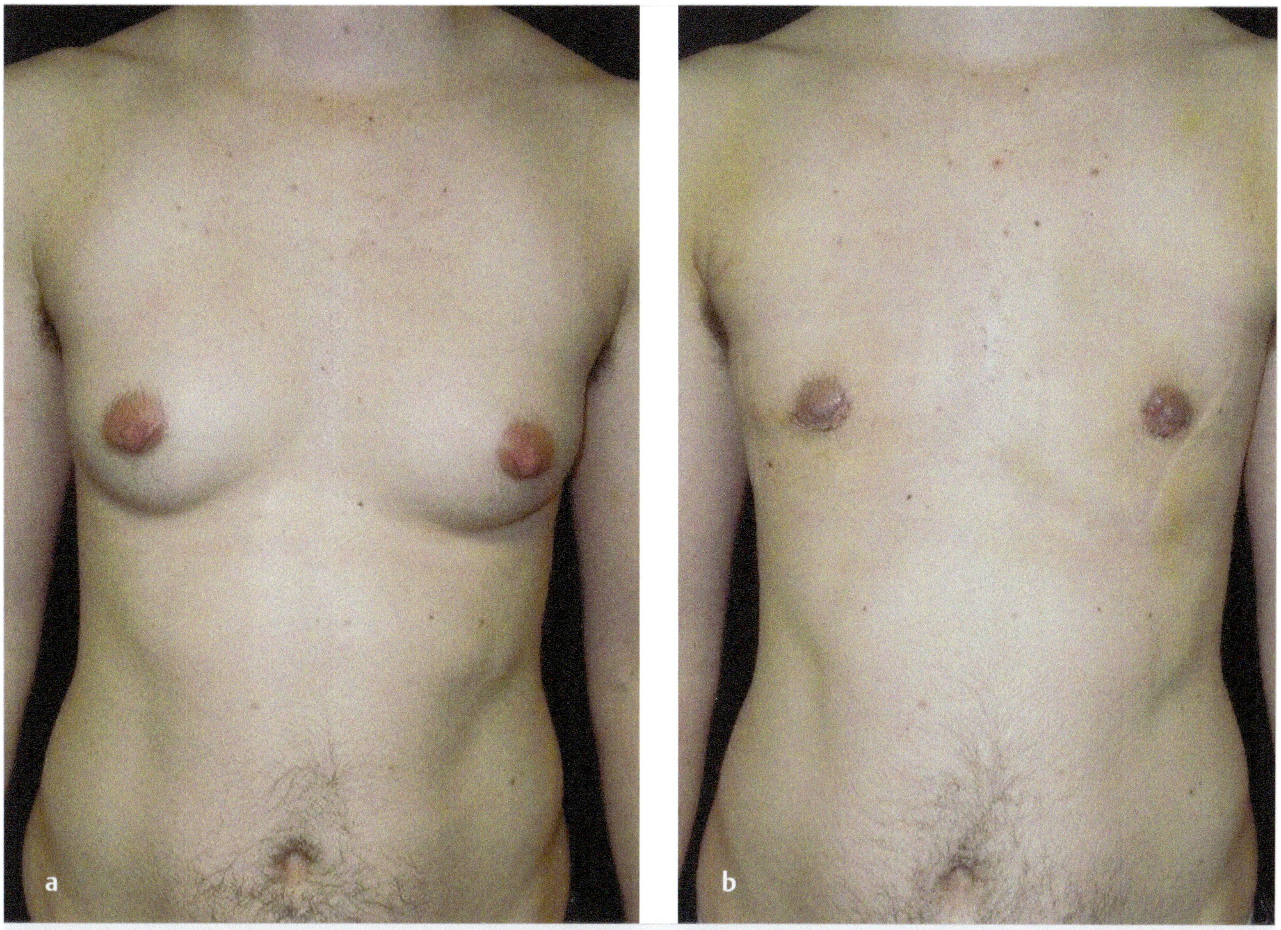

Fig. 21.3 (a) Pre- and (b) postoperative pictures of limited incision mastectomy in a trans man.

surgery include the aesthetic contouring of the chest by removal of breast tissue and excess skin, reduction and repositioning of the NAC when necessary, release of the IMF when necessary, liposuction of the chest, and, when possible, minimization of chest scars and preservation of nipple sensitivity.[24]

Before chest surgery is performed, preoperative breast imaging (mammogram or ultrasound) may be considered depending upon patient age, personal and family history, and physical examination. The American Congress of Obstetricians and Gynecologists recommends annual mammograms beginning at age 40. Earlier and additional testing may be warranted in high-risk individuals.

Chest surgery in trans men may present an aesthetic challenge due to breast volume, breast ptosis, NAC size and position, degree of skin excess, and potential loss of skin elasticity. In addition, concomitant obesity can increase the difficulty of achieving satisfactory contour, particularly in the subaxillary region. Breast binding may necessitate significant amounts of skin removal. Several surgical methods are utilized, and the choice of technique depends upon the skin quality and elasticity, the degree of breast ptosis, and the position of the NAC.[24] In addition, preservation of subcutaneous fat on the mastectomy skin flaps, preservation of the pectoralis and serratus fascia, release of the IMF and sternal attachments, and contouring of the lateral chest wall are also important components of chest surgery and chest wall contouring.

Small, nonptotic breasts can often be treated with periareolar incisions ("limited incision"). In these cases, the nipple may be reduced by a wedge resection of the lower pole, but the areola is not repositioned. A small amount of tissue is left beneath the NAC to preserve viability (▸ Fig. 21.3). Circumareolar ("purse-string") combined with vertical or horizontal incisions with free nipple-areola grafts can be used for larger breasts with mild ptosis requiring smaller amounts of skin removal. The vertical or horizontal extensions may assist with reducing postoperative areolar spread and distortion, but may result in a less aesthetically camoflouged scar as compared to the IMF (▸ Fig. 21.4). Finally, traditional transverse IMF incisions ("double incision") with free nipple-areola grafts may better serve individuals with larger breast volumes and increased breast ptosis requiring large amounts of skin removal (▸ Fig. 21.5). This approach facilitates excision of redundant skin. It is not uncommon to extend the incision laterally, into the axilla. Some surgeons extend the medial aspect of the incision across the midline in order to reduce medial "dog-ear" (▸ Fig. 21.6). Although crossing the midline produces a less aesthetic scar, contour improvement and reduced discrepancy between upper and lower incision lengths may make this approach desirable. When free nipple graft (FNG) is chosen for thinner subjects, a small dermoglandular pedicle is added to achieve a natural-appearing fullness under the nipple areola (▸ Fig. 21.7; also depicted is the authors' incision design for FNG).

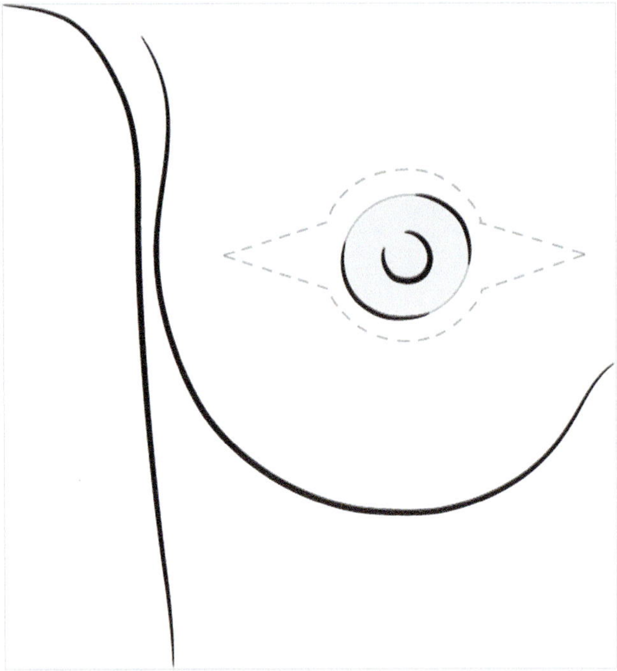

Fig. 21.4 Incision for limited skin redundancy.

Nipple reduction is commonly employed, often in conjunction with free nipple-areola grafts. FNGs necessitate thinning of the nipple to enable graft survival. In addition, liposuction is frequently used for both chest wall contouring and discontiguous undermining of the IMF and lateral chest wall. While free nipple-areola grafts are the most common technique for nipple transposition, some surgeons maintain the NAC on a dermoglandular pedicle. While this technique may preserve sensation to the NAC, it may also lead to residual breast fullness. Patients should understand that they may have fullness using this technique. This residual fullness may be reduced at a secondary surgical setting with direct excision or liposuction. The pedicle will be less noticeable in obese subjects, but these individuals usually have larger breasts and longer nipple-to-IMF distances. For some surgeons, the decision to utilize an FNG may be based upon the distance from the nipple to the IMF. When this distance exceeds 6–7 cm, an FNG may be preferable so as to prevent secondary contour deformities related to the bulk of the dermoglandular pedicle.[25]

For patients on hormone therapy, testosterone is discontinued 2 weeks prior to surgery. The patient is marked in the upright position. The relevant reference points include the IMF, the midbreast meridian, the lateral border of the pectoralis major muscle, the axillary tail of the breast, midline, and the anticipated position of the NAC (▶ Fig. 21.8). Alternatively, only the new nipple positions are marked standing and all other incisions are marked in a supine position after draping.

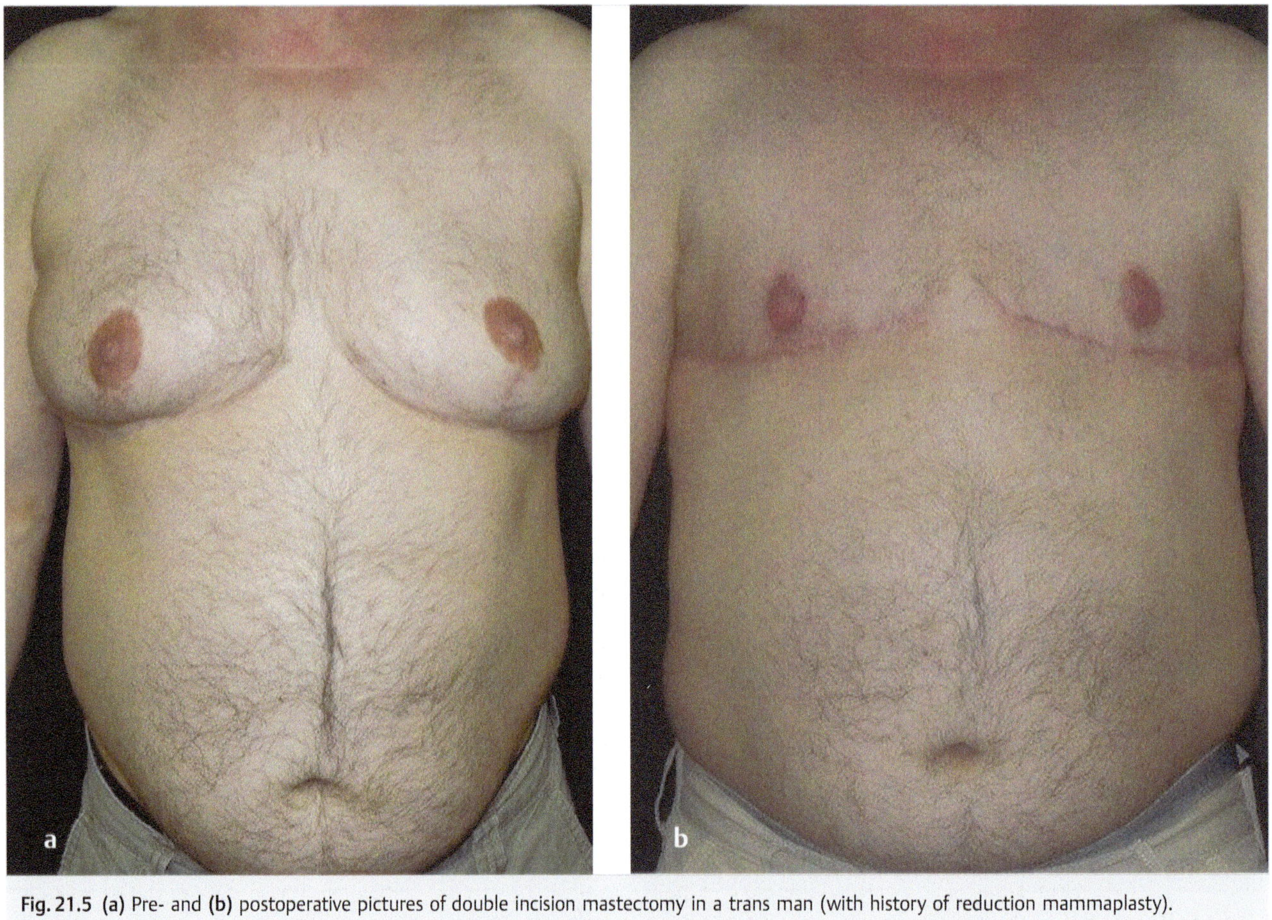

Fig. 21.5 (a) Pre- and (b) postoperative pictures of double incision mastectomy in a trans man (with history of reduction mammaplasty).

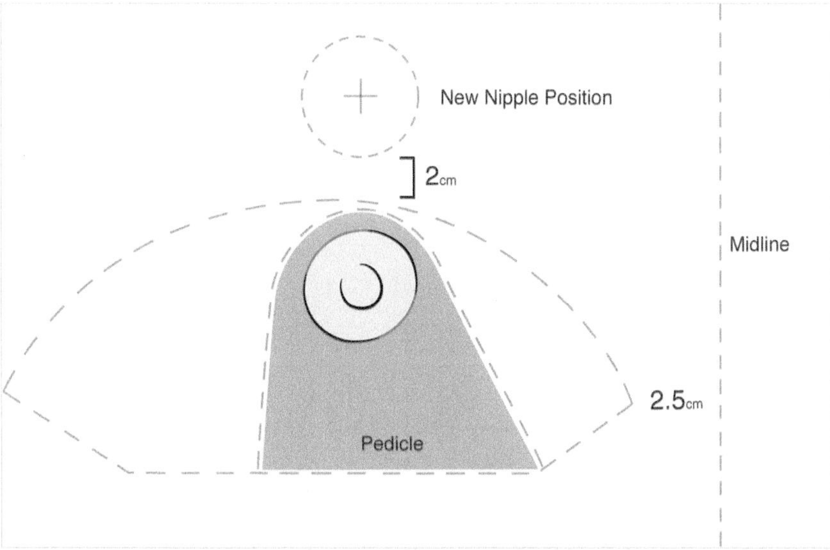

Fig. 21.6 Preop markings for breast reduction (subcutaneous mastectomy) with nipple transposition on a pedicle.

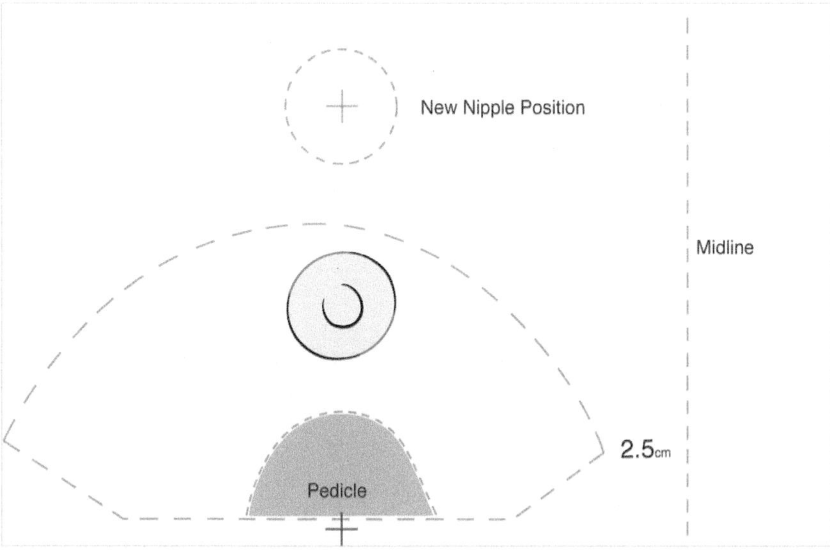

Fig. 21.7 Markings for free nipple graft with an inferior pedicle to augment the nipple contour.

Prior to surgery, sequential compression devices are placed and intravenous antibiotics are administered. Following induction of general anesthesia, chemoprophylaxis for venous thromboembolism is administered subcutaneously (either fractionated or unfractionated heparin depending upon institutional policies). With each of the operative techniques, the patient is positioned supine, with the arms abducted on foam rests with flexion at the elbow, and a lower body forced-air warming blanket is placed. Draping should allow access to the surgical field from both above and below the upper extremity. In addition, the patient is positioned and secured in anticipation of flexing the back of the operating table in order to assess symmetry and guide placement of the nipple-areola grafts. The reference points are tattooed with methylene blue to aid with intraoperative identification (▶ Fig. 21.9). If free nipple-areola grafts are to be performed, the NAC is resized to a diameter of 2.5–3.0 cm. In addition, if a nipple reduction is required, a wedge resection of the lower pole of the nipple may be performed. The nipple-areola grafts are harvested, defatted, and placed in moist gauze sponges for later use. When a skin resection is planned, regardless of the technique, the anticipated area of skin resection is incised in order to facilitate breast removal. The skin flaps are developed at the junction between the breast tissue and the subcutaneous fat at the level of the breast capsule. The medial dissection of the breast stops at the sternal border, and the perforating branches of the internal mammary artery are preserved, if possible. The lateral dissection proceeds subcutaneously over the serratus muscle, with preservation of the serratus fascia, and the breast is reflected off the chest wall, with preservation of the pectoralis fascia (▶ Fig. 21.10). Liposuction of the IMF, the lateral chest, and the axillary tail is performed. Some surgeons place fibrin sealant in the cavity. The patient is placed in a semi-Fowler position, and the skin flaps are tailored and inset in a layered fashion over a 15 French closed suction drain. Following resection, the breast tissue is marked and sent to pathology for routine examination. Additionally, some surgeons choose to weigh the specimen intraoperatively.

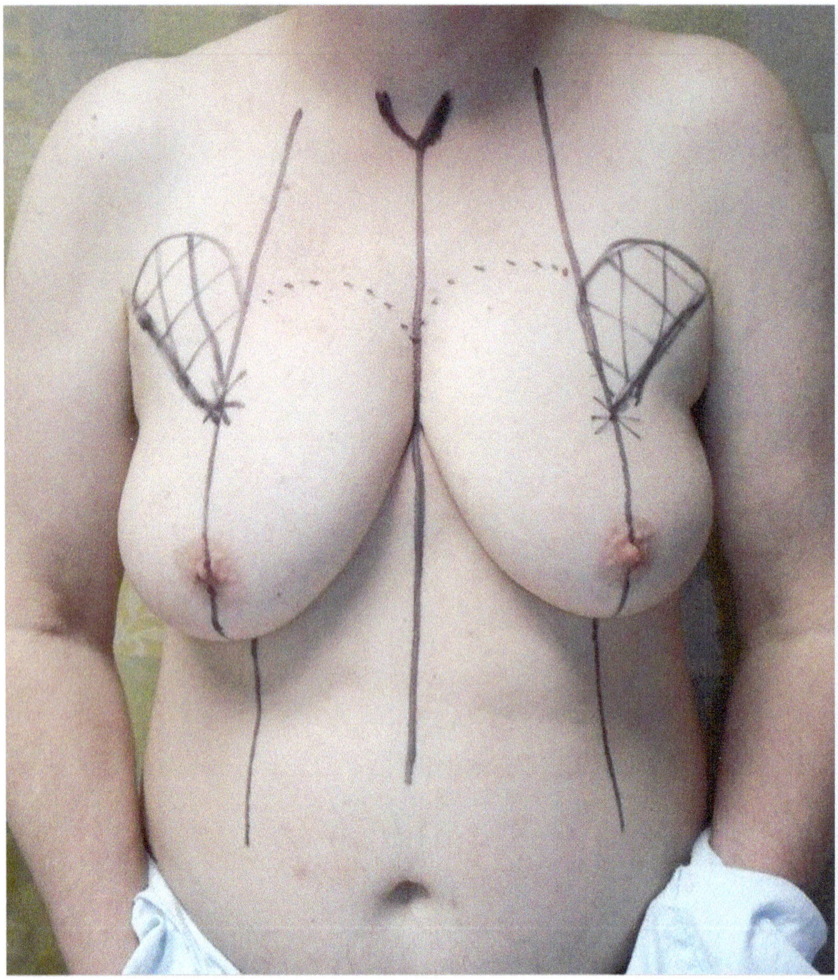

Fig. 21.8 Preoperative markings in a patient undergoing mastectomy.

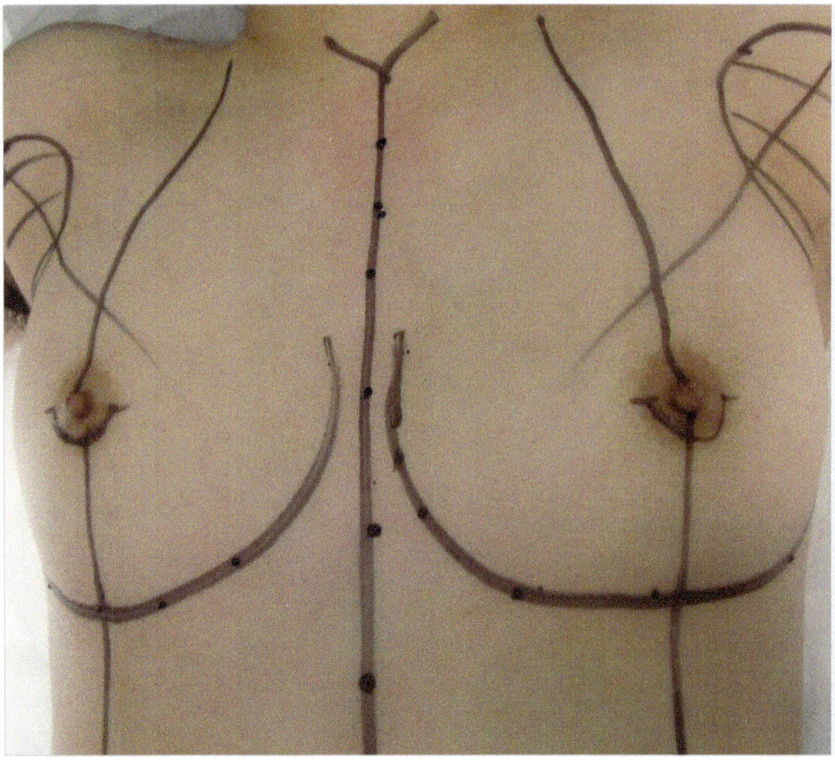

Fig. 21.9 Intraoperative markings during chest surgery using methylene blue to aid in identification of reference points.

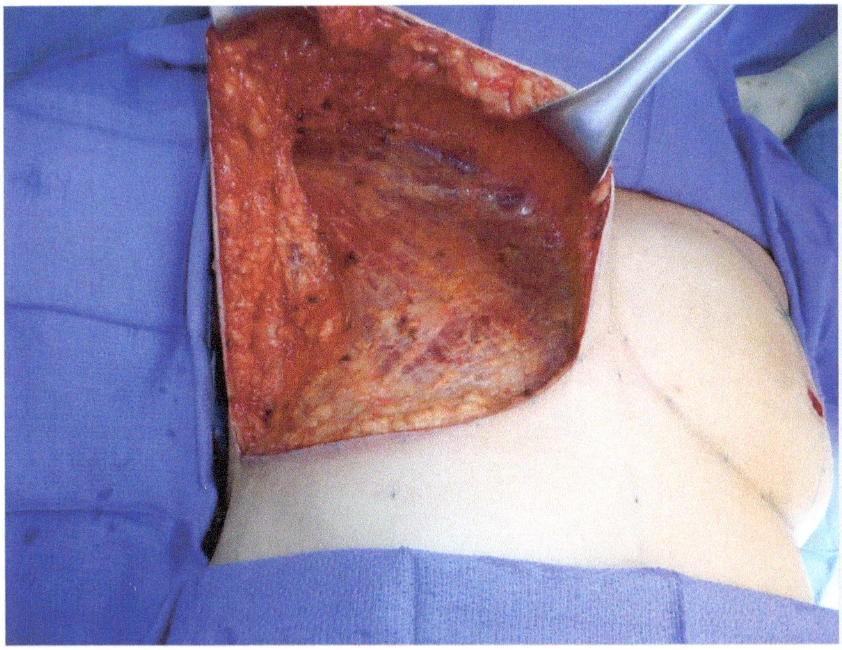

Fig. 21.10 Completion of mastectomy with preservation of pectoralis and serratus fascia.

There are no universally established guidelines for nipple position and areolar diameter in trans men. Some believe there is a tendency to create areolas that are too large and placed too high and medial on the chest wall.[26,27] Atiyeh et al proposed a mathematical formula for determining the ideal position for nipple placement in men after massive weight loss using the umbilicus–anterior axillary fold apex distance and the umbilicus–supersternal notch distance.[28] In addition, McGregor and Whallett reported on their technique for nipple-areola placement.[29] They suggest suturing threads at key points: the midclavicular position as the vertical axis, the midline axis of the sternum as the horizontal axis, and the suprasternal notch. The midline axis of the sternum is determined from a point on the upper arm midway between the elbow crease and the apex of the anterior axillary fold. The sutures are pulled along their axes. The point at which the sutures intersect is chosen for the nipple site. A 2-cm disk at this site is de-epithelialized for reception of the nipple-areolar graft. However, according to Monstrey et al, "absolute measurements can be misleading."[24]

In our experience, clinical judgment is best in positioning the NAC in trans men. In general, the nipple-areola is positioned medial to the lateral border of the pectoralis major muscle, approximately 1–2 cm above the inferior insertion of the pectoralis major muscle. While specifics regarding nipple placement may vary,[26,30] placement falls within the parameters suggested in ▶ Fig. 21.11. In obese individuals, the border of the pectoralis may be difficult to define. Final adjustments to nipple position may be performed at the time of wound closure.

In general, markings are made in a standing position. For the double-incision approach, the authors' preference is to place the lower chest incision at the IMF in order to remove breast tissue at this level. However, some surgeons place the lower chest incision at the lower border of the pectoralis muscle. If an inferior pedicle nipple transposition is planned, the areola is sized to 25 mm, and the pedicle is elevated deep to the level of the breast capsule. The pedicle is then de-epithelialized and can

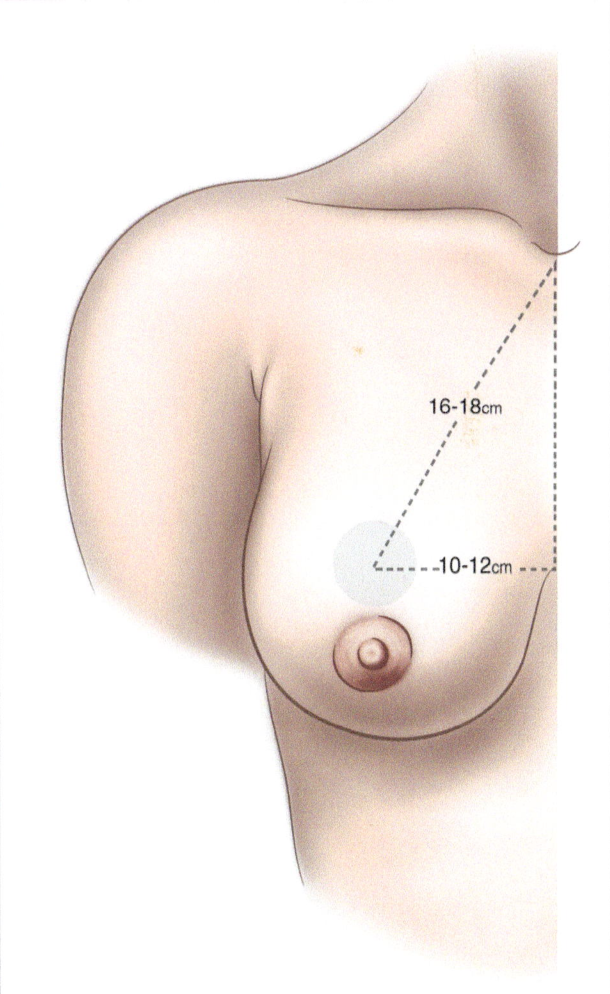

Fig. 21.11 Nipple position on a male chest.

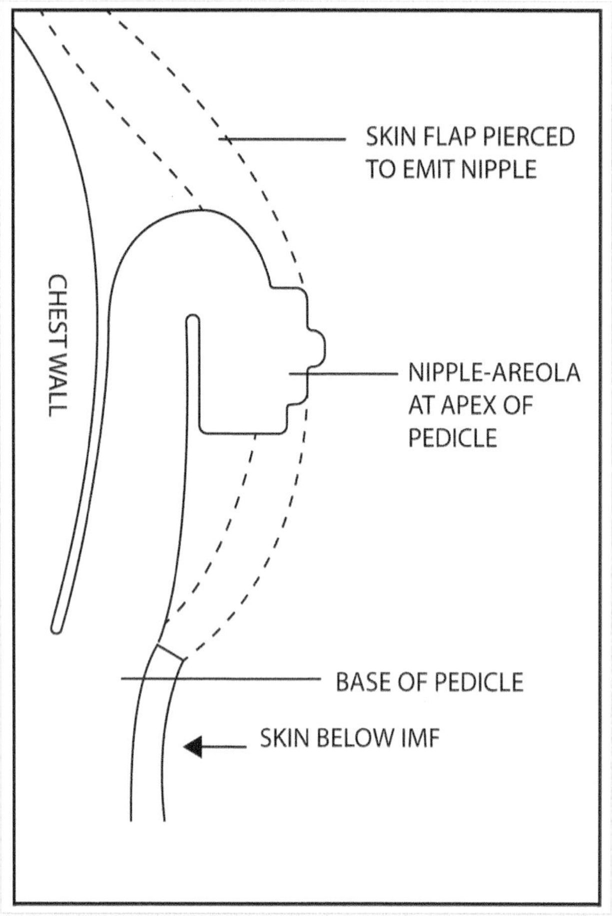

Fig. 21.12 Pedicle dissection.

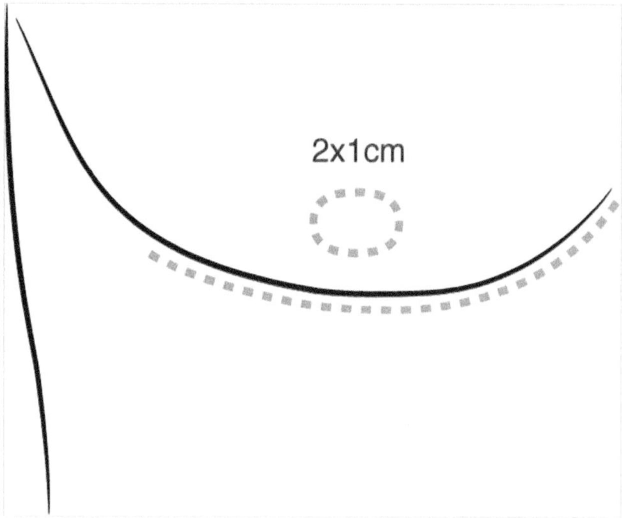

Fig. 21.13 Design for opening to admit nipple on a pedicle (full-thickness excision).

be sutured to the pectoralis fascia underlying the planned nipple position. The base of the pedicle is left in continuity with the underlying fascia (▶ Fig. 21.12). Alternatively, some authors describe disruption of the IMF so as to improve subsequent chest contour, but this maneuver may compromise the flap circulation.[31]

Following development of the pedicle, the upper incision is made down to the level of the breast capsule. Dissection proceeds superiorly and medially to the pectoralis fascia and laterally to the fascia overlying the serratus anterior muscle.

Prior to wound closure, liposuction of the chest wall may be performed for additional contouring. This it typically performed in the lateral chest or subaxillary region and/or the lower chest/upper abdomen/midline region. Most often a closed-suction drain is placed, and some surgeons also use fibrin sealant.

Final adjustments to nipple position are performed at the time of wound closure with the patient in a semi-Fowler position. The nipple position can be adjusted so that the inferior border of the areola is approximately 2–2.5 cm above the IMF and equal distance from the midline and sternal notch. These measurements may vary based upon common asymmetries in chest wall dimensions. When a pedicle technique is used, a 2 × 1-cm full-thickness ellipse of skin is excised in the chest flap (▶ Fig. 21.13). Due to flap tension, the ellipse becomes circular upon final inset. The nipple-areola is sutured with a single layer of interrupted, buried, absorbable sutures. In pedicle procedures, when a nipple reduction is required, it is performed at a secondary setting utilizing a three- or four-pointed star-shaped excision (▶ Fig. 21.14). When FNGs are used, the grafts are defatted and inset on a dermal bed. Fixation of the nipple graft is accomplished with a bolster dressing sutured over petrolatum gauze and an absorbant cotton pad. A compression wrap with elastic bandages is then placed.

Examples of several chest surgeries are provided. ▶ Fig. 21.15 shows a 27-year-old trans man before and 9 months after pedicle reduction. ▶ Fig. 21.16 shows a 24-year-old trans man before and 6 months after chest surgery using the FNG technique. Finally, ▶ Fig. 21.17 shows a 20-year-old trans man and 6 months post chest surgery using the inferior pedicle technique.

Chest surgery is generally performed as an outpatient procedure, unless the patient is traveling or has other medical comorbidities. Following surgery, an elastic compression wrap remains in place for 4–6 days. In addition, closed suction drains are placed bilaterally, and patients are instructed to monitor and record output. Discharge medications include an oral narcotic or non-narcotic alternative for analgesia, an antibiotic, a stool softener, and an antinausea medication. Patients are encouraged to ambulate as soon as possible. Patients can bathe, but not shower, until dressings are removed. Lifting is limited to 10–15 lb (4.5–6.8 kg) for several weeks, and patients sleep with their back elevated for 1 week after surgery. At an office visit 4–6 days after surgery, dressings are changed, bolster dressings are removed from the NACs, and local care with a topical antimicrobial ointment is initiated. The compression wrap is continued for 3 weeks after surgery, followed by a compression shirt for an additional 3 weeks. Drains are removed when output is less than approximately 30 mL per 24-hour period. It is recommended that patients stay locally for approximately 1 week after surgery before travel. For patients on hormone therapy, testosterone can be restarted a few days following surgery.

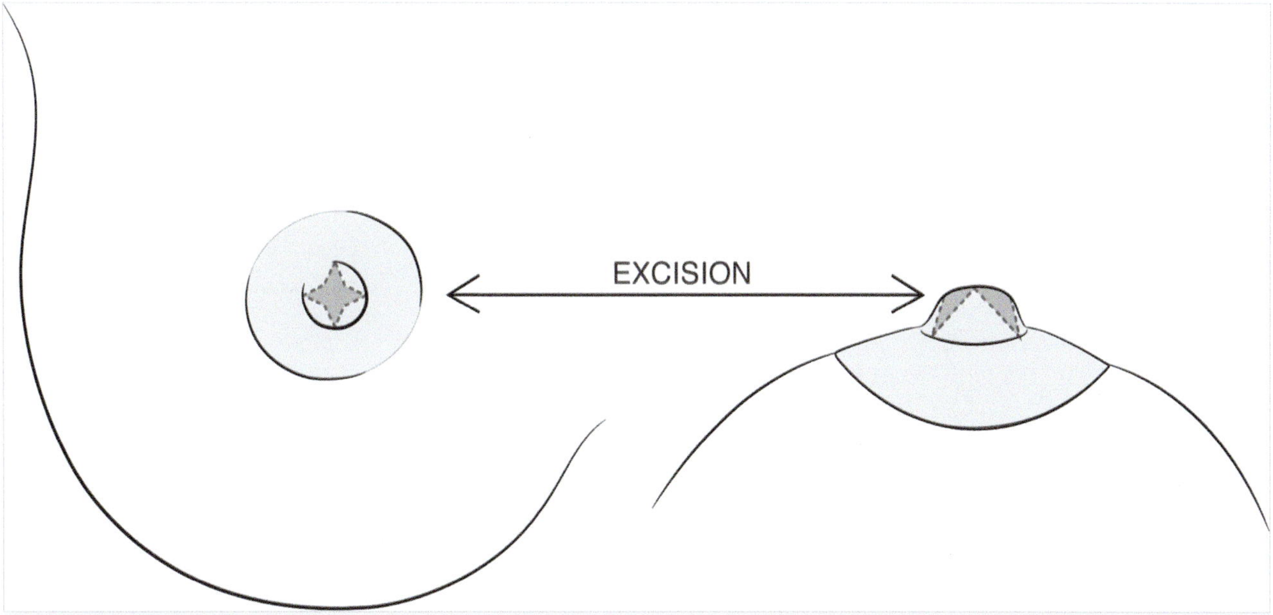

Fig. 21.14 Nipple reduction method.

21.3.4 Third-Party Payer Coverage

Although far from universal, insurance benefits for mastectomy/chest reconstruction are more common than coverage for augmentation mammaplasty. Many insurance providers follow the WPATH SOC and request referral letters from mental health providers before providing precertification for surgery.

21.4 Long-Term Postoperative Care

21.4.1 Trans Women

Trans women with no known increased risk of breast cancer should follow screening guidelines recommended for cis women.[5] Trans women at increased risk for breast cancer may need additional testing. There are no large randomized trials to evaluate adverse effects of hormone therapy on breast tissue in trans women.[14] Albeit rare, several cases of breast carcinoma in trans women have been reported in the literature.[32] Interestingly, in contrast to cis women, the cases of breast cancer in trans women occurred at younger ages and after relatively short spans of estrogen therapy and showed similarities with breast cancer in cis men.[32] Still, because many carcinomas are estrogen receptor–positive, it is possible that exogenous hormone therapy may increase cancer risk.[10] Studies investigating the risks of estrogen therapy on breast carcinoma in postmenopausal cis women are conflicting.[33,34] Furthermore, these studies are not readily translatable to the transgender population, where individuals often receive higher doses of estrogen and may have higher testosterone levels. Some believe that as the transgender community increases and ages, the incidence of breast carcinoma will increase as well.[35]

The best method for screening trans women who have undergone augmentation mammaplasty is not yet determined. Options include mammography, ultrasonography, and magnetic resonance imaging (MRI). In general, mammography is used for screening and is be performed in conjunction with regular self and clinical breast examinations. However, mammograms have been found to be less sensitive for detecting malignancies in cis women with implants compared to those without implants. In a study of 137 augmented and 684 nonaugmented women who had been diagnosed with breast cancer as well as 10,533 augmented women and 974,915 nonaugmented women without breast cancer, breast augmentation was found to decrease sensitivity of mammography (45% versus 66.8%; $p = 0.008$).[36] This study did not include transgender women. Recommendations regarding breast implant evaluation should follow FDA guidelines.

21.4.2 Trans Men

The incidence of breast cancer following mastectomy in trans men is thought to be low.[37] There are no guidelines as to how, when, or whether trans men who have undergone chest surgery should be screened for breast cancer. The American Cancer Society states that cis women who have undergone bilateral mastectomies should not need further mammograms.[38] There are no recommendations for radiologic examination for trans men. In the authors' experience, annual physical examination following mastectomy is recommended. Additional imaging studies are based upon clinical findings.

Bilateral mastectomy does not completely eliminate the risk of developing breast cancer. Katayama et al reported on a trans man who developed breast cancer 12 years after mastectomy and hysterectomy with bilateral salpingo-oophorectomy.[39] The patient had been receiving testosterone therapy continuously for 15 years. Pathological examination revealed a tumor with androgen and estrogen receptor expression, suggesting that testosterone therapy may have played a role in tumor development. Furthermore, Nikolic et al described a 43-year-old

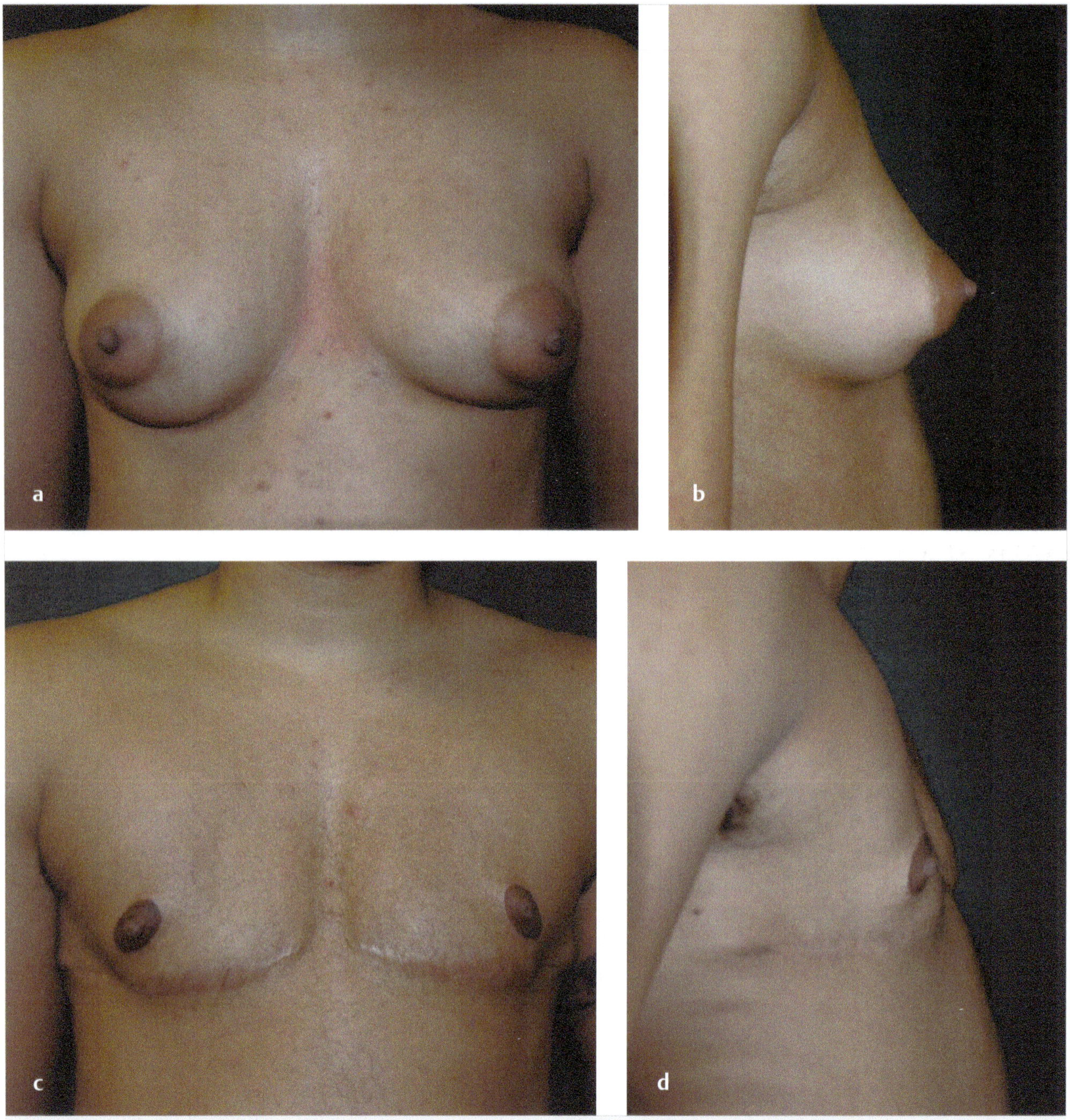

Fig. 21.15 Preoperative **(a)** anterior and **(b)** lateral views of patient undergoing inferior pedicle reduction; 9-month postoperative **(c)** anterior and **(d)** lateral views.

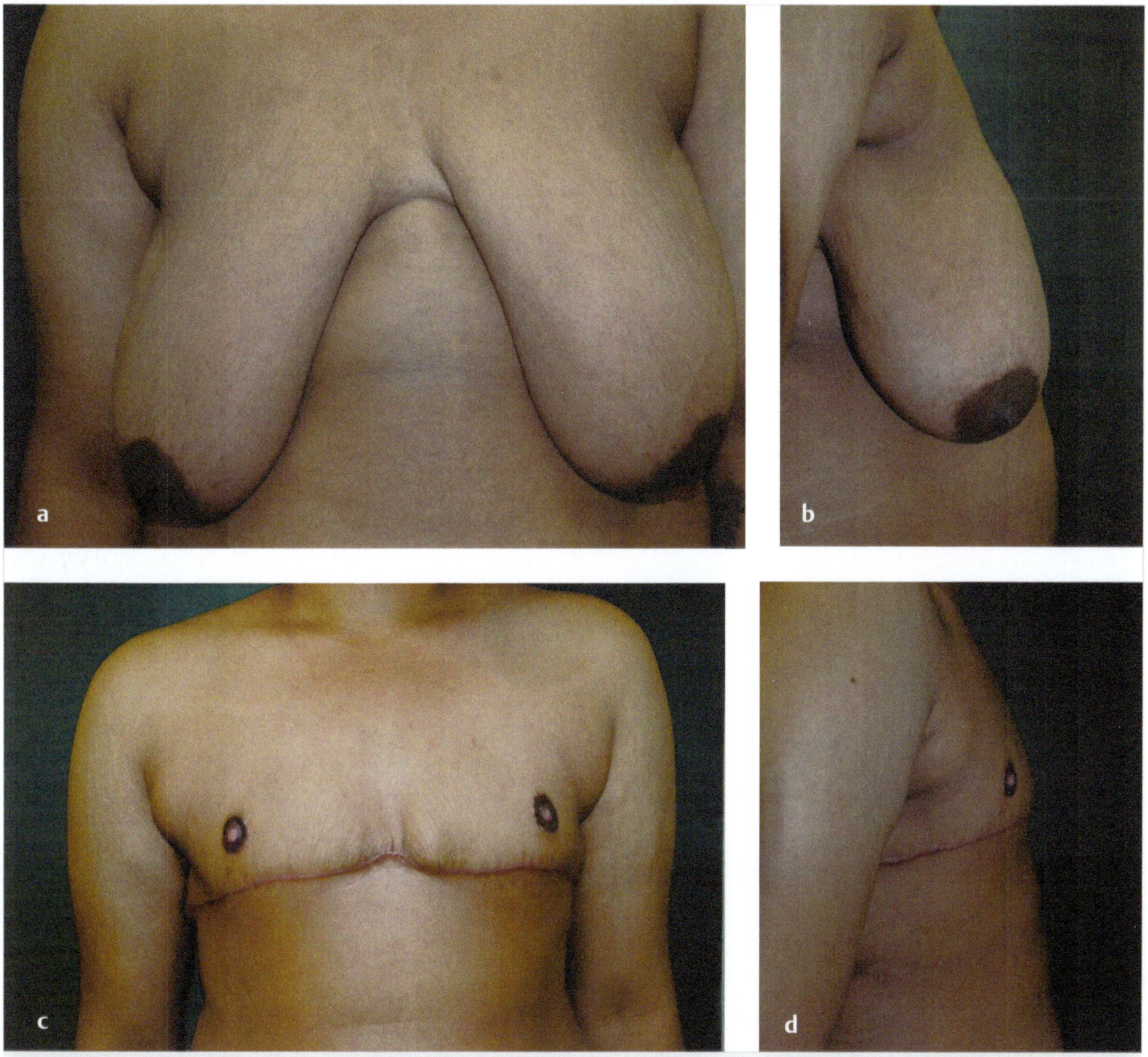

Fig. 21.16 Preoperative **(a)** anterior and **(b)** lateral views of patient undergoing free nipple graft reduction; 6-month postoperative **(c)** anterior and **(d)** lateral views.

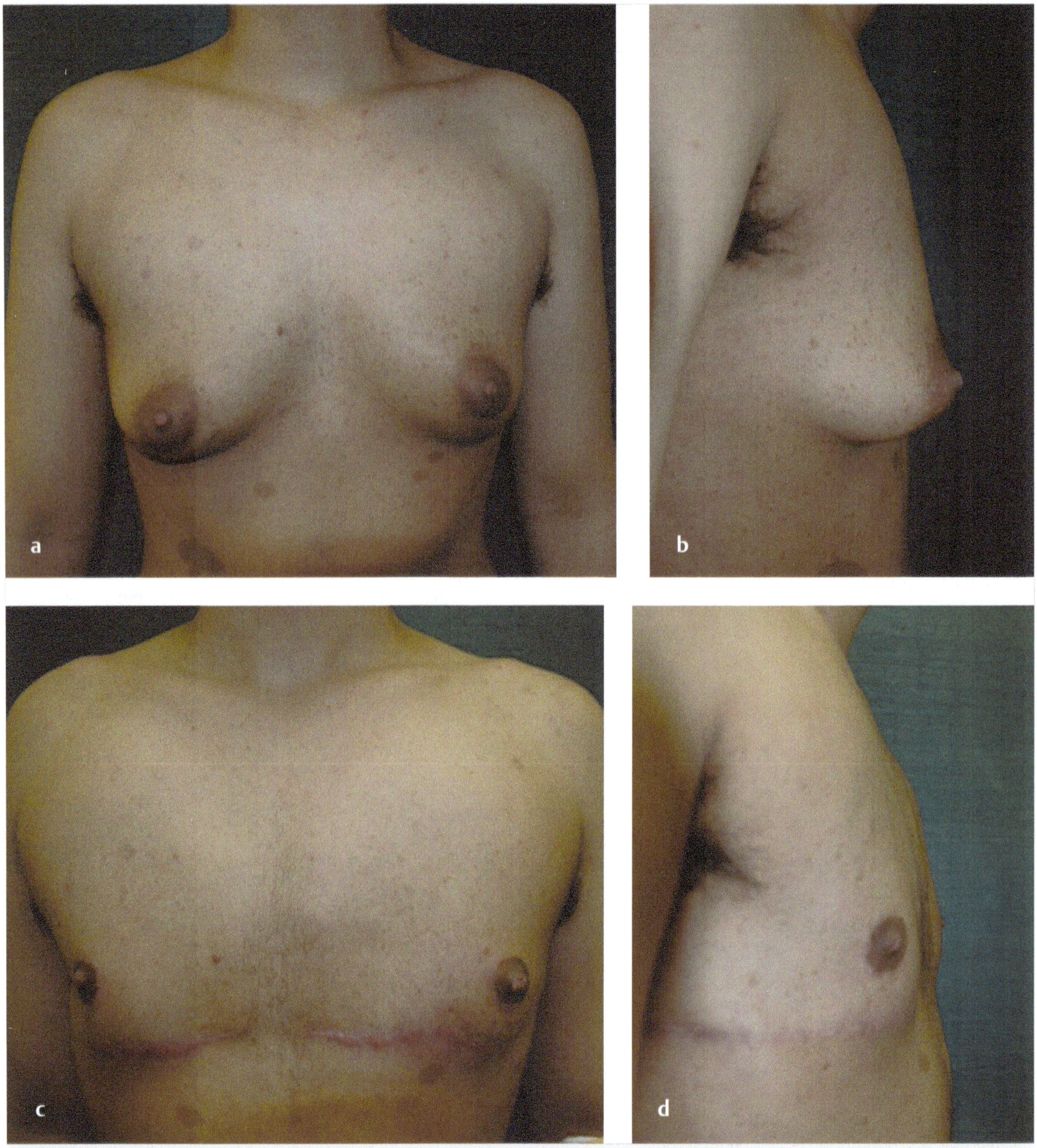

Fig. 21.17 Preoperative (a) anterior and (b) lateral views of patient undergoing inferior pedicle reduction; 6-month postoperative (c) anterior and (d) lateral views.

trans man who underwent gender confirmation surgery, including a total abdominal hysterectomy with bilateral salpingo-oophorectomy as well as bilateral nipple-sparing subcutaneous mastectomy.[40] Pathologic analysis was unremarkable. Before genital and chest surgery, breast ultrasound and mammogram and lung radiology were also unremarkable. The patient had been on testosterone for approximately 2.5 years. One year post mastectomy, the patient presented with a left areolar mass and was diagnosed with invasive ductal carcinoma (estrogen and progesterone receptor negative, Her 2/neu receptor positive) with spread to the left axillary lymph nodes and lung metastases. These cases illustrate that continued vigilance is necessary.

21.5 Management of Complications

21.5.1 Augmentation Mammaplasty Complications

Acute complications following augmentation mammaplasty, although uncommon, include hematoma, seroma, and infection. Additionally, some patients experience increased pain based upon placement of the implant in the subpectoral location. Other complications include capsular contracture, breast asymmetry, asymmetry of the IMF, implant displacement or leak, and an unsatisfactory cosmetic appearance. Patients should be counseled as to the need for implant replacement/exchange within 20 years following surgery if a problem occurs.

There are several reasons for revision after augmentation mammaplasty. In a 10-year retrospective study, Forster et al identified 24 trans women who underwent reoperation (either implant replacement or removal) at the University Hospital, Zurich, Switzerland.[41] Aesthetic indications included size ($n = 11$, 45.8%), asymmetry/malposition ($n = 15$, 7.8%), and shape ($n = 1$, 4.1%), while medical indications included capsular contracture ($n = 7$, 29.1%), and capsular contracture and size ($n = 1$, 4.1%).

21.5.2 Mastectomy/Chest Reconstruction Complications

Complications following mastectomy/chest surgery can be divided into acute complications and secondary revisions. Acute complication rates are reported between 11 and 33% and include, but are not limited to, hematoma, seroma, infection, delayed healing, and loss of nipple graft.[24,42,43,44] Reported reoperation rates for acute complications range from 4.3 to 10.4%.[42,43,44] Hematoma is the most commonly reported reason for reoperation in the acute postoperative period.[42]

Many patients also require later revisions for aesthetic reasons. Rates for aesthetic correction vary between 9.0 and 40.4%,[24,42,43,44] vary with the technique used, and may be more common in patients who had acute complications.[42] The need for correction ranges from 1.4 to 19.6% for scars, 5.5to 28% for chest contour, and 2.0 to 13.0% for the nipple-areola. In a retrospective review of 404 mastectomies in 202 trans men, Cregten-Escobar et al found that in general, the larger the breast, the large the incision and scar required, while on the other hand, the smaller the scars, the higher risk of hematoma.[44]

In the authors' opinion, obesity is correlated with the need for subsequent revisions. Most often, this relates to secondary excisions of redundant axillary tissue ("dog ears"). However, revisions are occasionally needed in thin individuals as well.

21.6 Conclusion

Augmentation mammaplasty and mastectomy/chest surgery can play an important role in alleviating gender dysphoria in some transgender and gender-diverse individuals. Care should be taken to ensure that individuals interested in such surgery are appropriate candidates. Surgeons should be familiar with the framework recommended in the WPATH SOC and work closely with the health care team to ensure optimal care. Individuals who decide to pursue surgery must fully understand the risks, benefits, and limitations of surgery before proceeding.

Key Points

- For breast augmentation, recognize (1) the anatomic differences between the patient and cis women (pectoralis major muscle, skin envelope, areolar size) and (2) the effects of estrogen on breast growth. In addition, these anatomic differences may require adjustments in the inframammary crease.
- For chest surgery (subcutaneous mastectomy), recognize the relevant anatomic considerations when choosing technique (skin elasticity and degree of breast ptosis).
- For both trans men and trans women, follow breast cancer screening guidelines (i.e., imaging studies and genetic testing) based upon patient history, family history, and physical examination.

References

[1] Hage JJ. Medical requirements and consequences of sex reassignment surgery. Med Sci Law. 1995; 35(1):17–24

[2] World Professional Association for Transgender Health. Standards of Care for the Health of Transsexual, Transgender, and Gender Nonconforming People. 7th Version. URL: https://s3.amazonaws.com/amo_hub_content/Association140/files/Standards of Care V7 - 2011 WPATH (2)(1).pdf. WPATH; 2012. Accessed July 23, 2019

[3] Javed A, Lteif A. Development of the human breast. Semin Plast Surg. 2013; 27(1):5–12

[4] Wierckx K, Gooren L, T'Sjoen G. Clinical review: Breast development in trans women receiving cross-sex hormones. J Sex Med. 2014; 11(5):1240–1247

[5] Hembree WC, Cohen-Kettenis P, Delemarre-van de Waal HA, et al. Endocrine Society. Endocrine treatment of transsexual persons: an Endocrine Society clinical practice guideline. J Clin Endocrinol Metab. 2009; 94(9):3132–3154

[6] Dahl M, Feldman JL, Goldberg JM, Jaberi A, et al. Physical aspects of transgender endocrine therapy. Int J Transgenderism. 2006; 9(3/4):111–134

[7] Moore E, Wisniewski A, Dobs A. Endocrine treatment of transsexual people: a review of treatment regimens, outcomes, and adverse effects. J Clin Endocrinol Metab. 2003; 88(8):3467–3473

[8] Tangpricha V, Ducharme SH, Barber TW, Chipkin SR. Endocrinologic treatment of gender identity disorders. Endocr Pract. 2003; 9(1):12–21

[9] Gooren LJ. Clinical practice. Care of transsexual persons. N Engl J Med. 2011; 364(13):1251–1257

[10] Gooren LJ, Giltay EJ, Bunck MC. Long-term treatment of transsexuals with cross-sex hormones: extensive personal experience. J Clin Endocrinol Metab. 2008; 93(1):19–25

[11] Wallace PM, Rasmussen S. Analysis of adulterated silicone: implications for health promotion. Int J Transgenderism. 2010; 12(3):167–175

[12] Orentreich N, Durr NP. Proceedings: Mammogenesis in transsexuals. J Invest Dermatol. 1974; 63(1):142–146
[13] Asscheman H, Gooren L. Hormone treatment in transsexuals. J Psychol Human Sex. 1993; 5(4):3:9–54
[14] Maycock LB, Kennedy HP. Breast care in the transgender individual. J Midwifery Womens Health. 2014; 59(1):74–81
[15] Levy A, Crown A, Reid R. Endocrine intervention for transsexuals. Clin Endocrinol (Oxf). 2003; 59(4):409–418
[16] Seal LJ, Franklin S, Richards C, Shishkareva A, Sinclaire C, Barrett J. Predictive markers for mammoplasty and a comparison of side effect profiles in transwomen taking various hormonal regimens. J Clin Endocrinol Metab. 2012; 97 (12):4422–4428
[17] Narins RS, Beer K. Liquid injectable silicone: a review of its history, immunology, technical considerations, complications, and potential. Plast Reconstr Surg. 2006; 118(3) Suppl:77S–84S
[18] Chasan PE. The history of injectable silicone fluids for soft-tissue augmentation. Plast Reconstr Surg. 2007; 120(7):2034–2040, discussion 2041--2043
[19] Kanhai RC, Hage JJ, Mulder JW. Long-term outcome of augmentation mammaplasty in male-to-female transsexuals: a questionnaire survey of 107 patients. Br J Plast Surg. 2000; 53(3):209–211
[20] Kanhai RC, Hage JJ, Asscheman H, Mulder JW. Augmentation mammaplasty in male-to-female transsexuals. Plast Reconstr Surg. 1999; 104(2):542–549, discussion 550--551
[21] Laub D. Discussion: augmentation mammaplasty in male-to-female transsexuals. Plast Reconstr Surg. 1999; 104(2):550–551
[22] Weigert R, Frison E, Sessiecq Q, Al Mutairi K, Casoli V. Patient satisfaction with breasts and psychosocial, sexual, and physical well-being after breast augmentation in male-to-female transsexuals. Plast Reconstr Surg. 2013; 132 (6):1421–1429
[23] Grynberg M, Fanchin R, Dubost G, et al. Histology of genital tract and breast tissue after long-term testosterone administration in a female-to-male transsexual population. Reprod Biomed Online. 2010; 20(4):553–558
[24] Monstrey S, Selvaggi G, Ceulemans P, et al. Chest-wall contouring surgery in female-to-male transsexuals: a new algorithm. Plast Reconstr Surg. 2008; 121(3):849–859
[25] Silfen R, Ritz M, Southwick G. Use of pedicled local flaps for male chest augmentation and reshaping. Plast Reconstr Surg. 2006; 117(5):1447–1451, discussion 1452--1454
[26] Beer GM, Budi S, Seifert B, Morgenthaler W, Infanger M, Meyer VE. Configuration and localization of the nipple-areola complex in men. Plast Reconstr Surg. 2001; 108(7):1947–1952, discussion–1953
[27] Lindsay WR. Creation of a male chest in female transsexuals. Ann Plast Surg. 1979; 3(1):39–46
[28] Atiyeh BS, Dibo SA, El Chafic AH. Vertical and horizontal coordinates of the nipple-areola complex position in males. Ann Plast Surg. 2009; 63(5):499–502
[29] McGregor JC, Whallett EJ. Some personal suggestions on surgery in large or ptotic breasts for female to male transsexuals. J Plast Reconstr Aesthet Surg. 2006; 59(8):893–896
[30] Shulman O, Badani E, Wolf Y, Hauben DJ. Appropriate location of the nipple-areola complex in males. Plast Reconstr Surg. 2001; 108(2):348–351
[31] Hammond DC. Surgical correction of gynecomastia. Plast Reconstr Surg. 2009; 124(1) Suppl:61e–68e
[32] Gooren LJ, van Trotsenburg MA, Giltay EJ, van Diest PJ. Breast cancer development in transsexual subjects receiving cross-sex hormone treatment. J Sex Med. 2013; 10(12):3129–3134
[33] Stefanick ML, Anderson GL, Margolis KL, et al. WHI Investigators. Effects of conjugated equine estrogens on breast cancer and mammography screening in postmenopausal women with hysterectomy. JAMA. 2006; 295(14):1647–1657
[34] Rossouw JE, Anderson GL, Prentice RL, et al. Writing Group for the Women's Health Initiative Investigators. Risks and benefits of estrogen plus progestin in healthy postmenopausal women: principal results from the Women's Health Initiative randomized controlled trial. JAMA. 2002; 288 (3):321–333
[35] van Trotsenburg MAA. Gynecological aspects of transgender healthcare. Int J Transgenderism. 2009; 11(4):238–246
[36] Miglioretti DL, Rutter CM, Geller BM, et al. Effect of breast augmentation on the accuracy of mammography and cancer characteristics. JAMA. 2004; 291 (4):442–450
[37] Lawrence A. Transgender health concerns. In: Meyer IH, Northridge ME, eds. The Health of Sexual Minorities: Public Health Perspectives on Lesbian, Gay, Bisexual and Transgender Populations. New York, NY: Springer; 2007:437–505
[38] American Cancer Society. Having a mammogram after you've had breast cancer surgery. URL: http://www.cancer.org/cancer/breast-cancer/screening-tests-and-early-detection/mammograms/having-a-mammogram-after-youve-had-breast-cancer-surgery.html. Updated October 9, 2017. Accessed July 23, 2019
[39] Katayama Y, Motoki T, Watanabe S, et al. A very rare case of breast cancer in a female-to-male transsexual. Breast Cancer. 2016; 23(6):939–944
[40] Nikolic DV, Djordjevic ML, Granic M, et al. Importance of revealing a rare case of breast cancer in a female to male transsexual after bilateral mastectomy. World J Surg Oncol. 2012; 10:280
[41] Forster NA, Künzi W, Giovanoli P. The reoperation cascade after breast augmentation with implants: what the patient needs to know. J Plast Reconstr Aesthet Surg. 2013; 66(3):313–322
[42] Kaariainen M, Salonen K, Helminen M, Karhunen-Enckell U. Chest-wall contouring surgery in female-to-male transgender patients: a one-center retrospective analysis of applied surgical techniques and results. Scand J Surg. 2017; 106(1):74–79
[43] Berry MG, Curtis R, Davies D. Female-to-male transgender chest reconstruction: a large consecutive, single-surgeon experience. J Plast Reconstr Aesthet Surg. 2012; 65(6):711–719
[44] Cregten-Escobar P, Bouman MB, Buncamper ME, Mullender MG. Subcutaneous mastectomy in female-to-male transsexuals: a retrospective cohort-analysis of 202 patients. J Sex Med. 2012; 9(12):3148–3153

22 Nipple Areolar Procedures and Aesthetics

Steven G. Woodward and Matthew P. Jenkins

Summary

An integral part of breast surgery is to preserve or re-create the natural appearance of the breast. Attaining quality aesthetic results after breast surgery is an important factor in physical appearance and psychological body image, which affects patients' quality of life after breast surgery. A key factor in the aesthetics of breast surgery is the preservation, recreation, and reconstruction of the nipple areolar complex (NAC). Factors that affect the aesthetics of the NAC include location, orientation, angulation, size, shape, color, and symmetry. To improve aesthetic results after breast surgery, several procedures have been developed to address the NAC. This chapter will review the anatomy, embryology, and physiology of the NAC, including the milk-secreting system, lymphatic drainage, innervation, and vascular supply. Furthermore, it will discuss the "ideal breast," describing the proportions and relative placement of the NAC on the breast that is associated with the greatest aesthetic result in the literature. Finally, primary pathology of the NAC, including inverted nipple and nipple hypertrophy, are discussed with surgical approaches for correction.

Keywords: nipple, areola, aesthetics, surgery

22.1 Introduction

An integral part of breast surgery is to preserve or re-create the natural appearance of the breast. Attaining quality aesthetic results after breast surgery is an important factor in physical appearance and psychological body image, which affects patients' quality of life after breast surgery.[1] A key factor in the aesthetics of breast surgery is the preservation, re-creation, and reconstruction of the nipple areolar complex (NAC).[2,3] Several factors affect the aesthetics of the NAC, including location, orientation, angulation, size, shape, color, and symmetry. Several primary pathologies of the NAC affect its aesthetic appearance, including inverted nipple and nipple hypertrophy; these have been studied in order to develop better surgical techniques for correction.

22.2 Nipple Areola Complex Anatomy

22.2.1 Embryology, Structure, Development

The NAC is a central breast structure that consists of the areola, which is distinguished from the rest of the surrounding breast tissue by its distinct change in skin pigment, as well as the nipple itself. The physiologic purpose of the NAC is to deliver milk, produced in the mammary glands of the breast, to an infant. The normal color of the areola can range from lighter to darker skin tones and can span the spectrum of pink to red to brown or nearly black, depending on the underlying skin color of the individual. Typically it is paler in those with lighter skin tones and darker in those with darker skin tones, but the pigment differs from that of the surrounding breast skin. Many believe this color difference makes it more visible and draws the attention of an infant attempting to breastfeed.

The breast tissue and makeup can be divided into parenchymal tissue and stromal tissue. In utero, the parenchymal tissue forms a system of branching ducts, which develop into secretory acinar cells and eventually form the lactiferous ductal system. The stromal tissue develops into the fatty breast tissue, which provides an environment for proper development of the ductal system. This system slowly develops in utero in conjunction with proliferation of mesoderm. The proliferation of mesoderm causes eversion of the nipples at the skin level shortly after birth. This is the same time in development when the change in pigmentation of the NAC occurs. Further development of erectile tissue within the NAC causes nipple protrusion.[4] In the mature breast the NAC contains Montgomery's glands, or areolar glands, which are large sebaceous glands that secrete a lubricating fluid to prevent chafing during breastfeeding.[5] These glands then open at Montgomery's tubercles, which are small raised papules on the areola. The milk-secreting system consists of glandular lobes containing cells that secrete milk into lactiferous sinuses, which empty into the lactiferous ducts, which secrete the milk through the nipple when stimulated (▶ Fig. 22.1).[5,6] It is important to note that the overlying skin is continuous with the ducts, which has oncologic implications and allows malignancy to travel from within the ducts to the overlying skin.

22.2.2 Lymphatic Drainage

There are four major lymphatic drainage pathways of the breast, including two deep lymphatic systems and two superficial lymphatic systems. The primary lymphatic drainage of the NAC is Sappey's plexus, a complex, subareolar lymphatic system that is in communication with one of the superficial drainage pathways. This superficial plexus then communicates with one of the deeper lymphatic systems, the glandular plexus, which runs with the lactiferous ducts. These lymphatic pathways eventually drain into the axillary lymph node system. The skin and glandular tissue have the same embryonic origin and therefore the same lymphatic drainage pathway. This is what enables breast surgeons to inject subcutaneous radiotracer or methylene blue in the subareolar or periareolar tissue and trace this to the axillary sentinel node in breast cancer surgery.[7]

22.2.3 Innervation

The nerve supply to the NAC is of particular importance, as the sensitivity plays a major role in morbidity and patient satisfaction after breast surgery. In several cadaveric studies, the nerve supply of the NAC has been dissected in order to understand its cutaneous innervation better.[8,9] The majority of the contribution to the sensory innervation of the NAC comes from lateral

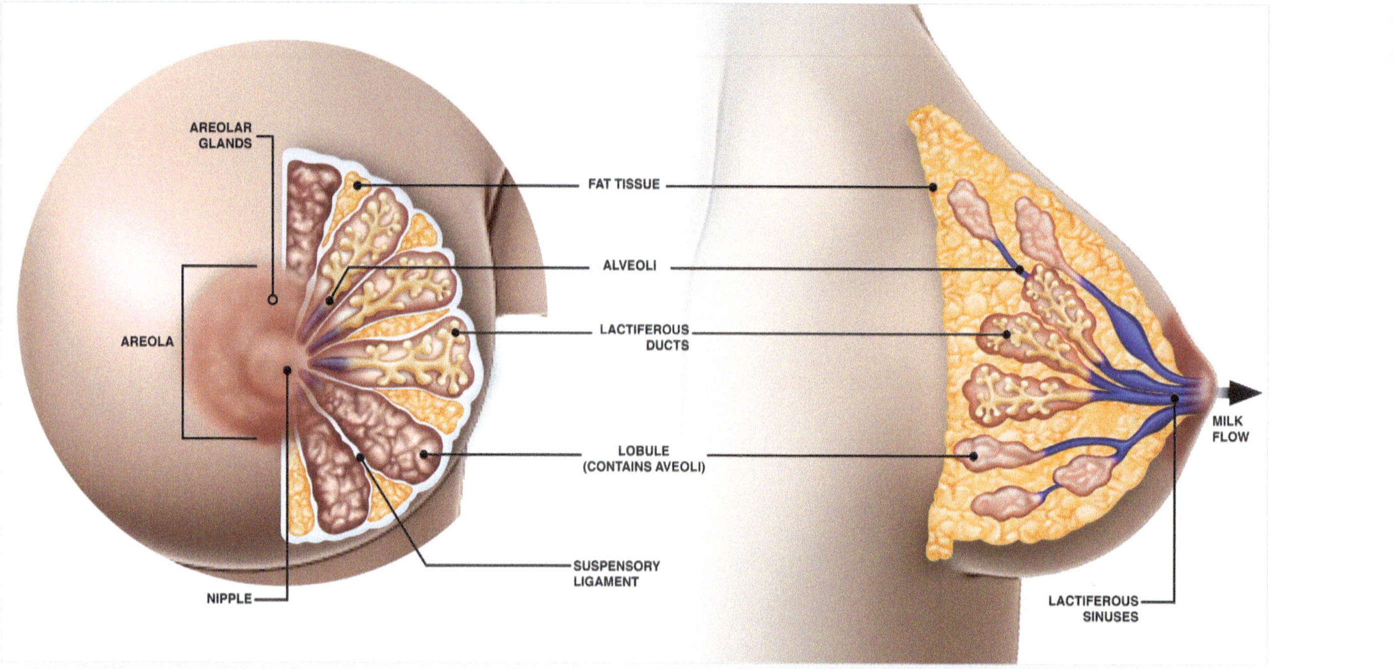

Fig. 22.1 Milk secreting system and ductal anatomy of the breast.

and anterior cutaneous branches of the second through fifth intercostal nerves (▶ Fig. 22.2). These studies have demonstrated that the most consistent of these contributions originates from the fourth intercostal nerve, specifically the lateral cutaneous branch; however, the anterior cutaneous branches of the third and fourth intercostal nerves were also highly consistent.

22.2.4 Blood Supply

The blood supply to the NAC generally has contributions from the internal thoracic artery (internal mammary artery), intercostal arteries, and lateral thoracic artery (▶ Fig. 22.3). Studies have been made in order to understand better the contribution of each arterial system to the NAC so as to guide better surgical techniques. In one particular cadaveric study, van Deventer dissected the arterial anatomy of 27 female breasts and found that the most consistent contribution to the NAC was the internal thoracic artery (100%), followed by the anterior intercostal arteries (74%) and the lateral thoracic artery (70%).[10] In a separate study that reviewed thoracic computed tomography (CT) angiograms to identify arterial supply to the NAC, Stirling et al found that perforating branches from the internal thoracic artery contributed to NAC blood supply in 81.8% of patients, followed by lateral thoracic contribution in 23.5% of patients and anterior intercostal artery contributions in 15.9% of patients.[11] Other studies have also described minor contributions directly from other arterial systems, including the axillary artery and posterior intercostal arteries. Given that the NAC receives blood supply from multiple sources, one would think it is a highly vascularized structure with collateral supply if needed during surgery. Iris et al analyzed breast magnetic resonance imaging (MRI) in order to understand with what frequency the NAC was receiving blood from multiple zones or arterial systems rather than from one arterial system. They found that in 58% of patients, blood supply came from one general breast zone (medial, lateral, central, superior, or inferior), with the great majority coming from medial perforating vessels. Only 42% of patients had NAC blood supply come from multiple zones, with the vast majority being medial and lateral perforating branches.[12] This suggests that the majority of the blood supply to the NAC comes from medial perforating vessels from the internal thoracic artery, as well as some contribution from lateral perforating vessels from the long thoracic artery and intercostal arteries. Knowledge of the origin and direction from which the NAC receives its blood supply can better direct surgical approach and dissection in order to avoid disrupting NAC perfusion, which could lead to necrosis and nipple loss during surgery.

22.3 The Ideal Nipple Areola Complex

22.3.1 General Principles

In regard to reconstruction and preservation of the NAC, one must keep several general principles in mind to have an aesthetically successful surgery. First and foremost, it is important to remember that every patient is different and will have certain preferences for the desired outcome. Therefore, it is important to discuss this and set these expectations with the patient prior to surgery.[13] Some texts have described a technique in which the patient is able to partake in the positioning of the NAC by using markers or stickers to designate possible placement in the preoperative setting. This allows the patient to see several possible positions and choose what they believe is the most aesthetically pleasing prior to surgery. The patient and

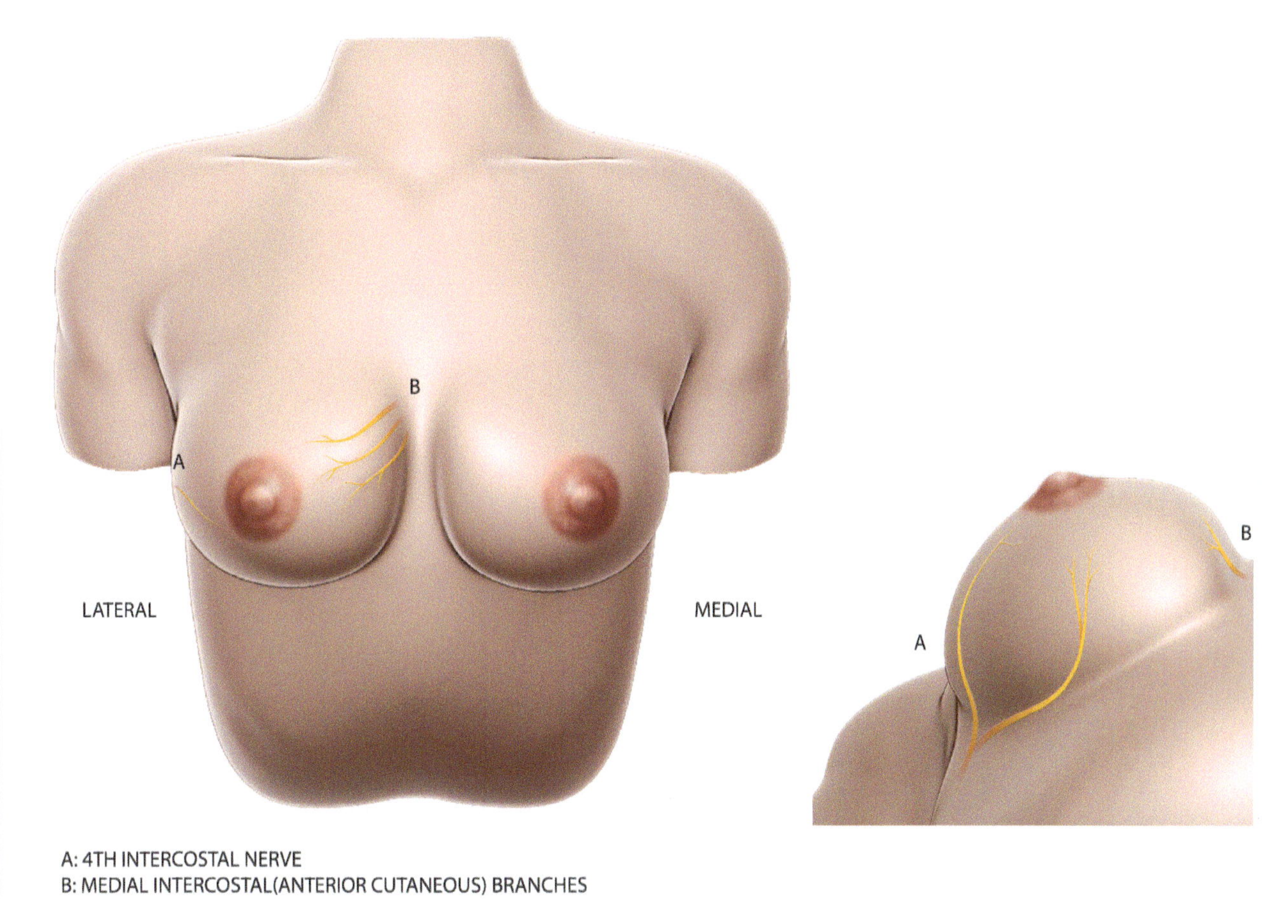

Fig. 22.2 Cutaneous innervation of the nipple areolar complex.

the surgeon can use this technique to find the ideal NAC placement and proportions together, which optimizes aesthetic outcomes.[4]

It should also be noted that any aesthetically pleasing outcome will incorporate and maintain symmetry between the breasts. This symmetry should incorporate parameters including color, texture, size, projection, angulation, placement, and relative proportions. In a unilateral reconstruction, the contralateral breast and NAC should be used as a template for the reconstruction. In bilateral reconstruction, symmetry of the NAC should be of highest consideration.[13]

22.3.2 Nipple Areolar Complex Placement

There have been several studies to determine the ideal position of the NAC relative to maintained landmarks on the breast and chest. One such study by Lewin et al used a questionnaire with several different NAC placements for the general public to determine which was the most aesthetically pleasing. In this survey it was determined that the ideal placement of the NAC was in a 40:60 ratio in the X dimension and a 50:50 ratio in the Y dimension as described in the representative figure (▶ Fig. 22.4). This can be described as the NAC being placed evenly between the upper and lower pole of the breast and placed more toward the lateral border of the breast in a 40:60 ratio compared to medially. Another study performed by Mallucci and Branford analyzed key characteristics of breast aesthetics in models and found that one key factor in NAC placement was a 45:55 ratio from upper pole to lower pole.[3] In a study by Beckenstein, the ideal nipple parameters were determined anatomically by analyzing males of ideal body weight. It was found in this study that the ideal nipple position was approximately 20 cm from the sternal notch and 18 cm from the midclavicular line. The mean nipple-to-nipple distance in these males was 21 cm.[14]

22.3.3 Nipple Characteristics

There are several parameters that must be determined in reconstructing the nipple itself. The nipple represents the apex of the breast, and several studies have studied the ideal ratio of breast-to-areola and nipple-to-areola proportions. It has been suggested that the ideal areola-to-breast proportion is 1:3–1:4, while the ideal nipple-to-areola proportion is 1:3.[4] In their study Mallucci and Branford further characterized the ideal nipple to have an angulation upwards of approximately 20° from the nipple median. This angulation is in the setting of a slightly concave slope of the upper pole of the breast and slightly

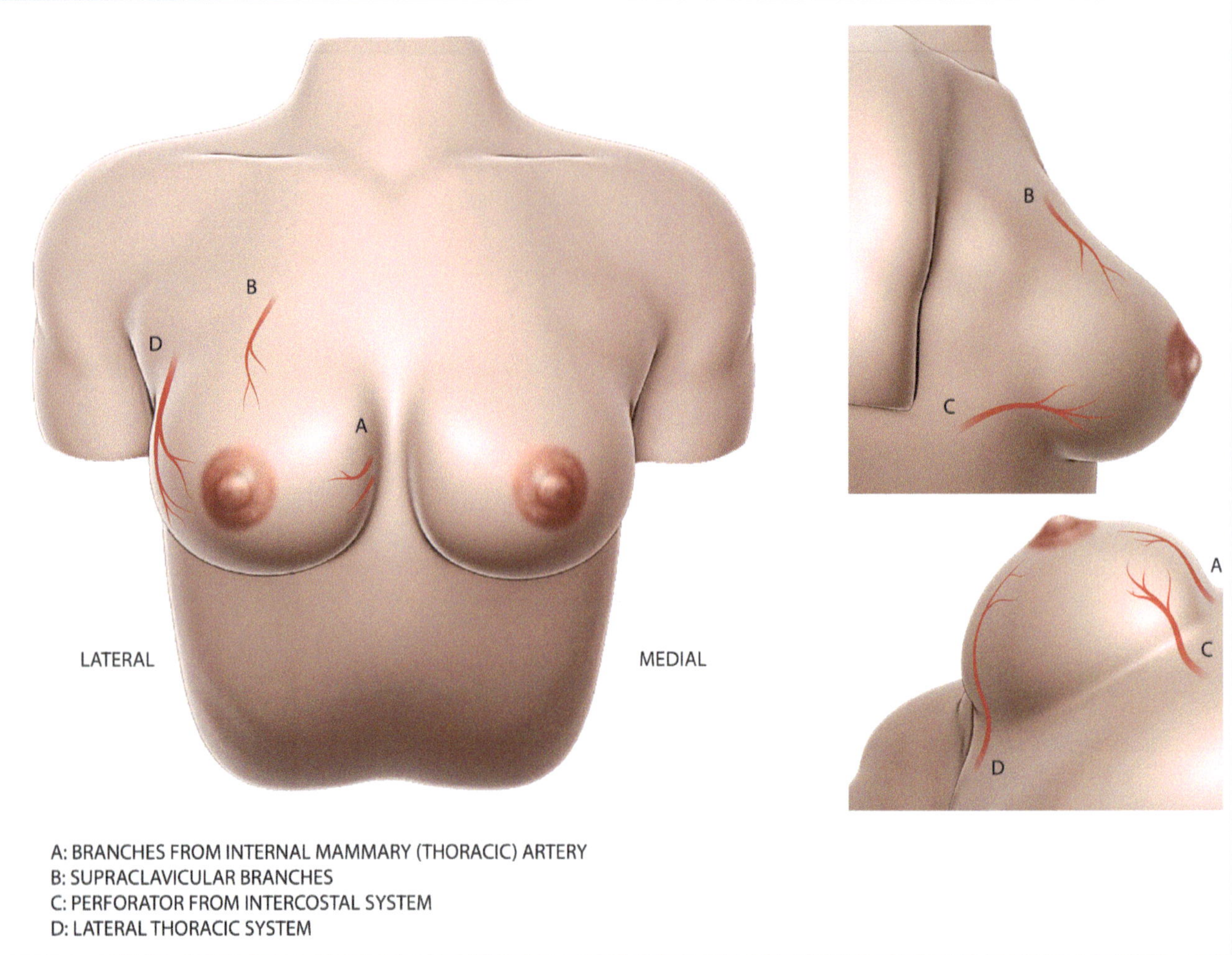

Fig. 22.3 Blood supply of the nipple areolar complex.

convex lower pole of the breast.[3] In Beckenstein's study of the ideal male nipple, he found that the average areolar diameter is approximately 2.8 cm with ranges from 2.5–3.0 cm.[14]

22.4 Nipple Areolar Complex Pathology and Reconstruction

Many NAC pathologies that have been studied in the literature with the goal of developing and guiding surgical technique for reconstruction. These defects can cause morbidity and negatively impact breastfeeding, sexuality, and patients' self-confidence secondary to aesthetic dissatisfaction. The more common pathologies described include inverted nipple and nipple hypertrophy.

22.4.1 Inverted Nipple

Inverted nipple can be described as a condition in which part of or the entire nipple is located below the level of the areola. It was first described in the 1800s, and since its first description there have been many identified causes including congenital, infectious, inflammatory, trauma, previous surgery, and oncologic. The most common of these is congenital, with an incidence of 3.26% and the majority being bilateral defects. This defect is typically caused by anatomically shortened ducts, which cause retraction of the nipple inward at their attachment points, leading to nipple inversion.[15] Han and Hong devised a grading system for inverted nipple in order to characterize this process and assess the role for surgical correction (▶ Fig. 22.5).[16] Grade I nipple inversion has minimal fibrosis and is easily pulled out manually, maintaining its projection without traction. Han and Hong describe that Grade I nipples can be treated with a simple purse-string suture behind the neck of the nipple. In Grade II inversion the nipple can be manually pulled out but not as easily as in Grade I, and the nipple does not maintain its projection, as it tends to retract without continued traction. In a Grade II repair, they describe releasing the fibrous tissue deep to the NAC in the vertical direction, while identifying and preserving lactiferous ducts, until the nipple can be easily everted and maintain projection without traction. An intradermal purse-string suture can then be placed deep to the nipple to help maintain its projection. In Grade III nipple inversion the nipple is severely inverted and retracted, it is difficult to

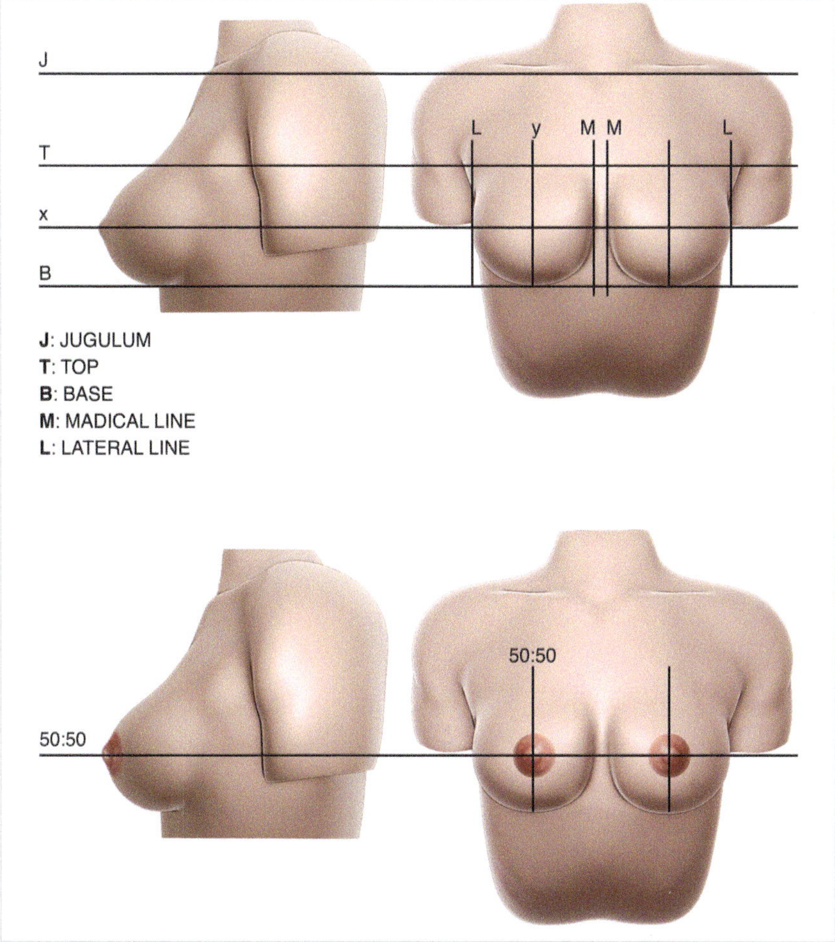

Fig. 22.4 Nipple areolar complex placement on the X and Y axes.

pull out, and it promptly retracts once everted. For a Grade III repair Han and Hong describe elevating deepithelialized flaps at the 10, 2, and 6 o'clock positions and dissecting the tissue beneath the nipple to release the fibrosis until the nipple easily everts. Once this is accomplished, the dermal flaps are turned down beneath the nipple and sutured together to give bulkiness to the nipple. A purse-string suture can then be placed below the nipple to help maintain its projection.[16] There have been many surgical techniques described in the literature for correction of nipple inversion. Like those of Han and Hong, most of these techniques fall into two categories: (1) creating flaps to maintain nipple protrusion and (2) placing sutures deep to the nipple to maintain its projection after traction. There is no consensus on which technique is preferred. Both of these techniques are used in conjunction with nipple traction. Continued nipple traction can be used either in the perioperative setting to maintain nipple projection while the surgical repair heals or as conservative therapy in the absence of surgery. When traction is used as conservative therapy, devices or sutures are used to maintain nipple projection and apply traction for a period of time up to several months to correct nipple inversion.[17]

22.4.2 Nipple Hypertrophy

There is no current definition for nipple hypertrophy (macrothelia), although it is often described within Asian populations. Most experts use the previously discussed parameters of the NAC in the setting of the "ideal breast" as a guideline in assessing hypertrophic nipple. This is in conjunction with patient preference and satisfaction with NAC aesthetics. Several techniques have been described for surgical correction of nipple hypertrophy. Many techniques describe taking a crescent- or triangular-shaped full-thickness wedge excision from the nipple (▶ Fig. 22.6). This can be done in several (usually 2–4) sections of the nipple to maintain symmetry. Once these sections are excised, the defects can be sutured together, resulting in a reduced nipple size. These sections can be marked in the preoperative setting and engineered for each patient in order to reduce the nipple diameter or height appropriately. Some authors describe the planned reduction typically being more than one-ninth and less than one-sixth of the diameter of the native nipple.[18,19] Other techniques have been described in the literature in which the anterior portion of the nipple is excised in a fashion that creates lateral flaps, which can then be sutured together in order to leave a smaller, more aesthetically pleasing nipple.[20] There is no strong evidence on which techniques minimize morbidity; however, one must keep the foregoing principles and anatomy in mind in order to avoid asymmetry, decreased nipple sensation, infection, delayed wound healing, and nipple loss/necrosis.

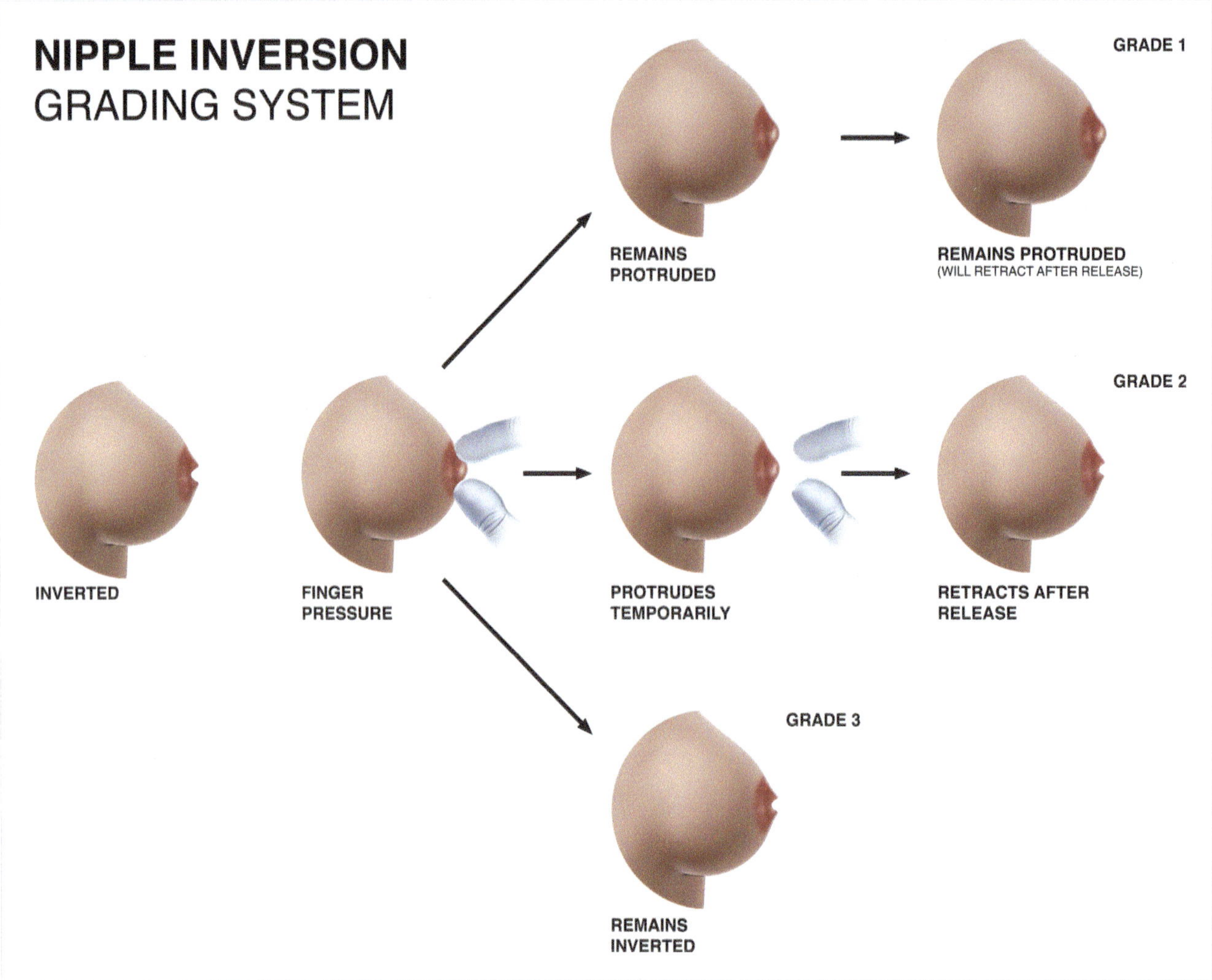

Fig. 22.5 Nipple inversion grading system.

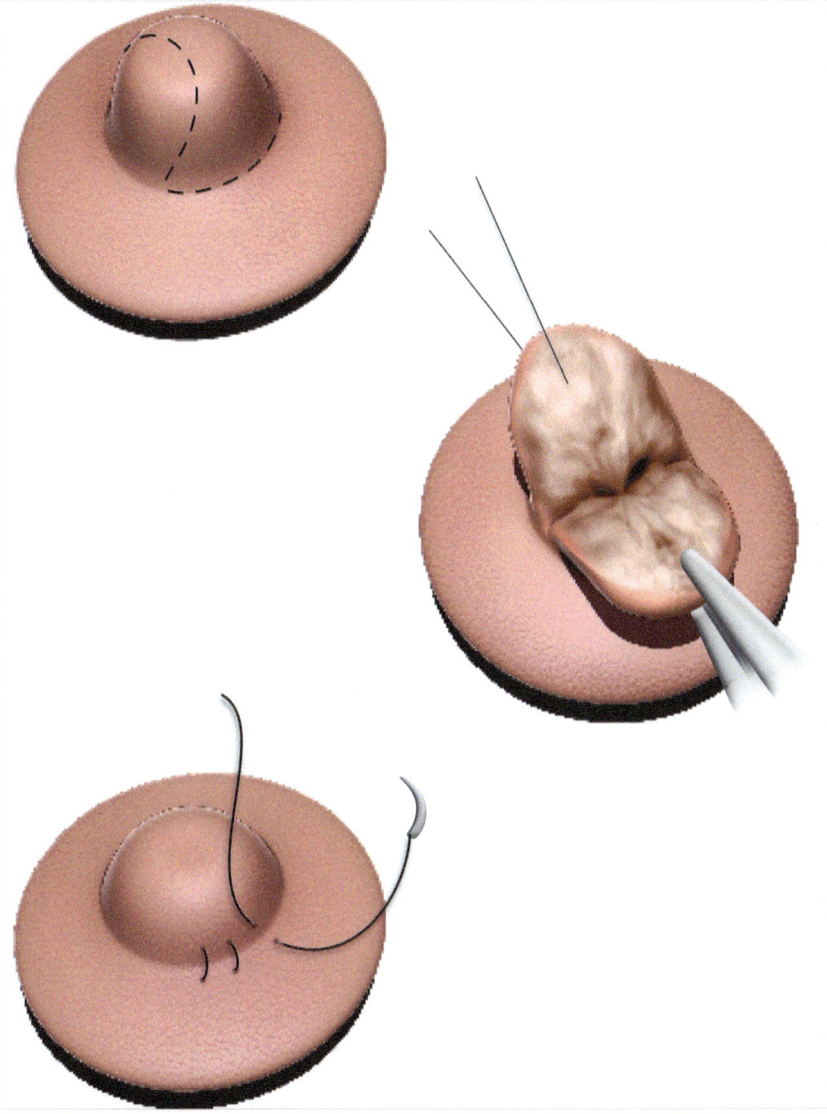

Fig. 22.6 Nipple hypertrophy reconstruction, wedge technique.

Key Points

- Preserving, re-creating, and reconstructing the nipple areolar complex are key factors in the aesthetics of breast surgery.
- A detailed knowledge of blood supply and innervation of the nipple areolar complex is essential in aesthetic breast surgery.
- The ideal nipple position is approximately 20 cm from the sternal notch and 18 cm from the midclavicular line.
- Inverted nipple and nipple hypertrophy are two of the more common conditions relating to the nipple areolar complex aesthetics, and multiple techniques have been proposed for correcting them.

References

[1] Kim MS, Sbalchiero JC, Reece GP, Miller MJ, Beahm EK, Markey MK. Assessment of breast aesthetics. Plast Reconstr Surg. 2008; 121(4):186e–194e

[2] Lewin R, Amoroso M, Plate N, Trogen C, Selvaggi G. The aesthetically ideal position of the nipple-areola complex on the breast. Aesthetic Plast Surg. 2016; 40(5):724–732

[3] Mallucci P, Branford OA. Concepts in aesthetic breast dimensions: analysis of the ideal breast. J Plast Reconstr Aesthet Surg. 2012; 65(1):8–16

[4] Shiffman MA, ed. Nipple-Areolar Complex Reconstruction: Principles and Clinical Techniques. Cham, Switzerland: Springer International Publishing; 2018

[5] OpenStax CNX. Anatomy and Physiology of the Female Reproductive System. URL: http://cnx.org/contents/9cccba49-6490-4e5b-a366-9991b7dbc56c@5 Accessed July 23, 2019

[6] Nicholson BT, Harvey JA, Cohen MA. Nipple-areolar complex: normal anatomy and benign and malignant processes. Radiographics. 2009; 29(2):509–523

[7] Fregnani JHTG, Macea JR. Lymphatic drainage of the breast: from theory to surgical practice. Int J Morphol. 2009; 27(3):873–878

[8] Schlenz I, Kuzbari R, Gruber H, Holle J. The sensitivity of the nipple-areola complex: an anatomic study. Plast Reconstr Surg. 2000; 105(3):905–909

[9] Jaspars JJ, Posma AN, van Immerseel AA, Gittenberger-de Groot AC. The cutaneous innervation of the female breast and nipple-areola complex: implications for surgery. Br J Plast Surg. 1997; 50(4):249–259

[10] van Deventer PV. The blood supply to the nipple-areola complex of the human mammary gland. Aesthetic Plast Surg. 2004; 28(6):393–398

[11] Stirling AD, Murray CP, Lee MA. The arterial supply of the nipple areola complex (NAC) and its relations: an analysis of angiographic CT imaging for breast pedicle design. Surg Radiol Anat. 2017; 39(10):1127–1134

[12] Seitz IA, Nixon AT, Friedewald SM, Rimler JC, Schechter LS. "NACsomes": A new classification system of the blood supply to the nipple areola complex

(NAC) based on diagnostic breast MRI exams. J Plast Reconstr Aesthet Surg. 2015; 68(6):792–799

[13] Farhadi J, Maksvytyte GK, Schaefer DJ, Pierer G, Scheufler O. Reconstruction of the nipple-areola complex: an update. J Plast Reconstr Aesthet Surg. 2006; 59(1):40–53

[14] Beckenstein MS, Windle BH, Stroup RT, Jr. Anatomical parameters for nipple position and areolar diameter in males. Ann Plast Surg. 1996; 36 (1):33–36

[15] Durgun M, Ozakpinar HR, Selçuk CT, Sarici M, Ceran C, Seven E. Inverted nipple correction with dermal flaps and traction. Aesthetic Plast Surg. 2014; 38 (3):533–539

[16] Han S, Hong YG. The inverted nipple: its grading and surgical correction. Plast Reconstr Surg. 1999; 104(2):389–395, discussion 396--397

[17] Li W, Wu Y, Deng Y, Zhang P, Ren GS. An adjustable-traction technique for correction of inverted nipples. Ann Plast Surg. 2016; 76(1):29–33

[18] Yu Y, Wei L, Shen Y, Xiao W, Huang J, Xu J. Windmill flap nipple reduction: a new method of nipple plasty. Aesthetic Plast Surg. 2017; 41(4):788–792

[19] Lee EI, Withers EH. Geometric nipple reduction technique: an approach to management of nipple hypertrophy. J Plast Reconstr Aesthet Surg. 2014; 67 (9):1301–1303

[20] Sim H, Sung S. Nipple reduction with the Chullo-Hat technique. Aesthet Surg J. 2015; 35:154–160

23 Marketing a Cosmetic Breast Surgery Practice through Social Media Outlets

Heather J. Furnas

Summary
This chapter offers tools to draw an audience through online tools, engage them, and attract them to your practice. Each component of a digital presence builds up the others. Strategy, A/B testing, and understanding your audience can make the difference between engagement or being ignored. The success of your website, social media presence, search engine optimization, and video creation can be measured through analytics. When used well, digital strategies will make a difference in building your cosmetic breast surgery practice.

Keywords: social media, digital marketing, search engine optimization, (SEO), advertising, promotion, patient education, digital analytics, Google AdWords, Google Analytics, social media, website

23.1 Introduction

Getting the word out that you're an expert in cosmetic breast surgery is important to nourish the growth of your practice. The most effective, efficient, and affordable way to market yourself is online, with social media and through your website. To see results, you need to know what platforms to use, how to maximize the reach of your posts, how to generate new content constantly, how to create good videos, and how to measure the return on investment. Whatever you post, using the best keywords and maximizing the metadata behind your online content will help you get noticed. Enticing people to connect with you online is an art, but if you can find your voice, and if people pay attention to you, you'll be successful at marketing your cosmetic breast surgery practice. You can pull people into your practice with a podcast, blog, guest blog, videos, eBooks, and social media, and you can push people your way through online ads with AdWords, display ads, search ads, social media ads, email marketing, and webinars. Whatever digital strategy you use, track all your efforts with digital analytics, and then adjust what you do. After that, it's up to you to deliver what patients are hoping for.

23.2 Leveraging Digital Strategies and Social Media

You may be a highly skilled cosmetic breast surgeon who gets great results, but unless people know who you are, you may not have as many patients as you'd like. A great reputation and word of mouth used to be sufficient to sustain the mature surgeon's practice, but today, people can confirm their friends' recommendations by searching for your online reviews and looking for before-and-after photos on your website. Even if you ignore your online presence, people may be talking about you on Yelp, Google Plus, and Facebook, and they might be trolls, angry patients, or unscrupulous competitors. So, if you've been sitting on the sideline watching the digital world fly by, it's time to join the conversation and take control of your online presence.

Traditional media, such as television, radio, and print, can play a role in your marketing efforts, but today most people search the Internet to find out about a procedure, locate a doctor near them, and check that surgeon's results and reputation. Consequently, when used well, digital media can be the most powerful marketing tool you can use to communicate your qualifications to potential patients. An effective online presence incorporates several platforms to cross-fertilize each other, including your website, your social media presence, and your reviews. Each needs to be strong in order to support the others effectively.

23.3 Website

A website has a huge advantage over social media platforms because *you* own all the content. Everything you post on social media, including all text, images, and videos, belongs to the social media parent company. If a company fails, becomes insignificant, or transforms into a music platform, as MySpace did, all your content goes with it. Your website is your Fort Knox, a home for all your valuable content. Your treasures might include a great bio; information about your practice; your photo gallery; embedded videos; books you've written; your social media platforms; your blog; and your media page, which can provide links to articles you've authored, TV shows you've appeared in, and podcasts you've created or participated in.

While social media networks allow personal connection and immediacy, your website allows greater depth and a large array of content. A social media post is like handing out brochures to a crowd. People may grab one as they walk by, and maybe they'll read it, but once the brochures are gone that day, they're difficult to find. A website is a like a library where a patient can look at your before-and-after photos, study your bio, and read about your practice week after week. The content will be there until you update it.

When you do update your website, or if you're starting from scratch, write down why you're doing so. The website designer is like the architect, but you're the one who's going to occupy it, so only you can accurately articulate the purpose (▶ Fig. 23.1). The more time you devote to developing your website purpose, flow, and design, the more effective it will be.

Next, write down the characteristics of your target audience. As a cosmetic breast surgeon, you'll obviously be targeting women, but identify other factors, such as ethnicity, level of education, age range, and geographic region. And don't forget men seeking breast/chest contouring. Although cosmetic breast surgery is largely a procedure performed on women, chest

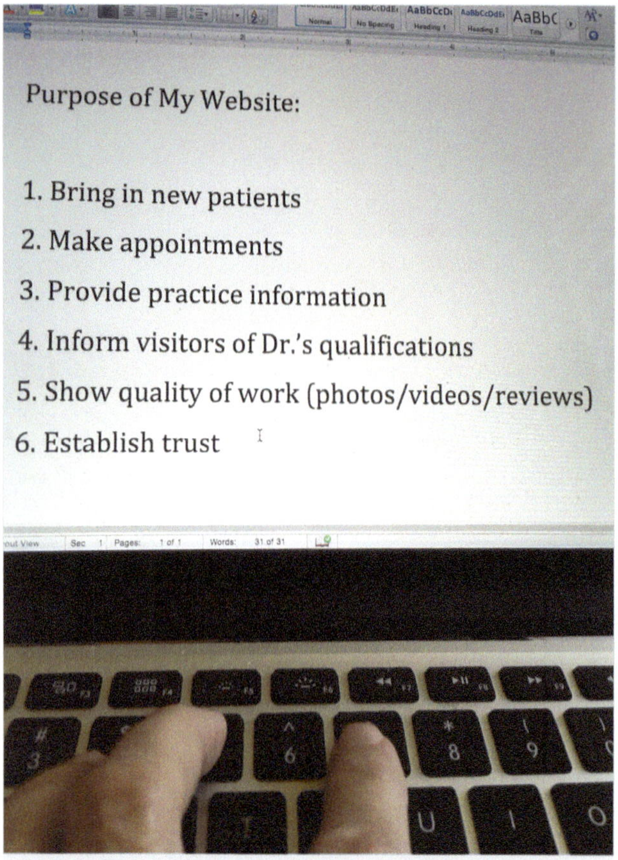

Fig. 23.1 Write down the purpose of your website.

contouring and breast reduction for gynecomastia are growing in popularity, with over 30,000 male breast reductions performed in 2016, a number that had risen nearly 200% in 20 years.[1]

Once you've established your target audience, design the website for them, not for you. Use a color scheme that will appeal to them, even if it's not your personal favorite choice. Avoid clutter, make navigation easy, and create logical flow throughout your website. The patient looking at a text description of a breast augmentation should be directed, without having to search, to related videos and to the photo gallery (▶ Fig. 23.2).

23.3.1 Before-and-After Photos

One of the biggest reasons potential patients visit a plastic surgeon's website is to view the photo gallery. The best photos feature good lighting and the absence of distractions such as clothing, jewelry, or a busy background. Potential patients are looking for good surgical results, especially in patients who looked like them before surgery and ended up with results that they hope to achieve. Increase the value of your gallery by telling each patient's story; give the potential new patient a reason to spend more time on your website. Include details, such as the patient's age, her height and weight, whether she's a mom, and the difference surgery made in her life. Some surgeons include the breast implant brand name and reference number, but that will be of little interest compared with the patient's story (▶ Fig. 23.3). The longer visitors linger over your website, the more likely they'll become your patients.

23.3.2 Text

Although it is often said in the search engine optimization (SEO) world that "content is king," if a page is only full of dense information about procedures, visitors are likely to search elsewhere. Limit the amount of text on a page and write at a sixth-grade reading level. Break up the page with eye-grabbing images and use subheadings for a visual break. Write in a simple style with short sentences and cut out unnecessary words. For example, "It is important to remember that you should always look for a board-certified plastic surgeon" should be shortened to: "Choose a board-certified plastic surgeon." After holding the reader's attention for a moment, reward her with an image. Be succinct but provide valuable information.

23.3.3 Choosing a Font

Nothing is more frustrating for a website visitor than coming across font that's difficult to read. Make the font large enough, and use strong contrast, such as black on white. If you choose white on black, make the font size larger than you'd use with black on white. Use common, browser-safe fonts. Browsers can use only those fonts stored on the computer or phone the viewer is using, so unusual fonts will be substituted with common ones. Arial, Times New Roman, and Verdana are examples of browser-safe fonts (▶ Fig. 23.4).

23.3.4 Images

The shortcut to developing an array of images is to pay for an array of stock photos. That's a great option when you're starting out, but off-the-rack photos give themselves away with their sterility, and viewers will spend little time looking at them. To make your website more authentic and a better reflection of you, arrange your own professional photo shoot. Show your office in action. A photo of your reception area with nobody in it gives the impression that you're not busy. Get some volunteers to stand in as staff and a patient or two, and let the scene come to life. You may be able to find patients willing to participate as models. Your own images can capture the culture of your practice in a way that stock photos can't (▶ Fig. 23.5).

23.3.5 Home Page

Eschew long, dramatic, musical introductions on your home page. Your visitors want to see before-and-after images, not a Hollywood movie, so don't waste their time. They're coming to your website for a reason, so usher them directly to where they want to go.

While you might think of the home page as the front door through which every visitor enters, online searches often direct visitors to secondary or tertiary pages. Every page can be a landing page, so each should have your logo in the top left corner or top center, and when clicked, it should direct the visitor to the home page. All pages should include your phone number, your clickable social media icons, and a search box for easy navigation. Take a tour of your website as if you were a visitor. If photos and videos take a long time loading, ask your webmaster to reduce the file size. Embedded videos should be well edited and short.

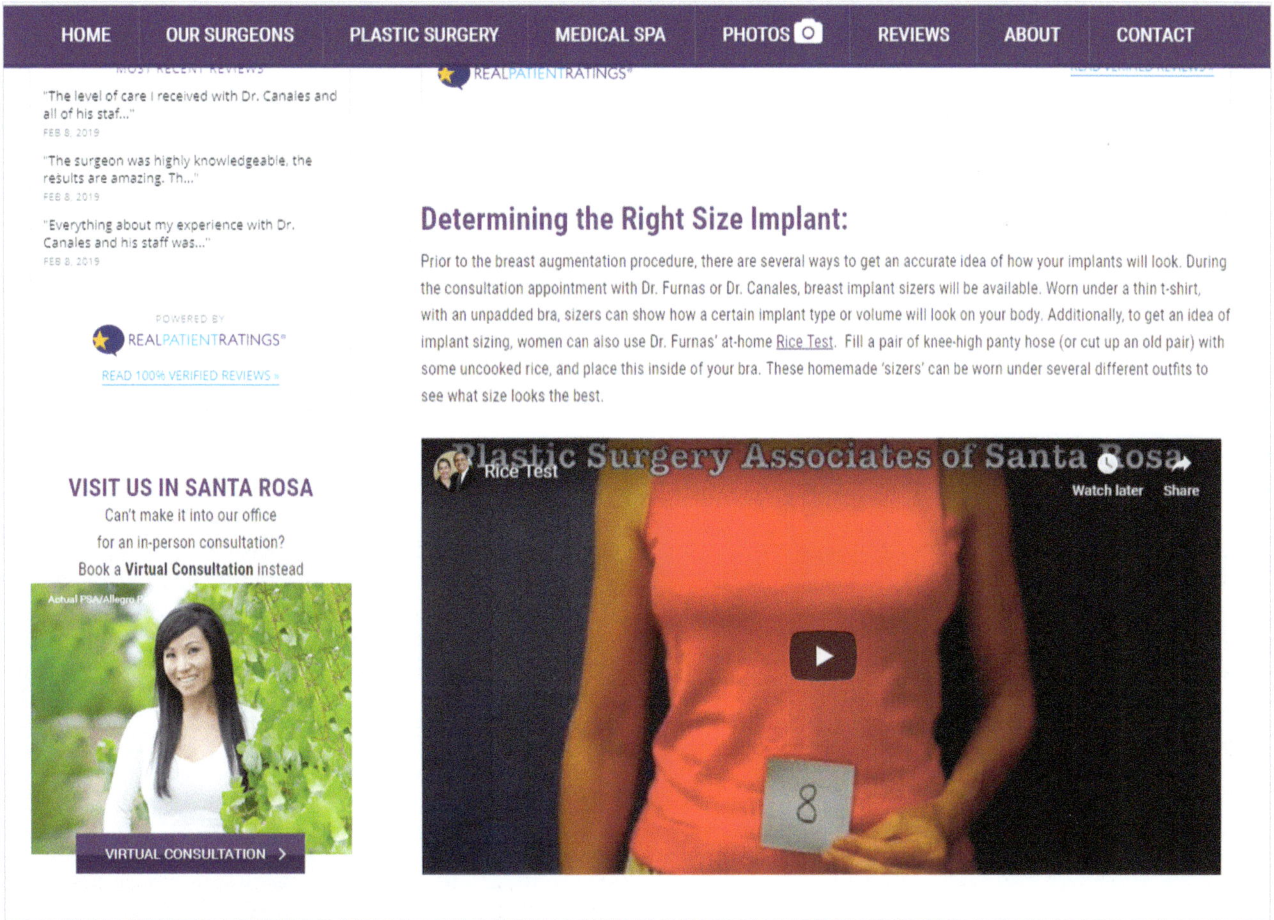
HOME
OUR SURGEONS
PLASTIC SURGERY
MEDICAL SPA
PHOTOS
REVIEWS
ABOUT
CONTACT
"The level of care I received with Dr. Canales and all of his staf..."
FEB 8, 2019
"The surgeon was highly knowledgeable, the results are amazing. Th..."
FEB 8, 2019
"Everything about my experience with Dr. Canales and his staff was..."
FEB 8, 2019
POWERED BY
REALPATIENTRATINGS
READ 100% VERIFIED REVIEWS »
VISIT US IN SANTA ROSA
Can't make it into our office
for an in-person consultation?
Book a Virtual Consultation instead
VIRTUAL CONSULTATION >
Determining the Right Size Implant:
Prior to the breast augmentation procedure, there are several ways to get an accurate idea of how your implants will look. During the consultation appointment with Dr. Furnas or Dr. Canales, breast implant sizers will be available. Worn under a thin t-shirt, with an unpadded bra, sizers can show how a certain implant type or volume will look on your body. Additionally, to get an idea of implant sizing, women can also use Dr. Furnas' at-home Rice Test. Fill a pair of knee-high panty hose (or cut up an old pair) with some uncooked rice, and place this inside of your bra. These homemade 'sizers' can be worn under several different outfits to see what size looks the best.
Plastic Surgery Associates of Santa Rosa
Rice Test
Watch later
Share
8

Fig. 23.2 Integrate related information about cosmetic breast surgery so the website visitor can find everything you have to offer without having to search.

23.3.6 Credentialing the Doctors

Somewhere on the home page, display the logos of the prestigious societies you belong to, the educational institutions where you received your education and training, and the seals of the awards you've received. A recognizable logo may make a bigger impression on a website visitor than a five-paragraph biography (▶ Fig. 23.6).

23.3.7 Social Media Icons

A key component of digital strategy is connectability, so your website should connect to your social media platforms and vice versa. Place the icons in a readily visible area, such as at the top of the page, and show them on every page of your website. The website pages that don't include before-and-after photos should be sharable on social media. If you have a blog on your website, make sure the featured image appears in social media shares.

23.3.8 Contact Form

Include an easy-to-find, easy-to-fill-out contact form. A contact form without staff support, however, is useless. Your patient coordinator should check online inquiries frequently to convert the curious website visitor into a patient with an appointment.

23.3.9 Media Page

Let people know about scientific articles you've written by creating a media page, since potential patients may not otherwise know of your expertise. Include instances in which you've been featured in the mainstream media. Your website media page serves as a library for visitors to browse through, while your social media feed serves as a news outlet to broadcast what's new (▶ Fig. 23.7).

23.3.10 Extend a Welcome Invitation

If you're hosting an event or planning a Facebook Live broadcast, create a pop-up announcement for your website. To capture the interested visitor with a burning question about a procedure, consider a live-chat service. Live-chat services typically function after hours to gather a visitor's specific interest, name, phone number, and email so that your office staff can make contact and set up an appointment.

23.3.11 Maintenance

Go through your website periodically, especially as it gets updated, and solicit feedback from volunteers to search for broken links, confusing navigation, misspellings, and grammatical

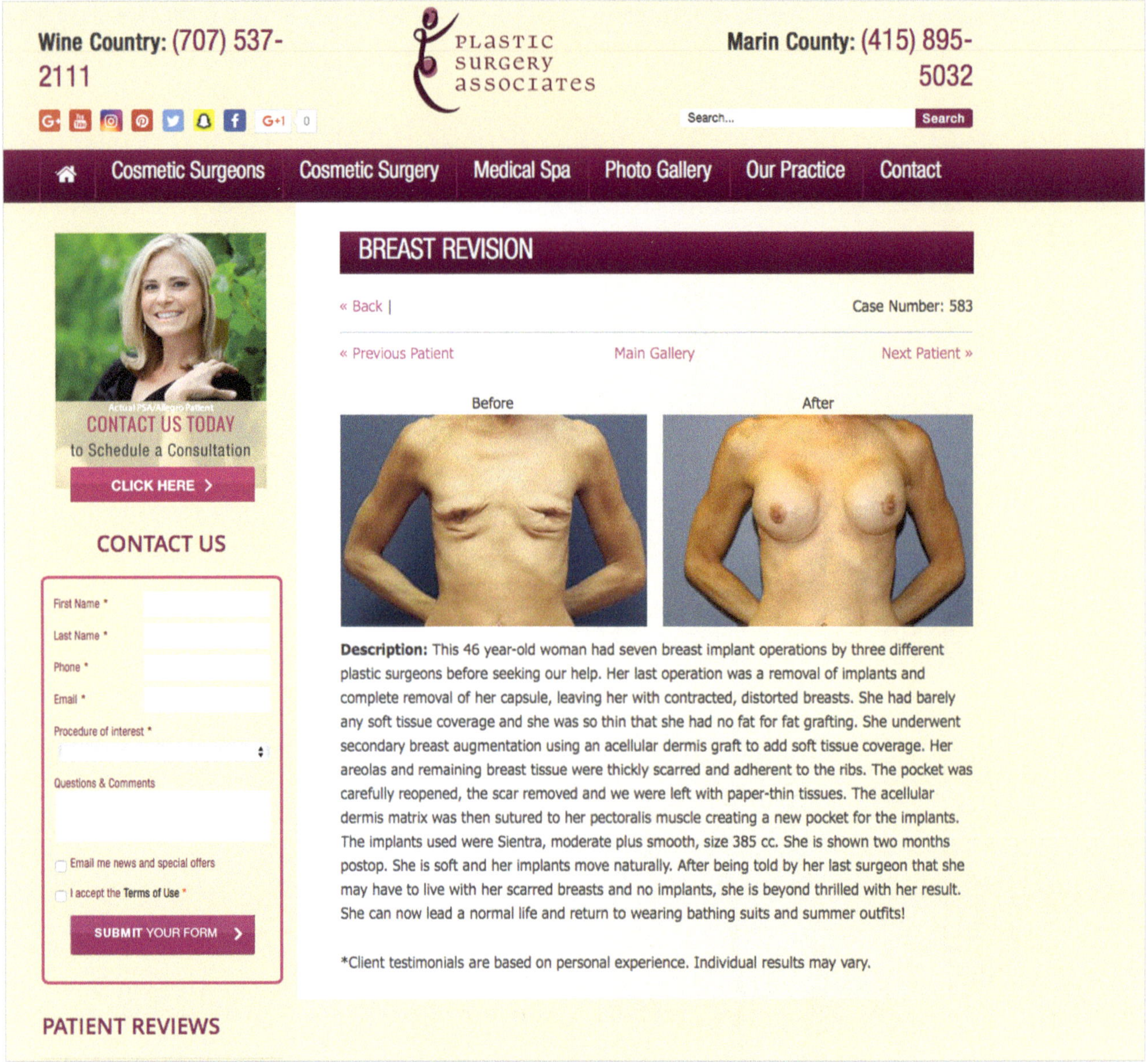

Fig. 23.3 Good before-and-after photos invite greater interest when accompanied by the patient's story.

errors. View your website on different devices, from mobile phones to a 27-inch desktop screen, to make sure it looks good in all dimensions. Around half of website traffic is now through mobile devices.[2] Adaptability across different devices is called *responsive web design*. To do a quick test, go to a large screen, such as your laptop or desktop computer, and resize your browser window to mimic the screen sizes of smaller devices. On your mobile phone, change from portrait to landscape views, and see how it looks. If your website looks like an image from an orbiting satellite, it's not responsively designed. Cross-device adaptability is particularly important now that so much of Internet traffic is on mobile phones.[2]

Update your content and keep the visual appearance current, crisp, and clean. A good webmaster will help keep your website updated with advances in the user experience. For example, virtual reality (VR), augmented reality (AR), and machine learning that allows searches by images are folding into the digital landscape.

23.3.12 Search Engine Optimization

No matter what or where you post, think in terms of search engine optimization (SEO). A *search engine* is the software that combs the World Wide Web for information to fulfill a search, such as Google or DuckDuckGo. *Web crawlers*, or *spiders*, are Internet bots that examine different websites seeking authoritative sources to answer an Internet user's search. The results are indexed and displayed on search engine results pages (SERP). Because the web crawlers are looking for well-used terms in fulfilling searches, they have their feelers out for *keywords*.

A breast augmentation is a procedure in which a breast implant is inserted beneath the breast through a small incision. The implant can be filled with salt water (saline) or silicone gel. It can be round or shaped. And the shell of the implant can be smooth or textured. Consult with a board certified plastic surgeon to find out the best approach for you.

A breast augmentation is a procedure in which a breast implant is inserted beneath the breast through a small incision. The implant can be filled with salt water (saline) or silicone gel. It can be round or shaped. And the shell of the implant can be smooth or textured. Consult with a board certified plastic surgeon to find out the best approach for you.

A breast augmentation is a procedure in which a breast implant is inserted beneath the breast through a small incision. The implant can be filled with salt water (saline) or silicone gel. It can be round or shaped. And the shell of the implant can be smooth or textured. Consult with a board certified plastic surgeon to find out the best approach for you.

Fig. 23.4 Fonts should be browser-safe and easy to read with high contrast and suitable font size (top). White-on-black type (middle) should be in a larger size than black-on-white type. Do not use fonts that are hard to read, not found on many computers or phones, or in colors that do not contrast much with their background (bottom).

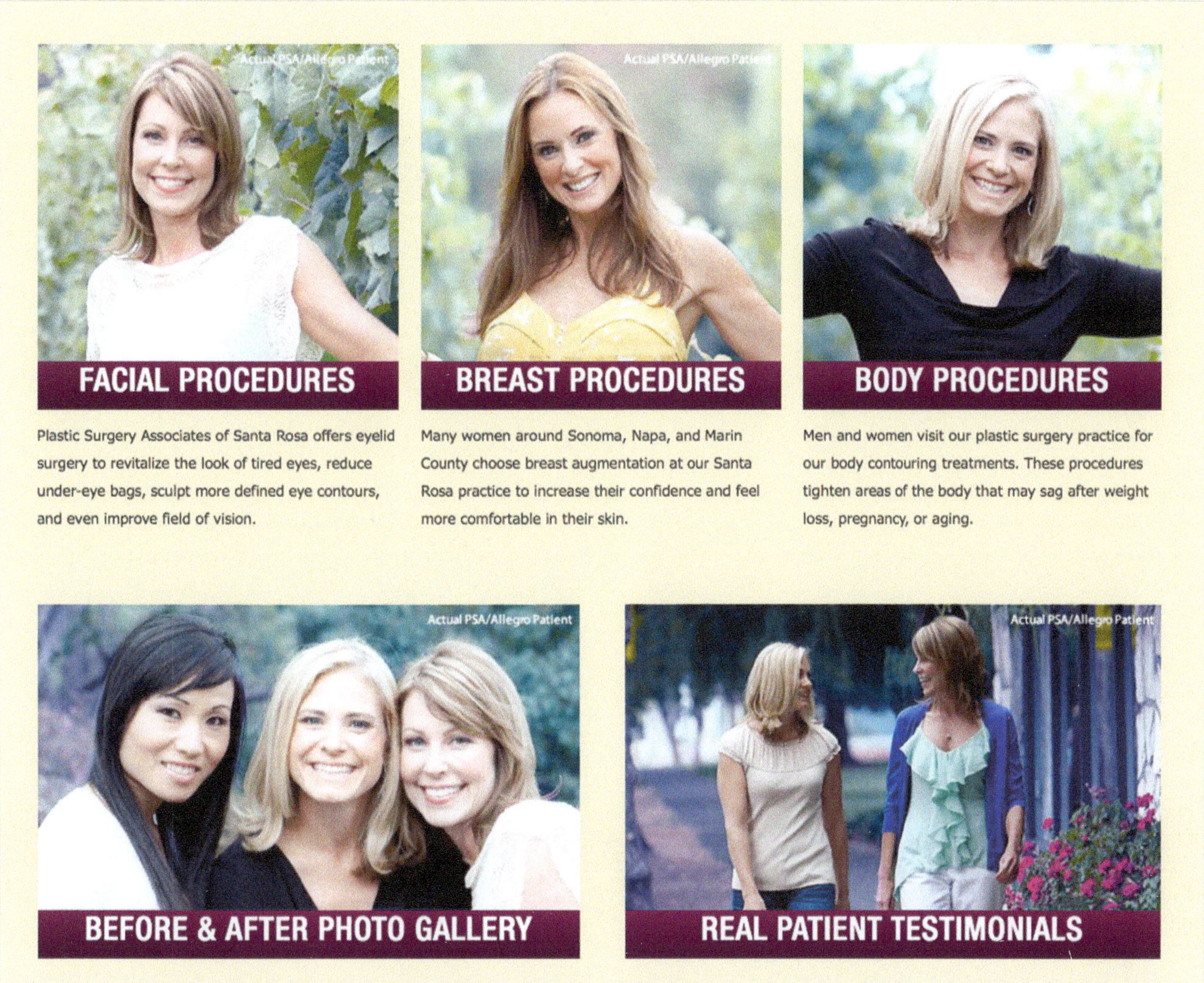

Fig. 23.5 Photos taken in your practice increase the chances that website visitors will pay attention to them.

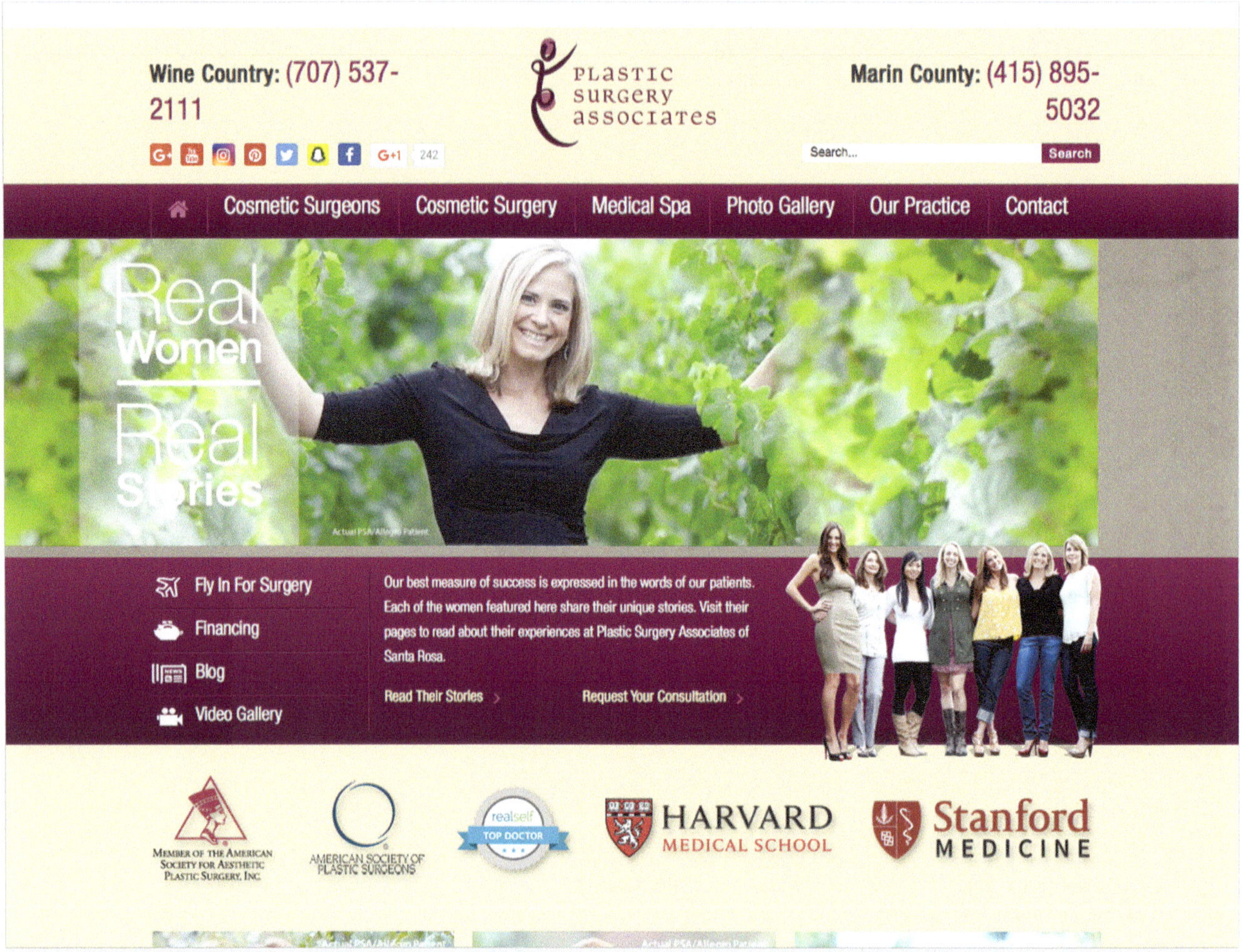

Fig. 23.6 Professional society, award, and university logos can convey a doctor's training and expertise at a quick glance.

Keywords

A keyword isn't limited to a word; it can be a phrase, like "breast augmentation cost." Imagine what people type into a search bar. Those frequently entered words and phrases are *keywords*. Use only the keywords that are truly pertinent to your content, since Google doesn't reward those who game the system.

Metadata

Metadata is information about data. A digital image is associated with information about its size and the date of creation. Such information is invisible to a website visitor, but to web crawlers, this metadata, which includes alternate text and descriptions of images and videos with topical keywords, enhances the authority of a document.[3]

23.4 Social Media

Social media are defined as "interactive computer-mediated technologies that facilitate the creation and sharing of information, ideas, career interests and other forms of expression via virtual communities and networks."[4] Among the most prominent social media are Facebook, Instagram, Snapchat, Pinterest, YouTube, and Twitter. Other examples include RealSelf, blogs, forums, photo and video sharing apps, review websites, social gaming, and virtual worlds. All of these entities enable you to connect your content with others.

23.4.1 Why Use Social Media?

Why should you be on social media outside of your personal life? Just as you did with your website, write down the reasons.[5] Even though the purpose may seem obvious (Get more patients!), breaking it down into specifics can help you focus what, where, and how you post (▶ Fig. 23.8).

After you've defined your goals, identify your target audience. Describe the patients you hope to attract. Your breast augmentation patients may be in their 20 s and 30 s, while your mastopexy patients may be in their 30 s, 40 s, and 50 s. Those different groups may favor different social media apps, so develop a plan for each one.

Just as important as creating posts that your audience wants to see is providing a variety of offerings. Posting information about a breast augmentation, then scenes from an office event,

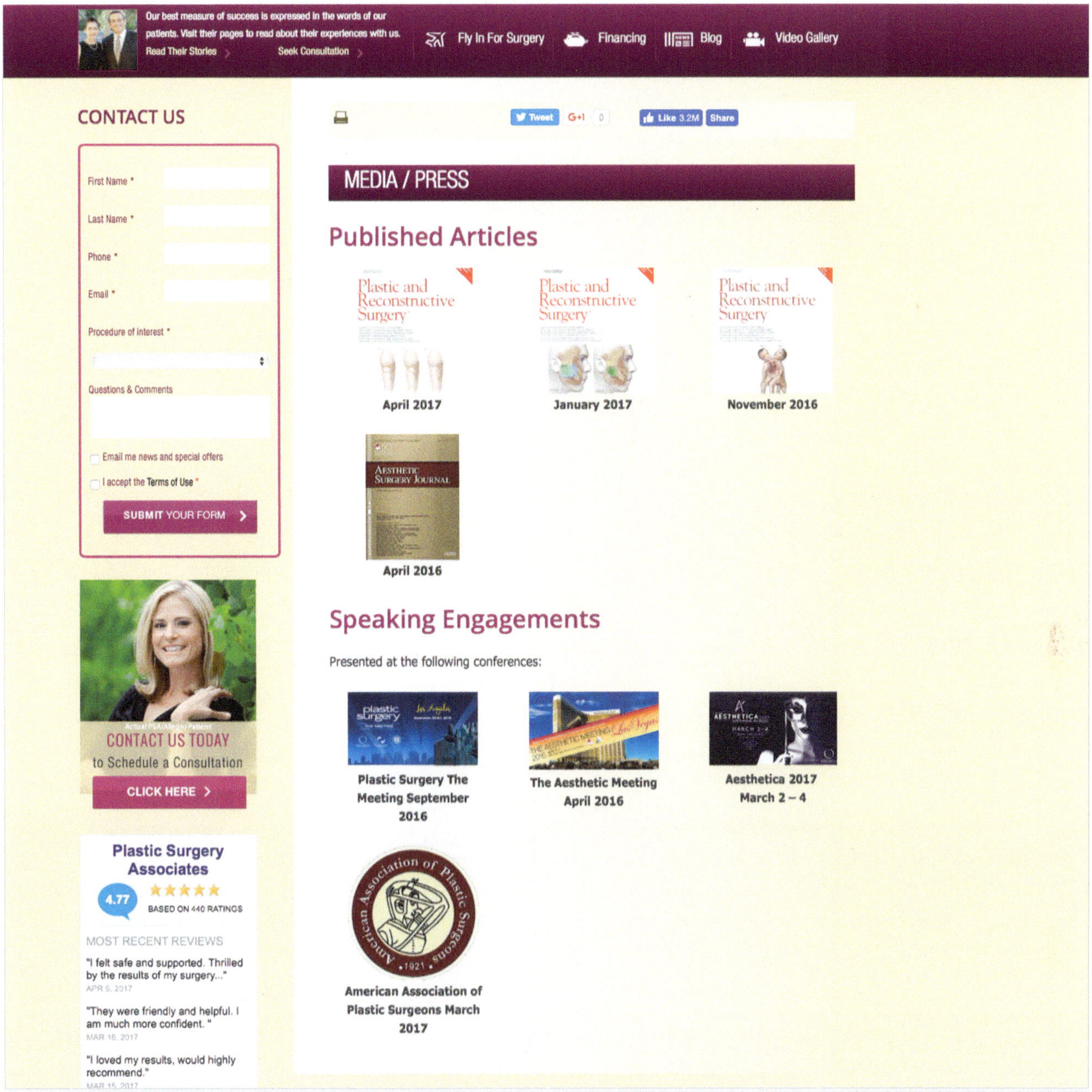

Fig. 23.7 A media page acts as a library to showcase your contributions to the field and your authority as a thought leader in cosmetic breast surgery.

then a photo of you with colleagues at a meeting will add depth to your social media presence and give potential patients a sense of who you are. Their trust in you will develop as they see the evidence that you're nice, that you're caring, and that you're an expert in cosmetic breast surgery.

23.4.2 How to Use Social Media Apps

After opening accounts on the social media apps that you'll be using, organize your profile to attract an audience. Your profile page is like your living room. People will visit, look at the pictures, read your bio, and search anything else you display. As with a medical chart, you're in control of how much it'll help you. The more areas you leave blank, the more people will ignore you. Facebook has a different format for personal and business pages.[6] Business pages have options for such things as a virtual tour of your office.

Another social media option with a different business model is RealSelf.com, which is specifically designed to connect providers of cosmetic surgery and treatments with potential patients. There are significant fees to boost your local visibility in your target areas of interest, such as breast augmentation or mastopexy, but you can answer patient questions, post photos and videos, and create a profile page to attract potential patients without paying a fee. As with any marketing expense, it is important for you to truly track the source of your leads and the revenue generated from each marketing effort.

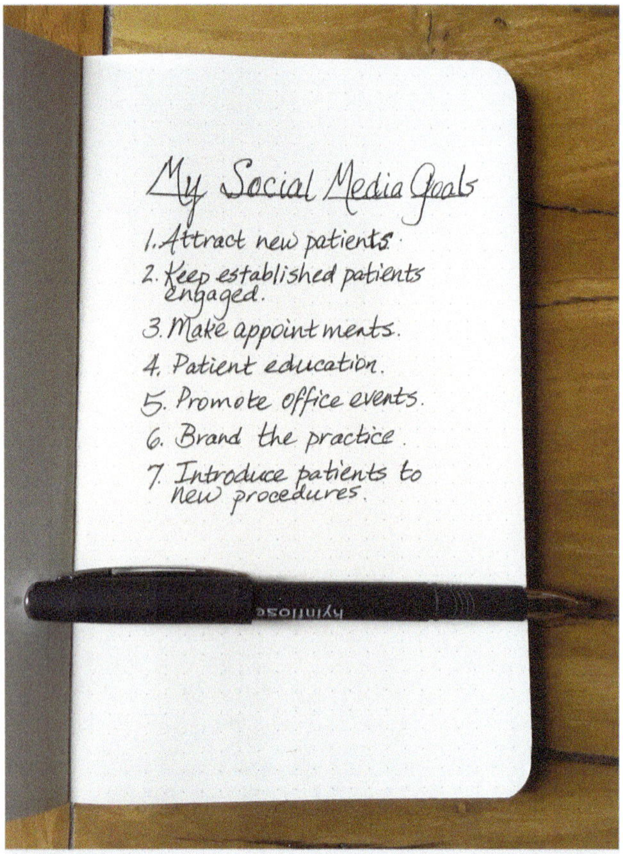

Fig. 23.8 Articulate your social media goals. Measurable goals allow you to track your performance.

Username/Handle

After opening a social media app account, choose a username that reflects who you are. A *username*, sometimes called *handle*, is your identification on that app. Make it easy for people to find you by using your name, and emphasize that you're a doctor by using the prefix *Dr.* or the initials *M.D./D.O.* after your name. For example, my Twitter username is *@drheatherfurnas*. Save informal names for your personal accounts.

Photos

Load up a profile photo that conveys professionalism, and, if available, a header photo that spans the top of the page. The header can add dimension to your profile. Surgeons often use photos of themselves scrubbed in surgery.

Link

Include your practice website link so that people can find out more about you. Remember, no social media app, including a Facebook business page, offers the depth of information that your website can. You can engage patients on social media, but ultimately you want them to visit your website, fill out a contact form, and make an appointment.

Maintain Separate Personal and Professional Accounts

Your friends want to see you with your hair down, on vacation, with your family, but they may not want to see your latest video on breast augmentation. On the other hand, you may not want potential patients looking for a good cosmetic breast surgeon to see photos of you drinking beer with your college buddies in face paint at a football game. A professional social media account, particularly a Facebook business page, can be used to give information about your practice, directions to your office, announcements of upcoming events, and photos of you and your staff in action. If you set up an Instagram business account, you can set up a Contact button for potential patients.[7]

YouTube Channel

While the public is less likely to comment or "like" YouTube posts compared with Facebook or Instagram, YouTube is a great place to display your professional videos without storing them on your website. In terms of number of users, YouTube is second only to Facebook.[8] Virtually all social media apps encourage video posts, but a YouTube channel enables you to organize videos in playlists. Don't forget: YouTube is owned by Google, which many people use for searches.

23.4.3 How to Choose Which Platform to Use

Each platform has its own culture, rules, and follower demographics. For example, at the time of this writing, YouTube and Twitter had a male-dominated user audience, and Facebook, Instagram, Snapchat, and Pinterest were female-dominated. Snapchat's audience was, on average, younger than Facebook's, but Facebook, Snapchat, and Instagram all invited engagement. A specific app may be more popular in some countries than others or even in different parts of the same country. Do an online search to find the most recent data applicable to your patients' demographics and geographic region. Even better, poll your own patients to find what apps they use and how frequently they use them.[8]

Once you've figured out the best social media apps to use to attract patients, choose no more than three to start. Learn about each app's culture by looking at different posts. Search for other plastic surgeons with a lot of followers, a lot of posts, and a lot of engagement. How are the posts that get a lot of engagement different from those that don't? Once you have a feel for the culture, start posting and let your personality come through. Expect to make mistakes, such as spelling errors and phrasing that you regret, but soon you'll find your voice.

Not all of your posts will necessarily appear on the newsfeed of your followers. An application's algorithm may restrict the appearance of your posts. Facebook's algorithm is notorious for limiting the percentage of followers who see a user's posts. You can promote a post for a fee, called *boosting*, to make it visible to more of your followers. You can also create an ad, but the Facebook algorithm controls eligibility. Nudity and sexually suggestive poses, among other qualities, are cause for rejection for both ads and boosting, making before-and-after breast photos ineligible for either.[9] Those restrictions limit Facebook's marketing flexibility for the cosmetic breast surgeon. Even though a quarter of the world's population is on Facebook, and there are clear benefits to using the app, you might want to consider using at least one other app as well. For example, Snapchat allows the cosmetic breast surgeon to show clinical photos and videos of breasts without restriction. Algorithms are constantly changing, so what works now may not work next month.

Review sites can be considered by some to be a form of social media. No matter how you categorize them, they should be on your radar. Potential patients are likely to search for your online reviews, and they'll be looking for recently posted ones, so ask happy patients to share their experiences, and then give them a link to post a review.

23.4.4 What Patients Want from Social Media

What *you* want to post on your website and on social media may not interest your target audience.[8] To attract patients to your practice, you need to catch their attention. If they like what they see, they'll be more likely to view your timeline, get to know you, visit your website, fill out a contact form, and request an appointment. It takes thought and planning to do all that through social media.

The key to success is to serve your target audience. If you're helpful, interesting, and entertaining, people will want to hear what you have to say. While your goal is to entice them to make an appointment, that won't happen if you post, "Over 5,000 breast augmentations performed. Call now for an appointment." That approach is like going to a party and pleading with people you don't know, "Please be my friend." You're sure to leave with no friends. On the other hand, if you show an interest in others and tell captivating stories, you'll probably get invitations to more parties. To figure out how to be popular on social media, pay attention to which of your posts get the most engagement. According to a survey of 100 patients, the three most popular types of posts among aesthetic surgery patients are contests for a free product or treatments, before-and-after photos, and information about the practice.[8]

Post Consistently

If you do your own social media posting, schedule at least 10 minutes to do so every day. You don't need to be the one posting, but if you give the responsibility to someone else, make sure the designated social media person captures your personality, posts ethically, and conveys the information you want to share. Review the posts, since you're responsible for your practice's entire presence in cyberspace. Frequent posting is appropriate on some apps, such as Twitter, while posting multiple times may annoy users of other apps, such as Facebook. Planning and scheduling posts using available software programs allows them to appear with appropriate frequency.

Engage with Others

Showing up on social media is like showing up at that cocktail party we just discussed. If you do all the talking, especially if you're always talking about yourself, and you ignore everyone else, your followers will lose interest. Similarly, if your posts are interesting, people will respond. Thank them and seize those opportunities to comment on and share or retweet others' posts.

Post Images

If you create a post without images, the chances are that few people will read it. Invest the time into creating good images to post about an upcoming or ongoing event, a staff's work anniversary celebration, before-and-after photos, or your latest article. For discretion, since social media are public, as well as to get by a specific app's censoring algorithms, paste shapes over nipples and genitalia. Uncensored clinical images are allowed on Snapchat and YouTube, since they both allow nudity "when the primary purpose is educational, documentary, scientific, or artistic" purposes and not pornography.[10,11] Pinterest considers the context that surrounds posted images (▶ Fig. 23.9).[12]

Videos are a powerful way to connect with the public, and they're growing in popularity. They're effective in creating a personal connection with your practice that text and images can't do. Most social media apps make posting videos easy. Venues with interactive videos, such as Snapchat and Facebook Live,[13] encourage a personal connection with viewers (Video 23.1).

Post Interesting Content

Show your personality, use stories and images, and post interesting content. Write for the audience, not for you. If you're posting a before-and-after photo, introduce it with text that's interesting, entertaining, or creates curiosity. For example, you could post, "Our doctors use a Keller funnel to insert implants with a no-touch technique." Alternatively you could shoot for greater audience engagement by asking, "How can our plastic surgeons insert breast implants without touching them?" Wait a day for people to respond, and then post: "How can our plastic surgeons insert breast implants without touching them? With a Keller funnel." Include a video with the answer to show how it's done. Look at the notifications on your social media app as well as the app's analytics. If no one's retweeting, liking, commenting, or sharing, you need to improve your posts. People who comment or ask questions about something you've posted have taken time to respond to you, so thank them and, if appropriate, answer their questions, ideally that same day. You never know who might be a potential patient.

Use Hashtags

A hashtag identifies a post's category, topic, or theme with the word immediately following a # symbol. If the topic is longer than one word, run them together and capitalize each. For example, including the hashtags #BreastAugmentation and #BreastImplants will identify your post in those categories. Apps that use them widely include Facebook, Twitter, and Instagram. For example, the post, "How can a plastic surgeon insert #BreastImplants during a #BreastAugmentation without touching them?" will get more traffic and be more easily found in a search than "How can a plastic surgeon insert breast implants during a breast augmentation without touching them?"

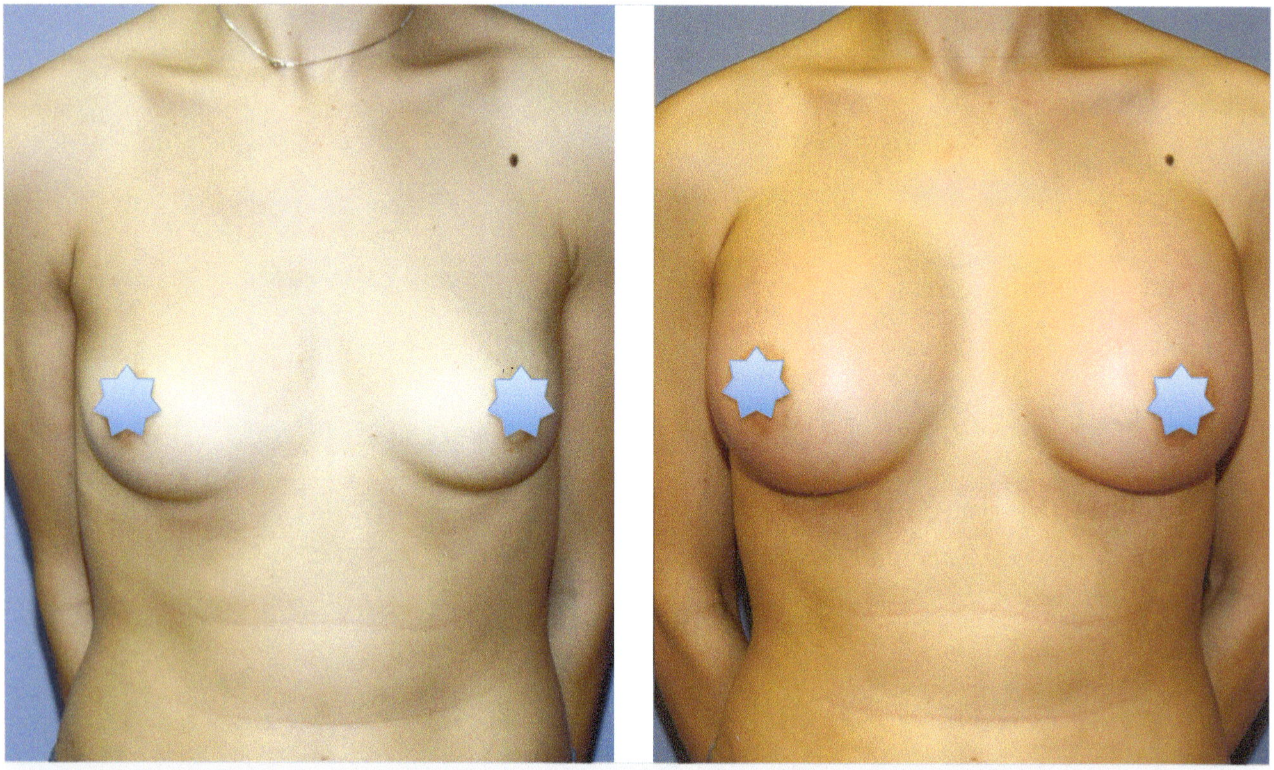

Fig. 23.9 Discreetly placed shapes make it possible to post clinical breast images on apps that do not allow visible nipples, though some apps, like Pinterest, consider the context.

How to Promote

If you provide thoughtful, informative, fun, and entertaining content in the majority of your posts, your audience will be more likely to pay attention to the occasional post announcing an event, a new treatment, a new product, or a limited-time Botox discount. When done infrequently, promotional posts can be viewed as helpful rather than annoying. Frequent promotions, however, can make you look like an advertiser rather than a thought leader. Just as people tolerate the occasional commercial while watching television, but if most of a half-hour program is devoted to hawking different fast food outlets and pharmaceuticals, the audience will leave. Rethink the type of content you're posting if you're not getting much engagement. It's possible you need to switch the focus from promoting your practice to being helpful and interesting to your target audience.

Contests

One of the most popular types of posts, besides before-and-after photos and information about the practice, is contests for a free product or treatment. For example, you can have a Halloween contest and ask followers to post a photo of themselves in their costumes. The person with the most likes can win a basket of products, a facial, a dinner with the staff, an iPad, or a gift certificate to your medical spa—just not a surgical procedure, which would be a violation of the codes of ethics of professional plastic surgery societies. Announcing the winner on social media, with her written consent, opens the door for further engagement.

23.4.5 A/B Testing Your Posts

Once you start posting, you can look at a social media network's analytics to view how much others are interacting with you through replies, "likes," retweets, and shares. All these interactions lumped together constitute *engagement*. While the analytics show your performance, they don't show you how to improve. To figure that out, you can use *A/B testing*, also called *split testing*.[5] To do A/B testing, create two posts that are identical in all but one variable, such as the image, the text copy, the app used, or the time of day. After choosing that single variable, create two different versions, and post both of them to see which gets more engagement. For example, you could post an announcement of an upcoming office event at the same time of day with the same image and the same copy, but vary the app. For example you could put the post on Facebook for version "A" and on Instagram for version "B." The next day, check which post got more engagement. Now you know which app gets more traffic for that type of post at that time of day on that day of the week.

23.4.6 Pay to Play

Newsflash: There is no free lunch. Facebook is the biggest social media network, and it's doing well for itself in the stock market. Remember that post-restricting algorithm we already discussed? That's their secret. They don't give away public exposure for free; you have to pay for it. To see what I'm talking about, if you're on Facebook, look at the analytics, and check out the reach of one of your posts. The *reach* indicates how many of your followers had your post appear on their newsfeed, even if they didn't actually see it, like it, share it, or comment on it. To get your post seen by more followers (but still not all!), give your post a *boost*.

Although physicians may recoil at the idea of plunking out money to advertise on social media, if you do so, you can reach a target audience in a way that radio, television, and print ads don't allow. Paying for Google AdWords may be an effective way to attract the audience that might already be looking for someone like you. You can create a Google Ad that appears when the Google AdWord is searched and/or when similar content is displayed. For example, potential patients may type in a search box, "How much does a breast augmentation cost?" and if you've paid for exposure to a targeted demographic, then your ad may appear on their screen. With Pay Per Click (PPC), also called Cost Per Click (CPC) ads, you're charged only when a person clicks on your ad. You can track your success by measuring the clickthrough rate to find out how many people clicked on your ad after it appeared on their screen.

To get the most out your advertising efforts, create a campaign: Decide how much you want to spend and define your goals. Possibilities might be to encourage people to fill out an online form to make an appointment or to get 50 people to attend your Valentine's Day event. Create individual campaigns for different purposes. For example, you might have one campaign for breast augmentation and another for breast reduction.

As you create your campaign, you can choose the type of device your ads will appear on, where on the screen they will appear, and whether they'll appear as text or as a video. Familiarize yourself with the process by watching the Google AdWords YouTube channel tutorials, and consider hiring an online marketing consultant.[14]

23.4.7 Measure Social Media Return on Investment

As with any marketing campaign, you need to measure the costs and benefits of your efforts to know whether it's worthwhile. Of course, some potential benefits can't be measured in dollars. Branding your practice is about creating trust and familiarity so that when someone recommends you, your name, your practice, and your personality will be familiar. While branding is hard to quantify, other aspects of your social media presence can be more easily measured. To understand the big picture of the impact of your efforts, your social media scorecard should include the following: tracking engagement; digital analytics; social media costs; and practice growth.

Tracking Engagement

Engagement is more important than number of followers. If it weren't, buying followers would be the key to success on social media. Engagement is the real measure of how much attention people are paying to you, much like looking at how many people are gathered around you at that cocktail party. If you're a great raconteur, you'll have a crowd. Look at an individual app's analytics page, and look at the number of replies, comments, shares, views, retweets, and likes you get.

To get a feel for how well you're doing, visit the feed of a colleague who's successful on social media. Look at the content of their posts, the type of post that gets the most engagement, whom they follow, and who's following them. If you're not doing as well, write down the differences, and challenge yourself to improve.

Digital Analytics

To follow the impact that social media, organic searches, ads, and other referral sources have on directing people to your website, use digital analytics. You can also find out where users are geographically, the type of device they're using, and much more. Google Analytics is one of the most accessible tools for digital analytics. To learn more about Google Analytics, visit their website and YouTube channel.[15,16]

Social Media Costs

Social media has potential benefits, but it's easy to overlook the costs. Facebook charges to boost a Facebook post, ads cost money, and social media posting takes time. If you spend time on it most days, and you're no good at it, it's a waste of time. You can hire a marketing person to do your social media posting, and you can send that person to nonmedical social media conferences to keep up with the most current trends, but you're still responsible for everything they post, as well as their salary and their training. If you outsource your social media, a person not working in your office is less likely to understand your personality and culture. Tracking your engagement and return on investment can help you figure out the best approach for your practice.

Once you've determined the app or apps that are best for your practice, the best solution may be to work as a team that includes a videographer, a photographer, a film editor, and someone who can create social media posts using the videos and images. This team might start with just you and one other person, and you can add more as your social media efforts grow (▶ Fig. 23.10).

Practice Growth

When your staff asks new patients how they found your practice, they should gather all possible platforms. Did a patient find you through an organic Google search, or did she also see your posts on Facebook and Instagram? Track this information and look at the monetary benefit the patient brought to the practice, such as one breast augmentation and four CoolSculpting cycles. Use this information to arrive at an approximate return on investment (ROI). Precision is elusive, since patients choose you by considering a variety of inputs, but an approximate number can give you an idea where your marketing dollars are best spent.[17]

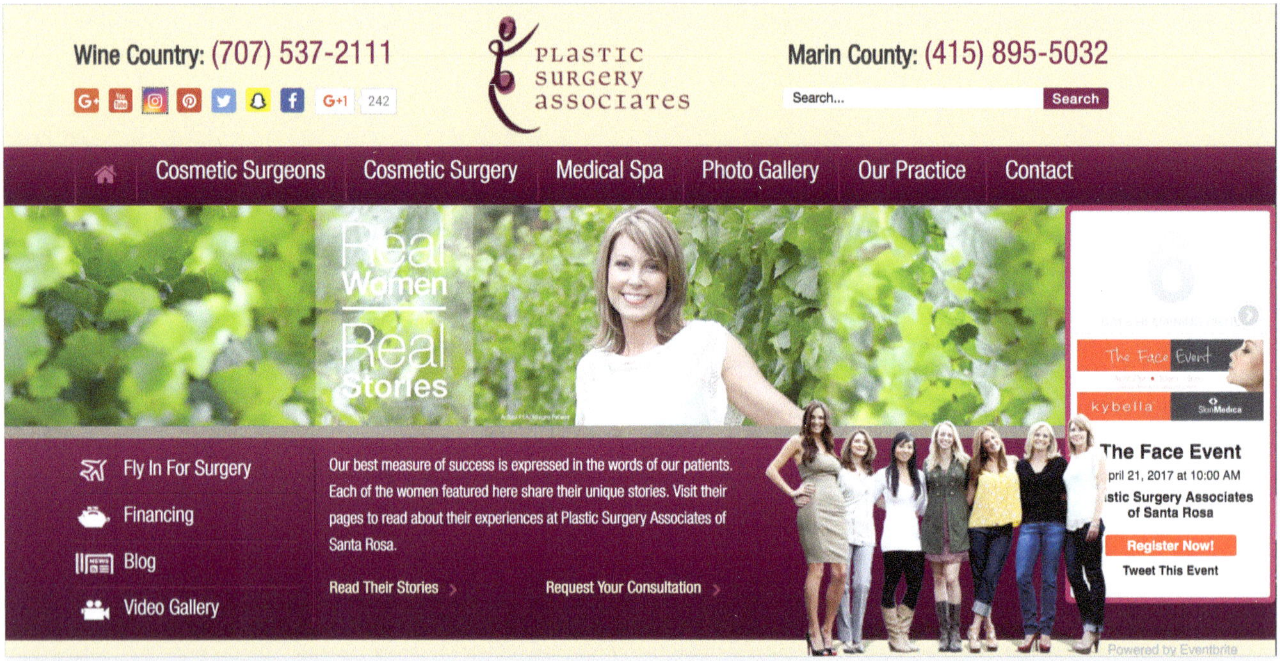

Fig. 23.10 You can use your website and your social media to announce upcoming events.

23.5 Conclusion

Unless you're able to harness a single platform with the frequency and magnetism of a television host, an individual platform may work best for the cosmetic breast surgeon when it's part of an online presence. Social media is a good tool, but its greatest utility is usually to drive your audience to your website, where they can fill out a contact form and make an appointment. On the other hand, without a social media presence, you're dependent on organic searches. If your website directs visitors to your social media apps, and vice versa, you'll appeal to a broader audience. The best digital strategy is to use social media to establish trust and familiarity. Fire on all cylinders by *pulling* people into your practice with a blog, guest blog, videos, eBooks, and social media, then *push* people your way through online ads with AdWords, display ads, search ads, social media ads, email marketing, webinars, and a RealSelf presence. Track all your efforts with digital analytics, and then adjust what you do.[18] After that, it's up to you to deliver what patients are hoping for.

References

[1] American Society for Aesthetic Plastic Surgery. 2016 Cosmetic Surgery National Data Bank Statistics. URL: https://www.surgery.org/sites/default/files/ASAPS-Stats2016.pdf Accessed July 23, 2019

[2] Clement J. Percentage of mobile device website traffic worldwide from 1st quarter 2015 to 1st quarter 2019. Statista. URL: https://www.statista.com/statistics/277125/share-of-website-traffic-coming-from-mobile-devices/ Updated May 3, 2019. Accessed July 24, 2019

[3] Brown JK. SEO: Why is metadata important? Practical Ecommerce. Available at: http://www.practicalecommerce.com/SEO-Why-Is-Metadata-Important. Updated November 19, 2018. Accessed July 24, 2019

[4] Wikipedia contributors. Social media. Wikipedia, The Free Encyclopedia. URL: https://en.wikipedia.org/w/index.php?title=Social_media&oldid=907536528. Updated July 23, 2019. Accessed July 24, 2019

[5] Aboulhosn S. Social media marketing tips for every platform. URL: http://sproutsocial.com/insights/social-media-tips/. July 16, 2019. Accessed July 24, 2019

[6] Create a free business Page in minutes. URL: https://www.facebook.com/business/pages/set-up. Accessed July 24, 2019

[7] Instagram Business Team. Make your business stand out with Instagram. URL: https://www.facebook.com/business/profiles. 2019. Accessed July 24, 2019

[8] Sorice SC, Li AY, Gilstrap J, Canales FL, Furnas HJ. Social media and the plastic surgery patient. Plast Reconstr Surg. 2017; 140(5):1047–1056

[9] Facebook. Advertising Policies. URL: https://www.facebook.com/policies/ads/?ref=u2 u. Accessed July 24, 2019

[10] YouTube Help. Nudity and sexual content policies. URL: https://support.google.com/youtube/answer/2802002?hl=en. Accessed July 24, 2019

[11] Snap Inc. Terms of Service. URL: https://www.snap.com/en-US/terms/. Effective: February 18, 2019. Accessed July 24, 2019

[12] Pinterest. Community Guidelines. URL: https://about.pinterest.com/en/community-guidelines. Accessed July 24, 2019

[13] Ente J. 5 Tips for Better Facebook Live Broadcasts. Available at: http://www.socialmediaexaminer.com/6-tips-for-better-facebook-live-broadcasts/. May 30, 2016. Accessed July 24, 2019

[14] YouTube channel: Google Ads. URL: https://www.youtube.com/user/learnwithgoogle. Accessed July 24, 2019

[15] Google Analytics Academy. Learn Analytics with Free Online Courses. URL: https://analytics.google.com/analytics/academy. Accessed July 24, 2019

[16] YouTube channel: Analytics Academy - Digital Analysis Fundamentals. Available at: https://www.youtube.com/playlist?list=PLI5YfMzCfRtZ8eV576YoY3-vlYrHjyVm_e. Accessed July 24, 2019

[17] Nazarian S. The return on investment of social media. Presented at the Women Plastic Surgeons' Enrichment Retreat, American Society of Plastic Surgeons. February 4, 2017. Newport Beach, California

[18] Smith L. Stanford Webinar: Introduction to growth hacking. Available at: https://www.youtube.com/watch?v=-LeKimVEi-Q. Accessed July 24, 2019

24 Breast Implant Illness

Jordan Kaplan and Rod J. Rohrich

Summary

The purpose of this chapter is to present the current state of scientific evidence related to the safety of silicone breast implants. "Breast implant illness" is a term used by women to describe a constellation of symptoms that they attribute to their breast implants. These self-identified women report systemic symptoms such as fatigue, chest pain, hair loss, headaches, chills, photosensitivity, rash, and chronic pain. At the present state, there is overwhelming evidence to support the safety of silicone breast implants. Ultimately the decision to obtain, keep, or remove breast implants is the choice of the patient. If a patient chooses to remove her breast implants, it is important to find a board-certified plastic surgeon with expertise in breast surgery. Ongoing studies are strongly encouraged in all areas from cancer detection to autoimmune disease as we strive for improved patient safety, patient awareness, and patient education. This chapter aims to delineate both the content and timing of all research and evidence as it pertains to the newly coined phrase "breast implant illness." To the best of our body of scientific knowledge to date, there have not been any concrete or evidence-based studies or peer reviewed data concerning the formation of a new syndrome- "silicone implant illness."

Keywords: breast implant, breast implant illness, breast augmentation, breast reconstruction

24.1 Introduction to Breast Implants

Today, nearly 300,000 breast augmentations and 100,000 breast reconstructions utilize breast implants annually in the United States.[1] Silicone gel–filled implants were first approved by the U.S. Food and Drug Administration (FDA) in 1962 by Cronin and Gerow. Since that time, few medical devices have been studied as closely for their safety profiles and associated adverse outcomes. Despite multiple generations of implant shells and gel fillers, the basic components remain as originally described.[2,3] See ▸ Table 24.1 for a description of differing characteristics among generations of silicone breast implants.

24.1.1 History of Breast Implant Safety Surveillance

In the early 1980s, just as third-generation silicone implants were being introduced, rising levels of consumer concern became evident in regard to the safety of silicone breast implants. As this was occurring, the FDA's new surveillance system began to identify frequent local complications associated with silicone implants. Breast implants became classified as higher-risk devices, which required premarket approval, and in light of this, manufacturers became responsible for providing data that supported the safety of these devices for patient use.[4] For more than 60 years there has been controversy as to the safety of these devices, with > 400 reports on various health conditions in association with breast implants.[5]

Ultimately, in 1992, the FDA determined that silicone implant manufacturers had not provided enough data to address consumer concerns adequately, and silicone implants were removed from the market. During this time the FDA required all breast implant manufactures to conduct core studies to assess overall implant safety profiles.[6,7,8,9,10] Seven years after the FDA moratorium on silicone implants, the Institute of Medicine (IOM) released a detailed report of the current literature, entitled *Safety of Silicone Breast Implants*, which ultimately concluded that local complications were of primary concern and, in order to comment definitively on systemic disease such as cancer or autoimmune disorders, further studies were needed, as there was a paucity of significant, well-controlled studies.[4]

The IOM report was the first step toward the return of silicone breast implants to the market in 2006. This report was instrumental in clarifying the scientific evidence, as well as identifying information gaps on the safety of these devices. Since the return of silicone implants, there has been ongoing research concerning their safety due in part to the FDA's stipulation that the two manufacturers of silicone breast implants at that time, Allergan Inc. (Dublin, Ireland) and Mentor Corp. (Minneapolis, MN), conduct large post-approval studies to guarantee that these potential long-term risks did not go unmonitored.[11,12]

24.1.2 Where Are We Now?

The extent of our knowledge on prior safety concerns has expanded since the FDA's decision to remove silicone breast implants from market.[4,13] Plastic surgeons must hold industry as well as one another accountable for the care of their patients by increasing awareness of evidence-based practices so that they can best inform their patients and the medical community on the safety of these devices.[12,14,15] Plastic surgeons, like all physicians, take an oath to "do no harm" and have a responsibility to inform their patients best on the safety of these devices

Table 24.1 Breast implant generations

Generation	Years of use	Unique characteristics	Changes in complication profile
1	1960s	Dacron patches on posterior wall	Capsular contracture and rupture
2	1972–1986	Thinner outer shell, less viscous gel filler, removal of Dacron patches	Increased incidence of gel leak
3	1980s	Thicker/reinforced outer shell (remains in current implants)	Decreased gel leak
4	2000s	Increased gel filler crosslinking to increase cohesiveness	Decreased gel leak with more natural feel
5	2000s	Increased crosslinking allowing for shaped implants	Increased rate of implant malrotation

and to listen with a kind ear when patients present with symptoms and complaints that have the potential to be associated with silicone breast implants. The information provided in this chapter reviews the current literature regarding the safety of silicone breast implants as well as the concerns that remain about these devices in light of recent consumer concern and social media reports about the possible existence of a "silicone breast implant illness" syndrome—an entity that currently has no clear definition but has been popularized by both health care providers and the media.

24.2 Cancer

The concern for potential carcinogenicity of silicone breast implants was initially sparked after the publication of a case series describing three women with breast implants diagnosed with cutaneous T-cell lymphoma in 1995.[16,17] To date there have been a myriad studies published in both Europe and North America investigating the potential association between these devices and malignancy, most with adequate sample size and long term follow-up.[12,18,19,20,21,22,23,24,25,26,27,28,29,30,31,32,33,34]

24.2.1 Breast Cancer

Because of breast implants' location, their use in oncologic reconstruction, and their potential to affect breast mammography adversely, the risk of breast cancer development in these patients is of upmost concern. There is extensive data refuting any association between these devices and an increased incidence of breast cancer, as many studies have shown that these patients have a lower incidence of primary breast cancer.[12,19,20,21,22,23,24,25,26,27,28,29,30,31,33,34,35,36,37,38,39] In 1999 the International Agency for Research on Cancer (IARC) published a report stating there was evidence to support a lack of breast carcinogenicity in women with silicone breast implants, and this was later backed by the IOM Committee on the Safety of Silicone Breast Implants.[36,40] Recent publications examining the incidence of breast cancer in patients with silicone breast implants include a meta-analysis by Noels and coworkers of results from 17 previously published articles.[39] Ultimately the authors found that breast implants are not associated with an increased incidence of breast cancer, and a 2016 review article by Balk and coworkers confirmed these findings.[23]

Box 24.1 Breast Cancer Key Points

- Large volume of literature looking at breast implants and the risk of breast cancer development.
- Their use in breast cancer reconstruction and location make this a major concern.
- The literature has overwhelmingly denied an association between breast implants and breast cancer.

24.2.2 Other Malignancies

Some reports describe an increased cancer risk among patients with cosmetic breast implants including brain, cervical, vulvar, and lung, in addition to nonmelanoma skin cancer.[4,12,41] However, the data do not support breast implants as being responsible for these findings.[4,13,42] Between 1999 and 2005 multiple independent scientific review boards concluded there is no excess risk of cancer of any type in women with silicone breast implants.[13,35,36,37,40] Since the release of these advisory reports, numerous studies have been conducted to better quantify the risk of breast and other types of cancer in women with breast implants.[12,19,20,21,22,23,28,29,34,35,36,37,38,39] Many have definitively concluded that their cancer incidence closely matches that of the general population.[19,20,21,22] However, in 2018, the largest study of patient safety and implant-specific outcomes for breast implants found that patients with Mentor Corp. silicone implants were 1.54 (95% CI: 1.42–1.68) times more likely to develop a cancer diagnosis compared to the general population.[12]

Brinton and coworkers reported a slight excess of cancer in patients with breast implants as a result of statistically significant increased risks for cervical, vulvar, and brain cancer as well as leukemia compared to the general public, but these patients showed no difference when compared to women who had undergone other plastic surgery procedures. It is important to recognize that the authors clearly state that this observed difference is likely due to both selection bias and lack of cancer diagnosis validation.[29] Additionally, multiple epidemiologic studies in the literature have found that women with breast implants have different patient demographics as well as lifestyle and/or reproductive characteristics compared to the general population, which may explain these findings.[43,44,45,46]

There is a breadth of literature concerning the risk of brain cancer in patients with breast implants, including a multitude of large-scale incidence studies as well as five mortality studies.[12,19,20,21,22,38,47,48,49,50] All but one study consistently failed to show an increased incidence of brain cancer or mortality from brain cancer in patients with breast implants. Such findings were explained by evidence that metastatic disease from distant sites is often not reflected in the diagnostic accuracy of death certificates in patients who die of brain cancer.[47]

Since McLaughlin's original paper in 2007, which concluded there is no credible evidence to support a causal relationship between breast implants and cancer, much of the literature on this topic remains consistent.[13] This is supported by a large, multicenter observational study published in 2017 that looked at long-term safety of women with Natrelle round silicone gel-filled breast implants. Their study population of 55,279 women, which represented an interim data set that was later fully reported on by Coroneos and coworkers, showed no excess risk for any cancer diagnoses including brain, cervical/vulvar, lung, or breast cancer.[12,51] Newly published literature found an increased incidence of melanoma in patients with Mentor Corporation breast implants compared to the general population.[12] However, the authors of that study do not suggest that silicone implants are responsible for these diagnoses of melanoma but rather that patients with breast implants may be more likely to have increased ultraviolet (UV) light exposure secondary to sunbathing or outdoor lifestyles. Because of this, physicians need to be aware of breast implant patients who present with suspicious skin lesions, as they may have placed themselves at risk for the development of such conditions. Despite some reports of an increased incidence of lung cancer in certain populations with breast implants, studies that examined characteristics of these patients found an elevated proportion of smokers in addition to various lifestyle differences as more likely culprits.

Box 24.2 Other Cancer Key Points

- Many studies have definitively concluded that the incidence of cancer in patients with breast implants closely matches that of the general population.[19,20,21,22]
- Studies that have found an increased incidence of cancer diagnoses explain that women with breast implants have different patient demographics as well as lifestyle and/or reproductive characteristics compared to the general population.[44,45,46,47]
- No increased risk of hematopoietic malignancy including multiple myeloma.[19,20,21,22,29]
- Increased incidence of lung cancer and non-melanoma skin cancer is attributed to patient factors including a higher prevalence of smokers as well as increased UV light exposure (sunbathing being the main risk factor).[12]
- Plastic surgeons should be aware that this patient population is likely to partake in such high-risk behaviors including smoking and sun bathing and therefore should actively participate in smoking cessation counseling and have a low threshold for referral to a dermatologist for suspicious skin lesions.

24.2.3 Breast Cancer Detection

In a report that looked at the safety of silicone breast implants, the IOM suggested that these devices may obstruct visualization of various parts of the breast and would affect the accuracy of routine screening mammography.[40] In response, multiple case series hypothesized that opaque breast implants may interfere with mammographic breast visualization as well as breast physical exam, ultimately delaying breast cancer diagnosis and causing worse prognosis for those affected.[52,53,54,55] In addition to the bias presented in most of these reports, many of the women included underwent screening mammography without utilization of the Eklund implant displacement technique.[56]

In the most recent article published on the effect breast implants have on mammogram outcomes, Kam and coworkers conclude there is no statistically significant difference between women with and without implants in regard to Breast Imaging Recording and Data System 0 score, callback exam, time to resolution of abnormal imaging, or cancer detection rate.[57] Additional studies have supported the conclusion that, although the sensitivity of screening mammography may be reduced by the presence of breast implants, this patient population does not present with more advanced stages of breast cancer or suffer from lower survival rates following diagnosis.[19,21,58,59,60,61]

Box 24.3 Breast Cancer Detection Key Points

- When utilizing proper techniques for breast imaging with breast implants there is no delay in cancer diagnosis or effect on breast cancer screening by means of mammography.[19,21,62,63,64,65]
- The Eklund implant displacement technique greatly improved the efficacy of screen mammography in patients with breast implants.[66]

24.3 Connective Tissue Disease

The FDA defines connective tissue disease (CTD) as any disorder that affects the connective tissue of the body either through genetic inheritance (fibromyalgia), autoimmune dysfunction (rheumatoid arthritis), or other types of exposure, as is the case with scurvy.[4] Additional examples of these conditions include scleroderma, Sjögren's syndrome, and systemic lupus erythematosus (SLE), in addition to many others. Because the incidence and prevalence of these conditions are quite low (fibromyalgia in 1,128 per 100,000 women and scleroderma in 3 per 100,000 women per year), a very large study of sufficient duration is required to conclude a causal relationship between breast implants and these diseases.[67,68]

24.3.1 Implant Rupture and Connective Tissue Disease

Implant rupture has traditionally been thought of as an important risk factor for the development of CTD in patients with breast implants. Two large scale studies published prior to 2007 confirmed that implant rupture does not place patients at increased risk of developing CTD.[69,70] One earlier study showed an increase in self-reported Raynaud's syndrome in patients with isolated extracapsular implant rupture (odds ratio = 4.2; 95% CI: 1.1–16.0) and "other CTD" (odds ratio = 2.7; 95% CI: 0.8–8.5). In this study the authors did not discern whether or not onset of symptoms was prior to breast augmentation.[71]

24.3.2 Historical Perspective and Current Evidence on Connective Tissue Disease

In the 1980s and early 1990s, anecdotal reports of CTD in women with breast implants were first published. Through 2004, data from all but one study unanimously concluded that there is no association between breast implants and CTD.[40,62,63,66,72,73,74,75,76]

Prior to recent reports, the only finding of a relationship between CTD and breast implants came from a large cohort study of female health professionals published in 1996.[64] Compared to women without breast implants, women with breast implants had a relative risk (RR) of 1.24 (95% CI: 1.08–1.41) for any self-reported combined CTD. For individual connective tissue disorders including rheumatoid arthritis, polymyositis/dermatomyositis, scleroderma, and Sjögren's syndrome, the relative risk of disease was slightly elevated but did not show statistical significance. Only 22.7% of self-reported CTD was confirmed in patients' medical records.[65] Additional evidence of overreporting and diagnostic biases was also evident in a cohort study that looked at CTD in 7,234 women in the United States with breast implants.[77] After examination of the medical record by rheumatologists deemed to be expert, only a minority of self-reports of CTD were declared as "likely," and the relative risk among women with breast implants was not significant for rheumatoid arthritis, scleroderma, or Sjögren's syndrome combined when compared to the general population.

Fryzek and coworkers compared 2,761 Danish women with breast implants to 8,807 women who had undergone reduction mammaplasty.[78] All outcomes were verified and based on thoroughly reviewed medical records. After a mean follow-up time of 13.4 years, the authors concluded that there was no significant increase in the incidence of any specific CTD or any of the CTDs combined for women with breast implants. Additionally, this study confirmed no difference between the two cohorts as it pertained to the incidence of fibromyalgia. Brinton and coworkers also found that women with breast implants were not at increased risk of developing fibromyalgia compared to those who underwent other types of plastic surgery procedures, although their data were self-reported.[77] That study did include a category of conditions termed "other disorders," for which they reported a risk ratio of 1.4 (95% CI: 0.8–2.6) prior to 1992 and 3.6 (95% CI: 1.9–7.0) for the period that followed, a period marked by widespread litigation in the United States, thereby supporting the authors' claim that these results were largely due to reporting bias among subjects. Additionally, and most importantly, no saline implant control cohort exists, as the data for these devices has not been released by the implant manufacturers. Therefore, a group that controls for patient demographics in women with saline breast implants cannot be compared to those with silicone implants.

It is important to recognize that, based on the evidence presented at the time, the 1999 IOM report found no "convincing evidence for atypical connective tissue or rheumatic disease or a novel constellation of signs and symptoms in women with silicone breast implants."[40] The authors of this report acknowledged that the study was underpowered and therefore would not have found an association had one existed. Following this report, Tugwell completed a systematic review per the request of a U.S. federal court-appointed national science panel to assist in evaluating expert testimony being presented in lawsuits brought against various breast implant manufacturers.[62] It too found no evidence of an association between breast implants and CTD, therefore discrediting the expert testimony that had been presented.

In May 2011, Lipworth, Holmich, and McLaughlin published a paper titled "Silicone Breast Implants and Connective Tissue Disease: No Association," with the intention of clarifying remaining claims regarding breast implants and CTD.[79] Of note, the authors of this editorial were paid consultants of the implant manufacturers and concluded that these claims were a byproduct of "unprecedented large-scale product liability litigation" rather than sound scientific evidence. In it they cite 18 large-scale cohort studies, 11 case-control studies, and 13 additional independent meta-analyses and critical reviews, all of which unequivocally refute an association between breast implants and CTD. It showed a small increased risk of self-reported CTDs in women with breast implants (RR 1.24; 95% CI: 1.08–1.41). The relative risk for each individual CTD, including rheumatoid arthritis, polymyositis/dermatomyositis, scleroderma, or Sjögren's syndrome were all slightly elevated but not statistically significant. A later study found that only a small fraction of diagnoses could be confirmed.[65]

Early reports of expert evidence reviews including a National Science Panel Report published in 1998, the 1999 IOM report, and a 2011 FDA review all supported that there was no evidence to link silicone breast implants with an increased incidence of connective tissue disease.[4,40,80] They did recognize that there were limitations to the existing evidence and further investigation was warranted. A 2017 article, discussed previously, reported that after looking at 55,279 women with breast implants over a 5-year follow-up period, silicone gel–filled implants had no increased risk of any connective tissue disease compared to national norms or those with saline implants.[51] All reported instances of adverse events were confirmed with the diagnosing physician to prevent inaccurate diagnoses based solely on patient reported symptoms. However, in the largest and most comprehensive epidemiologic study of patient safety and implant-specific outcomes for breast implants in the literature, studying nearly 100,000 patients (including the 55,279 in the aforementioned study) over a 7-year follow-up period, Coroneos and coworkers found that there were multiple connective tissue disorders for which diagnoses exceeded double that of the general population—conclusions that were contradictory to the interim analysis just discussed.[12] These included Mentor patients with Sjögren's syndrome (standardized incidence raio [SIR]: 8.14; 95% CI: 6.24–10.44), scleroderma (SIR: 7.00; 95% CI: 5.12–9.34), and rheumatoid arthritis (SIR: 5.96; 95% CI: 5.35–6.62). Additionally, the large study showed an increased risk of developing multiple sclerosis and myositis, although both at rates less than twice that of the general population. Data for Allergan implants had a 7-year follow-up period, were based on physician-confirmed diagnoses, and had an excellent follow-up rate. Patients who underwent revision of prior breast reconstruction with Allergan implants had incidence ratios greater than 2.0 for scleroderma, Sjögren's syndrome, and both dermatomyositis and polymyositis at 7-year follow-up. Finally, Coroneos and coworkers reported 500 autoimmune events in the silicone implant cohort compared to five events in those with saline devices. These results are congruent with the largest meta-analysis to date, written by Balk and coworkers, which pooled outcomes from 32 observational studies as well as a recent review article published in 2018 that found a statistically significant association between silicone breast implants and autoimmune/rheumatic disorders, Sjögren's syndrome, systemic sclerosis, and sarcoidosis.[23,81]

In response to the media craze that ensued following publication of the study by Coroneos and coworkers, the FDA released a statement to address the findings discussed above.[12] In it they urge both the public and health care providers to view their conclusions with caution, as the study has major shortcomings. While the author's analysis was sound, the processes used for data collection were designed by the various implant manufacturers and not without inconsistency and bias; Coroneos and coworkers themselves recognized these conclusions, as do Colwell and Mehrara in a recently published editorial.[82] Binita Ashar, of the FDA's Center for Devices and Radiological Health, reminded readers that the current evidence "does not conclusively demonstrate an association" and that "more evaluation is required."[83] Colwell and Mehrara highlight that the authors analyze a much smaller group of patients (< 34,000 vs. 99,993) for 7 years despite previous data concerns of poor follow-up and issues with data acquisition. The Mentor reported data had a 2-year follow-up rate of 24% and a 7-year follow-up rate of only 20%, both of which were drastically lower than those of the Allergan data set. Moreover, in addition to poor follow-up, a large subset of data was patient reported and had no physician confirmation. It is not surprising that the patient reported-data provided by Mentor ultimately had the greatest association with rare adverse health events; which were not upheld through the analysis of 25,219 Allergan patients. Outcomes were compared to "normative" populations and thus failed to control for many confounding variables. These methodological flaws prohibit any definitive conclusions to be reached from this article.

In summary, recent data suggest that, although this view was originally refuted, breast implants *may* have an association with CTD, a fact that must be explicitly communicated to patients interested in pursuing breast reconstruction or augmentation with silicone breast implants. Governing bodies such as the IOM and FDA strongly reaffirm that breast implants are overwhelmingly safe devices with a low overall risk of developing such conditions. We as plastic surgeons have a responsibility to advise our patients judiciously of these potential risks and look proactively for those who may present with symptoms indicating they require further evaluation. We must put our patients' best interest first, which starts by actively listening to their desires as well as their concerns and working together to ensure patient safety and satisfaction.

Box 24.4 Connective Tissue Disease Key Points

- Prior to 2004 all but one study concluded that there is no association between breast implants and CTD.[41,79,80,81,82,83,84,85,86]
- Implant rupture does not increase patients' risk of being diagnosed with CTD or other rheumatologic conditions.[87,88]
- An interim analysis of the LPAS database looked at 55,279 patients with breast implants with at least 5 year follow-up found no increased risk of any CTD compared to national norms or saline implants.[52]
- Final analysis of the same data was published in 2018 and found an association between[12]
  - Mentor implants and Sjögren's syndrome, scleroderma, and rheumatoid arthritis (SIR > 2.0) and multiple sclerosis and myositis (SIR < 2.0).
  - Allergan implants and Sjögren's syndrome, dermatomyositis and polymyositis (SIR > 2.0).
  - Results match those of two large review articles written in 2016 and 2018.[23,89]
- No saline implant cohort control exists, as this data has not been released by implant manufacturers, so current studies are not able to control for patient demographics in women with breast implants.
- Despite recent articles showing an association between silicone breast implants and certain CTDs, plastic surgeons and the FDA still regard breast implants as safe devices for patient use.

24.4 Mental Health

Plastic surgeons must consider how our work affects patients' psychiatric well-being. Breiting and coworkers found that women with breast implants had a higher self-reported rate of psychotropic medication use, which included both antidepressants and anxiolytics.[18] Although not diagnostic, they concluded that, despite there being no association between breast implants and depression, increased use of these medications warrants further investigation as to how breast implantation affect psychopathology.[23]

Coroneos and coworkers found no association between breast implants and the rate of suicide in the United States; a conclusion that opposed that of previous literature.[12,48,49,50,84,85,86] These conclusions were highlighted by Singh and cowrokers, who stated that the suicide rate (10.6 events per 100,000 person-years) was not significantly higher than that of the national norm.[51] While literature prior to this supported an association, it remained unclear whether or not it represented a causal link or whether it was secondary to an increased prevalence of prior underlying psychopathology.[90] This relationship may reflect other important underlying factors including socioeconomic status, self-esteem, psychological distress, and psychotherapy among individuals undergoing treatment with breast implants.[4,12,23] This is highlighted in the Danish breast implant mortality study, which showed that women undergoing cosmetic breast implantation had a higher prevalence of previous hospitalization for psychiatric illness compared to those undergoing either reduction mammaplasty or other types of cosmetic surgery.[49]

Box 24.5 Mental Health Key Points

- Patients with breast implants had a higher self-reported rate of psychotropic medication use, which included both antidepressants and anxiolytics, although they did not report increased levels of clinical depression.[18]
- Multiple studies prior to 2007 reported two- to threefold increased rates of suicide among women with breast implants, but these women had a higher prevalence of previous hospitalization for psychiatric illness.[49,50,51,91,92,93]
- Recent studies by Singh and coworkers and Coroneos and coworkers found no association between breast implants and the rate of suicide.[12,52]

24.5 Neurologic Disease

In the early 1990s, multiple case reports and case series described patients with silicone breast implants who had subsequently developed various neurologic symptoms or disorders. These conditions included multiple sclerosis, "multiple sclerosis type syndrome," both motor and peripheral neuropathies, and "atypical neurological disease syndrome." In response to these reports, three large population-based cohort studies examining the possible association between breast implants and neurologic conditions were conducted.[94,95,96] All three studies failed to report an association between these devices and the aforementioned conditions.[13] To the best of our knowledge, no new epidemiologic evidence has emerged since McLaughlin reached this conclusion in 2007.

Box 24.6 Neurologic Disease Key Points

- Three large population-based studies have all failed to report an association between silicone breast implants and neurologic conditions.[95,96]
- Patient-specific characteristics among women who undergo procedures with silicone breast implants are responsible for any excess risk of neurologic disease in that patient population.

24.6 Offspring Effects

Early case reports of isolated adverse health outcomes in children born to mothers with silicone breast implants were published in the mid 1990s. Such conditions included difficulty swallowing, irritability, nonspecific rashes, and fatigue, among other symptoms.[88,89,99,100,101,102] These studies lacked a control group in addition to having apparent selection bias, as many of these children were born to families with a history of scleroderma and esophageal dysmotility.

To date, four large-scale epidemiologic studies have analyzed health outcomes among children born to mothers with silicone breast implants, all of which concluded there is no evidence to suggest a causal relationship. Kjøller and coworkers compared 939 children born to women with silicone breast implants to 3,906 children of mothers who had undergone breast reduction surgery between 1977 and 1992.[103] After a mean follow-up of 5.5 years they observed a higher than expected rate of esophageal disorders in children born to women with breast implants compared to the general population. However, this excess was also observed in those who had undergone breast reduction surgery and among children born prior to their mothers' breast implant surgery. In a follow-up study they observed higher than expected rates of esophageal disorders for children born before ($O/E = 2.0$; 95% CI: 1.3–2.8) but not after ($O/E = 1.3$; 95% CI: 0.5–2.9) maternal breast implant surgery with similar excess seen both before ($O/E = 2.1$; 95% CI: 0.5–2.9) and after ($O/E = 1.6$; 95% CI: 1.1–2.3) breast reduction surgery.[104] No excess of rheumatic disease was seen. Ultimately, they concluded that any observed increased risk of adverse health outcomes appears to be unrelated to breast implants, as these findings are evident among children born both before and after breast implant surgery as well as in children born to control mothers who underwent breast reduction surgery. A large retrospective cohort study examining 5,874 children born to Swedish women with breast implants supported the conclusions above.[91] The fourth and final study, conducted in Finland by Heminki and coworkers, sought to evaluate perinatal health outcomes in infants born to mothers with silicone breast implants, but it suffered from major methodological flaws that included inadequate controls as well as confounding variables.[92]

Additionally, women with breast implants after augmentation worry about their ability to safely breastfeed their children following surgery. In a study that looked at 5,736 live births following breast augmentation, 79.4% of women breastfed at least one child, with the most common complication being insufficient milk production in 20% of cases, a number that closely mirrors that of the general population.[93]

Box 24.7 Offspring Effects Key Points

- Four large-scale epidemiologic studies have concluded that there is no evidence to suggest a causal relationship between silicone breast implants and adverse health outcomes in newborns.
- Any increased risk of adverse health outcomes was unrelated to silicone breast implants, as those findings were evident in both children born before and children born after their mothers underwent breast implant surgery.
- 79.4% of women are able to breast feed following breast augmentation with silicone breast implants which mirrors that of the general population.

24.7 Breast Implant Removal (Explantation): What You Need to Know

Implant removals are not all created equal; as there are a variety of degrees of capsulectomy/capsulotomy currently performed today. Defining the terminology is critical, since confusion exists even among plastic surgeons.

24.7.1 En Bloc Explantation

In en bloc explantation, the surgeon leaves the capsule tissue intact on the breast implant and removes the capsule and implant as one unit. Most surgeons prefer to perform en bloc implant removal through an inframammary fold incision, since visualization is challenging through a periareolar or transaxillary approach. Increasingly, patients desiring explanation request en bloc resection, since they believe it leads to less "contamination." However, many surgeons prefer to perform an anterior capsulectomy with the implant and leave the base of the capsule intact to avoid potential complications of posterior capsulectomy (e.g., pneumothorax or chest wall injury), especially if the patient has very thin chest wall musculature.

24.7.2 Explant with Total Capsulectomy

Surgeon removes the implants and then removes all capsule tissue. This is not done en bloc (i.e., as one piece) necessarily.

24.7.3 Explant with Partial Capsulectomy

Surgeon removes the implants and then removes a portion of the capsule tissue.

24.7.4 Open Capsulotomy

The capsule or scar tissue surrounding the implant is released surgically and left in the patient. Typically, this is done by scoring the tissue with electrocautery. In cases of capsular contracture, an acellular dermal matrix material may be used as a spacer to prevent recurrent capsular contracture.

In cases of anaplastic large-cell lymphoma (ALCL), patients require an en bloc removal of the breast implant and surrounding capsule on all sides as one piece. En bloc implant and capsule removal requires a skilled plastic surgeon with experience, as removal of the capsule off the chest wall has inherent risks. Particularly for patients who have capsules that are adherent to their chest wall, great care must be taken to avoid inadvertent injury to underlying chest wall structures, as this may lead to pneumothorax.

The literature describes clinical outcomes in patients who undergo explantation for symptoms of physician-confirmed diagnosis of rheumatic disease and other autoimmune conditions. A 1997 Canadian study compared 100 patients who presented for explantation surgery to 100 plastic surgery patients who had no prior exposure to breast implants.[105] The authors divided the explant cohort into three groups. Group 1 had no diagnosis of rheumatic disease or autoimmune disease, and they demonstrated a greater than 80% improvement in physical symptoms and a 93% improvement in psychological well-being following their explantation surgery. Group 2 had diagnosed rheumatic disease with no evidence of autoimmune disease, and these patients showed a small window of improvement in symptoms, with recurrence between 6 and 12 months following surgery. Group 3 had physician-confirmed autoimmune disease, and they showed no improvement in symptoms with explantation or improvement in autoantibody levels. In fact, these patients showed ultimate clinical deterioration.

Implant explanation has recently become an area of focus, as patients have growing concerns regarding potential adverse health effects of silicone breast implants. Women who believe their implants have caused them harm have every right to pursue explanation. It is the job of plastic surgeons to support their patients as they make this difficult decision by offering sound medical advice, just as we do for breast implantation surgery.

Box 24.8 Breast Implant Explantation Key Points

- Not all explanation surgeries are created equal, and most patients undergoing breast implant explantation do not require total en bloc capsulectomy.
- Plastic surgeons must support their patients who desire to have their breast implants removed and do so in a safe manner that best fits the patient's needs.
- Whether formally diagnosed with an autoimmune condition or not, patients have variable response to symptom alleviation following breast implant explantation.

24.8 Management of the Postexplant Breast Deformity

While patients seeking removal of their breast implants may be focused on explantation, plastic surgeons must address both explantation and secondary revision surgery at the time of consultation. In light of this, it is imperative to understand how both time and the breast implant cause structural changes to the breast footprint and overlying soft tissue. The expansive force of the implant can leave a residual deformity mirroring a postmastectomy patient, depending on the patient's preaugmentation breast characteristics and augmentation size. Contrary to popular belief, the breast implant does not only affect the overlying glandular tissue and breast skin but also affects the pectoralis muscle both in submuscular and subglandular breast augmentation.

The first step to any successful explantation and revision reconstruction is detailed patient education. Patients must be part of the decision-making process, and plastic surgeons must address all of these complex issues in an easy-to-understand fashion. Once this is done, it is up to the plastic surgeon to perform a detailed patient assessment to allow for proper operative planning and decision making.

Secondary breast revision must focus on two key components: (1) soft tissue contouring and (2) volume restoration. Breast contouring must focus on reshaping the breast mound repositioning the nipple areolar complex (NAC). Degree of preoperative ptosis, amount of nipple elevation needed, diameter of areola, and thickness of native breast parenchyma all factor into this decision-making process. One of us (Rohrich) and coworkers utilize three main criteria to determine whether staging these procedures is necessary: (1) smoking status, (2) nipple elevation > 4 cm, (3) breast parenchyma thickness < 4 cm.[97]

Volume restoration becomes a difficult problem to fix, as some patients are not interested in implant exchange despite substitution of implant surface or fill characteristics. In light of this, autologous fat grafting for revision breast augmentation is seen as a viable and reliable option, a trend that has been gaining much popularity in recent years. Ideally it is performed at the time of explantation, but it too can be done in a delayed fashion. Fat grafting is not recommended prior to mastopexy.

Box 24.9 Management of the Post Explant Breast Deformity Key Points

- Plastic surgeons must be prepared to discuss management of the secondary breast deformity at the time of explant consultation.
- Revision breast surgery must focus on both volume restoration and breast shape contouring.

24.9 Conclusion

The purpose of this book chapter is to discuss the current state of scientific evidence related to the safety of silicone breast implants. It is the responsibility of all physicians, especially plastic surgeons, to put patient safety always first and to self-evaluate our practices critically as well as the industry partners who serve our patients. Few medical devices have undergone the degree of scrutiny and speculation that silicone breast implants have.

At the present state, there is overwhelming evidence to support the safety of silicone breast implants, a fact that is echoed in the FDA's updated position on their use. Ultimately the decision to obtain, keep, or remove breast implants is the choice of the patient, which that surgeons have a responsibility to uphold and support. If a patient chooses to remove her breast implants, it is important to find a board-certified plastic surgeon with expertise in breast surgery. It is then the job of the plastic surgeon to support the patient's decision by providing sound medical advice, which includes presenting patients with facts regarding health risks associated with silicone breast implants. The patient must come first; it is her body and therefore her ultimate decision as to what is best for her, as breast implantation is an elective medical decision. If a patient chooses to have her implants removed, she should consider having the entire capsule removed, unless the posterior capsule is adherent to the chest wall, which may increase the risk of pneumothorax. In cases of ALCL or ruptured implants with thick calcified capsule, a total capsulectomy is mandated.[98]

To the best of our body of scientific knowledge to date, there have not been any concrete or evidence-based studies or peer-reviewed data concerning the formation of a new syndrome-"breast implant illness."

References

[1] Cosmetic Surgery National Data Bank statistics. Aesthetic Surg J. 2017; 37 Suppl_2:1–29

[2] Calobrace MB, Capizzi PJ. The biology and evolution of cohesive gel and shaped implants. Plast Reconstr Surg. 2014; 134(1) Suppl:6S–11S

[3] Maxwell GP, Gabriel A. Breast implant design. Gland Surg. 2017; 6(2):148–153

[4] US Food and Drug Administration [FDA] Center for Devices and Radiological Health [CDRH]. FDA Update on the Safety of Silicone Gel-Filled Breast Implants. https://www.fda.gov/media/80685/download Published June 2011. Accessed December 9, 2019

[5] Nanayakkara PWB, de Blok CJM. Silicone gel breast implants: What we know about safety after all these years. Ann Intern Med. 2016; 164(3):199–200

[6] Stevens WG, Calobrace MB, Alizadeh K, Zeidler KR, Harrington JL, d'Incelli RC. Ten-year core study data for Sientra's Food and Drug Administration-approved round and shaped breast implants with cohesive silicone gel. Plast Reconstr Surg. 2018; 141 4S Sientra Shaped and Round Cohesive Gel Implants:7S–19S

[7] Hammond DC, Canady JW, Love TR, Wixtrom RN, Caplin DA. Mentor Contour profile gel implants: clinical outcomes at 10 years. Plast Reconstr Surg. 2017; 140(6):1142–1150

[8] Spear SL, Murphy DK, Allergan Silicone Breast Implant U.S. Core Clinical Study Group. Natrelle round silicone breast implants: core study results at 10 years. Plast Reconstr Surg. 2014; 133(6):1354–1361

[9] Stevens WG, Harrington J, Alizadeh K, Broadway D, Zeidler K, Godinez TB. Eight-year follow-up data from the U.S. Clinical trial for Sientra's FDA-approved round and shaped implants with high-strength cohesive silicone gel. Aesthetic Surg J. 2015; 35 Suppl 1:S3–10

[10] Cunningham B, McCue J. Safety and effectiveness of Mentor's MemoryGel implants at 6 years. Aesthetic Plast Surg. 2009; 33(3):440–444

[11] Maxwell GP, Gabriel A. The evolution of breast implants. Plast Reconstr Surg. 2014; 134(1) Suppl:12S–17S

[12] Coroneos CJ, Selber JC, Offodile AC, Butler CE, Clemens MW. US FDA breast implant postapproval studies: long-term outcomes in 99,993 patients. Ann Surg. 2019; 269(1):30–36

[13] McLaughlin JK, Lipworth L, Murphy DK, Walker PS. The safety of silicone gel-filled breast implants: a review of the epidemiologic evidence. Ann Plast Surg. 2007; 59(5):569–580

[14] Eaves FF, III, Rohrich RJ, Sykes JM. Taking evidence-based plastic surgery to the next level: report of the second Summit on Evidence-Based Plastic Surgery. JAMA Facial Plast Surg. 2013; 15(4):314–320

[15] Thoma A, Kaur MN, Hong CJ, Li YK. Methodological guide to adopting new aesthetic surgical innovations. Aesthet Surg J. 2015; 35(3):308–318

[16] Duvic M, Moore D, Menter A, Vonderheid EC. Cutaneous T-cell lymphoma in association with silicone breast implants. J Am Acad Dermatol. 1995; 32(6): 939–942

[17] Gidengil CA, Predmore Z, Mattke S, van Busum K, Kim B. Breast implant-associated anaplastic large cell lymphoma: a systematic review. Plast Reconstr Surg. 2015; 135(3):713–720

[18] Breiting VB, Hölmich LR, Brandt B, et al. Long-term health status of Danish women with silicone breast implants. Plast Reconstr Surg. 2004; 114(1): 217–226, discussion 227–228

[19] Friis S, Hölmich LR, McLaughlin JK, et al. Cancer risk among Danish women with cosmetic breast implants. Int J Cancer. 2006; 118(4):998–1003

[20] Pukkala E, Boice JD, Jr, Hovi S-L, et al. Incidence of breast and other cancers among Finnish women with cosmetic breast implants, 1970–1999. J Long Term Eff Med Implants. 2002; 12(4):271–279

[21] McLaughlin JK, Lipworth L, Fryzek JP, Ye W, Tarone RE, Nyren O. Long-term cancer risk among Swedish women with cosmetic breast implants: an update of a nationwide study. J Natl Cancer Inst. 2006; 98(8):557–560

[22] Brisson J, Holowaty EJ, Villeneuve PJ, et al. Cancer incidence in a cohort of Ontario and Quebec women having bilateral breast augmentation. Int J Cancer. 2006; 118(11):2854–2862

[23] Balk EM, Earley A, Avendano EA, Raman G. Long-term health outcomes in women with silicone gel breast implants: a systematic review. Ann Intern Med. 2016; 164(3):164–175

[24] Malone KE, Stanford JL, Daling JR, Voigt LF. Implants and breast cancer. Lancet. 1992; 339(8805):1365

[25] Park AJ, Black RJ, Sarhadi NS, Chetty U, Watson ACH. Silicone gel-filled breast implants and connective tissue diseases. Plast Reconstr Surg. 1998; 101(2): 261–268

[26] McLaughlin JK, Nyrén O, Blot WJ, et al. Cancer risk among women with cosmetic breast implants: a population-based cohort study in Sweden. J Natl Cancer Inst. 1998; 90(2):156–158

[27] Brinton LA, Malone KE, Coates RJ, et al. Breast enlargement and reduction: results from a breast cancer case-control study. Plast Reconstr Surg. 1996; 97(2):269–275

[28] Brinton LA, Lubin JH, Burich MC, Colton T, Brown SL, Hoover RN. Breast cancer following augmentation mammoplasty (United States). Cancer Causes Control. 2000; 11(9):819–827

[29] Brinton LA, Lubin JH, Burich MC, Colton T, Brown SL, Hoover RN. Cancer risk at sites other than the breast following augmentation mammoplasty. Ann Epidemiol. 2001; 11(4):248–256

[30] Bryant H, Brasher P. Breast implants and breast cancer—reanalysis of a linkage study. N Engl J Med. 1995; 332(23):1535–1539

[31] Deapen DM, Bernstein L, Brody GS. Are breast implants anticarcinogenic? A 14-year follow-up of the Los Angeles Study. Plast Reconstr Surg. 1997; 99 (5):1346–1353

[32] Gabriel SE, O'Fallon WM, Kurland LT, Beard CM, Woods JE, Melton LJ, III. Risk of connective-tissue diseases and other disorders after breast implantation. N Engl J Med. 1994; 330(24):1697–1702

[33] Kern KA, Flannery JT, Kuehn PG. Carcinogenic potential of silicone breast implants: a Connecticut statewide study. Plast Reconstr Surg. 1997; 100(3): 737–747, discussion 748–749

[34] Mellemkjaer L, Kjøller K, Friis S, et al. Cancer occurrence after cosmetic breast implantation in Denmark. Int J Cancer. 2000; 88(2):301–306

[35] European Committee on Quality Assurance and Medical Devices in Plastic Surgery. Consensus Declaration on Breast Implants, 23-6-2000. Paper presented at: European Committee on Quality Assurance (EQUAM). Tel Aviv, Israel: 4th Consensus Declaration; 2000

[36] International Agency for Research on Cancer. Surgical Implants and Other Foreign Bodies: IARC Monograph on the Evaluation of Carcinogenic Risks to Humans. Vol. 74.; 1999

[37] National Institutes of Health. Breast Implants: Status of Research at the National Institutes of Health. Amended report 3/24/2005. https://permanent.access.gpo.gov/lps87130/rev305BreastImplantsReport.pdf Accessed December 9, 2019

[38] Lipworth L, Tarone RE, Friis S, et al. Cancer among Scandinavian women with cosmetic breast implants: a pooled long-term follow-up study. Int J Cancer. 2009; 124(2):490–493

[39] Noels EC, Lapid O, Lindeman JHN, Bastiaannet E. Breast implants and the risk of breast cancer: a meta-analysis of cohort studies. Aesthet Surg J. 2015; 35 (1):55–62
[40] Bondurant S, Ernster V, Herdman R, eds. Safety of Silicone Breast Implants. Washington, DC: National Academies Press; 2000
[41] Deapen DM, Hirsch EM, Brody GS. Cancer risk among Los Angeles women with cosmetic breast implants. Plast Reconstr Surg. 2007; 119(7):1987–1992
[42] Brinton LA. The relationship of silicone breast implants and cancer at other sites. Plast Reconstr Surg. 2007; 120(7) Suppl 1:94S–102S
[43] Kjøller K, Hölmich LR, Fryzek JP, et al. Characteristics of women with cosmetic breast implants compared with women with other types of cosmetic surgery and population-based controls in Denmark. Ann Plast Surg. 2003; 50(1):6–12
[44] Cook LS, Daling JR, Voigt LF, et al. Characteristics of women with and without breast augmentation. JAMA. 1997; 277(20):1612–1617
[45] Brinton LA, Brown SL, Colton T, Burich MC, Lubin J. Characteristics of a population of women with breast implants compared with women seeking other types of plastic surgery. Plast Reconstr Surg. 2000; 105(3):919–927, discussion 928–929
[46] Fryzek JP, Weiderpass E, Signorello LB, et al. Characteristics of women with cosmetic breast augmentation surgery compared with breast reduction surgery patients and women in the general population of Sweden. Ann Plast Surg. 2000; 45(4):349–356
[47] McLaughlin JK, Lipworth L. Brain cancer and cosmetic breast implants: a review of the epidemiologic evidence. Ann Plast Surg. 2004; 52(2):115–117
[48] Brinton LA, Lubin JH, Murray MC, Colton T, Hoover RN. Mortality rates among augmentation mammoplasty patients: an update. Epidemiology. 2006; 17(2):162–169
[49] Jacobsen PH, Hölmich LR, McLaughlin JK, et al. Mortality and suicide among Danish women with cosmetic breast implants. Arch Intern Med. 2004; 164 (22):2450–2455
[50] Villeneuve PJ, Holowaty EJ, Brisson J, et al. Mortality among Canadian women with cosmetic breast implants. Am J Epidemiol. 2006; 164(4):334–341
[51] Singh N, Picha GJ, Hardas B, Schumacher A, Murphy DK. Five-year safety data for more than 55,000 subjects following breast implantation: comparison of rare adverse event rates with silicone implants versus national norms and saline implants. Plast Reconstr Surg. 2017; 140(4):666–679
[52] Fajardo LL, Harvey JA, McAleese KA, Roberts CC, Granstrom P. Breast cancer diagnosis in women with subglandular silicone gel-filled augmentation implants. Radiology. 1995; 194(3):859–862
[53] Silverstein MJ, Handel N, Gamagami P, et al. Breast cancer in women after augmentation mammoplasty. Arch Surg. 1988; 123(6):681–685
[54] Silverstein MJ, Handel N, Gamagami P, et al. Breast cancer diagnosis and prognosis in women following augmentation with silicone gel-filled prostheses. Eur J Cancer. 1992; 28(2):635–40
[55] Silverstein MJ, Gierson ED, Gamagami P, Handel N, Waisman JR. Breast cancer diagnosis and prognosis in women augmented with silicone gel-filled implants. Cancer. 1990; 66(1):97–101
[56] Eklund GW, Busby RC, Miller SH, Job JS. Improved imaging of the augmented breast. AJR Am J Roentgenol. 1988; 151(3):469–473
[57] Kam K, Lee E, Pairawan S, et al. The effect of breast implants on mammogram outcomes. Am Surg. 2015; 81(10):1053–1056
[58] Deapen D, Hamilton A, Bernstein L, Brody GS. Breast cancer stage at diagnosis and survival among patients with prior breast implants. Plast Reconstr Surg. 2000
[59] Hoshaw SJ, Klein PJ, Clark BD, Cook RR, Perkins LL. Breast implants and cancer: causation, delayed detection, and survival. Plast Reconstr Surg. 2001; 107(6):1393–1407
[60] Miglioretti DL, Rutter CM, Geller BM, et al. Effect of breast augmentation on the accuracy of mammography and cancer characteristics. JAMA. 2004; 291 (4):442–450
[61] Tang SSK, Gui GPH. A review of the oncologic and surgical management of breast cancer in the augmented breast: diagnostic, surgical and surveillance challenges. Ann Surg Oncol. 2011; 18(8):2173–2181
[62] Tugwell P, Wells G, Peterson J, et al. Do silicone breast implants cause rheumatologic disorders? A systematic review for a court-appointed national science panel. Arthritis Rheum. 2001; 44(11):2477–2484
[63] Wong O. A critical assessment of the relationship between silicone breast implants and connective tissue diseases. Regul Toxicol Pharmacol. 1996; 23 (1 Pt 1):74–85
[64] Hennekens CH, Lee IM, Cook NR, et al. Self-reported breast implants and connective-tissue diseases in female health professionals. A retrospective cohort study. JAMA. 1996; 275(8):616–621
[65] Karlson EW, Lee IM, Cook NR, Manson JE, Buring JE, Hennekens CH. Comparison of self-reported diagnosis of connective tissue disease with medical records in female health professionals: the Women's Health Cohort Study. Am J Epidemiol. 1999; 150(6):652–660
[66] Lamm SH. Silicone breast implants, breast cancer and specific connective tissue diseases: a systematic review of the data in the epidemiological literature. Int J Toxicol. 1998; 17(4):497–527
[67] Weir PT, Harlan GA, Nkoy FL, et al. The incidence of fibromyalgia and its associated comorbidities: a population-based retrospective cohort study based on International Classification of Diseases, 9th Revision codes. J Clin Rheumatol. 2006; 12(3):124–128
[68] Mayes MD, Lacey JV, Jr, Beebe-Dimmer J, et al. Prevalence, incidence, survival, and disease characteristics of systemic sclerosis in a large US population. Arthritis Rheum. 2003; 48(8):2246–2255
[69] Hölmich LR, Kjøller K, Fryzek JP, et al. Self-reported diseases and symptoms by rupture status among unselected Danish women with cosmetic silicone breast implants. Plast Reconstr Surg. 2003; 111(2):723–732, discussion 733–734
[70] Hölmich LR, Lipworth L, McLaughlin JK, Friis S. Breast implant rupture and connective tissue disease: a review of the literature. Plast Reconstr Surg. 2007; 120(7) Suppl 1:62S–69S
[71] Brown SL, Pennello G, Berg WA, Soo MS, Middleton MS. Silicone gel breast implant rupture, extracapsular silicone, and health status in a population of women. J Rheumatol. 2001; 28(5):996–1003
[72] Lipworth L, Tarone RE, McLaughlin JK. Silicone breast implants and connective tissue disease: an updated review of the epidemiologic evidence. Ann Plast Surg. 2004; 52(6):598–601
[73] Blackburn WD, Jr, Everson MP. Silicone-associated rheumatic disease: an unsupported myth. Plast Reconstr Surg. 1997; 99(5):1362–1367
[74] Downing D. Silicone gel breast implants: The UK Independent Review Group report. J Nutr Environ Med. 1998; 8:317–319
[75] Janowsky EC, Kupper LL, Hulka BS. Meta-analyses of the relation between silicone breast implants and the risk of connective-tissue diseases. N Engl J Med. 2000; 342(11):781–790
[76] Silverman BG, Brown SL, Bright RA, Kaczmarek RG, Arrowsmith-Lowe JB, Kessler DA. Reported complications of silicone gel breast implants: an epidemiologic review. Ann Intern Med. 1996; 124(8):744–756
[77] Brinton LA, Buckley LM, Dvorkina O, et al. Risk of connective tissue disorders among breast implant patients. Am J Epidemiol. 2004; 160(7):619–627
[78] Fryzek JP, Holmich L, McLaughlin JK, et al. A nationwide study of connective tissue disease and other rheumatic conditions among Danish women with long-term cosmetic breast implantation. Ann Epidemiol. 2007; 17(5):374–379
[79] Lipworth L, Holmich LR, McLaughlin JK. Silicone breast implants and connective tissue disease: no association. Semin Immunopathol. 2011; 33(3):287–294
[80] Diamond B, Hulka BS, Kerkvliet N, Tugwell P. Silicone breast implants in relation to connective tissue diseases and immunologic dysfunction: a report by a National Science Panel to the Honorable Sam C. Pointer Jr. (coordinating judge for the Federal Breast Implant Multidistrict Litigation).November 30, 1998
[81] Watad A, Rosenberg V, Tiosano S, et al. Silicone breast implants and the risk of autoimmune/rheumatic disorders: a real-world analysis. Int J Epidemiol. 2018; 47(6):1846–1854
[82] Colwell AS, Mehrara B. Editorial: US FDA breast implant postapproval studies—long-term outcomes in 99,993 patients. Ann Surg. 2019; 269(1):39–40
[83] Ashar B. Statement from Binita Ashar, M.D., of the FDA's Center for Devices and Radiological Health on agency's commitment to studying breast implant safety. https://www.fda.gov/NewsEvents/Newsroom/PressAnnouncements/ucm620589.htm Accessed December 9, 2019
[84] Lipworth L, Nyren O, Ye W, Fryzek JP, Tarone RE, McLaughlin JK. Excess mortality from suicide and other external causes of death among women with cosmetic breast implants. Ann Plast Surg. 2007; 59(2):119–123, discussion 124–125
[85] Brinton LA, Lubin JH, Burich MC, Colton T, Hoover RN. Mortality among augmentation mammoplasty patients. Epidemiology. 2001; 12(3):321–326
[86] Pukkala E, Kulmala I, Hovi SL, et al. Causes of death among Finnish women with cosmetic breast implants, 1971–2001. Ann Plast Surg. 2003; 51(4): 339–342, discussion 343–344
[87] Ferguson JH. Silicone breast implants and neurologic disorders. Report of the Practice Committee of the American Academy of Neurology. Neurology. 1997; 48(6):1504–1507
[88] Levine JJ, Ilowite NT. Sclerodermalike esophageal disease in children breastfed by mothers with silicone breast implants. JAMA. 1994; 271(3):213–216

[89] Levine JJ, Ilowite NT, Pettei MJ, Trachtman H. Increased urinary NO3 (−) + NO2− and neopterin excretion in children breast fed by mothers with silicone breast implants: evidence for macrophage activation. J Rheumatol. 1996; 23(6):1083–1087

[90] McLaughlin JK, Lipworth L, Tarone RE. Suicide among women with cosmetic breast implants: a review of the epidemiologic evidence. J Long Term Eff Med Implants. 2003; 13(6):445–450

[91] Signorello LB, Fryzek JP, Blot WJ, McLaughlin JK, Nyrén O. Offspring health risk after cosmetic breast implantation in Sweden. Ann Plast Surg. 2001; 46 (3):279–286

[92] Hemminki E, Hovi SL, Sevón T, Asko-Seljavaara S. Births and perinatal health of infants among women who have had silicone breast implantation in Finland, 1967–2000. Acta Obstet Gynecol Scand. 2004; 83(12): 1135–1140

[93] Jewell ML, Edwards MC, Murphy D, Schumacher A. Lactation outcomes in more than 3500 women following primary augmentation: 5-year data from the Breast Implant Follow-Up Study. Aesthetic Surg J. 2019; 39(8):875–883

[94] Nyrén O, McLaughlin JK, Yin L, et al. Breast implants and risk of neurologic disease: a population-based cohort study in Sweden. Neurology. 1998; 50 (4):956–961

[95] Winther JF, Bach FW, Friis S, et al. Neurologic disease among women with breast implants. Neurology. 1998; 50(4):951–955

[96] Winther JF, Friis S, Bach FW, et al. Neurological disease among women with silicone breast implants in Denmark. Acta Neurol Scand. 2001; 103 (2):93–96

[97] Rohrich RJ, Beran SJ, Restifo RJ, Copit SE. Aesthetic management of the breast following explantation: evaluation and mastopexy options. Plast Reconstr Surg. 1998; 101(3):827–837

[98] Clemens MW, Brody GS, Mahabir RC, Miranda RN. How to diagnose and treat breast implant-associated anaplastic large cell lymphoma. Plast Reconstr Surg. 2018; 141(4):586e–599e

[99] Levine JJ, Trachtman H, Gold DM, Pettei MJ. Esophageal dysmotility in children breast-fed by mothers with silicone breast implants. Long-term follow-up and response to treatment. Dig Dis Sci. 1996; 41(8):1600–1603

[100] Levine JJ, Lin H-C, Rowley M, Cook A, Teuber SS, Ilowite NT. Lack of autoantibody expression in children born to mothers with silicone breast implants. Pediatrics. 1996; 97(2):243–245

[101] Teuber SS, Gershwin ME. Autoantibodies and clinical rheumatic complaints in two children of women with silicone gel breast implants. Int Arch Allergy Immunol. 1994; 103(1):105–108

[102] Gedalia A, Cuéllar ML, Espinoza LR. Skin rash and anti-Ro/SS-A antibodies in an infant from a mother with silicone breast implants. Clin Exp Rheumatol. 1995; 13(4):521–523

[103] Kjøller K, McLaughlin JK, Friis S, et al. Health outcomes in offspring of mothers with breast implants. Pediatrics. 1998; 102(5):1112–1115

[104] Kjøller K, Friis S, Signorello LB, et al. Health outcomes in offspring of Danish mothers with cosmetic breast implants. Ann Plast Surg. 2002; 48(3):238–245

[105] Peters W, Smith D, Fornasier V, Lugowski S, Ibanez D. An outcome analysis of 100 women after explantation of silicone gel breast implants. Ann Plast Surg. 1997; 39(1):9–19

25 Appendix: Update on Breast Implant–Associated Anaplastic Large-Cell Lymphoma

Eric Weiss and Sameer A. Patel

With increasing public awareness and as time since implant placement progresses, more cases of breast implant–associated anaplastic large-cell lymphoma (BIA-ALCL) are being reported to the U.S. Food and Drug Administration (FDA). As of July 6, 2019, the FDA's Manufacturer and User Facility Device Experience (MAUDE) database contained 573 unique cases of BIA-ALCL, increased from 457 as of September 30, 2018, and included 33 reported deaths.[1] Of the 573, 67% were textured implants and 28% had an unknown implant type. Of the remaining 5% or 26 implants, which were reportedly nontextured, 7 had previously been exposed to textured implants, 7 had a previous exposure to an unknown type of breast prosthetic, and 12 had an altogether unknown history. Through network collaboration with other international plastic surgical societies, the American Society of Plastic Surgery was aware of 735 total unique cases of BIA-ALCL worldwide as of August 2019.[2] To date there are no known confirmed cases of BIA-ALCL in patients with strictly nontextured implants.

A recent study by Magnusson and coworkers among the 81 patients to date from Australia and New Zealand who have developed BIA-ALCL assessed the risk of developing BIA-ALCL among several different implant types.[3] It demonstrated an estimated incidence of 1:86,029 patients with Siltex (Mentor Worldwide LLC, Santa Barbara, CA) implants and a 16.5-fold higher risk with Biocell (Allergan Inc., Dublin, Ireland) and a 23.4-fold higher risk with Silimed polyurethane (Silimed Inc., Rio de Janeiro, Brazil). An analysis of the surface characteristics of the implants was performed, grading them from 1 to 4 using a combined surface area/roughness implant classification system developed by Jones and coworkers.[4] The Biocell and Silimed implants were characterized as grade 3 and 4, respectively, suggesting a potential correlation between degree of roughness and risk for developing cancer. While polyurethane implants have been banned in the Unites States for many years due to carcinogenic components, the Biocell implant is the most prevalent offender linked to BIA-ALCL worldwide, and Allergan's CA/CARE trial estimated its risk at 1:2,207.[2]

In mid-2019, following recalls in over 30 other countries, the FDA issued a recall on Biocell textured implants as well as expanders (despite no cases of BIA-ALCL from expanders having been reported to date).[5] While the recall was initially voluntary, it has since been revised to a Class 1 recall, the most serious type. Because the absolute risk of developing BIA-ALCL is low, it is not recommended that patients with Biocell implants have their implants removed. However, providers with shelved implants are mandated to return their unused supply. The FDA has more recently proposed requiring implant manufacturers to place a boxed warning on the product informing consumers of, among other things, the risk of BIA-ALCL.

Standardized clinical practice guidelines for BIA-ALCL have been updated by the National Comprehensive Cancer Network (NCCN) in 2019.[6] Patients who present with a new periprosthetic effusion 1 year or later following implant placement, or who present with a new breast mass, rash, ulceration, or axillary lymphadenopathy, should undergo initial evaluation with ultrasound. If ultrasound findings are equivocal, magnetic resonance imaging (MRI) is recommended. Fine-needle aspiration should be performed to sample as much periprosthetic fluid as possible, and masses should be biopsied. Specimens should undergo evaluation of cellular morphology, CD30 immunohistochemistry, and flow cytometry to characterize T cells. Additional biomarkers that may be relevant in distinguishing BIA-ALCL may include CD2, CD3, CD4, CD5, CD7, CD8, CD45, and anaplastic lymphoma kinase. When confirmed, patients should undergo preoperative evaluation with a positron emission tomography/computed tomography (PET/CT) scan. If systemic involvement is suspected, patients are recommended to undergo bone marrow biopsy.

Two methods of staging BIA-ALCL have been employed: a Lugano revision to the Ann Arbor staging system and a TNM staging system initially developed by MD Anderson in 2016. Due to the improved ability of TNM staging to characterize tumor morphology and behavior more accurately as well as predict survival and recurrence,[7] it is now the recommended system.

Optimal management remains removal of implant and complete surgical resection of capsule and associated masses, or en bloc capsulectomy. Adjuvant radiation therapy is recommended for incomplete resection, positive margins, or unresectable disease. Systemic adjuvant therapy is advised for nodal involvement or invasion beyond breast capsule, and first-line therapy includes combination anthracycline-based chemotherapy and brentuximab vedotin (Adcetris, Seattle Genetics, Bothell, WA). In patients who achieve a complete response, history and physical should be performed every 3 to 6 months for 2 years, and CT chest/abdomen/pelvis or PET scan should be considered every 6 months for 2 years.

References

[1] U.S. Food and Drug Administration. Center for Devices and Radiological Health. Medical device reports of breast implant–associated anaplastic large cell lymphoma. http://www.fda.gov/medical-devices/breast-implants/medical-device-reports-breast-implant-associated-anaplastic-large-cell-lymphoma. Updated 2019. Accessed Oct 24, 2019

[2] Clemens M. BIA-ALCL resources: by the numbers, and what they mean. https://www.plasticsurgery.org/for-medical-professionals/health-policy/bia-alcl-physician-resources/by-the-numbers. Updated 2019. Accessed December 9, 2019

[3] Magnusson M, Beath K, Cooter R, et al. The epidemiology of breast implant–associated anaplastic large cell lymphoma in Australia and New Zealand confirms the highest risk for grade 4 surface breast implants. Plast Reconstr Surg. 2019; 143(5):1285–1292

[4] Jones P, Mempin M, Hu H, et al. The functional influence of breast implant outer shell morphology on bacterial attachment and growth. Plast Reconstr Surg. 2018; 142(4):837–849

[5] U.S. Food and Drug Administration. Allergan recalls Natrelle Biocell textured breast implants due to risk of BIA-ALCL cancer. https://www.fda.gov/medical-devices/medical-device-recalls/allergan-recalls-natrelle-biocell-textured-breast-implants-due-risk-bia-alcl-cancer. Updated September 12, 2019. Accessed December 9, 2019

[6] Clemens MW, Jacobsen ED, Horwitz SM. 2019 NCCN consensus guidelines on the diagnosis and treatment of breast implant-associated anaplastic large cell lymphoma (BIA-ALCL). Aesthet Surg J. 2019; 39 Supplement_1:S3–S13

[7] Clemens MW, Medeiros LJ, Butler CE, et al. Complete surgical excision is essential for the management of patients with breast implant–associated anaplastic large-cell lymphoma. J Clin Oncol. 2016; 34(2):160–168

Index

Note: Page numbers set **bold** or *italic* indicate headings or figures, respectively.

Y

Z